Ch. PUBLIC LIBRARY
BUSINESS / SCIENCE / TECHNOLOGY
400 S. STATE ST.   60605

CHICAGO PUBLIC LIBRARY

R.. 56 28197

D0891800

RG   Maternal-fetal
558.5   endocrinology.
.T84
1994

$69.16

DATE			

BAKER & TAYLOR

Maternal-Fetal Endocrinology

Maternal-Fetal Endocrinology

SECOND EDITION

Dan Tulchinsky, MD
Professor of Obstetrics and Gynecology,
Director of Reproductive Endocrinology,
Boston University, Boston, MA
Director of Reproductive Endocrinology
and Fertility Services
The Malden Hospital
Malden, MA

A. Brian Little, MD
Professor and Chairman, McGill University
Department of Obstetrics and Gynecology
The Royal Victoria Hospital
Montreal, Quebec

W.B. SAUNDERS COMPANY
A Division of Harcourt Brace & Company
Philadelphia London Toronto Montreal Sydney Tokyo

W.B. SAUNDERS COMPANY
A Division of
Harcourt Brace & Company

The Curtis Center
Independence Square West
Philadelphia, Pennsylvania 19106

Library of Congress Cataloging-in-Publication Data

Maternal-fetal endocrinology/Dan Tulchinsky, A. Brian Little
[editors].—2nd ed.

p.   cm.

ISBN 0–7216–4232–2

1. Obstetrical endocrinology.   I. Tulchinsky, Dan.
   II. Little, A. Brian.   [DNLM: 1. Fetus—physiology.
   2. Hormones—physiology.   3. Pregnancy—physiology.
   WQ 205 M425 1994]

RG558.5.T84 1994   612.6′3—dc20

DNLM/DLC   93–9931

Maternal-Fetal Endocrinology, 2nd edition   ISBN 0–7216–4232–2

Copyright © 1994, 1980 by W.B. Saunders Company

All rights reserved. No part of this publication may be reproduced or transmitted in any form or by any means, electronic or mechanical, including photocopy, recording, or any information storage and retrieval system, without permission in writing from the publisher.

Printed in the United States of America.

Last digit is the print number: 9   8   7   6   5   4   3   2   1

R00966 28197

CHICAGO PUBLIC LIBRARY
BUSINESS / SCIENCE / TECHNOLOGY
400 S. STATE ST.   60605

Contributors

———

Robert L. Barbieri, M.D.
Kate Macy Ladd Professor of Obstetrics,
Gynecology, and Reproductive Biology,
Harvard Medical School; Chief,
Department of Obstetrics and
Gynecology, Brigham and Women's
Hospital, Boston, Massachusetts.
The Maternal Adenohypophysis

Reinhart B. Billiar, Ph.D.
Professor, McGill University Faculty of
Medicine, Department of Obstetrics
and Gynecology, Royal Victoria
Hospital, Montreal, Quebec, Canada.
*Pregnancy-Related Changes in the
Metabolism of Hormones*

Charlotte Laplante Branchaud, Ph.D.
Associate Professor of Paediatrics,
McGill University; Associate Professor
of Endocrinology, Montreal Children's
Hospital, Montreal, Quebec, Canada.
The Fetal Adrenal

Thomas A. Buchanan, M.D.
Associate Professor, University of
Southern California; Physician
Specialist, Los Angeles County/
University of Southern California
Medical Center, Los Angeles, California
*Endocrine Pancreas and Maternal
Metabolism*

Martin Dym, Ph.D.
Professor and Chairman, Department
of Anatomy and Cell Biology,
Georgetown University Medical Center,
Washington, District of Columbia.
The Fetal Gonad and Sexual Differentiation

Tommaso Falcone, M.D.
Assistant Professor, Department of
Obstetrics and Gynecology, McGill
University; Royal Victoria Hospital,
Montreal, Quebec, Canada.
*Placental Synthesis of Steroid Hormones;
Placental Polypeptides; Maintenance of
Pregnancy and The Initiation of Normal
and Premature Labor*

Delbert A. Fisher, M.D.
Professor Emeritus, Department of
Pediatrics and Medicine, University of
California at Los Angeles, Los Angeles,
California; Harbor-UCLA Medical
Center, Torrance, California.
*The Ontogenesis of Thyroid Function and
Actions*

Peter D. Gluckman, M.D.
Head Department of Pediatrics, School
of Medicine, University of Auckland,
Auckland, New Zealand
*The Human Fetal Hypothalamus and
Pituitary Gland; The Maturation of*

Neuroendocrine Mechanisms Controlling the Secretion of Fetal Pituitary Growth Hormone, Prolactin, Gonadotropin, and Adrenocorticotropin-Related Peptides

George T. Griffing, M.D.
Professor of Medicine, University of Missouri; Director of Endocrinology, Diabetes, and Metabolism and Co-Director of Cosmopolitan International Diabetes Center, Columbia, Missouri.
The Maternal Adrenal Cortex

Melvin Grumbach, M.D., D.M. (hon)
Edward B. Shaw Professor of Pediatrics and Emeritus Chairman, Department of Pediatrics, University of California, San Francisco, California.
The Human Fetal Hypothalamus and Pituitary Gland; The Maturation of Neuroendocrine Mechanisms Controlling the Secretion of Fetal Pituitary Growth Hormone, Prolactin, Gonadotropin, and Andrenocorticotropin-Related Peptides

Michael M. Kaplan, M.D.
Private Practice Specializing in Thyroid Diseases.
The Maternal Thyroid and Parathyroid Glands

John L. Kitzmiller, M.D.
Clinical Professor of Obstetrics, University of California, San Francisco, California; Director of Maternal-Fetal Medicine, Good Samaritan Hospital, San Jose, California.
Endocrine Pancreas and Maternal Metabolism

Rosemary D. Leake, M.D.
Professor, UCLA School of Medicine, Los Angeles, California; Chairperson, Department of Pediatrics, Harbor-UCLA Medical Center, Torrance, California.
The Fetal-Maternal Neurohypophyseal System

A. Brian Little, M.D.
Professor and Chairman, Department of Obstetrics and Gynecology, McGill University, and The Royal Victoria Hospital, Montreal, Quebec, Canada.
Placental Synthesis of Steroid Hormones;

Placental Polypeptides; Maintenance of Pregnancy and the Initiation of Normal and Premature Labor

James C. Melby, M.D.
Professor of Medicine and Director of Endocrinology, Diabetes, and Metabolism, Boston University, Boston, Massachusetts.
The Maternal Adrenal Cortex

Francis Mimouni, M.D.
Associate Professor of Pediatrics, Obstetrics, and Gynecology, University of Pittsburgh; Associate Director and Clinical Director, Division of Neonatology, Magee Women's Hospital, Pittsburgh, Pennsylvania.
Perinatal Mineral Metabolism

Thomas J. Moore, M.D.
Associate Professor of Medicine, Harvard Medical School; Director, Cardiac Risk Reduction Center, Endocrine-Hypertension Division, Brigham and Women's Hospital, Boston, Massachusetts.
The Renin—Angiotensin—Aldosterone System and Vasopressin

Beverley E. Pearson Murphy, M.D., Ph.D.
Professor of Medicine, Obstetrics and Gynecology, and Psychiatry, McGill University; Senior Physician, Obstetrician and Gynecologist, Montreal General Hospital, Montreal, Quebec, Canada.
The Fetal Adrenal

Mary E. Norton, M.D.
Assistant Professor of Obstetrics and Gynecology, Tufts University and New England Medical Center, Boston, Massachusetts.
Endocrine Pancreas and Maternal Metabolism

Bahij S. Nuwayhid, M.D., Ph.D.
Professor, Obstetrics-Gynecology and Physiology, McGill University, Montreal, Quebec; Director, Maternal-Fetal Medicine Program, McGill University and Director, Obstetrics, Royal Victoria Hospital, Montreal, Quebec, Canada.
Hypertension in Pregnancy

Lauri J. Pelliniemi, M.D.
Associate Professor, Laboratory of
Electron Microscopy, University of
Turku, Turku, Finland.
The Fetal Gonad and Sexual Differentiation

Daniel H. Polk, M.D.
Associate Professor, Department of
Pediatrics, University of California at
Los Angeles, Los Angeles, California;
Harbor-UCLA Medical Center,
Torrance, California.
*The Ontogenesis of Thyroid Function and
Actions*

Martin Post, D.V.M., Ph.D.
Associate Professor of Paediatrics,
University of Toronto; Director,
Neonatology Research, Hospital for
Sick Children, Toronto, Ontario,
Canada.
*The Influence of Hormones of Fetal Lung
Development*

Edmond W. Quillen, Ph.D.
Associate Professor, Obstetrics-
Gynecology and Physiology, McGill
University, Montreal, Quebec; Research
Scientist, Royal Victoria Hospital,
Montreal, Quebec, Canada.
Hypertension in Pregnancy

Ellen W. Seely, M.D.
Assistant Professor of Medicine,
Harvard Medical School; Director of
Clinical Research, Endocrine-
Hypertension Division, Brigham and
Women's Hospital, Boston,
Massachusetts.
*The Renin—Angiotensin—Aldosterone
System and Vasopressin*

Barry T. Smith, M.D., F.R.C.P.C.
Professor of Paediatrics, Department of
Obstetrics and Gynecology, University
of Toronto; Associate Paediatrician in
Chief, Hospital for Sick Children;
Pediatrician in Chief, Mount Sinai
Hospital, Toronto, Ontario, Canada.
*The Influence of Hormones on Fetal Lung
Development*

Mark A. Sperling, M.D.
Professor and Chairman, Department
of Pediatrics, University of Pittsburgh,
School of Medicine; Pediatrician in
Chief, Children's Hospital of
Pittsburgh, Pittsburgh, Pennsylvania.
*Carbohydrate Metabolism: Insulin and
Glucagon; Newborn Adaptation:
Adrenocortical Hormones and
Adrenocorticotropic Hormone*

Reginald C. Tsang, M.B.B.S.
Professor, Department of Pediatrics,
Obstetrics, and Gynecology, University
of Cincinnati Medical Center;
Attending Staff at Children's Hospital
Medical Center and University Hospital
Medical Center; Consultant, Good
Samaritan Hospital and Christ Hospital;
Affiliate Staff, Bethesda Hospital;
Consultant, Jewish Hospital, Cincinnati,
Ohio.
Perinatal Mineral Metabolism

Dan Tulchinsky, M.D.
Professor of Obstetrics and Gynecology,
Director of Reproductive
Endocrinology, Boston University,
Boston, Massachusetts; Director of
Reproductive Endocrinology and
Fertility Services, The Malden Hospital,
Malden, Massachusetts.
*Postpartum Lactation and Resumption of
Reproductive Functions*

Gerson Weiss, M.D.
Professor and Chairman, UMD–New
Jersey Medical School; Chief of Service,
Department of Obstetrics and
Gynecology, UMDNJ–University
Hospital, Newark, New Jersey;
Consultant, Booth Memorial Hospital,
Flushing, Queens, New York.
The Maternal Ovaries

Koji Yoshinaga, B.S., M.S., Ph.D.
Adjunct Professor, Department of
Anatomy and Cell Biology, Georgetown
University School of Medicine,
Bethesda, Maryland.
Endocrinology of Implantation

Preface

——

It became clear in 1989 that the first edition of *Maternal-Fetal Endocrinology* had been received very well but that certain areas had become outdated. With this in mind, the authors of the first edition were contacted. The majority of the original authors have maintained and updated the substance and content of the first edition. New authors have been added as well, which has resulted in a new flavor overall.

It is hoped that this book will act as a stimulus and reference for all levels of students, including the investigator at one end of the spectrum and the thoughtful clinician at the other.

DAN TULCHINSKY
A. BRIAN LITTLE

Contents

———

Placental Synthesis of Steroid Hormones

Tommaso Falcone and A. Brian Little

The placenta synthesizes large quantities of steroids during pregnancy. The most important products of secretion are progesterone for the maintenance of pregnancy, estrogen for the growth of the reproductive tract, and both for the metabolic changes that accompany pregnancy. Large amounts of progesterone are secreted into the maternal circulation, but fetal concentrations of progesterone, which also originate in the placenta, are higher than maternal levels. Estrogens are secreted into the maternal circulation largely as a result of the placental conversion of maternal and fetal adrenal steroid precursors. Estriol, the unique estrogen of pregnancy, which is produced in increasing amounts during gestation,[85] is converted by the placenta largely from 16 α-hydroxylated C19 fetal androgen sulfate precursors (16-OH-dehydroepiandrosterone sulfate [DHS]). The reasons for the extensive fetal production and metabolism of the steroids is not understood, and much of the knowledge of the maternal activity, including alterations in maternal metabolism and reproductive tract, have been learned from studies carried out some years ago.[32, 44–46, 53, 75, 82, 85, 86]

As implantation takes place and human chorionic gonodotropin (hCG) begins to be secreted by the invading blastocyst into the circulation, the life of the corpus luteum is extended. Without a conceptus present, the life of the corpus luteum cannot be extended indefinitely,[7] which suggests an unknown contribution from the placenta and fetus as they develop to maintain the corpus luteum. However, the corpus luteum has a limited life span, and it starts to regress after the first trimester.

The placenta is not an autonomous steroid-secreting organ, as it requires precursors for both estrogen and progesterone secretion. The concept of the fetal and maternal adrenal precursors for estrogen and maternal cholesterol for progesterone synthesis by the placenta have been catalogued by the terms *maternal fetoplacental unit* and *fetoplacental unit*. These terms define this important relationship but may have inhibited the thought required to resolve the controls and importance of these complex steroid synthetic interactions.

MEDIATORS OF STEROID SYNTHESIS

Lipoprotein Precursors

High-density lipoprotein cholesterol (HDL-C) is not metabolized efficiently by these tissues.[18, 19, 25, 91, 92] Plasma low-density lipoprotein cholesterol (LDL-C) is the principal source of cholesterol for steroidogenesis in the placenta,[25, 91, 92] as it is in the fetal adrenal[18] and the corpus luteum.[19] Three-fourths of the total cholesterol in normal human plasma is contained in LDL particles. When LDL-C binds to specific receptors localized on the cell surface, the particle is taken up by endocytosis[16] (Fig. 1–1). Apoproteins (Apo B100) located on the surface of the LDL-C particle bind to membrane-bound receptors. Inside the cell, the endocytosed

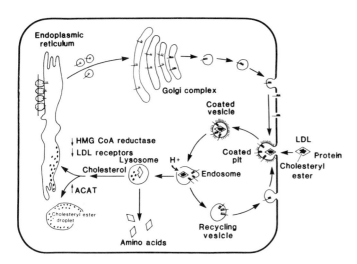

FIGURE 1–1. Route of the LDL receptor in mammalian cells. The receptor begins life in the endoplasmic reticulum from which it travels to the Golgi complex, cell surface, coated pit, endosome, and back to the surface. HMG CoA reductase = 3-hydroxy-3-methylglutaryl CoA reductase; ACAT = acyl-CoA; cholesterol acyltransferase. Vertical arrows indicate the direction of regulatory effects. (From Brown MS, Goldstein JL. A receptor-mediated pathway for cholesterol homeostasis. Science 1986;232:34. With permission from the Nobel Foundation.)

LDL-C is fused with acid lipase–containing liposomes, which leads to hydrolysis of the cholesterol esters, generating unesterified esters.[16] The apoprotein component is also digested off as amino acids, which are dispersed through the cytoplasm.

Human trophoblast, fetal adrenal, and corpus luteum cells have membrane-bound low-capacity, high-affinity binding sites for LDL.[25] The receptor number is regulated by the cellular demand for cholesterol.[17] Primate studies have shown that estrogens may play a role in regulating receptor-mediated uptake of LDL.[3, 39] This has not been shown in humans.

The LDL receptor is a glycoprotein present in coated pits on the cell surface. As with other receptors that participate in endocytosis, the receptors are recycled. The coated pits invaginate in a cyclical pattern whether or not LDL is present and bound to the receptor. The LDL receptor bound to LDL-C is dissociated within the endosome and returns to the surface. The receptor life span is 20 hours[16] (see Fig. 1–1).

Cells that actively synthesize steroid hormones have high concentrations of LDL-C receptors. The number of such receptors per unit weight in the fetal adrenal is greater than the human placenta.[25] The LDL-C receptors in the placenta are on the microvilli.[5] The LDL-C circulating in maternal blood binds to the syncytiotrophoblast to provide LDL for the fetus and precursor for progesterone biosynthesis secretion to the fetus and mother. The LDL-C receptors are present as early as 6 weeks' gestational age.[5] Expression of the LDL receptor gene is greatest in the first trimester.[31] This is at the time of the highest potential growth rate of placental steroidogenesis.[31]

De novo cholesterol synthesis in the placenta contributes little to progesterone synthesis.[38, 92, 95] A striking example of this is the report of a pregnancy in a woman with hypobetalipoproteinemia caused by familial lipoprotein deficiency.[67] Maternal circulating LDL-C was extremely low during pregnancy. Neonatal LDL-C concentration was also abnormal. The levels in the newborn were consistent with a heterozygote state. In this patient, maternal circulating concentrations of progesterone and estradiol were subnormal throughout pregnancy. Estriol was subnormal from 30 weeks' gestation onward (Fig. 1–2). The low levels could be predicted on the basis of the maternal/fetal LDL-C contribution to the steroid synthesis. Progesterone is almost exclusively derived from maternal LDL precursors and was therefore of very low circulating concentration throughout gestation. Placental estradiol is derived equally from maternal and fetal adrenal dehydroepiandrosterone (DHA) (which were converted from maternal and fetal circulatory LDL-C). These steroids were also low throughout gestation. Estriol, which is almost exclusively produced from fetal precursors, was normal up to 30 weeks' gestation; thereafter it appeared that the demand of the fetal adrenal for LDL-C to synthesize DHS was not met by the low LDL-C as a result of the heterozygote state of the fetus for hypobetalipoproteinemia. This was probably the source of the subnormal estriol levels after 30 weeks' gestation. Spontaneous labor, however, began at term, and a normal 3370-g baby girl was born.

Progesterone in this case appeared to be derived almost entirely from the maternal placental synthesis from LDL-C. Neither de novo cholesterol synthesis by the placenta nor HDL-C uptake could compensate for the lack of circulating maternal LDL-C. Estradiol and estrone are derived equally (50 : 50) from fetal and maternal precursors, whereas estriol is mostly (90%) from fetal precursors.[75] Therefore estriol was not adversely affected. The umbilical cord plasma concentrations of cortisol and DHS were normal. Cultured fetal adrenal cells have high rates of de novo cholesterol synthesis and steroidogenesis when maintained in a medium deprived of LDL.[55] In the presence of excess LDL-C in vivo, the fetal adrenal derives cholesterol largely from plasma LDL-C.[18, 65] Presumably in this instance cortisol and DHS were maintained in the fetus by a contribution from fetal adrenal cholesterol de novo synthesis.

Fetal LDL-C decreases progressively as gestation progresses. Much of this decrease is likely associated with its marked increased utilization by the fetal adrenal for steroidogenesis of steroids, such as DHS. DHS production in the fetus rises to reach a maximum of 100 to 200 mg per day at term. There is an inverse relation between LDL-C and DHS concentra-

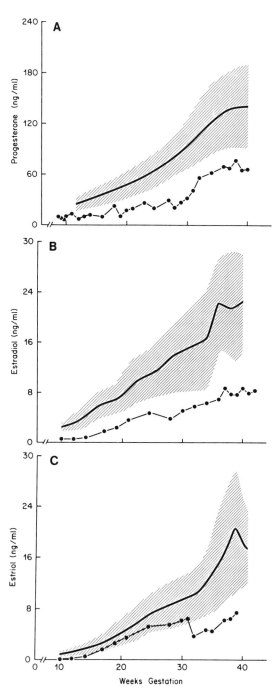

FIGURE 1–2. Serum levels of progesterone (*A*), estradiol (*B*), and estriol (*C*), throughout pregnancy in a woman with homozygous hypobetalipoproteinemia. Values for the patient are indicated by the solid circles; values for normal women during gestation (hatched area) are means ± 1 SD. To convert values for progesterone, estradiol and estriol to nanomoles per liter, multiply by 3.179, 3.676 and 3.472. (From Parker CR, Illingworth DR, Bissonnette JL, Carr BR. Endocrine changes during pregnancy in a patient with homozygous hypobetalipoproteinemia. N Engl J Med 1986;314:557. With permission.)

tions in the umbilical cord plasma associated with the increased DHS as gestation progresses.[67] This suggests that LDL-C in fetal plasma is regulated by the rate of utilization of LDL-C by the fetal adrenal. Fetal LDL-C is derived mostly by cholesterol synthesis in the fetal liver rather than from maternal sources.[11, 20]

The overwhelming evidence supports the concept that maternal LDL-C is the major precursor of both progesterone and estrogen placental and adrenal steroid synthesis in the mother. Fetal LDL-C acts similarly for adrenal steroidogenesis in the fetus during normal human pregnancy.

Steroidogenic Enzymes

Most of the cytochromes of the enzymes involved in steroid biosynthesis (Fig. 1–3) in both the placenta and the fetal adrenal belong to a family of genes known as cytochrome P450. In vivo the syncytial trophoblast is the major site of expression of the steroidogenic enzymes.[61] The first step in conversion of cholesterol is by P450 side-chain cleavage to form pregnenolone. Conversion of cholesterol to pregnenolone by the P450 side-chain cleavage enzyme is the rate-limiting step in steroid synthesis. This step occurs in the mitochondria. Pregnenolone can be converted to 17-α-hydroxypregnenolone (17-OH-pregnenolone) by the P450 17-α-hydroxylase enzyme. This enzyme has two activities: 17-α-hydroxylase and C17-20 lyase. The latter enzyme metabolizes 17-OH-pregnenolone to dehydroepiandrosterone (DHEA). This enzyme present in the endoplasmic reticulum is only minimally active[49] or inactive in placental tissue but is active in the fetal adrenal. Pregnenolone, 17-OH-pregnenolone, and DHEA can be converted to progesterone, 17α-hydroxyprogesterone, and androstenedione, respectively, by 3β-hydroxysteroid dehydrogenase and Δ5-Δ4-isomerase. These interconversions are mediated by enzyme(s) that are present in both mitochondrial and microsomal fractions. These enzymes are not part of the cytochrome P450 group and are not appreciably active in the fetal adrenal gland, although they are present in excess in the placenta and are not rate limiting. The

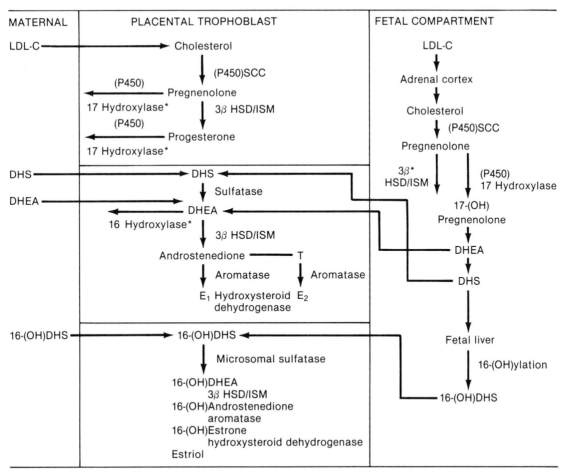

*Inactive

FIGURE 1–3. Steroid biosynthesis in the adrenal cortex. The major secretory products are underlined. The enzymes for the reactions are numbered on the left and at the top of the chart, with the steps catalyzed shown by the shaded bars. (1) (P450) SCC = cholesterol 20,22-hydroxylase:20,22 desmolase activity; (2) 3β-HSD/ISM = 3β-hydroxysteroid dehydrogenase: Δ^5-oxosteroid isomerase activity; (3) (P450) c21 = 21α-hydroxylase activity; (4) (P450) c11 = 11β-hydroxylase activity; (5) (P450) c17 = 17α-hydroxylase activity; (6) (P450) c17 = 17,20 lyase/desmolase activity; (7) sulfokinase.

contribution of peripheral pregnenolone to progesterone synthesis is minimal.[46]

Luteal Placental Shift

Estrogen and progesterone are important in the maintenance of human pregnancy. Although the corpus luteum and placenta are the major contributors to steroid synthesis, the embryo itself also may play an early role.[34, 50] For example, the 7-day rabbit embryo has been shown to synthesize androgens and estrogens.[34] These steroids appear to affect the implantation site.[50] Nuclear receptors for both estrogen and progesterone are present in two-fold higher concentration in implantation sites of the endometrium of 6-day pregnant rats.[50] These locally produced steroids may play a role in implantation. No such human data have yet been reported.

There is a period of time in early gestation when the corpus luteum is essential for the maintenance of pregnancy. The transfer of pregnancy maintenance and predominant estrogen and progesterone secretion from the corpus luteum to the placenta is called the *luteal placental shift* (LPS).

In humans, it appears that until the seventh week, the corpus luteum is necessary for pregnancy maintenance.[24] Lutectomy performed in early pregnancy (less than 7 weeks' gestation) resulted in a substantial number of spontaneous abortions.[24] To what extent the corpus luteum secretion is obligatory for early pregnancy is difficult to assess. A pregnancy that continued to term was reported in a woman with premature ovarian failure who received oocyte donation but no additional early pregnancy estradiol or progesterone support.[41] Moreover, there is a comparative difference among primates in the dynamics of this shift.[21, 29, 35] In the rhesus monkey, this shift may occur as early as 1 week after implantation.[35] In the baboon and the human, there is a more prolonged period of luteal dependence.[21, 24, 29]

In nonhuman primates,[21, 29] serum progesterone levels fall in the face of rising serum chorionic gonadotropin (CG) levels and reach a nadir at the time of maximal CG secretion. This could be the result of a limited ability of the corpus luteum to synthesize progesterone.

Several human studies have also demonstrated a fall in progesterone between the fifth and ninth week of pregnancy,[23, 57] whereas others have not[85] (Fig. 1–4). Serum estrogens show a continuous rise that follows the initial rise of hCG,[23, 57, 85] which may reflect a capacity for increasing synthesis by the corpus luteum at this time.

Serum androstenedione and testosterone also increase and follow a pattern similar to estrogen[23, 81] in early pregnancy. The rise of testosterone may be partially due to increased

sex hormone–binding globulin (SHBG), which is the result of estrogen stimulation of the liver. However, free testosterone also increases above nonpregnant levels in the third trimester.[8] DHEA and DHS levels are lower than in the nonpregnant woman. This is due to the increased metabolic clearance by the placenta and maternal liver.[32]

Progesterone

Placental progesterone synthesis is independent of fetal precursors (see Fig. 1–3; Fig. 1–5). LDL-C is transported to the trophoblast and binds to the receptor on the membrane surface. After endocytosis occurs, the vesicles fuse with lysosomes, and hydrolysis occurs; cholesterol is then liberated. Within the mitochondria, cholesterol side-chain cleavage and hydroxylation by cytochrome P450 enzyme complex takes place. Pregnenolone is then transformed by 3β-hydroxysteroid dehydrogenase/Δ5-Δ4-isomerase to progesterone. Placental 17β/20α-hydroxysteroid dehydrogenase converts estrone to estradiol and progesterone to 20α-dihydroprogesterone.[49] Equilibrium, however, favors progesterone and estradiol.

Most of the secreted progesterone goes into the maternal circulation (90%), but fetal plasma concentrations are higher than maternal.[87] The placenta at term produces about 210 mg of progesterone each day with a wide variation and a metabolic clearance rate (MCR) of about 2100 L per day.[44] The luteal-phase production is 15 to 20 mg per day and an MCR of about 2500 L per day.[43] Splanchnic and extrasplanchnic tissues contribute in a ratio of 40:60 to the MCR of progesterone in the nonpregnant state.[45, 47] The maternal plasma progesterone concentration rises in a linear fashion from 40 to greater than 175 ng/mL from the first to the third trimester[86] (see Fig. 1–5). Progesterone plasma levels change in early pregnancy and are characterized by cyclic pulsation.[60] It is unclear if this pulsation is due to episodic secretion, alterations in metabolic clearance rate, or changes in volumes of distribution. For example, there appears to be a decrease in progesterone levels after meals.[60] This is probably the result of a change in the MCR of progesterone as a result of increased

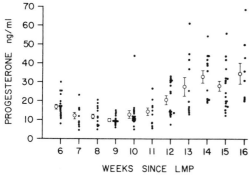

FIGURE 1–4. Mean serial progesterone values in early pregnancy in three women show a decline from the sixth to the ninth weeks after the last menstrual period. The mean at the nadir of 10 ng/ml at 9 weeks is followed by a steady rise. (From Mishell DR, Thorneycroft IH, Nagata Y, et al. Serum gonadotropin and steroid patterns in early human gestation. Am J Obstet Gynecol 1973;117:631. With permission.)

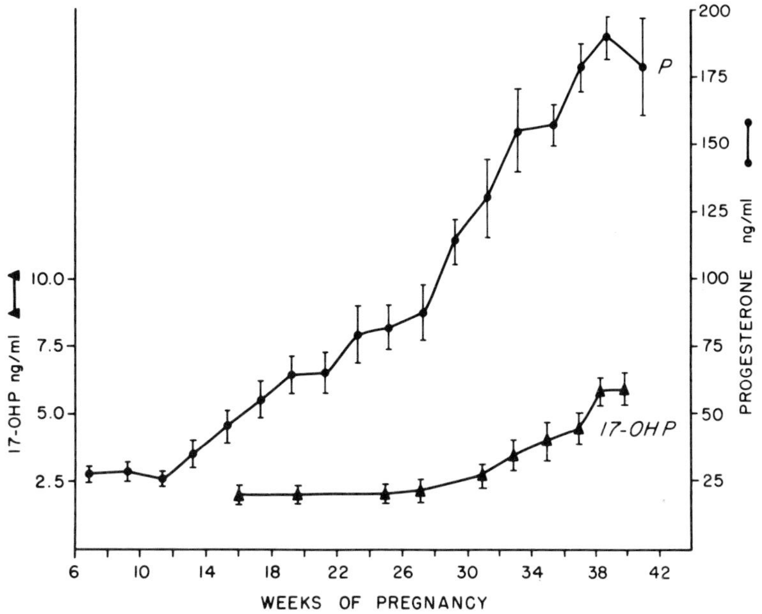

FIGURE 1–5. Progesterone and 17α-hydroxyprogesterone mean plasma levels during human pregnancy. (From Tulchinsky D, Hobel CJ, Yeager E, Marshall JR. Plasma estrone, estradiol, estriol, progesterone and 17-hydroxyprogesterone in human pregnancy—normal pregnancy. Am J Obstet Gynecol 1972; 112:1095. With permission.)

hepatic blood flow after meals. This phenomenon also occurs in nonpregnant women, in whom it may be the result of uninhibited splanchnic clearance.[60] No trend is seen with gestational age, suggesting that the variability in progesterone circulating concentration is not associated in a major way with either the corpus luteum or the trophoblast. There is no significant change in the relative concentrations of circulating estrogen and progesterone preceding the onset of labor in every case, although there is evidence for such a change in some cases.

The human placenta is rich in β-adrenergic receptors, which can be found as early as 10 weeks' gestation. These are present at term in high concentrations.[73, 89] The localization of the β receptors on the human placenta shows them to be closer to the fetal than to the maternal circulation.[89] β₂-agonist administration during placental explant perfusion results in increased adenyl cyclase and progesterone secretion in vitro.[42] Perfusion experiments with placental explants have also shown that intracellular calcium is necessary for placental progesterone production,[42] by the demonstration that placental explants incubated with β₂-adrenergic agonists (isoproterenol or terbutaline), LDL-C, and a calcium ionophore failed to show the expected cyclic adenosine monophosphate (cAMP) accumulation and progesterone production.[42] In placental monolayer culture, it has also been shown that luteinizing hormone–releasing hormone (LH-RH) has an inhibitory effect on progesterone secretion.[15] Therefore progesterone secretion is modulated at the cellular level of the placenta. The roles of cyclic nucleotides, β-adrenergic stimulation, neuropeptides, and growth factors in vivo remain to be determined.

Nonhuman primate studies in vivo and human placental tissue studies in vitro have shown a possible role for estrogen on progesterone synthesis.[3, 4, 39] Immunocytochemical studies on cultured human placental syncytiotrophoblasts have identified an estrogen receptor in the nuclei of these cells.[13] Because conditions associated with reduced estrogens, however, such as the presence of anencephaly, fetal death, placental sulfatase deficiency, or aromatase deficiency, are not associated with a decline in progesterone production, the role for such estrogen control is unknown. Androgens also have an inhibitory effect on progesterone synthesis in vitro.[13] No controlled in vivo studies have been performed in the human for obvious ethical reasons.

The syncytiotrophoblast has intracellular progesterone receptors. Progesterone has an important regulatory function on steroid and protein hormone synthesis in the placenta.[26] The output of certain peptide hormones, such as corticotropin-releasing hormone (CRH), and hCG production can be modulated by the addition of progesterone to placental tissue culture.[2, 40] Increasing concentrations of progesterone in vitro decreases CRH output from the placenta.[40] The addition of RU486 (a 19 norsteroid progesterone receptor antagonist) to culture of syncytiotrophoblast cells has resulted in an impaired output of hCG, human placental lactogen (hPL), and progesterone.[26] This effect was reversed by the addition of increasing amounts of progesterone. Therefore the abortifacient action of RU486 may not be limited to its effect on the endometrium, as previously reported.[26]

The very limited 17-hydroxylase activity in the placenta results in the failure of 17-hydroxyprogesterone to increase in the circulation until late pregnancy (about 30 weeks' gestation), when an increase is seen as a result of fetal precursors[85] (see Fig. 1–5).

Placental Estrogens

Placental estrogen production during pregnancy is largely a result of the conversion of maternal and fetal adrenal precursors (see Fig. 1–3; Fig. 1–6). Maternal and fetal DHS serve as precursors for DHA and placental production of estrogens. In both maternal and fetal circulation, the major form of this adrenal androgen is its sulfated form. It has been shown that in nonpregnant female adults, one-third

of circulating DHA is derived (hydrolyzed) from DHS,[37] whereas in the term pregnancy, 40% is derived from DHS.[9] No data exist on the fetus. In vitro studies of the fetal adrenal, however, have shown that the sulfated form is the major form of DHA produced, implying that the circulating unconjugated form is mostly derived from its conjugated form.[78] Maternal and fetal DHA/DHS contribute equally to formation of estrone and 17β-estradiol (50:50); more than 90% of the estriol formed, however, is derived from fetal 16α-(OH)-DHA.[75] In hypobetalipoproteinemia, the maternal compartment contributes little to placental steroid synthesis, but estriol is normal; however, both estrone and 17β-estradiol are substantially decreased (see Fig. 1–2).

At term, the metabolic clearance of DHA is increased twofold[10] and DHS eightfold[32] over the nonpregnant states. This increase in metabolic clearance is partly the result of its major conversion to estrogens by the placenta. Placental conversion of DHS to estradiol accounts for approximately 35% of total clearance.[54] In pregnancy, maternal DHA/DHS is 16α-hydroxylated by the maternal liver.[53, 54] This also contributes substantially to the increased metabolic clearance of DHA/DHS in pregnancy. This 16-α-hydroxy DHA/DHS is converted by the placenta to estriol. Loss to the fetus and excretion as unaltered DHS contribute little to the metabolic clearance.[54] The DHA/DHS production by the maternal adrenal does increase slightly in pregnancy, whereas DHA/

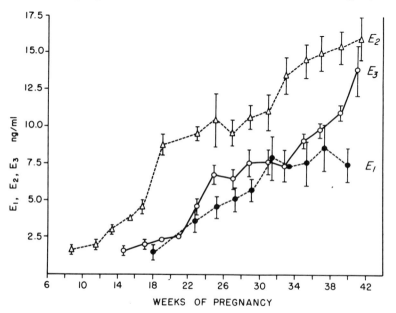

FIGURE 1–6. Mean plasma estrogen levels during human pregnancy. (From Tulchinsky D, Hobel CJ, Yeager E, Marshall JR. Plasma estrone, estradiol, estriol, progesterone and 17-hydroxyprogesterone in human pregnancy—normal pregnancy. Am J Obstet Gynecol 1972;112:1095. With permission.)

DHS production by the fetal adrenal increases markedly throughout pregnancy.

The fetal contribution to placental estrogen synthesis by DHA/DHS is the result of a low expression of the microsomal 3β-hydroxysteroid dehydrogenase, Δ5-Δ4-isomerase in the fetal adrenal. Consequently, DHA and pregnenolone (and their sulfated derivatives) are the principal secretory products of the fetus. The DHS is then 16-α-hydroxylated in the fetal liver. The circulating DHS is desulfated by sulfatase and converted by the placenta to estradiol, and the 16-α-hydroxylated DHS is converted to estriol. Estriol is quantitatively the predominant circulating estrogen in pregnancy.

Fetal C_{19} precursors are hydrolyzed by steroid sulfatase in the placenta before entering the pathway catalyzed by microsomal 3β-hydroxysteroid dehydrogenase, Δ5-Δ4-isomerase. Steroid sulfatase is a microsomal enzyme in the placenta. Using light and electron immunocytochemistry and in situ hybridization, the sulfatase has been localized to the endoplasmic reticulum of the syncytiotrophoblast and is absent in the cytotrophoblast.[71] Sulfatase deficiency results in lack of conversion of DHS to DHA (Fig. 1–7). As a result, the circulating umbilical cord sulfated estrogen precursors are of high concentration.[63] The production of estrogens from DHA remains intact. Thus estrone and estradiol are synthesized in low normal amounts,[63] but estriol is markedly reduced. Because the placenta lacks 16-hydroxylase activity it cannot form estriol from estrone or estradiol directly. The absence of steroid sulfatase is an X-linked genetic disorder associated with ichthyosis.

After desulfation, DHA is converted by 3β-hydroxysteroid dehydrogenase/Δ5-Δ4-isomerase to androstenedione. This enzyme is present in placental microsomes and mitochondria.[70] Both activities of this enzyme in the placenta (oxidation and isomerase) are nicotinamide-adenine dinucleotide/reduced nicotinamide-adenine dinucleotide (NAD/NADH) dependent.[80] The dehydrogenase or isomerase activity of the enzyme uses the appropriate pregnene (e.g., pregnenolone) and androstene (e.g., DHA) steroids as alternative, competitive substrates but of different affinity.[80]

These C_{19} steroids DHA and 16α hydroxy dehydroepiandrosterone DHA are then aromatized to C_{18} estrogens. Purification and characterization of the aromatase from human placenta have shown it to have the properties of a cytochrome P450 with an amino acid composition resembling other P450 enzymes.[36] It occurs primarily in the endoplasmic reticulum of the syncytiotrophoblast layer, and it is therefore consistent with the generation of estrogen primarily in the placental villi.[12] In choriocarcinoma cell lines, cytotrophoblast-like cells express a high degree of aromatase component antigen,[12] which may be a manifestation of the normal development of cytotrophoblast into syncytiotrophoblast but in an abnormal dedifferentiated state.

The products of the estrone pathway are estrone (from androstenedione) or 16-α-hydroxyestrone (from 16-α-hydroxy androstenedione). It appears that androstenedione and 16-α-hydroxy androstenedione are aromatized at separate but linked sites in placental microsomes[65] (Fig. 1–8). Aromatization by the placenta of C_{19} steroids is very efficient. It is estimated that all of the androstenedione entering a trophoblast is aromatized.[52] Therefore none enters the fetal circulation. Indeed, in a case of placental aromatase deficiency, the fetoplacental unit released sufficient free androgens to masculinize a female fetus and virilize the mother.[74] This is one likely explanation for the clinical observation that few androgen-secreting tumors in pregnancy masculinize the fetus, unless the tumor is producing a nonaro-

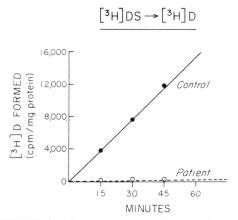

$$[^3H]DS \rightarrow [^3H]D$$

FIGURE 1–7. Failure of placental sulfatase deficient tissue to cleave tritiated (³H) DHS to DHA compared with control placenta. (From Osathanondh R, Canick J, Ryan KJ, Tulchinsky D. Placental sulfatase deficiency: A case study. J Clin Endocrinol Metab 1976;43:208. With permission.)

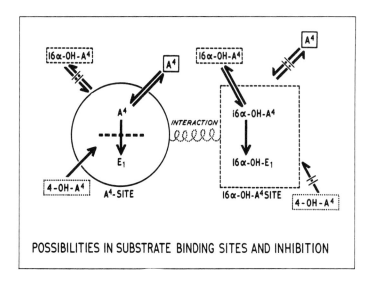

POSSIBILITIES IN SUBSTRATE BINDING SITES AND INHIBITION

FIGURE 1–8. Diagrammatic illustration of the sites proposed for aromatization of androstenedione (A^4) and 16α-hydroxyandrostenedione (16α-OH-A^4) in human placental microsomes. One site binds A^4 and 4-hydroxyandrostenedione (4-OH-A^4) but not 16α-OH-A^4. The other binds 16α-OH-A^4 but not A^4 or 4-OH-A^4. Noncompetitive inhibition is exerted through some interaction between the sites. (From Purohit A, Oakey RE. Evidence for separate sites for aromatization of androstenedione and 16 alpha-hydroxyandrostenedione in human placental microsomes. J Steroid Biochem 1989;33:439. With permission.)

matizable androgen. Most pharmacologic androgens are nonaromatizable (e.g., danazol).

The 17β-hydroxysteroid dehydrogenase (also named 17β-hydroxyoxidoreductase) converts estrone and 16-hydroxy estrone to estradiol and estriol, respectively. The 17β-hydroxysteroid dehydrogenase also has 20α-hydroxysteroid dehydrogenase activity.[79] Two kinetically distinct 17β-dehydrogenases exist: one with affinity for both estrogens and androgens and one with affinity solely for estrogens.[14] Estetrol is the 15-hydroxy derivative of estriol. Estradiol can be both 15-α and 16-α hydroxylated to form estetrol in the fetus but not the mother. Estetrol is transported into the maternal circulation.[84]

Control of estrogen production by the placenta appears to be mostly dependent on fetal precursors. In placental monolayer cultures, adding DHA/DHS and their 16α-hydroxy derivatives increases estrogen production.[15] Gonadotropin-releasing hormone (GnRH) and progesterone appear to have an inhibitory effect on estrogen synthesis by placenta in vitro.[15] The presence of GnRH in the placenta is another manifestation of the ubiquitous nature and variable action of such peptides, in this case of primary hypothalamic origin, which are not explained in physiologic terms as yet.

The human placenta at term secretes estrone, estradiol, and estriol into both the maternal and the fetal circulations. The total blood production rate of estradiol is approximately 10 to 25 mg per day and that of estriol is 40 to 50 mg per day at term. Much of the estrone in both the maternal and the fetal circulations is present as sulfate and has a low MCR in that form.[51] Of the unconjugated estrogenic steroids in serum, estradiol is present in highest concentration and has a relatively short half-life in blood (20 minutes). Estriol is present in maternal serum largely as a conjugated derivative, with only 10% being unconjugated. Unconjugated estriol is rapidly cleared, with a half-life similar to that of estradiol, of about 20 minutes.[86]

The general pattern of unconjugated estrogens in maternal plasma throughout pregnancy is illustrated in Figure 1–6. Steroid hormone values in serum do not change significantly during labor.[62]

Although there are marked fluctuations in serum levels of unconjugated estrogens during the day, there have been conflicting reports on whether a circadian rhythm exists.[22] Because both maternal and fetal adrenal steroids contribute to the precursor pools for estrogens and there is a circadian rhythm for maternal adrenal function, one might expect this to be reflected directly in the maternal adrenal contribution to estrogen precursors.

Estriol is conjugated by the maternal liver to glucuronide sulfate and to various mixtures of sulfoglucuronides. Some of these conjugated steroids are excreted in the bile to enter the enterohepatic circulation, where they are metabolized by intestinal flora and reabsorbed into the circulation, where they presumably exert their biologic effect and are reconjugated. This processing can be interfered with by changes in intestinal flora, such as after administration of antibiotics,[1] surgical colectomy, or colitis.[64]

CLINICAL APPLICATIONS

Estriol Measurement

It can be predicted that in disease states in which there is a nonfunctional or dysfunctional fetal adrenal, estriol formation will be altered. Anencephaly is associated with relative absence of the fetal zone of the adrenal cortex. Decreased adrenal androgen fetal precursors leads to a greatly decreased estriol output from the placenta.[52] Hydatidiform molar pregnancies are also associated with low estriol output. Estriol output can be increased by the administration of adrenocorticotropic hormone (ACTH) to the mother.[52]

In disorders in which fetal LDL-C precursors are decreased, as in hypobetalipoproteinemia and placental sulfatase deficiency, as discussed earlier, the lack of lipoprotein for androgen production and enzyme for sulfate cleavage lead to a decrease in estriol production. Glucocorticoid administration to the mother, such as that administered to promote fetal lung maturation or for intercurrent disease, e.g., rheumatoid arthritis, also results in a decrease in circulating estriol[76, 77] production by suppression of maternal and fetal ACTH and adrenal precursors.

Estriol measurements were used extensively in the past as a test of fetal well-being. In complications of pregnancy, such as hypertension, urinary estriol levels are low, fetal plasma levels of DHS are low, placental conversion to estrogen is low, and fetal plasma LDL-C is high.[68] Fetal plasma cortisol, however, is unchanged. This therefore reflects a reduced secretory activity of the fetal adrenal zone but a normal secretion by the neocortex[68] and thus the availability of substrate; i.e., LDL-C is not the limiting step. Urinary estriol levels in clinical practice, however, have been supplanted by other tests, such as fetal heart rate monitoring and biophysical profile.[90] Estradiol production fol-

lowing labeled DHS administration has also been used as an investigative tool for assessing uteroplacental function, but it has never reached clinical use.[54]

Interpretation of plasma or urinary estriol levels is made difficult because of a wide range of normal values that vary with gestational age, making a single measurement relatively uninterpretable.[83] The formation of estriol is further influenced by maternal ingestion of medications (e.g., antibiotics, steroids), maternal medical problems (renal, liver, and bowel disease), and fetal problems (anencephaly), which do not predict fetal outcome.[83]

Many studies have shown conflicting results in the use of urinary estriol tests in high-risk pregnancies in patients with pregnancy complications, such as hypertension, diabetes, and post dates gestational age. Such tests did not significantly alter pregnancy outcome.[6, 27, 28, 72] Estetrol measurements are subject to the same limitations as estriol[84] but have never been widely used.

The measurement of urinary estrogens after the infusion of exogenous substrate with either DHS (DHS loading test) or DHA has been suggested as an alternative method for studying fetal and placental function.[58, 88] Maternal DHS, however, is not a good precursor for estriol.[30] The rise in serum estradiol is measured at 1 hour and in serum estetrol at 4 hours after infusion. Although some predicable patterns can be determined,[88] it has never been extensively used.

Progesterone Measurement

Progesterone measurements are not clinically useful as a measure of fetal well-being. The fetus may die in utero without a change in progesterone levels, and progesterone is not affected in cases of anencephaly or placental sulfatase deficiency.[87]

Serum progesterone levels have been used for the diagnosis of ectopic pregnancy.[56, 94] Several authors have reported that many patients with abnormal intrauterine pregnancies as well as most patients with an ectopic pregnancy have progesterone levels less than 15 ng/mL[56, 94] at a time when patients with a normal intrauterine pregnancy had a 95% confidence interval of 17.4 to 44.4 ng/mL.[33, 54] Moreover, it has been shown that serum progesterone is the single most reliable predictor of pregnancy viability among a group of six potential predictors of outcome (serum estradiol, relaxin, Ca-125, Schwangerschaft protein, and hCG) at the time of threatened abortion or early pregnancy ≤77 days.[93] Nonetheless, further confirmatory reports will be required before the value of a progesterone level in patients with a suspected ectopic pregnancy can be determined.

REFERENCES

1. Adlercreutz H, Martin F, Tikhanen MJ, Pulkkinen M. Effect of ampicillin administration on the excretion of twelve estrogens in pregnancy urine. Acta Endocrinol 1975;80:551.
2. Ahmed NA, Murphy BEP. The effects of various hormones on human chorionic gonadotropin production in early and late placental explant cultures. Am J Obstet Gynecol 1988;159:1220.
3. Albrecht ED, Henson MC, Pepe GS. Regulation of placental low density lipoprotein uptake in baboons by estrogen. Endocrinology 1991;128:450.
4. Albrecht ED, Pepe GS. Placental steroid hormone biosynthesis in primate pregnancy. Endocrinol Rev 1990;11:124.
5. Alsat E, Bouali Y, Goldstein S, et al. Low-density lipoprotein binding sites in the microvillus membranes of human placenta at different stages of gestation. Mol Cell Endocrinol 1984;38:197.
6. Arias F, Zamora J. Antihypertensive treatment and pregnancy outcome in patients with mild chronic hypertension. Obstet Gynecol 1979;53:489.
7. Auletta FJ, Flint AP. Mechanisms controlling corpus luteum function in sheep, cows, nonhuman primates and women especially in relation to the timing of luteolysis. Endocrine Rev 1988;9:88.
8. Bammann BL, Coulam CB, Jiang NS. Total and free testosterone during pregnancy. Am J Obstet Gynecol 1980;137:293.
9. Belisle S, Osathanondh R, Tulchinsky D. The effect of constant infusion of unlabeled dehydroepiandrosterone sulfate on maternal plasma androgens and estrogens. J Clin Endocrinol Metab 1977;45:544.
10. Belisle S, Schiff I, Tulchinsky D. The use of constant infusion of unlabeled dehydroepiandrosterone for the assessment of its metabolic clearance rate, its half life and its conversion into estrogens. J Clin Endocrinol Metab 1980;50:117.
11. Belknap WM, Dietschy JM. Sterol synthesis and low density lipoprotein clearance *in vivo* in the pregnant rat, placenta and fetus. J Clin Invest 1988;82:2077.
12. Bellino FL, Lobo JO. Estrogen synthetase (aromatase) in cultured human term placental cells and neoplastic human trophoblast. Steroids 1987;50:73.
13. Billiar RB, Pepe GS, Albrecht ED. Immunocytochemical identification of the estrogen receptor in the nuclei of cultured human syncytiotrophoblast cells (abstr). Presented at the Society for Gynecologic Investigation, San Antonio, Texas, 1991.
14. Blomquist CH, Lindemann NJ, Hakanson EY. 17 Beta-hydroxysteroid and 20 alpha-hydroxysteroid dehydrogenase activities of human placental microsomes: kinetic evidence for two enzymes differing in substrate specificity. Arch Biochem Biophys 1985;239:206.
15. Branchaud CL, Goodyer CG, Lipowski LS. Progesterone and estrogen production by placental monolayer cultures: effect of dehydroepiandrosterone and luteinizing hormone-releasing hormone. J Clin Endocrinol Metab 1983;56:761.
16. Brown MS, Goldstein JL. A receptor-mediated pathway for cholesterol homeostasis. Science 1986;232:34.
17. Brown MS, Kovanen PT, Goldstein JL. Receptor-mediated uptake of lipoprotein cholesterol and its utilization for steroid synthesis in the adrenal cortex. Recent Prog Horm Res 1979;35:215.
18. Carr BR, Parker CR Jr, Milewich L, et al. The role of low density, high density and very low density lipoproteins in steroidogenesis by the human fetal adrenal gland. Endocrinology 1980;106:1854.
19. Carr BR, Sadler RK, Rochelle DB, et al. Plasma lipoprotein regulation of progesterone biosynthesis by human corpus luteum tissue in organ culture. J Clin Endocrinol Metab 1981;52:875.
20. Carr BR, Simpson ER. Cholesterol synthesis by human fetal hepatocytes: effect of lipoproteins. Am J Obstet Gynecol 1984;150:551.
21. Castracane VD, Goldzilha QW. Timing of the luteal-placental shift in the baboon (Papio cynocephalus). Endocrinology 1986;118:506.
22. Compton AA, Kirkish LS, Parra J, et al. Diurnal variations in unconjugated and total plasma estriol levels in late normal pregnancy. Obstet Gynecol 1979;53:623.
23. Corker CS, Michie E, Hobson B, Parboosingh J. Hormonal patterns in conceptual cycles and early pregnancy. Br J Obstet Gynaecol 1976;83:489.
24. Csapo AI, Pulkkinen MO, Wiest WG. Effects of lutectomy and progesterone replacement therapy in early pregnant patients. Am J Obstet Gynecol 1973;115:759.
25. Cummings SW, Hatley W, Simpson ER, Ohashi M. The binding of high and low density lipoproteins to human placental membrane fractions. J Clin Endocrinol Metab 1982;54:903.
26. Das C, Catt K. Antifertility actions of the progesterone antagonist RU486 include direct inhibition of placental hormone secretion. Lancet 1987;2:599.
27. Dorley SL, Depp R, Socol ML, et al. Urinary estriols in diabetic pregnancy: a re-appraisal. Obstet Gynecol 1984;64:469.
28. Duenhoelter JH, Whalley PJ, MacDonald PC. An analysis of the utility of plasma immunoreactive estrogen measurements in determining delivery time of gravidas with a fetus considered at high risk. Am J Obstet Gynecol 1976;125:889.
29. Ellenwood WE, Stanczyk FL, Lazur JJ, Novy MJ. Dynamics of steroid biosynthesis during the luteal placental shift in rhesus monkeys. J Clin Endocrinol Metab 1989;69:348.
30. Fraser IS, Leask R, Fufe J. Plasma estrogen response to dehydroepiandrosterone sulfate injection in normal and complicated late pregnancy. Obstet Gynecol 1976;47:152.
31. Furuhashi M, Seo H, Mizutani S, et al. Expression of low density lipoprotein receptor gene in human placenta during pregnancy. Mol Endocrin 1989;3:1252.
32. Gant NF, Hutchinson HT, Sitteri PK, MacDonald PC. Study of the metabolic clearance rate of dehydroepiandrosterone sulfate in pregnancy. Am J Obstet Gynecol 1971;111:555.

33. Gelder MS, Boots LR, Younger JB. Use of a single random serum progesterone value as a diagnostic aid for ectopic pregnancy. Fertil Steril 1991;55:497.

34. George FW, Wilson JD. Estrogen formation in the early rabbit embryo. Science 1978;199:200.

35. Goodman AL, Hodgen GD. Corpus luteum-conceptus-follicle relationships during the fertile cycle in rhesus monkeys: pregnancy maintenance despite early luteal removal. J Clin Endocrinol Metab 1979;48:469.

36. Hall PF, Chen S, Nakajin S, et al. Purification and characterization of aromatase from human placenta. Steroids 1987;50:37.

37. Haning RV, Chabot M, Flood CA, et al. Metabolic clearance rate (MCR) of dehydroepiandrosterone sulfate (DS), its metabolism to dehydroepiandrosterone, androstenedione, testosterone and dihydrotestosterone, and the effect of increased plasma DS concentration in DS MCR in normal women. J Clin Endocrinol Metab 1989;69:1047.

38. Hellig H, Gotterereau D, Lefebvre Y, Bolte E. Steroid production from cholesterol. I. Conversion of plasma cholesterol to placental progesterone in humans. J Clin Endocrinol Metab 1970;30:624.

39. Henson MC, Babischkin JS, Pepe GJ, Albrecht ED. Effect of the antiestrogen ethamoxytrophetol (MER-25) on placental low density lipoprotein uptake and degradation in baboons. Endocrinology 1988; 122: 2019.

40. Jones SA, Brooks AN, Challis JRG. Steroids modulate corticotropin releasing hormone production in human fetal membranes and placenta. J Clin Endocrinol Metab 1989;68:825.

41. Kapetanakis E, Pantos KJ. Continuation of a donor oocyte pregnancy in menopause without early pregnancy support. Fertil Steril 1990;54:1171.

42. Kasugai M, Kato H, Iriyama H, et al. The roles of Ca and adenosine 3', 5' monophosphate in the regulation of progesterone production by human placental tissue. J Clin Endocrinol Metab 1987;65:122.

43. Lin TJ, Billiar RB, Little B. Metabolic clearance rate of progesterone in the menstrual cycle. J Clin Endocrinol Metab 1972;35:879.

44. Lin TJ, Lin SC, Erlenmeyer F, Kline IT, et al. Progesterone production rates during the third trimester of pregnancy in normal women, diabetic women and women with abnormal glucose tolerance. J Clin Endocrinol Metab 1972;34:287.

45. Little B, Billiar RB, Bougas J, Tait JF. The splanchnic clearance rate of progesterone in patients with cardiac disease. J Clin Endocrinol Metab 1973;36:1222.

46. Little B, Billiar RB, Halla M, et al. Pregnenolone production in pregnancy. Am J Obstet Gynecol 1971; 111:505.

47. Little B, Billiar RB, Rahman SS, Johnson WA, et al. *In vivo* aspects of progesterone distribution and metabolism. Am J Obstet Gynecol 1975;123:527.

48. Little B, Di Martinis J, Nyholm B. The conversion of progesterone to Δ4-pregnene-20α-ol, 3-one by human placenta *in vitro*. Acta Endocrinol (Copenh) 1959; 30:530.

49. Little B, Shaw A. The conversion of progesterone to 17 α-hydroxy-progesterone by human placenta *in vitro*. Acta Endocrinol 1961;36:455.

50. Logeat F, Sartor P, Vattai MT, Milgrom E. Local effect of the blastocyst on estrogen and progesterone receptors in the rat endometrium. Science 1980;207:1083.

51. Loriaux DL, Ruder HJ, Knab DR, Lipsett MB. Estrone sulfate, estrone, estradiol and estriol plasma levels in human pregnancy. J Clin Endocrinol Metab 1972; 35:887.

52. MacDonald PC, Siiteri PK. Origin of estrogen in women pregnant with an anencephalic fetus. J Clin Invest 1965;44:465.

53. Madden JD, Gant NF, MacDonald PC. Studies of the kinetics of conversion of maternal plasma dehydroisoandrosterone sulfate to 16-α-hydroxy-dehydroisoandrosterone sulfate, estradiol and estriol. Am J Obstet Gynecol 1978;132:392.

54. Madden JD, Siiteri PK, MacDonald PC, Gant NF. The pattern and rates of metabolism of maternal plasma dehydroisoandrosterone sulfate in human pregnancy. Am J Obstet Gynecol 1976;125:915.

55. Mason JI, Rainey WE. Steroidogenesis in the human fetal adrenal. A role for cholesterol synthesized de novo. J Clin Endocrinol Metab 1987;64:140.

56. Matthews CP, Coulson PB, Wild RA. Serum progesterone levels as an aid in the diagnosis of ectopic pregnancy. Obstet Gynecol 1986;68:390.

57. Mishell DR, Thorneycroft IH, Nagata Y, et al. Serum gonadotropin and steroid patterns in early human gestation. Am J Obstet Gynecol 1973;117:631.

58. Nagey DA, Pupkin MJ, MacKenna J. A physiologic model of the dehydroepiandrosterone to estrogen conversion system in the fetoplacental unit. Am J Obstet Gynecol 1976;125:249.

59. Nahoul K, Daffos F, Forestier F, Scholler R. Cortisol, cortisone and dehydroepiandrosterene sulfate levels in umbilical cord and maternal plasma between 21 and 30 weeks of pregnancy. J Steroid Biochem 1985;23:445.

60. Nakajima ST, McAuliffe T, Gibson M. The 24 hour pattern of the levels of serum progesterone and immunoreactive human chorionic gonadotropin in normal early pregnancy. J Clin Endocrinol Metab 1990;71:345.

61. Naville D, Ushijima K, Ralph MM, Mason JI. Expression of steroidogenic enzymes in primary cultures of human villous trophoblast (abstr). Presented at the Society for Gynecologic Investigation, San Antonio, Texas, 1991.

62. Okada DM, Tulchinsky D, Ross JW, Hobel CJ. Plasma estrone, estradiol, estriol, progesterone and cortisol in normal labor. Am J Obstet Gynecol 1974;119:502.

63. Osathanondh R, Canick J, Ryan KJ, Tulchinsky D. Placental sulfatase deficiency: a case study. J Clin Endocrinol Metab 1976;43:208.

64. Osathanondh R, Fencl M, Schiff I, et al. Reduced urinary and serum total estriol levels in pregnancies after colectomy. Obstet Gynecol 1979;53:664.

65. Parker CR Jr, Carr BR, Simpson ER, MacDonald PC. Decline in the concentration of low density lipoprotein cholesterol in human fetal plasma near term. Metabolism 1983;32:919.

66. Parker CR, Illingworth DR, Bissonnette JL, Carr BR. Endocrine changes during pregnancy in a patient with homozygous familial hypobeta lipoproteinemia. N Engl J Med 1986;314:557.

67. Parker CR, Simpson ER, Billeimer DW, et al. Inverse relation between low density lipoprotein cholesterol and dehydroisoandrosterone sulfate in human fetal plasma. Science 1980;208:512.

68. Parker RC, Hankins GDV, Carr BR, et al. The effect of hypertension in pregnant women on fetal adrenal function and fetal plasma lipoprotein-cholesterol metabolism. Am J Obstet Gynecol 1984;150:263.

69. Purohit A, Oakey RE. Evidence for separate sites for aromatisation of androstenedione and 16 hydroxyan-

drostenedione in human placental microsomes. J Steroid Biochem 1989;33:439.

70. Rabe T, Brandstetter K, Kellerman J, Runnebaum B. Partial characterization of placental 3-β hydroxysteroid dehydrogenase, Δ4-5 isomerase in human term placental mitochondria. J Steroid Biochem 1982; 17:427.

71. Salido EC, Yen PHG, Barajas L, Shapiro LJ. Steroid sulfatase expression in human placenta: immunocytochemistry and in situ hybridization study. J Clin Endocrinol Metab 1990;70:1564.

72. Schneider JM, Olson RW, Curet LB. Screening for fetal and neonatal risk in the postdate pregnancy. Am J Obstet Gynecol 1978;131:473.

73. Schocken DD, Garon MG, Lefkowitz RJ. The human placenta—a rich source of β adrenergic receptors: characterization of the receptors in particulate and solubilized preparations. J Clin Endocrinol Metab 1980;50:1082.

74. Shozu M, Akasofu K, Harada T, Kubota Y. A new cause of female pseudohermaphroditism placental aromatase deficiency. J Clin Endocrinol Metab 1991;72:560.

75. Siiteri PK, MacDonald PC. Placental estrogen biosynthesis during human pregnancy. J Clin Endocrinol Metab 1966;26:751.

76. Simmer HH, Dignam WJ, Easterling WE, et al. Neutral C_{19} steroids and steroid sulfates in human pregnancy. III. Steroids 1966;8:179.

77. Simmer HH, Tulchinsky D, Gold EM, et al. On the regulation of estrogen production by cortisol and ACTH in human pregnancy at term. Am J Obstet Gynecol 1974;119:283.

78. Solomon S, Bird CE, Ling W, et al. Formation and metabolism of steroid in the fetus and placenta. Rec Progr Horm Res 1967;23:297.

79. Strickler RC, Tobias B. Estradiol 17β-dehydrogenase and 20α-hydroxysteroid dehydrogenase from human placental cytosol: one enzyme with two activities? Steroids 1980;36:243.

80. Thomas JL, Myers RP, Strickler RC. Human placental 3-β hydroxy-sene steroid dehydrogenase and steroid 5-4 ene-isomerase: purification from mitochondria and kinetic profiles, biophysical characterization of the purified mitochondrial and microsomal enzymes. J Steroid Biochem 1989;33:209.

81. Thorneycroft IN, Barberia JM, Ribeiro WO, Mishell DR. Serum androstenedione levels during normal and human menopausal gonadotropin induced human pregnancies. Am J Obstet Gynecol 1975;121:306.

82. Tulchinsky D. Placental secretion of unconjugated estrone, estradiol and estriol into the maternal and fetal circulation. J Clin Endocrinol Metab 1973;36:1079.

83. Tulchinsky D. The value of estrogen assays in obstetric disease. In: Klopper A, ed. Plasma hormone assays in evaluation of fetal well being. Edinburgh: Churchill Livingstone, 1976.

84. Tulchinsky D, Frigoletto F, Ryan KJ, Fishman J. Plasma estetrol as an index of fetal well-being. J Clin Endocrinol Metab 1975;40:560.

85. Tulchinsky D, Hobel CJ. Plasma human chorionic gonadotropin, estrone, estradiol, estriol, progesterone and 17-α hydroxyprogesterone in human pregnancy. Am J Obstet Gynecol 1973;117:884.

86. Tulchinsky D, Hobel CJ, Yeager E, Marshall JR. Plasma estrone, estradiol, estriol, progesterone and 17-hydroxyprogesterone in human pregnancy—normal pregnancy. Am J Obstet Gynecol 1972;112:1095.

87. Tulchinsky D, Ohada DM. Hormones in human pregnancy. IV. Plasma progesterone. Am J Obstet Gynecol 1975;121:293.

88. Tulchinsky D, Osathanondh R, Finn A. Dehydroepiandrosterone sulfate loading test in the diagnosis of complicated pregnancies. N Engl J Med 1976;294:517.

89. Whitsett JA, Johnson CL, Noguchi A, et al. β adrenergic receptors and catecholamine-sensitive adenylate cyclase of the human placenta. J Clin Endocrinol Metab 1980;50:27.

90. Williams. Techniques to evaluate fetal health. In: Cunningham FG, MacDonald PC, Gant NF, eds. Obstetrics, ed 18. Norwalk, CT: Appleton & Lange, 1989;307.

91. Winkel CA, Gilmore G, MacDonald PC, Simpson ER. Uptake and degradation of lipoproteins by human trophoblastic cells in primary culture. Endocrinology 1980;107:1892.

92. Winkel CA, Snyder JM, MacDonald PC, Simpson ER. Regulation of cholesterol and progesterone synthesis in human placental cells in culture by serum lipoproteins. Endocrinology 1980;106:1054.

93. Witt BR, Wolf GC, Wainwright CG, et al. Relaxin, Ca125, progesterone, estradiol, Schwangerschaft rotein, and human chorionic gonadotropin as predictors of outcome in threatened and non-threatened pregnancies. Fertil Steril 1990;53:1029.

94. Yeko TR, Gomel MJ, Hughes LH, et al. Timely diagnosis of early ectopic pregnancy using a single blood progesterone measurement. Fertil Steril 1987;48:1048.

95. Zelewski L, Villee CA. The biosynthesis of squalene, lanosterol and cholesterol by minced human placenta. Biochemistry 1966;5:1805.

CHAPTER 2

Placental Polypeptides

Tommaso Falcone and A. Brian Little

The placental polypeptide hormones are characterized historically by their similarities to hormones of other endocrine systems. Both human luteinizing hormone (hLH) and human chorionic gonadotropin (hCG) have similar biologic activities. The β subunits of each that confer biologic activity are relatively similar: Of the 145 amino acids in β-hCG, 97 are identical to those of β-hLH, which has a total of 119 amino acids.[118] There are similar homologies between human growth hormone (hGH), human placental lactogen (hPL), and prolactin (PRL). Both hGH and hPL have 191 amino acids, of which 161 are identical, and 146 amino acids of PRL (total 198 amino acids) are identical with both hGH and hPL.[125, 126] Both hPL and hCG, despite their homology with their pituitary analogs, are sufficiently different from each other to express different antigenic determinants and thus can be readily distinguished and measured by radioimmunoassay. The subunits of gonadotropins and other pituitary hormones, however, generally have no biologic action, although they are often secreted as subunits.

The peptide hormones, which include gonadotropin-releasing hormone (GnRH), somatostatin, thyrotropin-releasing hormone (TRH), gastrin, vasoactive intestinal polypeptide (VIP), and nerve growth factor (NGF), have all been identified in the placenta along with the pituitary-like polypeptides adrenocorticotropic hormone (ACTH), thyroid-stimulating hormone (TSH), and follicle-stimulating hormone (FSH). These peptides can have endocrine, exocrine, and paracrine effects as well as acting as neurotransmitters. The presence in the placenta of nicotinic, cholinergic, and muscarinic system components has been reported,[167] but little or nothing is known of their physiologic activity. The placenta also synthesizes both met-enkephalin and leu-enkephalin[196] and related peptides (e.g., β-adrenergic receptors.[177]) Although far from proven, an attractive theory has been proposed for the origin of these brain-like peptides from the neural crest of the embryo:[146] As the placenta is considered to be similarly derived, it therefore would be similarly programmed.[147]

Different complex methods have been used to identify placental peptides, including immunoassay, bioassay, immunocytochemistry, synthesis, and physicochemical and amino-acid sequencing. Not all tests have been applied to all peptides presently identified, and more are being isolated all the time.

When it comes to possible endocrine and paracrine activities of placental peptides, the identity of the molecule itself, its receptor, and a demonstrable placental response are all necessary. These are far from proven or detailed as yet. Placental receptors for GnRH and opiates, however, have been identified. Proopiomelanocortin (POMC)-like mRNA is present in the ovary and placenta of rat and monkey; the POMC-like mRNA of the placenta and ovary is smaller than that in the pituitary and hypothalamus. The peptide is probably shortened at the 5′ end of the molecule. The expression of the gene is regulated by gonadotropins in the ovary but not in the placenta.[43] Also, the placental GnRH receptor when solubilized showed a band of molecular weight of 53,700 daltons on polyacrylamide gel equivalent to that of pituitary GnRH. The placental receptor, however, is markedly different in its low binding affinity and lack of specificity from that of the pituitary.[93]

HUMAN CHORIONIC GONADOTROPIN

A number of reviews have brought our accumulated knowledge up to date.[142, 172, 199] The placenta is the principal site of hCG synthesis and secretion. It is the hCG secretion from early trophoblast that prevents the lysis of the corpus luteum. The resulting persistent secretion of estrogen and progesterone maintain the endometrium for implantation and development of the blastocyst.

Distribution of Human Chorionic Gonadotropin

The syncytiotrophoblast is the site of secretion of hCG in the placenta, and hCG is secreted into both maternal and fetal compartments but much less (1%) into the fetus. Extracts of testes, urine, and pituitary in the absence of pregnancy contain substances with similar chromatographic, electrophoretic, and biologic characteristics of hCG.[37, 161] An hCG-like material is present in sperm[3, 8] and preimplanted blastocysts of mouse, rat, and rabbit.[207, 212] Material similar to hCG has been identified in the urine of women using the intrauterine device; as the ovum contains no such material,[7] this has been suggested as evidence that the blastocyst is the source of the hormone.[86] In general, except during pregnancy, values of hCG in the serum greater than 1 mIu/mL or β-hCG greater than 1.5 mIu/mL and α-hCG greater than 3.5 mIu/mL are pathologic in origin.[61]

In tumors of the testis (42% of those tested) and ovary (51%), hCG is found, but it is also found in pancreatic tumors (as high as 33% incidence), gastric adenocarcinoma (22%), lung carcinoma (9%), large bowel tumors (3%), and hepatoma (17%).[165]

Trophoblastic tumors are a well-known source of hCG, with widely differing ratios of α and β subunits.[200] Free α and β subunits and hCG in toto are used to monitor benign and malignant trophoblastic tumors and distinguish both from pregnancy. For example, β-hCG is markedly increased in hydatidiform mole, a generally benign trophoblastic tumor, and it is present in concentrations greater than the intact molecule of hCG itself. The ratio of β-hCG to hCG in urine is 3.7 in hydatidiform mole, and 1.8 in normal pregnancy, with the ratio to α-hCG of a lower magnitude in both.[62] However, in normal pregnancy sera, free β-hCG is usually not present or is found in extremely low concentrations.

Ectopic endocrine tumors also may secrete hCG, including embryonal carcinoma, teratoma, and seminoma and its ovarian equivalent, dysgerminoma.[95] Other tumors may also secrete hCG, including lung, adrenal, liver, and bladder.[66, 166]

Structure

Similar to other gonadotropins, hCG is a glycoprotein; it has a molecular weight of 39,000 daltons;[71] it is composed of two dissimilar subunits α and β, noncovalently linked. Neither α nor β subunit alone has biologic activity, but when recombined more than 80% of the hCG biologic activity can be restored.[5, 160] The hCG-α molecular weight of 16,000 daltons is almost identical to hLH-α and hFSH-α.[24] The hCG-β molecular weight of 23,000 daltons has 97 of 145 amino acids identical to hLH-β. Thirty percent of hCG is composed of carbohydrate. There are four asparagine-linked branched carbohydrate chains at the 52nd and 78th position in the α chain and at the 13th and 30th positions in the β chain; three short-serine-linked oligosaccharide units are on the β subunit. Asialo-hCG is almost as bioactive as hCG in vitro but not in vivo, as evidenced by more rapid disappearance from the blood. T½ is the time required for one-half of a quantity of a substance (hormone) to be eliminated at a rate proportional to its concentration (i.e., exhibits first-order kinetics).

The biosynthesis of hCG is by the placental trophoblast. The outer layer of the syncytium appears to be the site of biosynthesis, but the cytotrophoblast provides the stem cells for syncytial development. The syncytium, however, contains morphologic components for protein synthesis and secretion, including rough endoplasmic reticulum, Golgi complex, and mitochondria. The villus membrane is convoluted and contains microvilli. The microvilli contain vesicles and vacuoles of endocytosed material from the maternal circulation. The prehormones are synthesized from maternal amino acids in the rough endoplasmic reticulum and transformed into secretory granules in the Golgi apparatus. They are then packaged and converted into mature granules as they fuse with the cell membrane. Only small amounts reach the fetal circulation.[47, 49, 53, 190] Incubations of placental explants have been used to examine the control of hCG production. Production is increased by incubation with luteinizing hormone–releasing hormone (LH-RH),[113] cyclic adenosine monophosphate (cAMP), with and without phosphodiesterase inhibitors, and epidermal growth factor (EGF).[25] Trophoblast-derived interleukin-6 (IL-6) can also stimulate release of hCG by an IL-6 receptor in trophoblast tissue.[140] Quantitatively, it appears that IL-6 is as efficient as LH-RH analogs at stimulating hCG in vitro. Trophoblast-derived tumor necrosing factor-α (TNF-α) and IL-1 can stimulate the release of IL-6 from the trophoblast and thereby indirectly effect hCG release.[127] No increase, however, was observed with dibutaryl cyclic guanosine monophosphate (cGMP), insulin, cortisol, or epinephrine.[79, 92, 115] Inhibin and activin play an important role in regulating the release of hCG.[135] Progesterone appears to inhibit pulsatile hCG secretion in the first trimester placenta in vitro.[11]

The placenta and maternal sera and urine have varying concentrations of α and β subunits of hCG during pregnancy.[61, 129] The β subunit synthesis appears to be rate limiting for the intact hCG molecule, as it is in extremely low concentrations in the sera[61, 129] compared with the α subunit. The gene for hCG is on chromosome number 6.

Physiology

It has been described that hCG is present in the blastocyst[202] and is required to maintain secretion of progesterone by the corpus luteum[198] (but not 17α-hydroxyprogesterone). hCG can be detected 1 day after implantation.[94] Fetal circulating hCG is elevated at midgestation and decreases thereafter.[20] In the male fetus, peak concentrations of total testosterone are seen at 11 to 16 weeks' gestation simultaneous to hCG.[161] Peak concentrations of free testosterone, however, are also seen at term, at a time when circulating hCG levels are at their lowest in the male fetus.[20] The relationship of androgen secretion of the fetal testes and circulating hCG remains to be elucidated. The fetal synthesis of dehydroepiandrosterone (DHA) may also be controlled by hCG.[89, 90, 179] It is not clear if there is autoregulation of hCG secretion. hCG has also been shown to be synthesized by the fetal kidney.[130] There is still much to be learned about the physiology of hCG.

Patients with tumors that secrete hCG ectopically are recognized by signs and symptoms attributed to excess gonadotropin secretion.[66, 91] Precocious puberty results from excess hCG secretion in boys.[185] No symptoms are noted in some nonpregnant women with levels of hCG as high as in the first trimester.[199] Intact hCG has weak intrinsic TSH activity (about 1/4000 of purified pituitary TSH).[9] Goiter and hyperthyroidism may result in women as a result of high levels of circulating hCG, as in the presence of hydatidiform moles complicating pregnancy.[184] hCG can stimulate thyroid gland adenylate cyclase.[39]

Secretion of hCG prolongs the life of the corpus luteum and stimulates progesterone production through the adenylate cyclase system. This is maintained until the shift from corpus luteum to predominant progesterone secretion by placental synthesis occurs at about the 11th week of gestation. Steroidogenesis appears to be stimulated by hCG in the trophoblast of the placenta. Some degree of autoregulation between hCG and steroids in the syncytiotrophoblast is suggested by the finding of an hCG-specific adenyl cyclase stimulation in the placenta.[134] The FSH-like activity of hCG may influence fetal ovarian development. The immunosuppressive effect of hCG in the blastocyst at implantation is moot.

Clinical Application

Routinely available assays cannot distinguish between hLH and hCG, and therefore antisera directed to the β subunit of hCG is required for specificity and clinical utility. Serum concentrations of hCG reach peak values by 60 to 90 days of gestation and then progressively decline to reach a plateau by about 20 weeks' gestation. The half-life of hCG is 32 to 37 hours; it is secreted in pulses of 2 to 4 hours.[136, 163] The doubling time of hCG in the serum appears to vary with gestational age.[121, 123] In early pregnancies up to 6 weeks' gestation, it appears to be approximately 1.4 days,[123] whereas afterward it is approximately 3.5 days.[121] This time of doubling is used clinically in the diagnosis of ectopic pregnancy.

In an ectopic pregnancy, we can expect an abnormal (or slow) hCG rise. If less than a 66% increase in hCG concentration within a 2-day interval is observed, an ectopic pregnancy should be suspected.[105] Fifteen percent of normal intrauterine pregnancies, however, may have a similar hCG pattern. Conversely, 13% of ectopic pregnancies have an apparently normal increase in hCG. When levels of 6000 to 6500 mIU/mL are reached in the serum, a normal intrauterine gestational sac should be visualized by transabdominal ultrasonography in 94% of cases. Alternatively, absence of a gestational sac when the β-hCG is 6000 mIU/mL has a positive predictive value (for an ectopic pregnancy) of 86%.[105] By transvaginal ultrasonography, a gestational sac should be visualized with serum β-hCG concentrations of 1500 mIU/mL (approximately 35 days from the last menstrual period).[52] Decline of hCG after termination of pregnancy, whether a term pregnancy, ectopic, or abortion, follows a variable half-life (Table 2–1).

PLACENTAL LACTOGEN

Three reviews of placental lactogen[99, 142, 195] characterize the history of placental lactogen's discovery, the complexity of its nomenclature, the incompleteness of our knowledge of its comparative ontogeny, its relation to prolactin, the control of its secretion, and sketchiness of its ultimate physiologic action. The nomenclature confusion is historic and should be settled in favor of simple communication. Josimovich and MacLaren[102] called the growth hormone–like substance in the serum of pregnant women secreted by the placenta *human placental lactogen* (hPL) because of its lactogenic properties. Kaplan and Grumbach[108] used the name *chorionic growth hormone–prolactin* (CGP), when they studied a similar hormone from human and monkey placentas. Li,[125] when he first characterized the protein structure of the same hormone, called it *human chorionic somatomammotropin* (hCS). It is known to prepare the breast for lactation,[65, 102] to be transiently luteotropic,[101] and to synergize with CG in controlling the secretion of estrogen and progesterone in pseudopregnant rats.[98] Because its growth hormone activity is small, placental lactogen would seem the most appropriate name.

TABLE 2–1. Maximal Days to Resolution of Human Chorionic Gonadotropin

Normal delivery[136, 145]	16
Therapeutic abortion by suction curettage–first trimester[145, 189]	27
Surgery for ectopic pregnancy (salpingostomy or resection)[107]	24
Transvaginal methotrexate for ectopic pregnancy[197]	70
Molar pregnancy terminated by suction curettage[144, 145]	115
Molar pregnancy terminated by hysterectomy[144]	56

Comparative Distribution

The presence of placental lactogen has been demonstrated for members of Primates (human,[41, 205] rhesus monkey,[74, 108] and hamadryas baboon),[194] Artiodactyla (cow,[32, 35] goat,[56] sheep,[40, 56, 57, 80, 111, 194] and deer pig),[56] and Rodentia (rat,[14] mouse,[112, 194] hamster,[112, 194] guinea pig,[112, 194] chinchilla,[194] and vole[58]). It has been demonstrated to be absent in members of Perissodactyl (horse),[60] Lagomorpha conflictingly (rabbit),[112, 194] and Carnivora (dog[194] and ferret[59]). The placental lactogens from the human, rhesus monkey, baboon, goat, sheep, and rat have been purified and characterized biochemically.

Chemical Structure

Placental lactogens in sheep and humans have been identified to have approximately 190 amino acids in a single chain cross-linked by two sulfide bonds of cystine bridges.[63] hPL has a molecular weight of 22,308 daltons with 191 amino acids;[46] 85% are identical to hGH.[81] There is also close similarity to PRL, both ovine (oPRL) and human (hPRL).[27, 126] Of the circulating and placental hPL, about 3% is dimeric with a molecular weight of 45,000 daltons.[78, 174, 175] A large peptide precursor of hPL may also exist.[30, 34] The hPL is a major product of placental secretion, which accounts for at least 10% of placental protein production at term.[33, 44, 82] The hPL has been synthesized in a cell-free system of placental polyribosomes and mRNA. Term placentas have been shown to produce 4 times as much hPL as those from the first trimester as a result of increased transcription.[33, 132] Although this confirms the rising circulating concentration of hPL with increasing gestation, the amount released from individual placentas is varied.[191, 192]

The significance of "big-hPL" is not certain.[176] The hPL molecule is synthesized from a pro-hPL about 25 amino acids longer than the molecule itself, which is cleaved at the endoplasmic membrane before secretion.[180, 193] In bioassay and receptor-binding studies, hPL cross-reacts with both GH and PRL. The hPL has a high degree of binding with lactogenic receptors, which is equal to that of hGH, but a much weaker cross-reactivity with hGH of only 0.03% in the specific binding of human lymphocyte cultures. Human PRL has no activity in this system.[124] The hPL's biologic activity is presumed to be exerted through PRL and hGH receptors, as there are no specific hPL receptors. The molecular basis for hormone action by hPL after binding has not been defined.[15]

Secretion

The pattern of increased secretion of hPL in pregnancy is parallel to the increase in placental and fetal weight. It is synthesized by the syncytiotrophoblast of the placenta; it is not secreted by maternal or fetal pituitary, but ectopic tumor sources have been found.[206] It can be isolated from urine, serum, and amniotic fluid. The first trophoblast synthesis was identified by release of hPL into the medium of explant incubations,[73] then by amino acid incorporation into hPL protein in human placental organ culture. Further labeled hormone studies expanded these observations.[191, 192] Immunofluorescent antibody studies identified the syncytiotrophoblast as the site of hPL origin.[16] κ-Receptor agonists, such as dynorphin, stimulate the release of hPL.[4] The placenta is rich in κ opiate receptors.[23] Placentally produced somatostatin decreases with gestational age.[119] This may be partially responsible for the increase in hPL seen with increasing gestational age. The cytotrophoblast synthesizes somatostatin.[119]

The disappearance curve of hPL from the maternal circulation after delivery of the placenta has determined the half-life to be from 21 to 30 minutes.[169] Although the linearity of disappearance was questioned,[109] the half-life was confirmed at 20 minutes following intravenous infusion in nonpregnant subjects.[18] Assuming a volume of distribution of 7.2% body weight and a term plasma concentration of 1.15 μg/mL, the daily secretion was calculated to be 3 g, which agrees with the 0.5 to 3 g estimated.[109] The metabolic clearance rate has been calculated to be 173 L/day. The calculations vary according to whether one pool or two are used for the estimation.

The hPL can be determined as early as 12 days after fertilization or at the time of the first missed period, which is just after time of implantation.[19] The concentration of placental hPL remains constant (100 to 700 μg/g wet weight), and third-trimester production rate is 0.39 to 3 g per day. The rise in circulating concentration begins at the fifth week (menstrual age) and plateaus at 35 weeks of pregnancy. There appears to be no diurnal fluctuations, and plasma values at term may range from 3.3 to 25 μg/mL.[169, 173] There is a close correlation between maternal circulating and amniotic fluid concentrations.[26]

Physiology

The mechanism of action of hPL on target tissues is not known. The hPL has over 80% homology with hGH and 60% with hPRL. These homologies are consistent with the idea that these hormones are evolved from a common ancestor. There are no bioassays that are totally specific for hPL. Pigeon crop biologic assays continue to be used for standardization of hPL and prolactins.[13] Dose-growth responses with acidic hPL may also be used in growth hormone assays. Radioligand assays, which make use of the binding properties of hPL (human pituitary PRL and other chemically related lactogenic hormones) to cell membrane fractions of lactating pseudopregnant rabbit mammary glands treated with corticosteroids, have been described.[182]

The binding of hPL-like hPRL and hGH is not completely clarified because the use of acidic preparations has not been as extensively studied as alkaline preparations. It may be also that hPL is not critical for fetal survival, as at least one woman has been identified who had no measurable circulating hPL during pregnancy.[139] In the primate, hPL is known to bind to fetal placenta, lung, myocardium, and liver and maternal ovary.[103, 104, 156, 168]

Although it has less than 3% of hGH activity, hPL has been shown to promote growth in hypopituitary dwarfs, but doses 200-fold greater than hGH were required.[75] The hPL also stimulates somatomedin production,[171] which may account for its growth-promoting activity. Substrate availability or the growth of the fetus may be controlled by hPL action on somatomedin release.

The lactogenic activity of hPL is well documented in animal models but does not appear to be critical for the human.[65] The luteotropic activity of hPL has been demonstrated with the corpus luteum of animals but not humans.[70]

When hPL is given in amounts to achieve blood concentrations equivalent to those of term pregnancy, serum free fatty acids and glycerol are mobilized.[77] In pregnant and nonpregnant women, lipolysis is stimulated by hPL,[208] which is suppressed by puromycin and actinomycin-D, which suggests intermediary enzyme synthesis; the lipolysis has been shown to be at least partly due to a hormone-sensitive lipase.[48]

A major effect of hPL is on insulin and glucose metabolism. Following hPL infusion in nonpregnant women, the glucose tolerance is impaired in the presence of an augmented insulin response.[18] In hypophysectomized diabetic women, hPL infusion increased fasting blood glucose and glucose excretion and reduced glucose tolerance.[170]

The mechanisms for the rise in free fatty acids, decreased sensitivity to insulin, and increased circulating insulin, with reduced glucose tolerance following hPL infusion and in pregnancy, are not clearly understood. The glucose-sparing and lipolysis effects of hPL, particularly in fasting pregnant women, have been assumed to be the rationale for hPL function, to protect the fetus.[106] The fasting state is a stimulus for hPL. Decreased maternal glucose utilization would ensure a steady energy source for the fetus. There is also a GH-like positive nitrogen balance effect following infusion of hPL.[76, 100]

A paradox is that successful pregnancies have been described in which low or no hPL was detected.[36, 67, 139] There are other hPL effects in which there is conflict between animal and human data. An example is the effect on milk production that is induced in the rhesus macaque by hPL but not in the human.[17, 64] There are other effects that are not well worked out, including those on calcium metabolism,[77] aldosterone excretion,[133] luteotropic effect, and erythropoietic effects.[96]

Assay and Normal Concentrations

It has not been proved that hPL circulates in any but the monomeric form, despite the identification of larger molecules in the purification process. There is no biologic standard for hPL; thus there are no bioassays specific for hPL. Pigeon crop stimulation measures the lactogenic component, and dose-growth response measurements may be made for the acidic-hPL growth component.[13, 99]

A series of modified radioimmunoassay procedures have been used to measure hPL,[102] including a rapid maternal serum test.[188] More recently, a radioligand receptor assay (RRA), which detects 1 ng/mL (0.2 ng/mL by radioimmunoassay [RIA]) and has some features that make it more valuable than RIA in some situations,[182] has been used.

Plasma concentrations rise from 0.3 to 5.4 µg/mL between the first and third trimester of pregnancy. The placenta contains 10 to 20 mg/100 g. There is about 300 µg per 24 hours excreted in the urine. Much less circulates in the fetus, with the cord blood concentration of 15.5 ng/mL. The amniotic fluid contains 0.5 ng/mL at term but has a much higher concentration in the first trimester.[102] The overall secretion at term is on the order of 3 g per 24 hours.[169] The circulating concentration during pregnancy roughly parallels the growth in placental mass.

Abnormal Values

The measurement of hPL is used rarely in the clinical evaluation of abnormal pregnancy. Values below 4 µg/mL at greater than 30 weeks' gestation have been designated as being in the "fetal danger zone."[186] In multiple gestation and in diabetic pregnancies, in which the placentas are larger, higher values are observed. The fetal danger zone has been set higher in diabetes (5 µg/mL). In intrauterine growth retardation, maternal hypertension, and preeclampsia, lowered values are observed.[110, 187] In threatened abortion, falling levels indicate the fetus is no longer viable, and in trophoblastic neoplasia, hydatidiform mole, and choriocarcinoma, low levels are found in the serum. These tests are generally not used clinically, as there are other methods of demonstrating fetal jeopardy that are available and sensitive (e.g., ultrasonography and fetal nonstress monitoring).

ENDOGENOUS OPIOIDS

β-Endorphin appears to be unchanged during pregnancy (15.6 ± 13.3 pg/mL) compared with nonpregnant controls (12.9 ± 1.9 pg/mL). In late labor, it rises (70.3 ± 8.2 pg/mL) and peaks during delivery (113 ± 13.3 pg/mL).[69] There are conflicting results,[116, 143] which appear to relate to method of extraction and purification before radioimmunoassay. In nonpregnant women, pregnant women, and women in labor, there is no difference in the molar ratios of β-endorphin to β-lipotropin. β-Endorphin has been shown to be synthesized by the placenta, but its role in placental function, maternal secretion, or fetal secretion is not known. A close correlation between adrenocorticotrophic hormone (ACTH) and β-endorphin has been observed in mother and fetus, suggesting a similar processing. ACTH, β-lipotrophic hormone, and β-endorphin are all derived from a parent hormone, proopiomelanocortin (POMC).

A wide range of opiate-like actions on the central nervous system occur, which include analgesia, tolerance and dependence, catalepsy, decreased blood pressure, increased or decreased body temperature, increased feeding, antidepressant and antipsychotic activity, alterations in learning and memory, decreased male sex behavior, changes in electroencephalography, increased seizure activity, and increased or decreased neuronal firing.[117, 141] None of these effects occur after intravenous administration but only when β-endorphin is infused into the third ventricle. Endorphins also stimulate the pituitary secretion of such hormones as PRL and inhibit gonadotropins.[157] Naloxone can inhibit these responses, possibly through the hypothalamus. It would be tempting to speculate that the elevated concentrations of β-endorphin in labor and delivery have important peripheral or neuroendocrine actions on labor and delivery, but the circulating β-endorphin does not cross the blood–brain barrier, and the circulating physiologic concentrations have little analgesic effect.[69]

Dynorphin, another endogenous opiate, appears to increase with gestation.[4] High concentrations are found in amniotic fluid and in maternal plasma in the third trimester,[201] which may have a regulatory role in hPL secretion.

HYPOTHALAMIC PEPTIDES IN THE PLACENTA

As more and more hormonally active peptides are identified, brain peptides are discovered in the placenta and gut and gut hormones in the placenta and brain. The placenta has been identified as having GnRH, TRH, somatostatin, and corticotropin-releasing hormone (CRH).

GnRH-like placental peptide has similarities and differences with pituitary GnRH.[115, 122, 137, 178] GnRH and GnRH precursor are synthesized by the cytotrophoblast.[114] Placental GnRH is immunologically and chemically identical to hypothalamic GnRH.[115] The best characterized peptide regulatory loop of the placenta involves GnRH.[21, 22] Placental GnRH stimulates hCG release through GnRH receptors present in trophoblast cell membranes. This receptor-mediated event is calcium dependent. GnRH-mediated hCG release can be inhibited by GnRH antagonists.[12] Estradiol and estriol potentiated, whereas progesterone reduced, the action of 8 br-cAMP on GnRH release from cultured placental cells[154] (Fig. 2–1). This then leads to a complete loop similar to the hypothalamic-pituitary-ovarian axis, i.e., GnRH, hCG, steroids. Opiate-receptor agonists inhibited the cAMP-induced GnRH release via high-affinity opioid receptors in placental cell membranes.

Insulin, VIP, prostaglandins, and epinephrine can also stimulate release of placental GnRH[155] (see Fig. 2–1). Inhibin has an inhibitory effect in GnRH secretion.[135, 153] This indirectly results in a suppressive effect in hCG secretion. This suppressive effect is seen only in the latter part of pregnancy.[135] Activin augments GnRH release and potentiates the GnRH-induced release of hCG.[153] Estriol increased and progesterone decreased the activin-mediated GnRH release.[154]

Placental CRH is identical to neuronal CRH in immunoreactivity and bioactivity.[181] It is synthesized primarily in the syncytiotrophoblast and intermediate cells of the placenta.[160] Others have suggested, however, that it is mainly

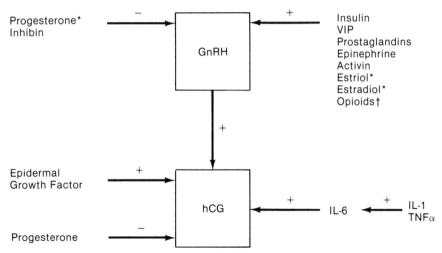

FIGURE 2–1. GnRH-mediated hCG release. *Estradiol and estriol potentiated, whereas progesterone reduced the action of 8 br-cAMP on GnRH release from cultured placental cells. †Opiate receptor agonists inhibited the cAMP-induced GnRH release via high-affinity opioid receptors in placental cell membranes.

derived from the cytotrophoblast.[151] CRH is present in large quantities in the last 5 weeks of pregnancy, at a time when cytotrophoblast cells are the least numerous. During pregnancy, CRH in maternal plasma and amniotic fluid levels are low until the last 5 weeks of pregnancy. At this time, there is a 20-fold increase in placental mRNA for CRH.[65a] This is reflected in placental tissue CRH concentration as well as maternal plasma levels.[38]

CRH immunoactivity (CRHi) has been measured to be present in maternal blood and undetectable in nonpregnant women.[68] Rising from 58 ± 18 pg/mL in the first trimester to 270 ± 68 pg/mL at term, it returns to undetectable levels by 24 hours later. The cord blood values (136 ± 16 pg/mL) correlate with the high maternal levels. The placenta may be a source of CRHi in the fetus, as the umbilical vein has a higher concentration than the umbilical artery.[68]

Maternal plasma ACTH rises with pregnancy but remains in the normal range.[120] The relative refractoriness of the maternal pituitary to a large rise in peripheral CRH concentrations has been attributed to the presence of CRH-binding protein, which masks the ACTH-releasing activity of CRH in late gestation.[128]

Maternal plasma levels of free cortisol, however, are high in the third trimester,[2] possibly due to the rise in ACTH that occurs. A small proportion of placental CRH in maternal plasma remains free of binding protein, or it is placentally derived. This binding protein allows large amounts of placental CRH to be synthesized and act as a local paracrine or fetal hormone with little maternal effect.

Despite elevated free cortisol and ACTH, placental CRH continues to increase with gestation. There are data to suggest that glucocorticoids have a positive feedback effect on placental CRH mRNA expression and CRH release.[97, 164] The implications of this positive feedback loop in parturition are obvious. The increase in CRH, which effects the fetal pituitary adrenal axis to produce increasing concentrations of glucocorticoid, which then have a positive feedback effect on placental CRH synthesis, may give credence to the theory of parturition that involves the fetal adrenal gland (see Chapter 18).

Progesterone has a negative effect on placental CRH release.[97] Prostaglandins, neurotransmitters, norepinephrine, acetylcholine, vasopressin, and angiotensin II all stimulate CRH release.[152]

Many of these neurotransmitters are directly synthesized by the placenta. Neuropeptide y is a 36–amino acid peptide synthesized by the cytotrophoblast, which acts directly on binding sites in the placenta to release CRH.[149]

The fetal placental interaction is also demonstrated in conditions that are associated with fetal stress. CRH is often elevated in abnormal pregnancies, such as those character-ized by intrauterine growth retardation or pre-term labor.[209]

Chorionic thyrotropin-releasing factor (TRF) appears to be different from pituitary TRF and has little known physiologic effect at present.[210, 211] Somatostatin-like activity has been identified in the cytotrophoblast (as well as in amniotic fluid) with a different structure than somatostatin itself.[119, 183] Because cho-rionic somatostatin decreases with gestation as somatomammotropin increases, it has been suggested that this may be a similar placental inhibitory mechanism.[204]

GROWTH FACTORS

A myriad of growth factors and their receptors have been identified in the placenta. These are potent mitogens for many cell types. They are responsible for growth and differentiation of trophoblastic tissue.

Transforming growth factor-α (TGF-α) and EGF are similar in structure and bind a com-mon receptor. TGF-α/EGF receptors are pre-sent on human trophoblast tissue.[42] Human placentas contain high levels of immunoreac-tive and receptor active TGF-α and TGF-α mRNA throughout gestation.[31] This suggests a possible autocrine/paracrine role. Consistent with this hypothesis are the low levels of both growth factors in maternal blood.[85] EGF recep-tors are found predominantly on the syncytio-trophoblast.[45]

EGF receptors have been found in the en-dometrium and decidua as well, although at approximately 1000 times less concentration[45] than in placenta. The human embryo, cul-tured in vitro, can produce TGF-α. This pro-duction becomes significant from day 5 after fertilization, which corresponds with the mor-ula to blastocyst transformation[84] (Fig. 2–2). Early human implantation sites (34 to 38 days from last menstrual period) obtained from hysterectomy specimens and ectopic pregnan-cies show immunohistochemical evidence of EGF and EGF-receptor localized to the tropho-blast (syncytiotrophoblast > intermediate tro-phoblast > cytotrophoblast).[87] Therefore there is evidence to support a role for these peptides (TGF-α and EGF) in embryo-uterine signaling

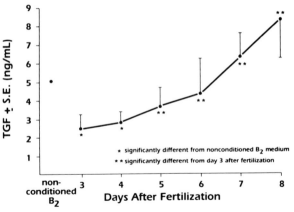

FIGURE 2–2. Concentrations of TGF-α activity (ng/ml ± SE) in nonconditioned culture media (B₂) and culture media of human embryos (n = 6) from days 3 to 8 after fertilization. (From Hemmings R, Langlais J, Falcone T, et al. Human embryos transforming growth factors activity and insulin-like growth factors II. Fertil Steril 1992;58:101–104. Reproduced with permission of The American Fertil-ity Society.)

for implantation. EGF is known to cause in-creased synthesis and release of hCG, hPL, and progesterone.[10, 138] Parathyroid hormone in-creases the number of biologically active EGF (epidermal growth factor) receptors during in vitro differentiation of human trophoblast cells[6] and therefore may play a role in tropho-blastic growth.

Insulin-like growth factors (IGF-I and -II) and endothelin are other peptides that are produced by the placenta that act via a para-crine or autocrine mechanism to regulate pla-cental growth.[50, 51, 203] IGF-I augments the stim-ulatory effect of EGF on hPL secretion but is not effective by itself.[28] It can also effect trophoblast cellular differentiation.[29]

INHIBIN

TGF-β, müllerian inhibiting substance, and in-hibin form another family of growth factors with structural homologies. Inhibin is a glyco-protein heterodimer joined by disulfide bonds. Two forms of β subunits have been isolated: αA and βB resulting in inhibin A and inhibin B. Homodimers of the β subunits form the activins (Fig. 2–3).

Two forms of inhibin are found, 31 and 58 kDa forms.[55] These different molecular weights are due to the cleavage of the double arginine residue on the α subunit resulting in

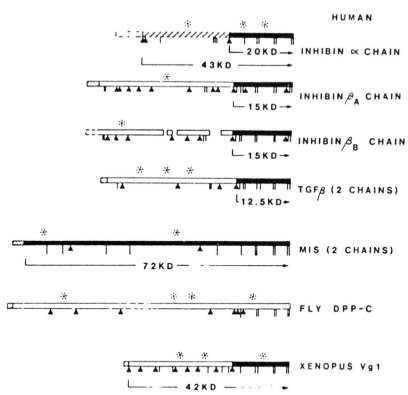

FIGURE 2–3. Schematic representation of the structure of human inhibin and related peptides. (From Healy DL., Polson D, Yohkachiya T, et al. Inhibin and related peptides in pregnancy. Bailliere's Clin Endocrinol Metab 1990;4:233. With permission.)

a shorter molecule (i.e., from 43 to 20 kDa). Serum inhibin concentrations rise in pregnancy to a peak at 11 weeks' gestation, then decline to a plateau from week 14 to week 25, and finally rise again to term[1] (Fig. 2–4). Serum inhibin levels in pregnancy are almost exclusively derived from the placenta. Women without ovaries who have achieved pregnancy by oocyte donation and embryo transfer demonstrated inhibin levels in early pregnancy no different from normal women.[131]

Inhibin α and βA subunits and GnRH show a similar localization in the human trophoblast.[156] Some of the cytotrophoblast cells hybridize to inhibin (α/βA), activin (βA/βA), and GnRH probes.[162]

There is a gestation-related increase of inhibin α subunit mRNA as well as βA and βB subunits.[150] Inhibin α and βA subunit mRNA are present as early as the first trimester. Inhibin βB subunit mRNA is detected only in term placentas; however, immunoreactive inhibin βB fluorescent material was also observed in early pregnancy in very small quantities.[150] In the decidua, however, there are high levels of inhibin βB subunit mRNA detected.[148] Inhibin α subunit is localized in the cytotrophoblast; inhibin βB subunit immunoreactivity was observed in the syncytial layer of the villi, and inhibin βA subunit was widely distributed.[150] The close anatomic relationship of inhibin, activin, and GnRH attests to the important interactions in a classic neuroendocrine fashion.[153, 154]

Inhibin selectively suppresses FSH release from the pituitary. In cultured human placental cells, activin increases the release of GnRH and progesterone and augments the release of hCG induced by GnRH.[153, 154] Activin alone does not increase the release of hCG.[153, 154] Some authors have shown that in vitro inhibin suppresses hCG secretion in term placenta.[135] Others using a different method did not confirm a direct effect of inhibin.[153] Inhibin, however, completely reversed the activin-induced GnRH and progesterone increase. Further, the

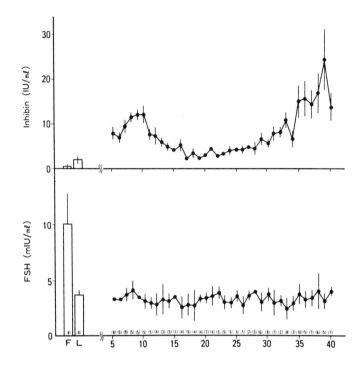

FIGURE 2–4. The average plasma inhibin and FSH concentrations in the midfollicular phase (F), in the midluteal phase (L), and during normal pregnancy. The numbers of subjects are indicated in parentheses. Values are the mean ± SE. (From Abe Y, Hasegawa Y, Miyamota K, et al. High concentrations of plasma immunoreactive inhibin during normal pregnancy in women. J Clin Endocrinol Metab 1990;71:133–137. With permission.)

activin-induced potentiation of GnRH effects on hCG secretion is also reversed by inhibin.[153, 154] Neither dimer affected hPL concentration. Curiously inhibin levels are substantially increased in patients with hydatidiform mole concomitantly with high levels of hCG.[83] This reflects on the complex nature of suppressing and stimulating factors in hCG secretion. Postevacuation, hCG levels can take up to 10 weeks to reach nonpregnant levels. Inhibin levels are similar to the early follicular phase within 10 days.[83]

PLACENTAL SPECIFIC PROTEINS

Placental specific proteins have been described and measured in a variety of situations. Apart from hPL and hCG, pregnancy-associated plasma proteins have been identified. Although no biologic function has been found for them as yet, they have been used for markers of fertilization and implantation, ongoing pregnancy,[54, 72] and small-for-gestational-age infants.[88]

REFERENCES

1. Abe Y, Hasegawa Y, Miyamota K, et al. High concentrations of plasma immunoreactive inhibin during normal pregnancy in women. J Clin Endocrinol Metab 1990;71:133.

2. Abou-Scemia AB, Pugeat M, Declaud H, et al. Increased plasma concentrations of N-terminal lipotrophin and unbound cortisol during pregnancy. Clin Endocrinol (Oxf) 1984;20:221.

3. Acevedo HF, Slifkin M, Pouchet GR, Rakhshan M. Identification of the beta subunit of choriogonadotropin in human spermatozoa. In: Troen P, Nankin HR, eds. The testis in normal and infertile men. New York: Raven Press, 1977;185.

4. Ahmed MS, Horst MA. Opioid receptors of human placental villi modulate acetylcholine release. Life Sci 1988;39:535.

5. Aloj SM, Edelhoch H, Ingham KC. The rates of dissociation and reassociation of the subunits of human chorionic gonadotropin. Arch Biochem Biophys 1973;159:497.

6. Alsat E, Mirlesse V, Fondacci C, et al. Parathyroid hormone increases epidermal growth factor receptors in cultured human trophoblast cells from early and term placenta. J Clin Endocrinol Metab 1991;73:288.

7. Asch RH, Fernandez EO, Magnasco LA, Pauerstein CJ. Demonstration of a chorionic gonadotropin-like substance in rabbit morulae. Fertil Steril 1978;29:444.

8. Asch RH, Fernandez EO, Pauerstein CJ. Immunodetection of a human chorionic gonadotropin-like substance in human sperm. Fertil Steril 1977;28:1258.

9. Azukizawa M, Kurtzman G, Pekary AE, Hershman JM. Comparison of the binding characteristics of bovine thyrotropin and human chorionic gonadotropin to thyroid plasma membrane. Endocrinology 1977;101:1880.

10. Bahn RS, Speeg FV, Assoli M, Rabin O. Epidermal growth factor stimulates production of progesterone in cultured choriocarcinoma cells. Endocrinology 1980;107:2121.

11. Barnea ER, Kaplan M. Spontaneous, gonadotropin

releasing hormone-induced and progesterone inhibited pulsatile secretion of human chorionic gonadotropin in the first trimester placenta in vitro. J Clin Endocrinol Metab 1989;69:215.

12. Barnea ER, Kaplan M, Naor Z. Comparative stimulatory effect of gonadotropin releasing hormone (GnRH) and GnRH agonist upon pulsatile human chorionic gonadotropin secretion in superfused placental explants: reversible inhibition by a GnRH antagonist. Hum Reprod 1991;6:1063.

13. Bates RW. Bioassay methods for prolactin in blood. In: Josimovich JB, Reynolds M, Cobo E, eds. Lactogenic hormones, fetal nutrition and lactation. New York: John Wiley & Sons, 1974:85.

14. Battaglia FC. The comparative physiology of fetal nutrition. Am J Obstet Gynecol 1984;148:850.

15. Baxter JD, MacLeod KM. Molecular basis of hormone action. In: Bondy DK, Rosenburg LE, eds. Metabolic control and disease. Philadelphia: WB Saunders, 1980:146.

16. Beck JS, Gordon RL, Donald D, Melvin JMO. Characterisation of antisera to a growth-hormone-like placental antigen (human placental lactogen): immunofluorescence studies with these sera on normal and pathological syncytiotrophoblast. J Pathol 1969;97:545.

17. Beck P. Lactogenic activity of human chorionic somatomammotropin in rhesus monkeys. Proc Soc Exp Biol Med 1972;140:183.

18. Beck P, Daughaday WH. Human placental lactogen: studies of its acute metabolic effects and disposition in normal man. J Clin Invest 1967;46:103.

19. Beck P, Parker ML, Daughaday WH. Radioimmunologic measurement of human placental lactogen in plasma by a double antibody method during normal and diabetic pregnancies. J Clin Endocrinol Metab 1965;25:1457.

20. Beck-Pecciz P, Padmanabhan V, Baggieri AM, et al. Maturation of hypothalamic-pituitary gonadal function in normal human fetuses: circulatory levels of gonadotropins, their common α subunit and free testosterone and discrepancy between immunological and biological activities of circulating FSH. J Clin Endocrinol Metab 1991;73:525.

21. Belisle S, Guivin GF, Bellabarba D, Lehour JG. Luteinizing hormone-releasing hormone binds to enriched human placental membranes and stimulates in vitro synthesis of bioactive human chorionic gonadotropin. J Clin Endocrinol Metab 1984;59:119.

22. Belisle S, Petit A, Bellabarba D, et al. Ca²⁺ but not membrane lipid hydrolysis, mediates human chorionic gonadotropin production by luteinizing hormone-releasing hormone in human term placenta. J Clin Endocrinol Metab 1989;69:31.

23. Belisle S, Petit A, Gallo-Payet N, et al. Functional opioid receptor sites in human placentas. J Clin Endocrinol Metab 1988;66:283.

24. Bellisario R, Carlsen RB, Bahl OP. Human chorionic gonadotropin; linear amino acid sequence of the alpha subunit. J Biol Chem 1973;248:6796.

25. Benveniste R, Speeg KV Jr, Carpenter G, et al. Epidermal growth factor stimulates secretion of human chorionic gonadotropin by cultured human choriocarcinoma cells. J Clin Endocrinol Metab 1978; 46:169.

26. Berle P. Pattern of the human chorionic somatomammotrophic (HCS) concentration ratio in maternal serum and amniotic fluid during normal pregnancy. Acta Endocrinol 1974;76:364.

27. Bewley TA, Li CH. Structural similarities between human pituitary growth hormone, human chorionic somatomammotropin and ovine pituitary growth hormone and lactogenic hormones. In: Josmovich JB, Reynolds M, Cobo E, eds. Lactogenic hormones, fetal nutrition and lactation. New York: John Wiley & Sons, 1974:19.

28. Bhaumick B, Bala RM. Synergistic effects of insulin like growth factor I and epidermal growth factor on placental lactogen secretion by human term placenta trophoblast cells in culture. Trophoblast Res 1991;5:171.

29. Bhaumick B, George D, Bala RM. Potentiation of epidermal growth factor induced differentiation of cultured human placental cells by insulin like growth factor I. J Clin Endocrinol Metab 1991;74:1005.

30. Birken S, Smith DL, Canfield RE, Boime I. Partial amino acid sequence of human placental lactogen precursor and its mature hormone form produced by membrane-associated enzyme activity. Biochem Biophys Res Commun 1977;74:106.

31. Bissonnette F, Cook C, Geoghegan T, et al. Transforming growth factor α and epidermal growth factor messenger ribonucleic acid and protein levels in human placentas from early, mid and late gestation. Am J Obstet Gynecol 1992;166:192.

32. Blank MS, Chan JSD, Friesen HG. Placental lactogens, new developments. J Steroid Biochem 1977; 8:403.

33. Boime I, Boguslawski S. Radioimmunoassay of human placental lactogen synthesized on ribosomes isolated from first trimester and third trimester placentae. FEBS Lett 1974;45:104.

34. Boime I, Boguslawski S, Caine J. The translation of a human placental lactogen mRNA fraction in heterologous cell free systems. The synthesis of a possible precursor. Biochem Biophys Res Commun 1975; 62:103.

35. Bolander FF, Ulberg LC, Fellows RE. Circulating placental lactogen levels in dairy and beef cattle. Endocrinology 1976;99:1273.

36. Borody IB, Carlton MA. Isolated defect in human placental lactogen synthesis in a normal pregnancy. Br J Obstet Gynaecol 1981;88:447.

37. Braunstein GD, Rasor J, Wade ME. Presence in normal human testes of a chorionic-gonadotropin-like substance distinct from human luteinizing hormone. N Engl J Med 1975;293:1339.

38. Campbell EA, Linton EA, Wolfe CDA, et al. Plasma corticotropin-releasing hormone concentrations during pregnancy and parturition. J Clin Endocrinol Metab 1987;63:1054.

39. Carayon P, Lefort G, Nisula B. Interaction of human chorionic gonadotropin and human luteinizing hormone with human thyroid and membranes. Endocrinology 1980;106:1907.

40. Chan JSD, Robertson HA, Friesen HG. Maternal and fetal concentrations of ovine placental lactogen measured by radioimmunoassay. Endocrinology 1978; 102:1606.

41. Chatterjee M, Munro HN. Structure and biosynthesis of human placental peptide hormones. Vit Horm 1977;35:149.

42. Chen CF, Kurachi H, Fujita Y, et al. Changes in epidermal growth factor receptor and its messenger ribonucleic acid levels in human placenta and isolated trophoblast cells during pregnancy. J Clin Endocrinol Metab 1988;67:1171.

43. Ching-Ling CC, Chang CC, Krieger DT, Bardin CW.

Expression and regulation of proopiomelanocortin-like gene in the ovary and placenta. Comparison with the testis. Endocrinology 1986;118:2382.

44. Chopra IJ, Sack J, Fisher DA. Circulating 3,3′,5′-triiodothryonine (reverse T_3) in the human newborn. J Clin Invest 1975;55:1137.

45. Clegini N, Rao CLV. Epidermal growth factor binding to human amnion, chorion, decidua and placenta from mid and term pregnancy: quantitative light microscopic autoradiographic studies. J Clin Endocrinol Metab 1965;61:529.

46. Cushard WG, Creditor MA, Canterbury JM, Reiss E. Physiological hyperparathyroidism in pregnancy. J Clin Endocrinol Metab 1972;34:767.

47. Dreskin RB, Spicer SS, Greene WB. Ultrastructural localization of chorionic gonadotropin in human term placenta. J Histochem Cytochem 1970;18:862.

48. Elliott JA. The effect of pregnancy on the control of lipolysis in fat cells isolated from human adipose tissue. Europ J Clin Invest 1975;5:159.

49. Enders AC. A comparative study of the fine structure of the trophoblast in several hemochorial placentas. Am J Anat 1965;116:29.

50. Fant ME, Munro HN, Moses AC. An autocrine/paracrine role for insulin like growth factors (IGFs) in the regulation of human placental growth. J Clin Endocrinol Metab 1986;63:499.

51. Fant ME, Nanu L, Word RA. A potential role for endothelin-1 in human placental growth: interactions with the insulin like growth factor family of peptides. J Clin Endocrinol Metab 1992;74:1158.

52. Fassum GT, Danajan V, Kletzky OA. Early detection of pregnancy with transvaginal ultrasound. Fertil Steril 1988;49:788.

53. Fawcett DW, Long JA, Jones AL. The ultrastructure of endocrine glands. Rec Prog Horm Res 1969;25:315.

54. Folkersen J, Grudzinskas JG, Hindersson P, et al. Pregnancy-associated plasma protein A: circulating levels during normal pregnancy. Am J Obstet Gynecol 1981;139:910.

55. Forage RG, Ring JM, Brown RW, et al. Cloning and sequence analysis of cDNA species coding for the two subunits of inhibin from bovine follicular fluid. Proc Nat Acad Sci USA 1986;83:3091.

56. Forsyth IA. Use of a rabbit mammary gland organ culture system to detect lactogenic activity in blood. In: Wolstenholme GEW, Knight J, eds. Lactogenic hormones. London: Churchill Livingstone, 1972;151.

57. Forsyth IA. The comparitive study of placental lactogenic hormones: a review. In: Josimovich JB, Reynolds M, Cobo E, eds. Lactogenic hormones, fetal nutrition and lactation. New York: John Wiley & Sons, 1974;49.

58. Forsyth IA, Blake LA. Placental lactogen (chorionic mammotrophin) in the field vole, Microtus agrestis, and the bank vole, clethrionomys glareolus. J Endocrinol 1976;70:19.

59. Forsyth IA, Jones EA. Organ culture of mammary gland and placenta in the study of hormone action and placental lactogen secretion. In: Balls M, Monnickendan MA, eds. Organ culture in biomedical research. London: Cambridge University Press, 1976;201.

60. Forsyth IA, Rossdale PD, Thomas CR. Studies on milk composition and lactogenic hormones in the mare. J Reprod Fertil 1975;23(suppl):631.

61. Franchimont P, Renter A. Evidence of alpha and beta-subunits of hCG in serum and urines of pregnant women. In: Margoulies M, Greenwood FC, eds. Structure-activity relationship of protein and polypeptide hormones. Amsterdam: Excerpta Medical Foundation, 1972;381.

62. Franchimont P, Renter A, Gaspard U. Ectopic production of hCG and its alpha and beta subunits. In: Martini L, James VHT, eds. Current topics in experimental endocrinology, Vol 3. New York: Academic Press, 1978;202.

63. Friesen H. Purification of a placental factor with immunological and chemical similarity to human growth hormone. Endocrinology 1965;76:369.

64. Friesen HG. Placental protein hormones and tissue receptors for hormones. In: Gluck L, ed. Modern perinatal medicine. Chicago: Year Book Medical Publishers, 1974:224.

65. Friesen HG. Lactation induced by human placental lactogen and cortisone acetate in rabbits. Endocrinology 1966;79:212.

65a. Frim DM, Emanuel RL, Robinson BG, et al. Characterization and gestational regulation of corticotropin releasing hormone messenger RNA in human placenta. J Clin Invest 1988;82:287.

66. Fusco FD, Rosen SW. Gonadotropin-producing anaplastic large-cell carcinomas of the lung. N Engl J Med 1966;275:507.

67. Gaede P, Trolle D, Pedersen H. Extremely low placental lactogen hormone (hPL) values in an otherwise uneventful pregnancy preceding delivery of a normal baby. Acta Obstet Gynecol Scand 1978;57:203.

68. Goland RS, Wardlaw SL, Stark RI, et al. High levels of corticotropin-releasing hormone immunoactivity in maternal and fetal plasma during pregnancy. J Clin Endocrinol Metab 1986;63:1199.

69. Goland RS, Wardlaw SL, Stark RI, Frantz AG. Human plasma beta-endorphin during pregnancy, labor, and delivery. J Clin Endocrinol Metab 1981;52:74.

70. Goldsmith LT, Hochman JA, Weiss G. Effect of human placental lactogen upon the human corpus luteum of late pregnancy. Gynecol Obstet Invest 1978;9:210.

71. Got R, Bourrillon R. Nouvelle methode de purification de la gonadotropine choriale humaine. Biochim Biophys Acta 1960;42:505.

72. Grudzinskas JG, Charnock M, Obiekwe BC, et al. Placental protein 5 in fetal and maternal compartments. Br J Obstet Gynaecol 1979;86:642.

73. Grumbach MM. Chorionic growth hormone-prolactin (CGP): secretion, disposition, biologic activity in man, and postulated function as the "growth hormone" of the second half of pregnancy. Ann NY Acad Sci 1968;148:501.

74. Grumbach MM, Kaplan SL. On the placental origin and purification of chorionic "growth hormone-prolactin" and its immunoassay in pregnancy. Trans NY Acad Sci 1964;27:167.

75. Grumbach MM, Kaplan SL. Clinical investigation. In: Pecile A, Muller EE, eds. Second International Symposium on Growth Hormone. New York: Excerpta Medica, 1971:382.

76. Grumbach MM, Kaplan SL, Abrams CL, et al. Plasma free fatty acid response to the administration of chorionic "growth hormone-prolactin." J Clin Endocrinol Metab 1966;26:478.

77. Grumbach MM, Kaplan SL, Vinik A. Human chorionic somatomammotropin. 2. Physiology: hormonal effects and 3. Measurement. In: Berson SA, Yalow RS, eds. Methods in investigative and diagnostic endocri-

nology, Vol 20. Amsterdam: North Holland, 1973: 797.

78. Hambley J, Grant DB. Apparent heterogeneity of serum chorionic somatomammotrophin on gel filtration. Acta Endocrinol 1972;70:43.

79. Handwerger S, Barrett J, Tyrey L, Schomberg D. Differential effect of cyclic adenosine monophosphate on the secretion of human placental lactogen and human chorionic gonadotropin. J Clin Endocrinol Metab 1973;36:1268.

80. Handwerger S, Crenshaw C, Maurer WF, et al. Studies on ovine placental lactogen secretion by homologous radioimmunoassay. J Endocrinol 1977;72:27.

81. Handwerger S, Sherwood LM. Comparison of the structure and lactogenic activity of human placental lactogen and human growth hormone. In: Josmovich JB, Reynolds M, Cobo E, eds. Lactogenic hormones, fetal nutrition and lactation. New York: John Wiley & Sons, 1975:33.

82. Haustraete F, Mous J, Peeters B, Rombauts W. The synthesis of human placental lactogen hormone (hPL) in a cell-free wheat germ system. Mol Biol Rep 1976;3:189.

83. Healy DL, Polson D, Yohkachiya T, et al. Inhibin and related peptides in pregnancy. Bailliere's Clin Endocrinol Metab 1990;4:233.

84. Hemmings R, Langlais J, Falcone T, et al. Human embryos produce transforming growth factors α activity and insulin-like growth factors II. Fertil Steril 1992;58:101.

85. Hirata Y, Moore GW, Bertagna C, Orth ON. Plasma concentrations of immunoreactive human epidermal growth factor (Urogastrone) in man. J Clin Endocrinol Metab 1980;50:440.

86. Hodgen GD, Chen HC, Dufau ML, et al. Transitory hCG-like activity in the urine of some IUD users. J Clin Endocrinol Metab 1978;46:698.

87. Hoffman GE, Drews MR, Scott RT, et al. Epidermal growth factor and its receptor in human implantation trophoblast: immunohistochemical evidence for autocrine/paracrine function. J Clin Endocrinol Metab 1992;74:981.

88. Howell RJS, Perry LA, Choglay NS, et al. Placental protein 12 (PP12): a new test for the prediction of the small-for-gestational-age infant. Br J Obstet Gynaecol 1985;92:1141.

89. Huhtaniemi IT, Korenbrot CC, Jaffe RB. hCG binding and stimulation of testosterone biosynthesis in the human fetal testes. J Clin Endocrinol Metab 1977;44:963.

90. Huhtaniemi IT, Korenbrot CC, Jaffe RB. Content of chorionic gonadotropin in human fetal tissues. J Clin Endocrinol Metab 1978;46:994.

91. Hung W, Blizzard RM, Migeon CJ. Precocious puberty in a boy with hepatoma and circulating gonadotropin. J Pediatr 1963;63:895.

92. Hussa RO, Pattillo RA, Ruckert ACF, Scheuermann KW. Effects of butyrate and dibutyryl cyclic AMP on hCG-secreting trophoblastic and non-trophoblastic cells. J Clin Endocrinol Metab 1978;46:69.

93. Iwashita M, Evans MI, Catt KJ. Characterization of a gonadotropin-releasing hormone receptor site in term placenta and chorionic villi. J Clin Endocrinol Metab 1986;62:127.

94. Jaffe RB, Lee PA, Midgley AR. Serum gonadotropin before, at the inception of, and following human pregnancy. J Clin Endocrinol Metab 1969;29:1281.

95. Javadpour N, McIntire KR, Waldmann TA. Human chorionic gonadotropin (HCG) and alpha-fetoprotein (AFP) in sera and tumor cells of patients with testicular seminoma: a prospective study. Cancer 1978;42:2768.

96. Jepson JH, Friesen HG. The mechanism of action of human placental lactogen on erythropoiesis. Br J Haematol 1968;15:465.

97. Jones SA, Brooks AN, Challis JRG. Steroids modulate corticotropin-releasing hormone production in human fetal membranes and placenta. J Clin Endocrinol Metab 1989;68:825.

98. Josimovich JB. Maintenance of pseudopregnancy in the rat by synergism between human placental lactogen and chorionic gonadotrophin. Endocrinology 1968;83:530.

99. Josimovich JB. Hormonal physiology of pregnancy: steroid hormones of the placenta, and polypeptide hormones of the placenta and pituitary. In: Gold JJ, Josimovich JB, eds. Gynecologic endrocrinology, ed 3. New York: Harper & Row, 1980:147.

100. Josimovich JB, Atwood BL. Human placental lactogen (HPL), a trophoblastic hormone synergizing with chorionic gonadotropin and potentiating the anabolic effects of pituitary growth hormone. Am J Obstet Gynecol 1964;88:867.

101. Josimovich JB, Atwood BL, Goss DA. Luteotrophic, immunologic and electrophoretic properties of human placental lactogen. Endocrinology 1963;73:410.

102. Josimovich JB, MacLaren JA. Presence in the human placenta and term serum of a highly lactogenic substance immunologically related to pituitary growth hormone. Endocrinology 1962;71:209.

103. Josimovich JB, Merisko K, Boccella L, Tobon H. Binding of prolactin by fetal rhesus cell membrane fractions. Endocrinology 1977;100:557.

104. Josimovich JB, Weiss G, Hutchinson DL. Sources and disposition of pituitary prolactin in maternal circulation, amniotic fluid, fetus and placenta in the pregnant rhesus monkey. Endocrinology 1974;94:1364.

105. Kadar N, Caldwell BU, Romero R. A method of screening for ectopic pregnancy. Obstet Gynecol 1981;58:162.

106. Kalkhoff K, Richardson BL, Beck P. Relative effects of pregnancy, human placental lactogen and prednisolone on carbohydrate tolerance in normal and subclinical diabetic subjects. Diabetes 1969;18:153.

107. Kamrava MM, Taymor ML, Berger MJ, et al. Disappearance of human chorionic gonadotropin following removal of ectopic pregnancy. Obstet Gynecol 1983;62:486.

108. Kaplan SL, Grumbach MM. Studies of a human and simian placental hormone with growth hormone-like and prolactin-like activities. J Clin Endocrinol Metab 1964;24:80.

109. Kaplan SL, Gurpide E, Sciarra JJ, Grumbach MM. Metabolic clearance rate and production rate of chorionic growth hormone-prolactin in late pregnancy. J Clin Endocrinol Metab 1968;28:1450.

110. Kelly AM, England P, Lorimer JD, Ferguson JC. An evaluation of human placental lactogen levels in hypertension of pregnancy. Br J Obstet Gynaecol 1975;82:272.

111. Kelly PA, Robertson HA, Friesen HG. Temporal pattern of placental lactogen and progesterone secretion in sheep. Nature (Lond) 1974;248:435.

112. Kelly PA, Shiu RPC, Friesen HG, Robertson HA. Placental lactogen levels in several species throughout pregnancy. Endocrinology 1973;92(suppl):A-233.

113. Khodr GS, Siler-Khodr TM. The effect of luteinizing

hormone-releasing factor on human chorionic gonadotropin secretion. Fertil Steril 1978;30:301.

114. Khodr GS, Siler-Khodr TM. Localization of luteinizing hormone releasing hormone in the human placenta. Fertil Steril 1978;29:523.

115. Khodr GS, Siler-Khodr TM. Placental luteinizing hormone-releasing factor and its synthesis. Science
1980;207:315.

116. Kimball CD, Chang CM, Huang SM, Houck JC. Immunoreactive endorphin peptides and prolactin in
umbilical vein and maternal blood. Am J Obstet Gynecol 1981;140:157.

117. Koob GF, Bloom FE. Behavioural effects of opioid
peptides. Br Med Bull 1983;38:89.

118. Krieger DT, Liotta AS, Brownstein MJ, Zimmerman
EA. ACTH, beta-lipotropin, and related peptides in
brain, pituitary, and blood. Rec Prog Horm Res
1980;36:272.

119. Kumasaka T, Nashi N, Jai Y, et al. Demonstration of
immunoreactive somatostatin-like substance in villi
and decidua in early pregnancy. Am J Obstet Gynecol
1979;134:39.

120. Laatikainen T, Virtanen T, Raisanen I, Salminen K.
Immunoreactive corticotropin releasing factor and
corticotropin in plasma during pregnancy, labor and
puerperium. Neuropeptides 1987;10:343.

121. Lagrew DC, Wilson EA, Jaured MJ. Determination of
gestational age by serum concentrations of human
chorionic gonadotropin. Obstet Gynecol 1983;62:37.

122. Lee JN, Seppala M, Chard T. Characterization of placental luteinizing hormone-releasing factor-like material. Acta Endocrinol 1981;96:394.

123. Lenton EA, Neal LM, Sulaiman R. Plasma concentrations of human chorionic gonadotropin from the
time of implantation until the second week of pregnancy. Fertil Steril 1982;37:773.

124. Lesniak MA, Gorden P, Roth J. Reactivity of nonprimate growth hormones and prolactins with human growth hormone receptors on cultured human
lymphocytes. J Clin Endocrinol Metab 1977;44:838.

125. Li CH. On the characterization of human chorionic
somatomammotropin. Ann Sclavo 1970;12:651.

126. Li CH, Dixon JS, Chung D. Primary structure of the
human chorionic somatomammotropin (HCS) molecule. Science 1971;173:56.

127. Li Y, Matsuzaki N, Masuhiro K, et al. Trophoblast
derived tumor necrosis factor-α induces release of
human chorionic gonadotropin using IL-1 and IL-6
receptor dependent system in the normal human
trophoblast. J Clin Endocrinol Metab 1992;74:184.

128. Linton EA, Behan DP, Saphier PN, Loury PJ. Corticotropin releasing hormone (CRH)-binding protein.
Reduction in the adrenocorticotropin releasing activity of placental but not hypothalamic CRH. J Clin
Endocrinol Metab 1990;70:1574.

129. Marshall JR, Hammond CB, Ross GT, et al. Plasma
and urinary chorionic gonadotropin during early human pregnancy. Obstet Gynecol 1968;32:760.

130. McGregor WG, Kuhn RW, Jaffe RB. Biologically active chorionic gonadotropin synthesis by the human
fetus. Science 1983;220:306.

131. McLachlan RI, Healy DL, Robertson DM, et al. Circulating immunoreactive inhibin in the luteal phase
and early gestation of women undergoing ovulation
induction. Fertil Steril 1987;48:1001.

132. McWilliams D, Callahan RC, Boime I. Human placental lactogen mRNA and its structural genes during
pregnancy: quantitation with a complementary DNA.
Proc Natl Acad Sci USA 1977;74:1024.

133. Melby JC, Dale SL, Wilson TE, Nichols AS. Stimulation of aldosterone secretion by human placental lactogen. Clin Res 1966;14:283.

134. Menon KMJ, Jaffe RB. Chorionic gonadotropin-sen-
sitive adenyl cyclase in human term placenta. J Clin
Endocrinol Metab 1973;36:1104.

135. Mersol-Barry MS, Miller KF, Choi CM, et al. Inhibin
suppresses human chorionic gonadotropin secretion
in term, but not first trimester placenta. J Clin Endocrinol Metab 1990;71:1294.

136. Midgley AR, Jaffe RB. Regulation of human gonadotropins. Disappearance of human chorionic gonadotropins following delivery. J Clin Endocrinol Metab
1968;28:1712.

137. Miyaki A, Sakumoto T, Aono T, et al. Changes in
luteinizing hormone-releasing hormone in human
placenta throughout pregnancy. Obstet Gynecol
1980;60:444.

138. Morris DW, Bhardwag D, Dabbagh LK, et al. Epidermal growth factor induces differentiation and secretion of human chorionic gonadotropin and placental
lactogen in human placenta. J Clin Endocrinol Metab
1987;65:1282.

139. Nielsen PV, Pedersen H, Kampmann EM. Absence of
human placental lactogen in an otherwise uneventful
pregnancy. Am J Obstet Gynecol 1979;135:322.

140. Nishino E, Matsuzaki N, Masuhico K, et al. Trophoblast derived interleukin 6 (IL-6) regulates human
chorionic gonadotropin release through IL-6 receptor on human trophoblasts. J Clin Endocrinol Metab
1990;71:436.

141. O'Donahue TL, Dorsa DM. The opiomelanotropi-
nergic neuronal and endocrine systems. Peptides
1982;3:353.

142. Osathanondh R, Tulchinsky D. Placental polypeptide
hormones. In: Tulchinsky D, Ryan KJ, eds. Maternal-
fetal endocrinology, ed 1. Philadelphia: WB Saunders, 1980:17.

143. Panerai AE, Martini A, DiGiulio AM, et al. Plasma
beta-endorphin, beta-lipotropin, and met-enkephalin
concentrations during pregnancy in normal and
drug-addicted women. J Clin Endocrinol Metab
1983;57:537.

144. Pastorfide GB, Goldstein DP, Kosasa T. The use of a
radioimmunassay specific for human chorionic gonadotropin in patients with molar pregnancy and
gestational trophoblastic disease. Am J Obstet Gynecol 1974;120:1025.

145. Pastorfide GB, Goldstein DP, Kosasa TS, Levesque L.
Serum chorionic gonadotropin activity after molar
pregnancy, therapeutic abortion and term delivery.
Am J Obstet Gynecol 1974;118:293.

146. Pearse AGE. The cytochemistry and ultrastructure of
polypeptide hormone-producing cells of the APUD
series and the embryologic, physiologic and pathologic implications of the concept. J Histochem Cytochem 1969;17:303.

147. Pearse AGE. The diffuse neuroendocrine system and
the APUD concept: related "endocrine" peptides in
brain, intestine, pituitary, placenta and Anuran cutaneous glands. Med Biol 1977;55:115.

148. Petraglia F, Calza L, Garuti GC, et al. Presence and
synthesis of inhibin subunits in human decidua. J
Clin Endocrinol Metab 1990;71:87.

149. Petraglia F, Calza L, Giardino L, et al. Identifcation
of immunoreactive neuropeptide-y in human placenta: localization, secretion and binding sites. Endocrinology 1989;124:2016.

150. Petraglia F, Garuti GC, Calza L, et al. Inhibin sub-

units in human placenta. Localization and messenger ribonucleic acid levels during pregnancy. Am J Obstet Gynecol 1991;165:750.

151. Petraglia F, Sawchenko PE, Rivier J, Vale W. Evidence for local stimulation of ACTH secretion by CRH in human placenta. Nature 1987;328:717.

152. Petraglia F, Sutton S, Vale W. Neurotransmitters and peptides modulate the release of immunoreactive CRH from human cultured placental cells. Am J Obstet Gynecol 1989;160:247.

153. Petraglia F, Vaughan J, Vale W. Inhibin and activin modulate the release of GnRH, hCG and progesterone from cultured human placental cells. Proc Natl Acad Sci USA 1989;86:5114.

154. Petraglia F, Vaughan J, Vale W. Steroid hormones modulate the release of immunoreactive GnRH from cultured human placental cells. J Clin Endocrinol Metab 1990;70:1173.

155. Petraglia F, Volpe AO, Genazzani AR, et al. Neuroendocrinology of the human placenta. Front Neuroendocrinol 1990;11:6.

156. Petraglia F, Woodruff TK, Bolticelli G, et al. Gonadotropin releasing hormone inhibin and activin in human placenta: evidence for a common cellular localization. J Clin Endocrinol Metab 1992;74:1184.

157. Pittaurey DE. βhCG dynamics in ectopic pregnancy. Clin Obstet Gynecol 1987;30:129.

158. Poindexter AN, Buttram VC Jr, Besch PK, Smith RG. Prolactin receptors in the ovary. Fertil Steril 1979;32:273.

159. Ragavan VV, Frantz AG. Opioid regulation of prolactin secretion evidence for a specific role of beta-endorphin. Endocrinology 1981;109:1769.

160. Rayford PL, Vaitukaitis JL, Ross GT, et al. Use of specific antisera to characterize biologic activity of hCG-beta subunit preparations. Endocrinology 1972;91:144.

161. Reyes FI, Boroditsky RS, Winter JSD, Faiman C. Studies on human sexual development. II. Fetal and maternal serum gonadotropin and sex steroid concentrations. J Clin Endocrinol Metab 1974;38:612.

162. Riley SC, Wallen JC, Herlich JM, Challis JRG. The localization and distribution of CRH in the human placenta and fetal membranes throughout gestation. J Clin Endocrinol Metab 1991;72:1001.

163. Robertson DM, Suginami H, Montes HH, et al. Studies on a human chorionic gonadotrophin-like material present in non-pregnant subjects. Acta Endocrinol 1978;89:492.

164. Robinson BG, Emanuel RL, Frim DM, Majzoub JA. Glucocorticoid stimulates expression of corticotropin releasing hormone gene in human placenta. Proc Natl Acad Sci USA 1988;85:5244.

165. Rochman H. Tumor associated markers in clinical diagnosis. Ann Clin Lab Sci 1978;8:167.

166. Rose LI, Williams GH, Jagger PI, Lauler DP. Feminizing tumor of the adrenal gland with positive "chorionic-like" gonadotropin test. J Clin Endocrinol Metab 1968;28:903.

167. Rowell PP, Rama Sastry BV. Human placental cholinergic system: depression of the uptake of alpha-aminoisobutyric acid in isolated human placental villi by choline acetyltransferase inhibitors. J Pharmacol Exp Ther 1981;216:232.

168. Saito T, Saxena BB. Specific receptors for prolactin in the ovary. Acta Endocrinol 1975;80:126.

169. Samaan N, Yen SCC, Friesen H, Pearson OH. Serum placental lactogen levels during pregnancy and in

170. trophoblastic disease. J Clin Endocrinol Metab 1966;26:1303.

170. Samaan N, Yen SCC, Gonzalez D, Pearson OH. Metabolic effects of placental lactogen (HPL) in man. J Clin Endocrinol Metab 1968;28:485.

171. Sara V, Hall V. Somatomedins and the fetus. Clin Obstet Gynecol 1980;23:765.

172. Saxena BB. Human chorionic gonadotropin. In: Fuchs F, Klopper A, eds. Endocrinology of pregnancy. Philadelphia: Harper & Row, 1983:50.

173. Saxena BN, Refetoff S, Emerson K, Selenkow HA. A rapid radioimmunoassay for human placental lactogen. Am J Obstet Gynecol 1968;101:874.

174. Schneider AB, Kowalski K, Sherwood LM. Identification of "big" human placental lactogen in placenta and serum. Endocrinology 1975;97:1364.

175. Schneider AB, Kowalski K, Sherwood LM. "Big" human placental lactogen: disulfide linked peptide chains. Biochem Biophys Res Commun 1975;64:717.

176. Schneider AB, Kowalski K, Sherwood LM. Chemical structure and biologic immunologic activity of "big" human placental lactogen. In: Pecile A, Muller EE, eds. Growth hormone and related peptides. Amsterdam: Excerpta Medica, 1976:327.

177. Schocken DD, Caron MG, Lefkowitz RJ. The human placenta—a rich source of beta adrenergic receptors: characterization of the receptors in particulate and solubilized preparations. J Clin Endocrinol Metab 1980;50:1082.

178. Seppala M, Wahlstrom T, Lehtovirta P, et al. Immunohistochemical demonstration of luteinizing hormone-releasing factor-like material in human syncytiotrophoblast and trophoblastic tumors. Clin Endocrinol 1980;12:441.

179. Serron-Ferre M, Lawrence CC, Jaffe RB. Role of hCG in the regulation of the fetal zone of the human fetal adrenal gland. J Clin Endocrinol Metab 1978;46:834.

180. Sherwood LM, Burstein Y, Schechter I. Primary structure of the NH$_2$-terminal extra piece of the precursor to human placental lactogen. Proc Natl Acad Sci USA 1979;76:3819.

181. Shibasaki T, Odagiri E, Shizume K, Ling N. Corticotropin-releasing factor–like activity in human placental extracts. J Clin Endocrinol Metab 1982;55:384.

182. Shiu RPC, Kelly PA, Friesen HG. Radioreceptor assay for prolactin and other lactogenic hormones. Science 1973;180:968.

183. Siler-Khodr TM. Hypothalamic-like peptides of the placenta. Sem Reprod Endocrinol 1983;1:321.

184. Silverberg J, O'Donnell J, Sugenoya A, et al. Effect of human chorionic gonadotropin on human thyroid tissue in vitro. J Clin Endocrinol Metab 1978;46:420.

185. Sklar CA, Conte FA, Kaplan SL, Grumbach MD. Human chorionic gonadotropin-secreting pineal germinoma and precocious puberty. Arch Dis Child 1983;9:743.

186. Spellacy WN. Human placental lactogen in high-risk pregnancy. Clin Obstet Gynecol 1973;16:298.

187. Spellacy WN, Buhi WC, Birk SA, McCreary SA. Distribution of human placental lactogen in the last half of normal and complicated pregnancies. Am J Obstet Gynecol 1974;120:214.

188. Spellacy WN, Buhi WC, McCreary SA. Measurement of human placental lactogen with a simple immunodiffusion kit (Plac Gest). Obstet Gynecol 1974;43:306.

189. Steier JA, Bergsjo P, Myking OL. Human chorionic gonadotropin in maternal plasma after induced abortion and removal of ectopic pregnancy. Obstet Gynecol 1984;64:391.

190. Steiner DF. Peptide hormone precursors: biosynthesis, processing and significance. In: Parsons, JA, ed. Peptide hormone. Baltimore: University Park Press, 1976:49.

191. Suwa S, Friesen H. Biosynthesis of human placental proteins and human placental lactogen (HPL) in vitro: I. identification of ^{3}H-labeled HPL. Endocrinology 1969;85:1028.

192. Suwa S, Friesen H. Biosynthesis of human placental proteins and human placental lactogen (HPL) in vitro. II. Dynamic studies of normal term placentas. Endocrinology 1969;85:1037.

193. Szczesna E, Boime I. mRNA-dependent synthesis of authentic precursor to human placental lactogen: conversion to its mature hormone form in ascites cell-free extracts. Proc Natl Acad Sci USA 1976;73:1179.

194. Talamantes F. Comparative study of the occurrence of placental prolactin among mammals. Gen Comp Endocrinol 1975;27:115.

195. Talamantes F, Ogren L, Markoff E, et al. Phylogenetic distribution, regulation of secretion, and prolactin-like effects of placental lactogens. Fed Proc 1980;39:2582.

196. Tan L, Yu PH. De novo biosynthesis of enkephalins and their homologues in the human placenta. Biochem Biophys Res Commun 1981;98:752.

197. Tulandi T, Atri M, Bret P, et al. Transvaginal intratubal methotrexate treatment of ectopic pregnancy. Fertil Steril 1992;58:98.

198. Tulsky AJ, Koff AK. Some observations on the role of the corpus luteum in early human pregnancy. Fertil Steril 1957;8:118.

199. Vaitukaitis JL. Immunologic and physical characterization of human chorionic gonadotropin (hCG) by tumours. J Clin Endocrinol Metab 1973;37:505.

200. Vaitakaitis JL. Glycoprotein hormones and their subunits—immunological and biological characterization. In: McKerns KW, ed. Structure and function of the gonadotropins. New York: Plenum Press, 1978:339.

201. Valette A, Desprat R, Cros J, et al. Immunoreactive dynorphine in maternal blood, umbilical vein and amniotic fluid. Neuropeptides 1986;7:145.

202. Varma SK, Dawood MY, Haour F, et al. Gonadotropin-like substance in the pre-implanted rabbit blastocyst. Fertil Steril 1979;31:68.

203. Wang CY, Daimon M, Shen SJ, et al. Insulin like growth factor I messenger ribonucleic acid in the developing human placenta and in term placenta of diabetics. Mol Endocrinol 1988;2:217.

204. Watkins WB, Yen SSC. Somatostatin in cytotrophoblast of the immature human placenta: localization by immunoperoxidase cytochemistry. J Clin Endocrinol Metab 1980;50:969.

205. Ways J, Markoff E, Ogren L, Talamantes F. Lactogenic response of mouse mammary explants from different days of pregnancy to placental lactogen and pituitary prolactin. In Vitro 1979;15:891.

206. Weintraub BD, Rosen SW. Ectopic production of human chorionic somatomammotropin by nontrophoblastic cancers. J Clin Endocrinol Metab 1971;32:94.

207. Wiley LD. Presence of a gonadotropin on the surface of pre-implanted mouse embryos. Nature 1974; 252:715.

208. Williams C, Coltart TM. Adipose tissue metabolism in pregnancy: the lipolytic effect of human placental lactogen. Br J Obstet Gynaecol 1978;85:43.

209. Wolfe CDA, Paterl SP, Linton EA, et al. Plasma CRH in abnormal pregnancy. Br J Obstet Gynaecol 1988;95:1003.

210. Youngblood WW, Humm J, Kizer JS. TRH-like immunoreactivity in rat pancreas and eye, bovine and sheep pineals and human placenta: non-identity with synthetic pyrogluhis-pro-NH$_2$ (TRH). Brain Res 1979;163:101.

211. Youngblood WW, Humm J, Lipton MA, Kizer JS. Thyrotropin-releasing hormone-like bioactivity in placenta: evidence for the existence of substances other than pyrogluhis-pro-NH$_2$ TRH) capable of stimulating pituitary thyrotropin release. Endocrinology 1980;106:541.

212. Zeilmaker GH, Verhamme CMPM. Luteotrophic activity of ectopically developing rat blastocysts. Acta Endocrinol 1978;88:589.

Pregnancy-Related Changes in the Metabolism of Hormones

Reinhart B. Billiar

In pregnancy-associated changes in the metabolism of hormones, the emphasis is on how such changes affect the concentrations of biologically active hormones in the maternal circulation. The method selected to analyze such changes, when possible, is primarily the metabolic clearance rates (MCRs) of hormones and factors that might alter the MCR and metabolism of the hormones during pregnancy. The MCR of a hormone is the sum of all its organ and tissue clearances.

STEROID HORMONES

Androgens

The largest change in the MCR of a steroid during pregnancy is that of dehydroepiandrosterone sulfate (DHEA SO_4). This is due to its very low clearance rate in the nonpregnant woman, whereas in pregnancy, the human placenta can actively metabolize DHEA SO_4. The placenta contains an active sulfatase so that DHEA SO_4 is converted to free DHEA, which can diffuse into the syncytiotrophoblasts, where it is actively metabolized by the 3β-hydroxysteroid dehydrogenase and aromatase activities to estrogen. Thus as the placenta increases in mass and the uteroplacental blood flow increases with advancing gestation, the metabolic clearance rate of DHEA SO_4 increases from 7 L per day in the nonpregnant woman to 63 L per day in the pregnant woman in the third trimester, associated with a steady increase throughout the latter half of gestation.[34]

Another significant change in the metabolism of DHEA SO_4 during pregnancy is an estrogen-induced increase in maternal hepatic 16α-hydroxylation.[41, 67] This results in an increase in the hepatic metabolism of DHEA SO_4 and accounts for approximately one-third of its MCR during the third trimester.[67] The overall rate of 16α-hydroxylation increases sufficiently to maintain an increase in the MCR of DHEA SO_4 in the immediate postpartum period.[12, 67] Because of the maternal metabolism, the conversion of DHEA SO_4 to estradiol occurring solely via the irreversible placental metabolism of DHEA SO_4 is a better reflection of placental activity than is the total MCR of DHEA SO_4. The conversion of DHEA SO_4 to estradiol, as measured in the maternal circulation, increases from about 5% in the first trimester to 5 to 25% in the second trimester to 25 to 40% in the third trimester.[42, 99] This increased conversion with gestational age is probably attributable to several factors, which include an increase in the uteroplacental perfusion and placental mass as well as changes in placental metabolism.[17, 26, 33–35] The conversion of DHEA to estradiol has been proposed as a test of placental function (see Chapter 1).

As would be expected, the placental conversion of androstenedione to estrogen also increases with advancing gestation, and the MCR of androstenedione increases from about 2000 L per day in the nonpregnant woman to approximately 2800 L per day in the pregnant woman in the third trimester.[23] The effect of pregnancy on the MCR of testosterone has not been studied extensively. In the first trimester of pregnancy, the levels of sex steroid–binding globulin (SBG) are increased,[78, 109] and the MCRs of both testosterone and 5α-dihydrotestosterone (DHT) are significantly decreased compared with those of nonpregnant women.[96] It is not clear, however, whether the changes in plasma binding of androgen remain elevated throughout gestation,[109, 113] and neither the MCR of testosterone nor DHT has been studied in the third trimester. The effect of a potential increase in placental metabolism of testosterone might offset changes in the plasma protein binding of testosterone on the overall metabolism (MCR) of testosterone during the third trimester (e.g., see under Estrogen). Because of the active metabolism of androgens by the placenta, several unique metabolites of androgens are present in the maternal circulation in much higher concentrations than in the nonpregnant woman; these may be biologically active, especially at or near the site of formation. For example, both 19-nor testosterone[90] (19-norT) (20 to 60 pg/mL) and 19-hydroxyandrostenedione (19-OHA)[75] are found in increasing concentrations in pregnancy. The concentrations of 19-OHA increase from about 225 pg/mL in the first trimester of pregnancy to 1500 pg/mL in the third trimester. Although 19-OHA has been reported to cause hypertension in animal models, there is no difference in its plasma concentration in the third trimester of women with normal pregnancy or pregnancies complicated by hypertension.[75] Both 19-norT and 19-OHA are believed to be formed by the aromatization pathway(s) of placental androgen metabolism.

Progestogens

The blood levels of progesterone increase throughout pregnancy, increasing from plasma levels of less than 1 and 10 ng/mL during the follicular and luteal phases of the menstrual cycle to approximately 100 ng/mL at term (see Chapter 1). Remarkably the plasma MCR of progesterone of about 2200 L per day does not significantly change over this wide range of progesterone production rates, which varies from approximately 2 mg per day during the follicular phase to 250 mg per day at term.[13, 59, 60] The half-lives of progesterone clearance from the circulation are the same in the nonpregnant woman and in the pregnant woman during the third trimester: an initial volume half-life of disappearance of 1.6 ± 0.2 minutes followed by the second integrated half-live of 19.3 ± 2.5 minutes.[60]

Even though a significant fraction, 40%, of circulating progesterone is tightly associated via noncovalent binding to the specific serum globulin protein transcortin (also termed *corticosteroid-binding globulin* [CBG]) and even though the CBG concentration under the influence of the high estrogen secretion rates of pregnancy is increased twofold to threefold in pregnancy,[93] the progesterone clearance rate is not changed during pregnancy. Increasing the CBG concentrations twofold to threefold by the administration of ethinyl estradiol to ovariectomized women also does not alter the MCR of progesterone but does decrease the MCR of cortisol by half, 306 ± 33 L per day to 136 ± 14 L per day, within several days of initiating the daily oral estrogen.[14] Also the lack of a correlation (inverse) between CBG levels and progesterone clearance is in agreement with the current concepts of a diminished emphasis of the role of plasma-binding proteins on the tissue distribution and metabolism of steroid hormones, especially progesterone.[70, 107]

The high levels of circulating estrogen of pregnancy do not alter the maternal tissues'

metabolism of progesterone. Consistent with this observation is the lack of an effect of the daily administration of the antiestrogen MER-25 on the MCR of progesterone in the third trimester of baboon pregnancy, although it did reduce the placental secretion of progesterone by about 50%.[48] Thus the high circulating levels of progesterone and estrogens of pregnancy do not alter the metabolic clearance of progesterone.

The MCR of progesterone in pregnant subjects with abnormal glucose tolerance tests did not differ from that of normal patients.[60] Also insulin-dependent diabetic pregnant women had similar progesterone MCRs whether or not they were treated with exogenous estrogen/progestin.[60]

The MCR of a hormone is the sum of all organ and tissue clearances; tissue clearance is the product of tissue extraction times blood flow rate. In humans, it has been estimated that about 60% of the overall MCR of progesterone is extrasplanchnic clearance.[63] At term, the uteroplacental blood flow is about 500 L per day[15]; so theoretically if 100% of the progesterone were removed, i.e., extracted, during its passage through the pregnant uterus, the MCR would increase 500 L per day, i.e., about 25%. This would have been measurable by the constant infusion technique. Direct sampling of uterine venous blood at both midterm and at term suggests that the uterine extraction of progesterone is negligible.[13] This is consistent with the lack of change in the MCR of progesterone during pregnancy. Indirect measurements suggest that approximately 50% of the progesterone secreted by the placenta into the fetus at midgestation is metabolized by the fetus (umbilical venous–arterial differences).[15]

In contrast to progesterone, the MCR of pregnenolone does increase during pregnancy, from about 2900 L per day at 12 weeks and 2700 L per day between 33 and 36 weeks to 4200 L per day between 37 and 39 weeks of gestation.[64] This increase in clearance rate can be attributed, at least in part, to the placental extraction of pregnenolone by its conversion to progesterone.[15, 48, 64] Thus the transfer constant (i.e., conversion) of pregnenolone to progesterone, as measured in the peripheral blood, is 7.3% in early pregnancy and increases to 25% in the third trimester. The placental enzyme 3β-hydroxysteroid dehydrogenase, which catalyzes the conversion of pregnenolone to progesterone, is not rate limiting for this in vivo conversion, so the increase during pregnancy is most likely due to the increased placental mass, with associated increased blood flow, of late pregnancy.[64] The daily administration of the antiestrogen MER-25 late in baboon pregnancy did not alter the in vivo placental conversion of pregnenolone to progesterone.[48]

Synthetic glucocorticoids have been administered during pregnancy in anticipation of premature delivery as a method of preventing neonatal respiratory distress syndrome.[62] Increasing the *sheep* placenta exposure to increased concentrations of glucocorticoid, natural or synthetic, alters the placental metabolism of progesterone by the induction of placental 17α-hydroxylase.[3] This results in an increase in the placental conversion of progesterone to 17α-hydroxyprogesterone (17α-OHP) and 17α, 20α-dihydroxypregn-4-en-3-one (17,20α-OHP), which is reflected in increased circulating levels of these steroids near term in the sheep.[3, 30] The plasma concentration of 17α,20α-OHP is also significantly higher during the third trimester of human pregnancy than in the first or second trimester of pregnancy or in nonpregnant women.[68] The plasma concentrations of this steroid, however, were significantly decreased in the third trimester of women who received four intramuscular doses of dexamethasone at 12-hour intervals compared with those who received placebo.[68] The decrease in maternal 17α,20α-OHP concentrations induced by administration of the synthetic glucocorticoid is believed to be due to a decrease in fetal adrenal activity mediated by glucocorticoid suppression of fetal pituitary adrenocorticotropic hormone (ACTH) secretion. Thus in the *human*, there is no evidence that glucocorticoids induce placental 17α-hydroxylase activity.

The increased production rate of progesterone during pregnancy provides the tissues with more substrate for the formation of metabolites. Some of these metabolites, such as ring A reduced metabolites and 21-hydroxylated derivatives (discussed later) may be biologically active; ring A metabolites are believed

to mediate progesterone's anesthetic and analgesic effects.[66] Thus increased levels of these progesterone metabolites may be responsible for the drowsiness and some behavioral effects associated with pregnancy.

Mineralocorticoids

11-Deoxycorticosterone

The blood levels of 11-deoxycorticosterone (DOC) are much higher in women in the third trimester of pregnancy than in nonpregnant women and are highly variable.[66, 74, 77] The source of these elevated DOC levels of pregnancy is not the adrenal gland but the peripheral 21-hydroxylation of progesterone, such as in the kidney.[16, 115] The extraadrenal 21-hydroxylase has been demonstrated by mRNA methods to be a different protein than the corresponding enzyme present in the adrenal.[69] Increased circulating estrogen stimulates extraadrenal 21-hydroxylase activity[16, 65] but does not change the MCR of DOC.[16] Therefore the increased levels of estrogen of pregnancy result in a specific increase in the maternal metabolism of progesterone to DOC. The physiologic significance of the conversion of progesterone to DOC, especially the high concentrations of DOC that are generated by progesterone during pregnancy, remains to be established. It is interesting to note that some of this conversion occurs in mineralocorticoid target tissues, e.g., the kidney.

Aldosterone

Plasma aldosterone concentrations increase steadily throughout gestation and fall rapidly after birth.[89] The MCR of aldosterone, approximately 1600 L per day, is the same in the pregnant woman as in the nonpregnant woman.[106] Because aldosterone extraction is about 90% by the splanchnic bed (i.e., almost all of it is removed from the circulation during its passage through the splanchnic bed) and because there is very little extrasplanchnic metabolism of aldosterone,[6] the lack of change in aldosterone MCR indirectly confirms that hepatic blood flow is not altered by pregnancy.[71] The pattern of aldosterone metabolism, however, is altered during pregnancy, with an increase in its conversion to aldosterone 18-glucuronide (splanchnic metabolism), a small increase in tetrahydroaldosterone formation (extrasplanchnic), and a small decrease in the splanchnic extraction from 90% in the nonpregnant woman to 77% in the pregnant woman during the third trimester.[105] The lack of a significant change in the MCR of aldosterone indicates that the steady increase in plasma aldosterone concentrations during pregnancy is due mainly to an increased adrenal secretion rate.

Estrogen

Estrogen concentrations in the maternal circulation increase steadily throughout gestation. Early in gestation, estradiol and estrone predominate, as the ovary is a major source of estrogen secretion, and the maternal adrenal is the major source of the androgen precursors, DHEA SO$_4$ and androstenedione, for placental estrogen formation. As the pregnancy continues, estriol becomes the principal estrogen as a result of placental conversion of the fetal precursor, 16α-hydroxydehydroepiandrosterone (16α-OHDHEA), to estriol (see Chapter 1). Also, as discussed earlier, there is an increase in the maternal 16 hydroxylation of DHEA. Thus as pregnancy advances, relatively more of the maternal androgen precursor for placental aromatization becomes 16α-OHDHEA.[34, 67] The maternal contribution of 16α-OHDHEA to placental estriol formation, however, is small compared with the fetal supply of 16α-OHDHEA.[42]

Estradiol binds with a relatively high affinity to the specific plasma globulin SBG. It has been suggested that the interaction of estradiol with SBG accounts, in part, for the difference in the MCR of estradiol in men and women; lack of a sex difference in the MCR of estrone, which does not bind to SBG; and the higher MCR of estrone than estradiol.[6] During pregnancy, the SBG concentrations increase twofold to threefold,[78, 113] and it might be expected that the MCR of estradiol would decrease during pregnancy. The MCR of estradiol, however, is the same in the woman in the third trimester of pregnancy as in the nonpregnant woman: 1350 L per day.[42] Studies of the metabolism of estradiol administered to pregnant women supports this conclusion of a lack of change in estrogen metabolism.[101] The absence of a change in estradiol MCR during the third trimester also supports the suggestion made with regard to androgens that either the SBG levels do not remain elevated throughout pregnancy or that factors, such as placental clearance, offset any effect of protein binding on the clearance rate of estradiol in late gestation. To my knowledge, the MCRs of estrone and estriol have not been studied in pregnancy. If their MCRs also remain unchanged during pregnancy, the clearance of estriol would be the most rapid of these three estrogens.[101]

An interesting feature of the placental secretion and metabolism of estrogens is the selective secretion of estradiol into the maternal circulation, whereas estrone is secreted into both the fetal and the maternal circulation.[43, 102, 110, 111] The mechanism(s) controlling this unique polarity of secretion of these closely related compounds is not known, but presumably the morphologic distribution of the enzyme 17β-hydroxysteroid dehydrogenase is a significant determinant.

Cortisol

The plasma concentration of cortisol steadily increases during pregnancy, starting near the end of the first trimester. The concentration of the cortisol-binding protein CBG increases twofold to threefold in pregnancy, and although the amount of cortisol bound to CBG increases throughout pregnancy, the concentration of unbound cortisol also increases.[93, 97, 113] Estrogen treatment of nonpregnant women similarly increases the plasma CBG concentrations. Although estrogen treatment of nonpregnant subjects significantly changes the half-life and decreases the MCR of cortisol, the half-life of cortisol is only slightly prolonged during pregnancy, and there is no significant difference in the MCR of cortisol in the pregnant woman in the third trimester compared with the nonpregnant woman.[11, 14, 113] Similar observations of a change in the MCR of cortisol during estrogen treatment of female baboons have been reported, and, similar to the human, there is an increase in CBG during baboon pregnancy without a change in the MCR of cortisol.[81, 82] The urinary pattern of cortisol metabolites changes only minimally during human pregnancy, supporting the observation of a lack of change in the MCR.[83] It is not known why the overall metabolism of cortisol is not changed during pregnancy in response to the high estrogen levels, which can invoke changes in cortisol metabolism in the nonpregnant woman or man.

The interconversions of cortisol and cortisone are, however, changed during pregnancy, with an increase in the overall conversion of cortisol to cortisone and a decrease in cortisone to cortisol.[11] In the baboon placenta, there is also a change with gestation in the placental interconversion of cortisol and cortisone.[79] At midgestation, the placental formation of cortisol predominates over cortisone, but at term the oxidation of cortisol to cortisone is favored. Although the placental enzymatic 11β-reduction of cortisone to cortisol appears to be present primarily in the decidual cells, the conversion of cortisol to cortisone is located in the trophoblastic cells and is modulated by the estrogen status of the pregnant baboon.[79, 80] Thus estrogen produced by the trophoblasts acts in an autocrine/paracrine manner to modulate trophoblastic metabolism of cortisol. Although it is well established that the term human placenta can actively metabolize cortisol to cortisone, it is not yet known if human placental cortisol-cortisone interconversion changes with gestational age.[80] This is of obvious importance with regard to the sources and concentrations of fetal corticoids at different stages of fetal development (see Chapter 14).

THYROXINE

Thyroxine (T_4) is present in the circulation bound to proteins: T_4 binding α globulin (TBG) (about 76%), albumin (9%), and prealbumin (PA) (15%).[45] The amount of free T_4 is present as only a small percentage (0.03%) of the total T_4. During pregnancy, the levels of TBG increase twofold to threefold during the first half of pregnancy and remain constant

thereafter; the concentrations of PA do not change.[45, 91] The increases in TBG during pregnancy can be attributed to the high levels of estrogen resulting from placental secretion that stimulate the liver synthesis of TBG and also produce an increase in the hepatic sialylation of TBG.[1, 91] Estrogen treatment, and presumably pregnancy, has no effect on the clearance of intact TBG other than by alteration of the degree of sialylation.[87] Thus the increased production rate of TBG during pregnancy results primarily from an increased hepatic secretion rate in conjunction with a reduced MCR of the more heavily sialylated forms of TBG.

During pregnancy, the total concentrations of both T_4 and triiodothyronine (T_3) are significantly elevated; T_4 increases before T_3.[45, 52, 72, 100] Free T_4 levels have been reported to be both significantly decreased and unchanged during pregnancy.[45, 52, 72, 100] Because the urinary levels, which presumably are a reflection of primarily free thyroid hormone serum concentrations, of both T_4 and T_3 are the same in pregnant as in nonpregnant women,[86] it is likely that the free hormone levels are unchanged by pregnancy.

Even though the TBG levels and total thyroid hormone concentrations are significantly increased during pregnancy, it is unclear if the MCRs of the hormones are changed. Thyroid-stimulating hormone levels are increased during normal pregnancy, as is thyroid size.[86] Thus an increase in the thyroid secretion rate may account solely for the increase in total T_4 and T_3 concentrations and the unchanged free thyroxine levels associated with pregnancy; that is, a decrease in the MCR of T_4 and T_3 may not be associated with the increase in TBG concentrations. The increase in TBG may cause a transient decrease in the free T_4 and T_3 levels, which may account for the increase in TSH levels and subsequent stimulation of the thyroid. That the clearance of T_4 from the circulation may not be changed during pregnancy is supported by the study of Dowling et al,[22] who measured T_4 turnover in seven nonpregnant women and eight normal pregnant women, gestational age 2.5 to 8 months. They reported only a slight, nonsignificant decrease in the fractional rate of degradation of T_4 in pregnant women. Initial disappearance rates, however, were not measured, nor were T_4 and T_3 specifically isolated and measured. Thus definitive studies of the MCRs of T_4 and T_3 (or half-lives) during human pregnancy have yet to be done.

The human placenta has the capability to metabolize T_4 and T_3; it can deiodinate the tyrosyl ring of both T_4 and T_3 and convert these active hormones to inactive derivatives.[53, 94] It has been suggested that this is part of the mechanism that keeps T_4 and T_3 from crossing the placenta to the fetus. The activity of the deiodination is highest early in pregnancy and steadily decreases with progression of gestation. Various complications of pregnancy studied do not appear to alter this placental activity.[117] There is a rapid decline in the activity of this enzyme as pregnancy progresses, and this may account for the apparent maintenance of a low uteroplacental extraction of thyroid hormones, which otherwise might be increased with an increasing blood flow to the pregnant uterus. Nevertheless, the placental inactivation of thyroid hormones may be important to the fetal metabolic economy.

POLYPEPTIDE HORMONES

Studies of changes in the metabolism of polypeptide hormones during pregnancy are less numerous and detailed than those of the steroid hormones. The availability for metabolic studies of sufficient quantities of purified polypeptide hormones is generally less than for the steroid hormones. With advances in isolation techniques, sensitive and specific radioimmunoassays, monoclonal antibodies, synthetic polymer techniques, and recombinant DNA methodology for producing polypeptides, more detailed information is becoming available with regard to polypeptide hormone metabolism and human pregnancy. It still remains difficult, however, to label polypeptides for studies to follow the metabolic fate of the specific hormones in a manner that is sufficiently sensitive for in vivo "tracer" studies and also is not a biohazard to the recipient of the labeled polypeptide (e.g., gamma radiation of iodinated polypeptides). Additionally,

it is conceivable that the method selected for labeling of the polypeptide might alter its distribution and metabolism, at least the metabolic rate compared with the endogenous, nonlabeled polypeptide hormone (see discussion of insulin growth factor-I (IGF-I) binding proteins). Also for full physiologic relevance, the chemical structure of the exogenously administered polypeptide hormone should be identical to that of the endogenous circulating hormone not only with respect to the amino acid polypeptide backbone, but also with regard to secondary modifications, such as specific glycosylation structures and sulfation (e.g., gonadotropins). Nevertheless, interesting developments with respect to polypeptide hormone metabolism and primate pregnancy have been reported and demonstrate the importance of studying polypeptide hormone metabolism for a complete understanding of hormonal activity and primate pregnancy.

Vasopressin-Oxytocin

The MCR of vasopressin measured in normotensive women late in pregnancy is approximately 3 L per minute compared with an MCR of 0.7 L per minute in the same women 8 to 10 weeks after normal delivery.[20] The MCRs were determined by a constant infusion of vasopressin at known infusion rates to achieve a steady state of plasma vasopressin concentrations, while the endogenous vasopressin secretion was suppressed by the infusion of normal saline and ingestion of water to ensure sufficiently low tonicities (approximately 270 mOsm/kg). The MCR of vasopressin at 6 to 8 weeks' gestation was the same as in nonpregnant women but reached maximal clearance by midgestation.[61] Increased renal blood flow apparently does not significantly contribute to the increase in clearance rate during pregnancy, as two women with single kidneys also had fourfold increases in the MCR of vasopressin during the third trimester.[20]

The mechanism for the increase in the MCR of vasopressin during pregnancy is not known with certainty. The human placenta is known to be able to metabolize vasopressin,[20] but women with twins or triplets had a similar

MCR of vasopressin during the third trimester as women with only a single fetus.[20] Cystine-aminopeptidase (vasopressinase), the enzyme that catalyzes the cleavage of the peptide bond between the N-terminal cystine and adjacent tyrosine in vasopressin and oxytocin, is undetectable in the circulation early in gestation but is measurable at about 14 weeks' gestation and increases to maximum levels at 36 weeks' gestation (from approximately 0.1 to 3 to 6 U per minute).[92] The vasopressinase is secreted by the syncytiotrophoblasts of the placental villi.[92] The increase in circulating concentrations of this degradative enzyme is probably an important component of the increase in the MCR of vasopressin during human pregnancy. This concept is supported by the observation of a parallel decrease in the MCR of vasopressin and circulating vasopressinase concentrations postpartum as well as the observation that the MCR of 1-deamino-8-D-vasopressin, which is resistant to inactivation by vasopressinase, is not altered by pregnancy.[61] The increase in the clearance rate of vasopressin in pregnancy may explain, in part, the decrease in the vasopressin response to changes in plasma osmolality observed in the woman in the third trimester of pregnancy compared with the nonpregnant woman.[61]

Similar to vasopressin, oxytocin is present in the circulation as the free hormone and not bound significantly to proteins. Renal clearance appears to be a major route of oxytocin metabolism and plasma clearance.[21] In contrast to vasopressin, the MCR of oxytocin of approximately 1.5 L per minute apparently does not change during pregnancy.[2, 21, 56, 95] Incubation of oxytocin with the plasma of pregnant women, however, does result in its rapid degradation by vasopressinase, whereas oxytocin is stable when incubated with plasma from men and nonpregnant women or cord blood, which are low in vasopressinase content.[56] Thus it might be expected that the clearance of oxytocin would be increased in pregnancy. The methods used to determine its clearance rate may be too variable to detect pregnancy-associated changes, or there may be a compensating decrease in the clearance by some other organ system(s) in pregnancy. These observations again emphasize the importance of in vivo measurements of polypeptide hormone metabolism in addition to in vitro studies.

Insulin, Insulin-like Growth Factor, and Growth Hormone

Insulin

In the third trimester of nondiabetic pregnancy, there is increased insulin resistance as evidenced by the hyperinsulinemia in response to glucose. Theoretically this response could be due to a change in the insulin clearance rate. Although the human placenta can metabolize insulin,[32] several studies of insulin pharmacokinetics indicate that the MCR, circulating half-life, and distribution space of insulin are not altered by pregnancy.[39, 55] Thus a change in metabolism does not appear to contribute to the insulin resistance of pregnancy. Because a major mechanism for the clearance of insulin from the peripheral circulation is suggested to be via binding of insulin to its receptor,[118] the pharmacokinetic results appear to be consistent with the suggestion that the insulin resistance of pregnancy is primarily at the postreceptor level.[55]

Gastrointestinal Polypeptide Hormones

Apparently the circulating half-lives of gastric inhibitory polypeptide, gut glucagon-like immunoreactivity, gastrin, pancreatic polypeptide, or glucagon are not altered by normal pregnancy or gestational diabetes.[49] The secretion response of these hormones to various metabolic stimuli may, however, be altered during pregnancy.[49]

Growth Hormone

Growth hormone (GH) in the nonpregnant woman is synthesized from one active gene (hGH-N) in the anterior pituitary and circulates as both a 20 and a 22 kD form.[19, 47] In the circulation, there are two GH binding proteins: a high-affinity, low-capacity and a low-affinity binding protein.[9, 58] The high-affinity binding protein, which corresponds to the extracellular domain of the cellular plasma membrane GH receptor,[58] accounts for 80 to 90% of the bound GH in the blood.[9] The GH bound to the high-affinity binding protein is cleared much more slowly from the circulation than is free GH, as tested in the rat.[7] Because the binding proteins may be a major regulator of the MCR of GH[7] and because the amount of plasma binding of GH is the same (about 25%) in pregnant women as in nonpregnant women,[9] the metabolism and MCR of GH are probably not altered by pregnancy.

The plasma pattern of GH, however, changes as gestation proceeds; in the nonpregnant woman and in the woman during early pregnancy, the 24-hour pattern is pusatile, but starting at the end of the first trimester it becomes less pulsatile until the levels are nonpulsatile and steady in the last trimester.[25] Also, GH levels increase in the third trimester of pregnancy. This increase is due solely to the placental syncytiotrophoblast cell secretion of a second form of GH, derived from a second GH gene (GH-V), in the absence of pituitary GH secretion.[19, 31, 47] Because the GH secreted by the pituitary and the GH secreted by the placenta differ in amino acid sequences at only 13 of 191 positions distributed throughout the GH molecule[98] and because the two GHs bind with equal affinity to the high-affinity binding protein of the plasma,[8] it seems likely that the metabolism and clearance rate of the placental GH circulating in the latter half of pregnancy is similar to the clearance rate of the GH in the woman during the first half of pregnancy and in the nonpregnant woman. This has not been, to my knowledge, directly measured.

The placenta also synthesizes and secretes another GH-like hormone, human placental lactogen (hPl) or chorionic somatomammotropin.[46] The MCR of about 170 L per day of this nonglycosylated hormone is similar in both nonpregnant and pregnant women.[54] hPl clearance from the circulation can be resolved into two exponential curves of half-lives of approximately 12 minutes and 55 minutes.[54] Only a small percentage of this hormone circulates complexed to other protein(s).[46] It can be concluded that the increasing plasma concentrations of hPl during pregnancy reflect increasing placental secretion rates.

Insulin-like Growth Factors

In the last trimester of pregnancy, maternal serum concentrations of IGF-I are elevated approximately threefold compared with nonpregnant serum concentrations, whereas IGF-II levels are unchanged, or only slightly increased, in the third trimester.[36, 44] Although it is known that the placenta or fetus can alter the maternal circulating levels of IGF-I and IGF-II in women and baboons,[19, 44, 84, 85] it is not known if changes in the clearance rates of the IGFs occur during gestation and thereby mediate changes in the total serum concentrations of IGF-I or IGF-II. In the circulation, the IGFs are present primarily complexed to IGF-binding proteins in a large 150-kD complex.[10, 37] The major binding protein of this complex is IGF-binding protein 3. (To date, six IGF-binding proteins have been identified.[88]) The free IGFs are cleared from the blood faster than the IGFs complexed to their binding proteins, and there is a good correlation between the blood concentration of IGF-I and IGF-binding protein 3.[37] The concentration of IGF-binding protein 3, which is regulated by GH, is also increased during pregnancy.[104] Thus the increase in IGF-I during the third trimester of pregnancy might result both from a combination of placental GH (GH-V) stimulation of IGF-I secretion and GH-V stimulation of an increase of IGF-binding protein 3, which might reduce the plasma clearance of IGF-I. Additionally, IGF-I might also be secreted by the placenta.[85] Direct measurements of IGF-I clearance in nonpregnant and pregnant women (or primate models) are not available, and indeed such studies might be difficult to conduct because the binding of derivatives (e.g., iodo-) of IGF-I to IGF-binding protein 3 in women during pregnancy appears to be different than to the same binding protein of nonpregnant women.[104]

The concentration of a second IGF binding protein, IGFBP-1, also increases during human gestation.[38, 76] This binding protein, which has a molecular weight of approximately 26 kD, is synthesized and secreted by the decidual tissue of pregnancy in both the human and the baboon.[28, 76] The decidual production of IGFBP-1 is believed to be regulated by the progesterone stimulation of the estrogen-primed decidua.[27, 76] Thus factors, e.g. fetectomy,[84, 85] that affect the circulating concentrations of growth hormone, progesterone, and estrogen during the third trimester of pregnancy might influence the circulating concentrations of the IGFs by effects both on their secretion rate and on their binding protein concentrations and thus clearance rates.

Luteinizing Hormone–Chorionic Gonadotropin

During the luteal phase and throughout pregnancy, the circulating concentrations of luteinizing hormone (LH) are low owing to the negative feedback action of estradiol and progesterone on its pituitary secretion. Yet substantial and increasing LH activity is required to "rescue" the human corpus luteum and to maintain its progesterone secretion throughout the first trimester for the maintenance of the pregnancy. This is achieved by the placental trophoblast synthesis and secretion of a different LH, human chorionic gonadotropin (hCG). The placental production of hCG is not subjected to the negative feedback action of gonadal steroids, and hCG has a much longer circulating time than LH. Thus high levels of hCG are achieved. The initial half-life for endogenous LH is 21 minutes but for hCG it is 11 hours.[116] This is followed by a much slower second clearance of half-life of 235 minutes for LH compared with 23 hours for hCG. The MCR of hCG is approximately 2 mL per minute/m² for both men and women.[112, 114] The clearance of the individual α and β subunits are much faster: about 6 minutes for the α subunit and 11 minutes for the β subunit.

A major pathway for the clearance of glycoproteins may be through their binding, internalization, and metabolism via a galactose-terminal glycoprotein hepatic membrane receptor–mediated mechanism.[4] The asialoprotein bound to the membrane receptor is internalized into the hepatocyte, where it is digested to amino acids by lysosomal proteolytic enzymes.[4] Thus once the terminal sialic acid residues have been removed from the oligosaccharide side chain of hCG, it is rapidly removed from the circulation and degraded in the liver; the half-life of 141 and 725 minutes for intact hCG in rats is increased to less than 1 minute with removal of 60% of the terminal sialic acid residues.[108] It had been suggested that the much longer half-life of hCG compared with LH might be attributed to the greater degree of glycosylation of hCG com-pared with LH. Although intact glycoproteins can be desialylated in vivo and cleared from the circulation via the galactose-terminal pathway,[50] removal of the sialic acid does not appear to occur efficiently in vivo,[51] and it is now believed that this is not a major pathway for the removal of intact hCG from the circulation.[57, 73] That is, the carbohydrate content cannot explain the large differences in the clearance rates of the hCG and LH.

A major route of the removal of hCG from the circulation appears to be by renal clearance, where hCG is metabolized to an immunoreactive β core polypeptide of molecular weight of approximately 10,000.[73] This peptide consists of the 6–40 and 55–92 amino acid sequences of the β subunit linked together by a disulfide bond and lacks the carboxyterminal region of the β subunit.[24] It is not further metabolized by proteolytic enzymes. The renal clearance as well as the clearance from the plasma of hCG appears to decrease with increasing concentrations of circulating hCG.[103] Thus because the plasma concentrations of hCG vary considerably throughout gestation, it is conceivable that the MCR of hCG is different at different times of pregnancy, but this has not been experimentally verified.

It has been observed that the terminal residue capping the galactose moiety of the asparagine-linked carbohydrate chain of LH is not sialic acid but rather a sulfate.[5] The sulfate does not alter the ability of LH to interact with its target-organ receptor, but its presence does alter the circulating half-life of LH, analogous to the presence or absence of a terminal sialic acid moiety.[5] It was suggested that "the presence of sulfate rather than sialylated oligosaccharides on bLH results in a shorter circulatory half-life. . . ."[5] Follicle-stimulating hormone (FSH), similar to hCG, has its asparagine-linked oligosaccharides also terminating with sialic acid,[40] and, also similar to hCG, it has a slower clearance rate (about one-half) than LH.[18] Thus the bioavailability of glycoproteins may be influenced in a major way by their circulatory half-life, which may be regulated by the specific galactose-capping moiety, i.e., sialic acid or sulfate. Presumably the sulfate is more readily removed by sulfatase than the terminal sialic acid is removed by neuraminidase, resulting in a more active utilization of the hepatic galactose-terminal oligosaccharide pathway for the removal of polypeptides such as LH. More recently, it has also been observed that the hepatic reticuloendothelial cells contain a receptor specific for the sulfate-4-galactose terminal sequence of LH.[29] This receptor pathway is also believed to contribute to the more rapid clearance of LH as compared with hCG and FSH.

REFERENCES

1. Ain KB, Mori Y, Refetoff S. Reduced clearance rate of thyroxine-binding globulin (TBG) with increased sialylation: a mechanism for estrogen-induced elevation of serum TBG concentration. J Clin Endocrinol Metab 1987;65:689.
2. Amico JA, Seitchik J, Robinson AG. Studies of oxytocin in plasma of women during hypocontractile labor. J Clin Endocrinol Metab 1984;58:274.
3. Anderson ABM, Flint ARF, Turnbull AC. Mechanism of action of glucocorticoids in induction of ovine parturition: effect on placental steroid metabolism. J Endocrinol 1975;66:61.
4. Ashwell G, Morrell AG. The binding of deglycosylated glycoproteins by plasma membranes of rat liver. Adv Enzmol 1974;41:99.
5. Baenziger JU, Kumar S, Brodbeck RM, et al. Circulatory half-life but not interaction with the lutropin/chorionic gonadotropin receptor is modulated by sulfation of bovine lutropin oligosaccharides. Proc Natl Acad Sci USA 1992;89:334.
6. Baird DT, Horton R, Longcope C, Tait JF. Steroid dynamics under steady-state conditions. Rec Progr Hormone Res 1969;25:611.
7. Baumann G, Amburn KD, Buchanan TA. The effect of circulating growth hormone-binding protein on the metabolic clearance, distribution, and degradation of human growth hormone. J Clin Endocrinol Metab 1987;64:657.
8. Baumann G, Davila N, Shaw MA, et al. Binding of human growth hormone (GH)-variant (placental GH) to GH-binding proteins in human plasma. J Clin Endocrinol Metab 1991;73:1175.
9. Baumann G, Shaw MA, Amburn K. Regulation of growth-hormone binding proteins in health and disease. Metabolism 1989;38:683.
10. Baxter RC, Martin JL. Structure of the Mr 140,000 growth-hormone-dependent insulin-like growth factor binding protein complex: determination by reconstitution and affinity labeling. Proc Natl Acad Sci USA 1989;86:6898.
11. Beitins IZ, Bayard F, Ances IG, et al. The metabolic clearance rate, blood production, interconversion and transplacental passage of cortisol and cortisone in pregnancy near term. Pediat Res 1973;7:509.
12. Belisle S, Osathanondh R, Tulchinsky D. The effect of constant infusion of unlabeled dehydroepiandrosterone sulfate on maternal plasma androgens and estrogens. J Clin Endocrinol Metab 1977;45:544.
13. Billiar RB, Jassani M, Little B. The metabolic clearance rate and uterine extraction of progesterone at midgestation. Endocr Res Comm 1974;1:339.
14. Billiar RB, Jassani M, Little B. Estrogen and the metabolism of progesterone in vivo. Am J Obstet Gynecol 1975;121:877.
15. Billiar RB, Jassani M, Saarikoski S, Little B. Pregnenolone and pregnenolone sulfate metabolism in vivo and uterine extraction at midgestation. J Clin Endocrinol Metab 1974;39:27.
16. Casey ML, MacDonald PC. Extraadrenal formation of a mineralocorticosteroid: deoxycorticosterone and deoxycorticosterone sulfate biosynthesis and metabolism. Endocr Rev 1982;3:396.
17. Clewell W, Meschia G. Relationship of the metabolic clearance rate of dehydroepiandrosterone sulfate to placental blood flow: a mathematical model. Am J Obstet Gynecol 1976;125:507.
18. Coble YD Jr, Kohler PO, Cargille CM, Ross GT. Production rates and metabolic clearance rates of human follicle-stimulating hormone in premenopausal and postmenopausal women. J Clin Invest 1969;48:359.
19. Daughaday WH, Rotwein P. Insulin-like growth factors I and II. Peptide, messenger ribonucleic acid and gene structures, serum, and tissue concentrations. Endocr Rev 1989;10:68.
20. Davison JM, Barron WM, Lindheimer MD. Metabolic clearance rates of vasopressin increase markedly in late gestation: possible cause of polyuria in pregnant women. Trans Assoc Am Phys 1987;100:91.
21. Dawood MY. Neurohypophyseal hormones. In: Fuchs F, Klopper A, eds. Endocrinology of pregnancy, ed 3. Philadelphia: Harper & Row, 1983;204.
22. Dowling JT, Appleton WG, Nicoloff JT. Thyroxine turnover during human pregnancy. J Clin Endocrinol Metab 1967;27:1749.
23. Edman CD, Toofanian A, MacDonald PC, Gant NF. Placental clearance rate of maternal androstenedione through estradiol formation: an indirect method of assessing uteroplacental blood flow. Am J Obstet Gynecol 1981;141:1029.
24. Endo T, Nishimura R, Saito S, et al. Carbohydrate structures of β-core fragment of human chorionic gonadotropin isolated from a pregnant individual. Endocrinology 1992;130:2052.
25. Eriksson L. Growth hormone in human pregnancy. Maternal 24-hour serum profiles and experimental effects of continuous GH secretion. Acta Obstet Gynaecol Scand 1989;147(suppl):1.
26. Everett RB, Porter JC, MacDonald PC, Gant NF. Relationship of maternal placental blood flow to the placental clearance of maternal plasma dehydroisoandrosterone sulfate through placental estradiol formation. Am J Obstet Gynecol 1980;136:435.
27. Fazleabas AT, Jaffe RC, Verhage HG, et al. An insulin-like growth factor-binding protein in the baboon (*Papio anubis*) endometrium: synthesis, immunocytochemical localization, and hormonal regulation. Endocrinology 1989;124:2321.
28. Fazleabas AT, Verhage HG, Waites G, Bell SC. Characterization of an insulin-like growth factor binding protein, analogous to human pregnancy-associated secreted endometrial α,-globulin, in decidua of the baboon (*Pabio anubis*) placenta. Biol Reprod 1989;40:873.
29. Fiete D, Srivastava V, Hindsgaul O, Baenziger J. A hepatic reticuloendothelial cell receptor specific for SO₄-4 gal NAcβ1, 4 Glc NAcβ1,2 Man α that mediates rapid clearance of lutropin. Cell 1991;67:1103.
30. Flint APF, Goodson JD, Turnbull AC. Increased concentration of 17α,20α-hydroxypregn-4-en-3-one in

maternal and foetal plasma near parturition in sheep. J Endocrinol 1975;67:89.

31. Frankenne F, Rentier-Delrue F, Scippo M-L, et al. Expression of the growth hormone variant gene in human placenta. J Clin Endocrinol Metab 1987; 64:635.

32. Freinkel N, Goodner CJ. Carbohydrate metabolism in pregnancy. I. The metabolism of insulin by human placental tissue. J Clin Invest 1960;39:116.

33. Fritz MA, Stanczyk FZ, Novy MJ. Relationship of uteroplacental blood flow to the placental clearance of maternal dehydroepiandrosterone through estradiol formation in the pregnant baboon. J Clin Endocrinol Metab 1985;61:1023.

34. Gant NF, Hutchinson HT, Siiteri PK, MacDonald PC. Study of the metabolic clearance rate of dehydroisoandrosterone sulfate in pregnancy. Am J Obstet Gynecol 1971;111:555.

35. Gant NF, Madden JD, Siiteri PK, MacDonald PC. The metabolic clearance rate of dehydroisoandrosterone sulfate. III. The effect of thiazide diuretics in normal and future pre-eclamptic pregnancies. Am J Obstet Gynecol 1975;123:159.

36. Gargosky SE, Moyse KJ, Walton PE, et al. Circulating levels of insulin-like growth factors increase and molecular forms of their serum binding proteins change with human pregnancy. Biochem Biophys Res Comm 1990;170:1157.

37. Gargosky SE, Owens PC, Walton PE, et al. Most of the circulating insulin-like growth factors -I and -II are present in the 150 Kda complex during human pregnancy. J Endocrinol 1991;131:491.

38. Giudice LC, Farrell EM, Pham H, et al. Insulin-like growth factor binding proteins in maternal serum throughout gestation and in the puerperium: effects of a pregnancy associated serum protease activity. J Clin Endocrinol Metab 1990;71:806.

39. Gray RS, Cowan P, Steel JM, et al. Insulin action and pharmacokinetics in insulin treated diabetics during the third trimester of pregnancy. Diab Med 1984;1:273.

40. Green ED, Baenziger JU. Asparagine-linked oligosaccharides on lutropin, follitropin, and thyrotropin. I. Structural elucidation of the sulfated and sialylated oligosaccharides on bovine, ovine, and human pituitary glycoprotein hormones. J Biol Chem 1988; 263:25.

41. Gurpide E, Giebenhain M, Stolee A, et al. Stimulation of 16α-hydroxylation of dehydroisoandrosterone sulfate by diethylstilbestrol. J Clin Endocrinol Metab 1973;37:867.

42. Gurpide E, Holinka C. Pregnancy-related changes in the metabolism of hormones. In: Tulchinsky D, Ryan KJ, eds. Maternal-fetal endocrinology. Philadelphia: WB Saunders, 1980:45.

43. Gurpide E, Marks C, de Ziegler D, et al. Asymmetrical release of estrone and estradiol derived from labeled precursors in perfused human placentas. Am J Obstet Gynecol 1982;144:551.

44. Hall, K, Emberg G, Hellem E, et al. Somatomedin levels in pregnancy: longitudinal study in healthy subjects and patients with growth hormone deficiency. J Clin Endocrinol Metab 1984;59:587.

45. Hamada S, Nakagawa T, Moi T, Torizuka K. Re-evaluation of thyroxine binding and free thyroxine in human serum by paper electrophoresis and equilibrium dialysis, and a new free thyroxine index. J Clin Endocrinol Metab 1970;31:166.

46. Handwerger S. The physiology of placental lactogen in human pregnancy. Endocr Revs 1991;12:329.

47. Hennen G, Frankenne F, Closset J, et al. A human placental GH: increasing levels during second half of pregnancy with pituitary GH suppression as revealed by monoclonal antibody radioimmunoassays. Int J Fertil 1985;30:27.

48. Henson MC, Pepe GJ, Albrecht ED. Transuterofetoplacental conversion of pregnenolone to progesterone in antiestrogen-treated baboons. Endocrinology 1987;121:1265.

49. Hornnes PJ, Kühl C. Gastrointestinal hormones and cortisol in normal pregnant women and women with gestational diabetes. Acta Endocrinol 1986; 277(suppl):24.

50. Hossner KL, Billiar RB. Plasma clearance and liver metabolism of native and asialotranscortin in the rat. Biochim Biophys Acta 1979;585:543.

51. Hossner KL, Billiar RB. Plasma clearance and organ distribution of native and desialylated rat and human transcortin: species specificity. Endocrinology 1981; 108:1780.

52. Hotelling DR, Sherwood LM. The effects of pregnancy on circulating triiodothyronine. J Clin Endocrinol Metab 1971;33:783.

53. Kaplan MM, Shaw EA. Type II iodothyronine 5'-deiodination by human and rat placenta in vitro. J Clin Endocrinol Metab 1984;59:253.

54. Kaplan SL, Gurpide E, Sciarra JJ, Grumbach MM. Metabolic clearance rate and production rate of chronic growth hormone-prolactin in late pregnancy. J Clin Endocrinol Metab 1968;28:1450.

55. Kühl C. Aetiology of gestational diabetes. Bailliere's Clin Obstet Gynaecol 1991;5:279.

56. Leake RD, Weitzman RE, Fisher DA. Pharmacokinetics of oxytocin in the human subject. Obstet Gynecol 1980;56:701.

57. Lefort GP, Stolk JM, Nisula BC. Evidence that desialylation and uptake by hepatic receptors for galactose-terminated glycoproteins are immaterial to the metabolism of human choriogonadotropin in the rat. Endocrinology 1984;115:1551.

58. Leung DW, Spencer SA, Cachianes G, et al. Growth hormone receptor and serum binding protein: purification, cloning and expression. Nature 1987; 330:537.

59. Lin TJ, Billiar RB, Little B. Metabolic clearance rate of progesterone in the menstrual cycle. J Clin Endocrinol Metab 1972;35:879.

60. Lin TJ, Lin SC, Erlenmeyer F, et al. Progesterone production rates during the third trimester of pregnancy in normal women, diabetic women, and women with abnormal glucose tolerance. J Clin Endocrinol Metab 1972;34:287.

61. Lindheimer MD, Barron WM, Davison JM. Osmoregulation of thirst and vasopressin release in pregnancy. Am J Physiol 1989;257:F159.

62. Little AB, and Collaborative Groups on Antenatal Steroid Therapy. Effect of antenatal dexamethasone administration on the prevention of respiratory distress syndrome. Am J Obstet Gynecol 1981;141:276.

63. Little B, Billiar RB, Bougas J, Tait JF. The splanchnic clearance rate of progesterone in patients with cardiac disease. J Clin Endocrinol Metab 1973;36:1222.

64. Little B, Billiar RB, Halla M, et al. Pregnenolone production in pregnancy. Am J Obstet Gynecol 1971;111:505.

65. MacDonald PC, Cutrer S, MacDonald SC, et al. Regulation of extraadrenal steroid 21-hydroxylase activ-

ity: increased conversion of plasma progesterone to deoxycorticosterone during estrogen treatment of women pregnant with a dead fetus. J Clin Invest 1982;69:469.
66. MacDonald PC, Dombroski RA, Casey ML. Recurrent secretion of progesterone in large amounts: an endocrine/metabolic disorder unique to young women? Endocr Revs 1991;12:372.
67. Madden JD, Siiteri PK, MacDonald PC, Gant NF. The pattern and rates of metabolism of maternal plasma dehydroisoandrosterone in human pregnancy. Am J Obstet Gynecol 1976;125:915.
68. Mahajan DK, Anderson G, Poole WK, et al. Changes in the concentration of 17α, 20α-dihydroxypregn-4-en-3-one during pregnancy, labor, and delivery and the effect of dexamethasone treatment during the third trimester of pregnancy. J Clin Endocrinol Metab 1983;57:585.
69. Mellon SH, Miller WL. Extraadrenal steroid 21-hydroxylation is not mediated by P450c21. J Clin Invest 1989;84:1497.
70. Mendel CM. The free hormone hypothesis: a physiologically based mathematical model. Endocr Revs 1989;10:232.
71. Munnell EW, Taylor HC Jr. Liver blood flow in pregnancy—hepatic vein catheterization. J Clin Invest 1947;26:952.
72. Nakagawa T, Matsumura K, Shinoda N, et al. A decrease in the equilibrium constant for the binding of thyroxine to TBG in pregnant women. Rad Med 1989;7:265.
73. Nisula BC, Blithe DL, Akar A, et al. Metabolic fate of human choriogonadotropin. J Steroid Biochem 1989;33:733.
74. Nolten WE, Lindheimer MD, Oparil S, Ehrlich EN. Desoxycorticosterone in normal pregnancy. I. Sequential studies of the secretory patterns of deoxycorticosterone, aldosterone, and cortisol. Am J Obstet Gynecol 1978;132:414.
75. Osawa Y, Ohnishi S, Yarborough C, et al. Serum levels of 19-hydroxyandrostenedione during pregnancy and at delivery determined by gas chromatography mass spectrometry. Steroids 1990;55:165.
76. Owens JA. Endocrine and substrate control of fetal growth: placental and maternal influences and insulin-like growth factors. Reprod Fertil Dev 1991;3:501.
77. Parker CR Jr, Everett RB, Quirk JG, et al. Hormone production in pregnancy in the primi-gravid patient. II. Plasma levels of deoxycorticosterone throughout pregnancy of normal women and of women who developed pregnancy-induced hypertension. Am J Obstet Gynecol 1980;138:626.
78. Pearlman WH, Crepy O, Murphy M. Testosterone-binding levels in the serum of women during the normal menstrual cycle, pregnancy, and the post-partum period. J Clin Endocrinol Metab 1967;27:1012.
79. Pepe GJ, Albrecht ED. Transuteroplacental metabolism of cortisol and cortisone during mid- and late gestation in the baboon. Endocrinology 1984;115:1946.
80. Pepe GJ, Albrecht ED. Regulation of the primate fetal adrenal cortex. Endocr Revs 1990;11:151.
81. Pepe GJ, Ehrenkranz RA, Townsley JD. The metabolic clearance and interconversion of cortisol and cortisone in pregnant and nonpregnant baboons. Endocrinology 1976;99:597.
82. Pepe GJ, Johnson DK, Albrecht ED. The effects of estrogen on cortisol metabolism in female baboons. Steroids 1982;39:471.
83. Peterson RE. Corticosteroids and corticotropins. In: Fuchs F, Klopper A, eds. Endocrinology of pregnancy, ed 3. Philadelphia: Harper & Row, 1983:112.
84. Putney DJ, Henson MC, Pepe GJ, Albrecht ED. Influence of the fetus and estrogen on maternal serum growth hormone, insulin-like growth factor-II, and epidermal growth factor concentrations during baboon pregnancy. Endocrinology 1991;129:3109.
85. Putney DJ, Pepe GJ, Albrecht ED. Influence of the fetus and estrogen on serum concentrations and placental formation of insulin-like growth factor I during baboon pregnancy. Endocrinology 1990;127:2400.
86. Rastogi GK, Sawhney RC, Sinha MK, et al. Serum and urinary levels of thyroid hormones in normal pregnancy. Obstet Gynecol 1974;44:176.
87. Refetoff S, Fang VS, Marshall JS, Robin NI. Metabolism of thyroxine-binding globulin in man. Abnormal rate of synthesis in inherited thyroxine-binding globulin deficiency and excess. J Clin Invest 1976;57:485.
88. Report on the nomenclature of the IGF binding proteins. Endocrinology 1992;130:1736.
89. Resnick LM, Laragh JH. The renin-angiotensin-aldosterone system in pregnancy. In: Fuchs F, Klopper A, eds. Endocrinology of pregnancy, ed 3. Philadelphia: Harper & Row, 1983:191.
90. Reznik Y, Herrou M, Dehennin L, et al. Rising plasma levels of 19-nortestosterone throughout pregnancy: determination by radioimmunoassay and validation by gas chromatography mass spectrometry. J Clin Endocrinol Metab 1987;69:1086.
91. Robbins J, Cheng S-Y, Gershengorn MC, et al. Thyroxine transport proteins of plasma. Molecular properties and biosynthesis. Rec Progr Hormone Res 1978;34:477.
92. Rosenbloom AA, Sack J, Fisher DA. The circulating vasopressinase of pregnancy: species comparison with radioimmunoassay. Am J Obstet Gynecol 1975;121:316.
93. Rosenthal HE, Slaunwhite WR Jr, Sandberg AA. Transcortin: a corticosteroid-binding protein of plasma. X. Cortisol and progesterone interplay and unbound levels of these steroids in pregnancy. J Clin Endocrinol Metab 1969;29:352.
94. Roti E, Fang SL, Green K, et al. Human placenta is an active site of thyroxine and 3,3′,5-triiodothyronine tyrosyl ring deiodination. J Clin Endocrinol Metab 1981;53:498.
95. Ryden G, Sjoholm I. The metabolism of oxytocin in pregnant and non-pregnant women. Acta Obstet Gynecol 1971;50:37.
96. Saez JM, Forest MG, Morera AM, Bertrand J. Metabolic clearance rate and blood production rate of testosterone and dihydrotestosterone in normal subjects, during pregnancy, and in hyperthyroidism. J Clin Invest 1972;51:1226.
97. Scott EM, McGarrigle HHG, Lachelin GCL. The increase in plasma and saliva cortisol levels in pregnancy is not due to the increase in corticosteroid-binding globulin levels. J Clin Endocrinol Metab 1990;71:639.
98. Seeburg PH. The growth hormone gene family: nucleotide sequences show recent divergence and predict a new polypeptide hormone. DNA 1982;1:239.
99. Siiteri PK, MacDonald PC. Placental estrogen biosynthesis during human pregnancy. J Clin Endocrinol Metab 1966;26:751.
100. Skjoldebrand L, Brundin J, Carlstrom A, Pettersson

T. Thyroid associated components in serum during normal pregnancy. Acta Endocrinol 1982;100:504.

101. Slaunwhite WR Jr, Kirdani RY, Sandberg AA. Metabolic aspects of estrogens. In: Greep RO, Astwood EB, eds. Handbook of Physiology. Section 7, Endocrinology. Vol II, Part 1. Washington, DC: American Physiological Society, 1973:485.

102. Slikker W Jr, Hill DE, Young JFL. Comparison of the transplacental pharmacokinetics of 17β-estradiol and diethylstilbestrol in the subhuman primate. J Pharmacol Exp Ther 1982;221:173.

103. Sowers JR, Pekary AE, Hershman JM, et al. Metabolism of exogenous human chorionic gondotropin in men. J Endocrinol 1979;80:83.

104. Suikkari AM, Baxter RC. Insulin-like growth factor (IGF) binding protein-3 in pregnancy serum binds native IGF-I but not iodo-IGF-I. J Clin Endocrinol Metab 1991;73:1377.

105. Tait JF, Little B. The metabolism of orally and intravenously administered labeled aldosterone in pregnant subjects. J Clin Invest 1968;47:2423.

106. Tait JF, Little B, Tait SAS, Flood C. The metabolic clearance rate of aldosterone in pregnant and non-pregnant subjects estimated by both single-injection and constant-infusion methods. J Clin Invest 1962;41:2093.

107. Tait JF, Tait SAS. The effect of plasma protein binding on the metabolism of steroid hormones. J Endocrinol 1991;131:339.

108. Van Hall EV, Vaitukaitis JL, Ross GT, et al. Effects of progressive desialylation on the rate of disappearance of immunoreactive HCG from plasma in rats. Endocrinology 1971;89:11.

109. Vermeulen A, Verdonck L, Van der Straeten M, Oué N. Capacity of testosterone-binding globulin in human plasma and influence of specific binding of testosterone on its metabolic clearance rate. J Clin Endocrinol Metab 1969;29:1470.

110. Waddell BJ, Albrecht ED, Pepe GJ. Utilization of maternal and fetal androstenedione for placental estrogen production at mid and late baboon pregnancy. J Steroid Biochem Mol Biol 1992;41:171.

111. Walsh SW, McCarthy MS. Selective placental secretion of estrogens into fetal and maternal circulations. Endocrinology 1981;109:2152.

112. Wehmann RE, Nisula BC. Metabolic and renal clearance rates of purified human chorionic gonadotropin. J Clin Invest 1981;68:184.

113. Westphal V. Steroid-protein interactions. Monographs on endocrinology. New York: Springer-Verlag, 1971:216;361.

114. Wide L, Johannisson E, Tillinger K-G, Diczfalusy E. Metabolic clearance of human chorionic gonadotropin administered to nonpregnant women. Acta Endocrinol 1968;59:579.

115. Winkel CA, Milewich L, Parker CR Jr, et al. Conversion of plasma progesterone to deoxycorticosterone in men, nonpregnant and pregnant women, and adrenalectomized subjects: evidence for steroid 21-hydroxylase activity in nonadrenal tissues. J Clin Invest 1980;66:803.

116. Yen SSC, Llerena O, Little B, Pearson OH. Disappearance rates of endogenous luteinizing hormone and chorionic gonadotropin in man. J Clin Endocrinol Metab 1968;28:1763.

117. Yoshida K, Suzuki M, Sakurada T, et al. Human placental thyroxine inner ring monodeiodinase in complicated pregnancy. Metabolism 1985;34:535.

118. Zeleznik AJ, Roth J. Demonstration of the insulin receptor in vivo in rabbits and its possible role as a reservoir for the plasma hormone. J Clin Invest 1978;61:1363.

CHAPTER 4

Endocrine Pancreas and Maternal Metabolism

Mary Norton

Thomas A. Buchanan

John L. Kitzmiller

The purpose of this chapter is to review the structure and hormones of the endocrine pancreas and their function during pregnancy. The effect of placental hormones on these processes is also considered. An understanding of metabolism during pregnancy requires an appreciation of maternal adaptation with reference to metabolic fuels and is essential in appreciating factors important in fetal growth and in managing pregnancies complicated by diabetes.

FUNCTIONAL ANATOMY OF THE PANCREATIC ISLETS

The islets of Langerhans are hundreds of thousands of small endocrine glands scattered throughout the exocrine pancreas (Fig. 4–1). They develop from epithelial cells of the outgrowing pancreatic ducts. First seen in the terminal and side buds of the primitive ducts, these epithelial cells multiply and enlarge to form *early islets*. These "primary islets" consist of a central mass of insulin-producing B cells surrounded by glucagon-producing A cells. The fetal B cells are capable of synthesizing and storing insulin by the 10th week of gestation.[117]

The islets constitute approximately 2 to 3% of the *adult pancreas*. They are composed of at least four cell types, each producing a different secretory product: A cells produce glucagon, B cells produce insulin, D cells produce somatostatin, and F cells produce pancreatic polypeptide (Table 4–1, Fig. 4–2). The cell types are not uniformly distributed throughout the pancreas. Rather the posterior head is the only portion containing pancreatic polypeptide (PP) secreting F cells and consists of 80% F cells, 17 to 20% B cells, and <0.5% A cells. The islets located in the tail, body, and anterior portions of the head are so-called PP-poor islets, containing 75% B cells, 20% A cells, and 3 to 5% D cells.[119]

Organized ultrastructural *relationships among the different types of islet cells* suggest a functional unit. The cell to cell contacts in heterocellular regions occur in areas of the islet that receive nerves and small vessels.[301] Gap junctions, membrane specializations thought to provide pathways for intercellular exchange of ions and small molecules, have been noted in pancreatic islets.[220] Studies have demonstrated the transfer of dye molecules, ions, and radiolabeled metabolites among B cells. A relationship between increased insulin secretion and increased gap junctions and junctional transfer among B cells has been suggested,[220] and such increased transfer has been documented in islets removed from rats during late pregnancy.[277] Precise mechanistic links, however, between increased junctional transfer and increased glucose-stimulated insulin secretion in pregnancy remain to be identified.

Hormones secreted by one islet cell type may alter the function of other cell types. Somatostatin suppresses insulin, glucagon, and PP secretion; insulin suppresses glucagon secretion; and glucagon stimulates insulin and

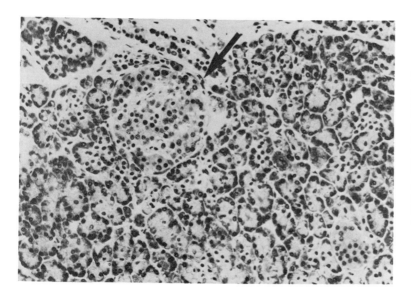

FIGURE 4–1. Photomicrograph of a section of a human pancreas. In the islet of Langerhans *(arrow)*, the A cells appear mainly in the periphery as large cells with dark cytoplasm. The remaining cells are primarily B cells. (From Kloppel G, Veld P, Stamm B, Heitz P. The endocrine pancreas. In: Kovacs K, Asa S, eds. Functional endocrine pathology. Cambridge, MA: Blackwell Scientific, 1991, 409.)

TABLE 4–1. Cell Types in Pancreatic Islets of Langerhans

Cell Types	Approximate Percentage of Islet Mass	Secretory Product
A cell	20	Glucagon, proglucagon
B cell	75	Insulin, C-peptide, proinsulin
D cell	3–5	Somatostatin
F cell (PP cell)	<2	Pancreatic polypeptide

From Karam JH, Salber PR, Forsham PH. Pancreatic hormones and diabetes. In: Greenspan FS, Forsham PH, eds. Basic and clinical endocrinology. E Norwalk, CT: Appleton-Century-Crofts,1987; 523.

somatostatin secretion. Thus regulation of islet function at the paracrine level may occur via direct intraislet processes. Paracrine regulation could occur via secretion of hormones into the interstitial space between cells, although evidence for this mechanism is lacking. It appears that the islet microcirculation may be involved in intraislet regulation of hormonal secretion. The islet microcirculation carries blood from the B cell–rich medulla to the A cell–rich cortex of the islet.[33] Perfusion of rat pancreatic arteries with potent anti-insulin serum leads to immediate and striking enhancement of glucagon secretion, suggesting that insulin within the islets maintains an ongoing inhibition of glucagon secretion.

Marked changes occur in the structure and function of the *maternal islets during pregnancy.* Islet cell hypertrophy and hyperplasia have been demonstrated in pregnant rats and in autopsy studies of pregnant women[307, 309] (Fig. 4–3). There appears to be a lesser increase in the number of A cells, so the ratio of B:A cells increases.[128] In human pregnancy, these

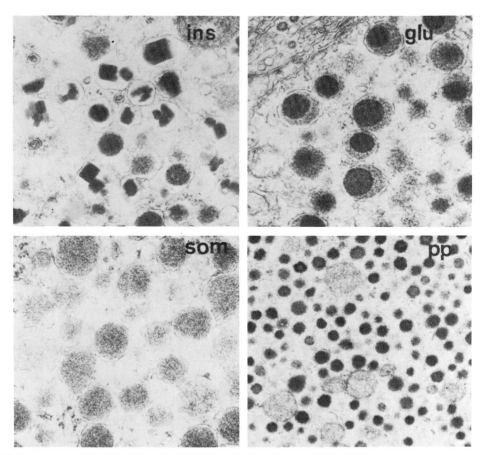

FIGURE 4–2. Ultrastructural appearance of the secretory vesicles of the four islet cell types in the adult human pancreas. glu = Glucagon (A) cells; ins = insulin (B) cells; pp = pancreatic polypeptide (F) cells; som = somatostatin (D) cells. (From Kloppel G, Veld P, Stamm B, Heitz P. The endocrine pancreas. In: Kovacs K, Asa S, eds. Functional endocrine pathology. Cambridge, MA: Blackwell Scientific, 1991, 397.)

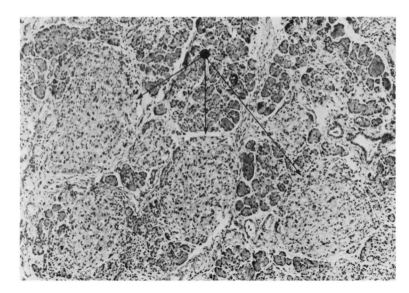

FIGURE 4–3. Photomicrograph of human pancreas with islets *(arrows)* demonstrating hyperplasia and hypertrophy. (From Kloppel G, Veld P, Stamm B, Heitz P. The endocrine pancreas. In: Kovacs K, Asa S, eds. Functional endocrine pathology. Cambridge, MA: Blackwell Scientific, 1991, 427.)

changes are not noted before the 20th week of gestation.[309] The islet changes of pregnancy may be related to direct effects of pregnancy hormones on the islets as well as to indirect effects of hormonally mediated insulin resistance and substrate changes on B cell structure and function. A full discussion of the effects of gestational hormones on the pancreas can be found later in this chapter.

ISLET HORMONES: REGULATION AND FUNCTION

Insulin

Synthesis, Secretion, and Clearance

From the standpoint of intermediary metabolism, insulin is the main secretory product of the endocrine pancreas. Insulin is a 5808 molecular weight protein consisting of 51 amino acids arranged in two peptide chains, the A and B chains, containing 21 and 30 amino acids. The chains are connected by two disulfide bridges. Insulin is synthesized in the rough endoplasmic reticulum of the B cells as the precursor peptide, preproinsulin. Soon after synthesis, preproinsulin is cleaved by microsomal enzymes to proinsulin. Further proteolytic cleavage at two sites along the proinsulin chain converts proinsulin to insulin plus a connecting peptide (C-peptide), which ap-

pears to be biologically inert. This final cleavage occurs either before or after transport to the Golgi apparatus, where secretory granules are packaged. Mature secretory granules contain equimolar amounts of insulin and C peptide as well as small quantities of unprocessed proinsulin.[157]

Insulin is secreted only by the B cells of the pancreas. Its secretion occurs under two general conditions: basal and stimulated. *Basal insulin secretion* is oscillatory, with a period of 9 to 14 minutes.[187, 286] The underlying periodicity of insulin release seems to be inherent to the B cells, perhaps modulated by neural mechanisms.[285] Hormonal inputs to the B cell (e.g., somatostatin) and nonglucose substrate concentrations may also affect basal insulin secretion rates.[90, 272, 276]

Stimulated insulin secretion has been studied most thoroughly in response to glucose, the most potent stimulus for insulin release. An acute rise in blood glucose above some threshold, usually in the range of 5.0 to 5.6 mM (90 to 100 mg/dL) in humans, stimulates a rapid (1 to 3 minute) *initial or first-phase release of stored insulin.* The magnitude of the acute insulin response increases in parallel with the magnitude of the hyperglycemic stimulus, up to a maximal effect at approximately 8.3 mM (150 mg/dL) above basal glucose.[196] Loss of the acute insulin response to glucose is one of the earliest signs of B cell dysfunction.[38] Continued hyperglycemia after an acute increase

TABLE 4–2. Tissue Distribution, Glucose K_m, and Function of Five Major Facilitated Glucose Transporters in Humans*

Transporter Isoform	Tissue Distribution	Glucose K_m (mM)	Primary Function
GLUT 1 Independent uptake	Ubiquitous (especially brain, placenta)	1–2	Insulin glucose
GLUT 2 Transporter; independent	Liver, kidney, gut, pancreatic B cell	15–20	Export insulin uptake
GLUT 3 Independent uptake	Ubiquitous (especially brain, kidney, placenta)	1–2	Insulin glucose
GLUT 4 Dependent uptake	Striated muscle adipose	2–10	Insulin glucose
GLUT 5	?	?	?

*GLUT 1 and GLUT 3 transporters mediate glucose uptake by insulin-independent tissues and may account for basal uptake in insulin-sensitive tissues as well. GLUT 2 transports glucose across a wide range of glucose concentrations. Thus GLUT 2 is expressed by liver (efficient glucose uptake, storage, and production at varied glycemia), pancreatic B cells (glucose sensing for insulin secretion across a wide range of glycemia), and gut/kidney epithelial cells (glucose export at the basolateral membrane after active transport into cells at the luminal membrane). GLUT 4 is the major insulin-sensitive transporter and mediates insulin-stimulated glucose uptake in fat and striated muscle.

Adapted from Thorens B, Charron MJ, Lodish HF. Molecular physiology of glucose transporters. Diab Care 1990; 13:209; and Kasanicki MA, Pilch PF. Regulation of glucose transporter function. Diab Care 1991; 13:219. With permission.

in glucose potentiates the release system and stimulates insulin synthesis, so additional insulin becomes available for a *second phase of insulin release*.[118] This second-phase response occurs as long as plasma glucose is elevated above a threshold level and normally lasts from 10 to 60 minutes after a single glucose injection.[41] Persistent hyperglycemia stimulates continued insulin release. Glucose-stimulated insulin synthesis, however, contributes little to released insulin until after 2 hours of hyperglycemia.[270] Because glucose stimulates only B and D cells, whereas amino acids stimulate A cells and glucagon secretion as well, the amount of insulin and other hormones released during a meal depends on the *ratio of ingested carbohydrate to protein*. Meals high in carbohydrate predominantly stimulate insulin release. Conversely, a protein meal results in relatively greater glucagon secretion because amino acids provoke insulin release less efficiently in the absence of high glucose levels but effectively stimulate glucagon-secreting A cells.[157]

Glucose-stimulated insulin release requires the *uptake of glucose by the B cell*. Because the plasma membrane is impermeable to polar molecules, such as glucose, the cellular uptake of glucose is accomplished by membrane-associated carrier proteins, called *glucose transporters*.[22, 159, 291] These specialized molecules transfer glucose across the lipid bilayer by facilitated diffusion, and they are chemically and functionally distinct from energy-dependent transporters that move glucose up a concentration gradient in the gut and kidney. Molecular studies have identified a family of facilitated glucose transporters consisting of at least five molecules with specific tissue localizations and functions[22, 29] (Table 4–2). One of these transporters, referred to as *GLUT 2*, is expressed by B cells but not by other islet cell types. Evidence that GLUT 2 is required for normal glucose sensing by B cells includes (1) its localization in B cells but not other islet cells; (2) its high Km (15 to 20 mM) for glucose, which allows intracellular sensing of glucose over a wide range of plasma concentrations; and (3) reduced expression of GLUT 2 in insulinoma cells, which are minimally sensitive to glucose,[291] and in the B-cells of at least one animal model of diabetes mellitus.[145]

Glucose-stimulated insulin secretion requires not only glucose uptake, but also *intracellular metabolism of glucose*. Adenosine triphosphate (ATP), which is produced during metabolism of glucose and related hexoses, is a likely link between hexose utilization by B cells and insulin release. An increase in the intracellular concentration of ATP results in the closure of ATP-dependent potassium channels in the B cell membrane.[62, 247, 266] The resultant reduction in outflow of potassium ions causes B cell depolarization, which in turn activates voltage-regulated calcium channels, allowing an influx of calcium into the B cell. Inositol triphosphate is also released in the B cell in response to glucose and may serve to mobilize stored calcium within the cell. *The increase in intracellular calcium appears to trigger insulin release.* Insulin release is mediated at least in part by a microtubular apparatus, which transports the granule-containing vacuoles to the cell surface. One theory states that mature insulin-containing granules in the B cell attach to microtubules that contract linearly in response to high intracellular calcium. This contraction causes ejection of the granules and release of the insulin, C peptide, and proinsulin that they contain.[107, 157] Glucose also elevates B cell cyclic adenosine monophosphate (cAMP), and this cAMP induction causes mobilization of calcium from mitochondrial compartments. Many nonglucose stimuli to insulin release also increase intracellular cAMP, and cAMP in itself is an important modulator of insulin release. Elevation of cAMP, however, does not stimulate insulin release in the absence of glucose[157] (Fig. 4–4).

Failure of glucose-stimulated insulin release is a common finding in hyperglycemic conditions. Evidence from isolated islets,[31] intact animals,[190, 191] and humans[133, 306] indicates that chronic exposure to hyperglycemia contributes to the reduction in glucose-stimulated insulin release. This *glucotoxicity* may be important in the pathogenesis of B cell failure in noninsulin-dependent diabetic patients.[257]

Numerous nonglucose substances may be involved in the regulation of insulin secretion (Table 4–3). These agents act by stimulating insulin secretion directly, by amplifying the B cell response to glucose, or by inhibiting insulin secretion. Glucose, however, is necessary in vitro for nonglucose regulators of insulin secretion to be effective. Some of the substances that amplify the effect of glucose on insulin release are gastrointestinal hormones (e.g., gastric inhibitory polypeptide). Those hormones are referred to as *incretins* because they appear to explain why glucose administered orally is a more potent insulin secretogogue than glucose administered intravenously, with a similar degree of hyperglycemia.[67]

Other facets of B cell regulation include input from the nervous system and the effects of other nonislet hormones. α_2-Adrenergic stimulation inhibits, whereas β-adrenergic stimulation enhances, insulin release. Norepinephrine and epinephrine stimulate both α-adrenergic and β-adrenergic receptors. The net effect on basal insulin secretion is small, but both hormones inhibit glucose-stimulated insulin release.[2, 244, 245] Norepinephrine also stimulates glucagon release, whereas acetylcholine stimulates both

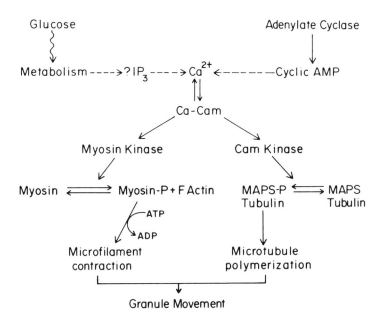

FIGURE 4–4. Role of Ca^{2+} in the stimulation of insulin secretion from pancreatic B cells (see text). The increase in cytosolic Ca^{2+} can be mediated by an influx of extracellular Ca^{2+} and an increase in inositol 1,4,5-P3 (IP3) or cAMP. The increase in cytosolic Ca^{2+} activates the two kinases, resulting in the phosphorylation of myosin and tubulin. The phosphorylation of these proteins is probably involved in the movement of insulin-containing granules to the plasma membrane and the release of insulin into the blood stream. (From Exton JP, Blackmore PF. Calcium-mediated hormonal responses. In: DeGroot LJ, ed. Endocrinology. Philadelphia: WB Saunders, 1989, 71.)

TABLE 4–3. Regulator of Insulin Release

Stimulators of Insulin Release
  Glucose, mannose
  Leucine
  Vagal stimulation
  Sulfonylureas
  Potassium

Amplifiers of Glucose-Induced Insulin Release
  Gastrin inhibitory polypeptide, cholecystokinin,
    secretin, gastrin
  β-adrenergic stimulation
  Arginine

Inhibitors of Insulin Release
  α-adrenergic stimulation
  Somatostatin
  Diazoxide, phenytoin, vinblastine, colchicine
  Prostaglandin E_1

Modified from Karam JH, Salber PR, Forsham PH, Pancreatic hormones and diabetes mellitus. In: Greenspan FS, Forsham PH, eds. Basic and clinical endocrinology. E Norwalk, CT: Appleton-Century-Crofts, 1986; 527. With permission.

insulin and glucagon release.[107, 222] Galanin inhibits B and D cells, whereas cholecystokinin stimulates B cell secretion.[75, 251] Central nervous system innervation is not a prerequisite for islet cell function. Rather, nervous input seems to synchronize islet secretion, to control activity of some non-B cells and to signal anticipated food intake.[171]

Once secreted, insulin has a half-life of 7 to 10 minutes in the circulation. The majority of *circulating insulin* is degraded by the liver, which removes on first pass approximately half of the insulin entering the portal circulation.[94] Skeletal muscle and kidney also have significant insulin-degrading activity. In addition, insulin is cleared by glomerular filtration and direct uptake from peritubular capillary blood in the kidneys.[161] Proteolytic enzymes that degrade insulin have been identified in both soluble and particulate fractions of human placental homogenates, and an ability to remove insulin from the circulation and degrade it has been demonstrated by both in vivo and in vitro studies of the metabolism of human placental tissue.[246] Both the half-life and degradation kinetics of insulin, however, are similar in pregnant and nonpregnant women, indicating that placental removal of insulin has little impact on overall insulin dynamics during pregnancy.[24, 43, 185, 201, 284]

Concentrations of insulin in the serum of overnight-fasted humans vary considerably. In lean normal individuals, concentrations are generally in the range of 5 to 15 μU/mL. Patients who are obese or who have other conditions associated with insulin resistance may have fasting insulin levels 2 to 3 times those of lean normal people. Postprandial insulin concentrations seldom rise above 50 to 70 μU/mL in lean normal people. Insulin-resistant subjects may have considerably higher postprandial insulin levels because, similar to fasting insulin, nutrient-stimulated insulin responses are related to the peripheral effectiveness of insulin. In general, the relationship between insulin action and glucose-stimulated insulin secretion is reciprocal,[15, 27, 39] the extra insulin secreted by insulin-resistant people serving to maintain normal glucose utilization rates. Disruption of this relationship between the magnitude of the insulin response and insulin action results in *hyperglycemia*.[25] The dynamics of insulin secretion are also important in the regulation of plasma glucose. After eating, peripheral insulin concentrations normally rise within 8 to 10 minutes and peak in 30 to 45 minutes, whereas postprandial glucose concentrations rise only slightly and return to baseline values within 90 to 120 minutes. Patients with impaired B cell function manifest a sluggish rise in plasma insulin,[79] and the resultant prolongation of postprandial hyperglycemia causes a delay in the return of plasma insulin levels to basal.

Actions of Insulin

The *actions of insulin are multiple* and include stimulation of glucose, ion, and amino acid uptake;[314] modification of rate-limited enzymes, such as glycogen synthetase and hormone-sensitive lipase;[68, 150] regulation of gene expression for some regulatory enzymes;[271] intracellular redistribution of proteins, such as one type of glucose transporter and the insulin-like growth factor II (IGF II) and transferrin receptors;[178] and promotion of cell growth[255] (Table 4–4). Many of these effects are cell or tissue specific. Further, some actions occur within seconds of insulin exposure, suggesting effects on existing membrane or cytoplasmic mediators of insulin action, whereas other effects require hours of insulin exposure and may occur through nuclear effects and alteration of protein synthesis. This discussion fo-

TABLE 4–4. Metabolic Effects of Insulin and Glucagon

Insulin	Glucagon
Liver	
Anabolic	Antianabolic
Promotes glycogen storage	Decreased glycogen synthesis
Increases synthesis of triglyceride, cholesterol, and very low density lipoprotein	
Promotes glycolysis	
Anticatabolic	Catabolic
Inhibits glycogenolysis	Increases glycogenolysis
Inhibits gluconeogenesis	Increases conversion alanine to glucose
Inhibits ketolysis	Increases ketogenesis
Muscle	
Promotes protein synthesis	
Increases amino acid transport	
Stimulates ribosomal protein synthesis	
Retards proteolysis	
Promotes glycogen synthesis	
Increases glucose transport	
Enhances activity of glycogen synthetase	
Inhibits activity of glycogen phosphorylase	
Fat	
Promotes triglyceride storage	Increases lipolysis
Induces lipoprotein lipase, increased uptake of free fatty acids	
Increases glucose transport into fat cell	
Inhibits intracellular lipolysis	

Modified from Karam JH, Salber PR, Forsham PH. Pancreatic hormones and diabetes mellitus. In: Greenspan FS, Forsham PH, eds. Basic and clinical endocrinology. E Norwalk, CT: Appleton-Century-Crofts, 1986; 528. With permission.

cuses on insulin's effects on carbohydrate, lipid, and protein metabolism in tissues specialized for energy storage, i.e., liver, skeletal muscle, and adipose tissue, where insulin serves an anabolic function.

Although elegant physiologic and molecular studies have greatly expanded our understanding of insulin's actions, the precise mechanisms by which insulin exerts its many effects have not been elucidated. As a first step, insulin must reach target cells from the blood stream. Studies of insulin concentrations in plasma and lymph, the latter reflecting insulin levels in the interstitial fluid, indicate that *transcapillary transport* is an important step in insulin action.[317] Once insulin reaches target cells, the hormone initiates its many biologic functions by *binding to cell membrane receptors*, which are ubiquitous in mammalian cells. The human insulin receptor is a glycoprotein consisting of two extracellular A chains, to which insulin binds, and two membrane spanning B chains, connected to the A chains by disulfide bonds.[77, 300] Insulin receptors are synthesized from a single gene located on chromosome 19 and are processed posttranslationally into the tetrameric structure shown in Figure 4–5. Binding of insulin to the extracellular A chains initiates a series of tyrosine phosphorylations *(autophosphorylations)* within the intracellular portions of the B chains.[256] The phosphorylation of the B chains initiates a cascade of tyrosine and serine phosphorylations of cytoplasmic proteins.[74, 224] Steps immediately distal to the protein phosphorylations are poorly understood, although some of the phosphorylations seem to be critical for insulin action.[57, 83] Additionally, there is a group of low-molecular-weight compounds generated in response to insulin that have been reported to affect the activity of several cellular enzymes in the same manner as insulin.[267] Additional work is needed to determine whether these compounds are obligate mediators of some of insulin's actions and, if so, how their generation is triggered.

In addition to protein phosphorylations, insulin binding initiates *internalization of the insulin-insulin receptor complex*, a process that may play a role in the regulation of insulin receptor density on the cell surface and thus sensitivity to ambient insulin concentrations.[13] Conditions associated with high insulin levels and low receptor binding include obesity and chronic exogenous overinsulinization. Conditions associated with low insulin levels and enhanced binding of insulin to receptors include chronic exercise and fasting. Hormones such as cortisol and progesterone decrease insulin binding to the receptor. That effect may be

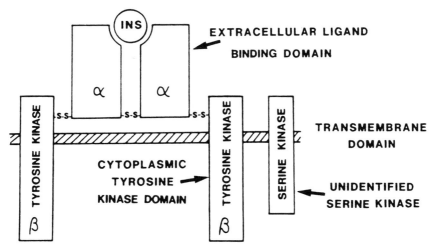

FIGURE 4–5. Schematic model of the insulin receptor kinase complex. (From Csaba G [ed]. Development of hormone receptors. Experientia 1987; 53(suppl):32.)

direct[262] or may result in part from the accompanying increase in circulating insulin levels.[157] Although reductions in the number of receptors on the cell surface may alter insulin action, only a small fraction (approximately 10%) of the normal complement of cell surface receptors is normally required for maximal insulin effect.[177] Thus most cases of impaired insulin action are related to defects distal to the receptor binding step *(postreceptor defects)*.

Insulin has two major *effects on glucose metabolism:* It suppresses glucose release from and promotes glucose storage by the *liver,* and it stimulates glucose uptake, metabolism, and storage by insulin-sensitive *peripheral tissues,* such as striated muscle and fat. Because glucose transport into the hepatocytes is largely independent of insulin, insulin's effect on hepatic glucose storage is thought to occur via direct enzyme modulation. Insulin causes glycogen accumulation in liver by stimulating glycogen synthase activity[236, 253] and by inactivating glycogen phosphorylase, the major regulator of glycogen breakdown. These effects are enhanced in a synergistic fashion by increased glucose flux into the liver, which is mainly dependent on glycemia. Insulin's suppression of gluconeogenesis may be due in part to direct enzyme effects in the liver.[96, 275] Evidence suggests, however, that insulin also modulates gluconeogenesis by controlling the blood-borne supply of substrates available for glucose synthesis.[1]

Insulin's effect on glucose transport into muscle and fat cells depends in large part on the ability of those cells to express the insulin-responsive glucose transporter, GLUT 4.[22, 159, 291] Most if not all human cells express one or both constitutive glucose transporter isoforms, GLUT 1 and GLUT 3. The presence of those constitutive transporters in the cell membrane is largely independent of insulin and accounts for glucose uptake by insulin-independent cells (e.g., neurons and erythrocytes). GLUT 1 and GLUT 3 may also contribute to basal glucose uptake by insulin-sensitive cells. In the presence of low insulin levels, most GLUT 4 transporters reside in cytoplasmic vesicles of insulin-sensitive cells (e.g., skeletal myocytes and adipocytes). In response to some signal from insulin, the vesicles move to the cell membrane, where *GLUT 4 transporters mediate glucose influx.* Thus expression of GLUT 4 appears to be the major determinant of a cell's ability to respond to insulin by increasing glucose uptake. Insulin regulates not only the subcellular localization of GLUT 4 (cytoplasm versus membrane), but also the synthesis of GLUT 4.[149] States of chronic insulin deficiency, such as untreated diabetes, are characterized by reduced GLUT 4 content of insulin-dependent cells and reduced action of insulin to stimulate glucose uptake. To date, molecular abnormalities of GLUT 4 transporters rarely have been identified in states of reduced insulin action. Therefore attention is being directed toward the coupling between binding of insulin to its receptor and translocation of GLUT 4 to identify possible cellular mechanisms of insulin resistance.

In addition to stimulating glucose transport, *insulin stimulates glucose metabolism* within insulin-sensitive cells. Stimulated pathways include glycogen synthesis[236, 253] and glucose oxidation.[46] In theory, a defect in stimulation of these intracellular pathways could cause a buildup of free glucose and a reduction in the gradient that favors glucose transport into cells. In normal tissues, however, it has been difficult to demonstrate a buildup of intracellular glucose during insulin stimulation, indicating that glucose transport rather than glucose metabolism is normally the rate-limiting step in insulin-mediated glucose uptake. Whether defects of intracellular glucose metabolism in disease states such as diabetes may be severe enough to contribute to insulin resistance remains controversial.

Insulin has *several effects on lipid metabolism.* The ones most relevant to pregnancy occur in fat cells, where insulin stimulates lipogenesis and suppresses free fatty acid (FFA) release, and in the liver, where insulin suppresses ketogenesis and stimulates triglyceride synthesis. In adipose tissue, insulin promotes lipogenesis by activating lipoprotein lipase,[37] a capillary endothelial enzyme that removes triglycerides from circulating lipoprotein particles and hydrolyzes them to fatty acids and glycerol, which are taken up by fat cells. Insulin also activates the uptake of glucose and its metabolism to glycerol-3-phosphate, the three-carbon backbone used for triglyceride synthesis in adipocytes. Insulin suppresses lipolysis by inhibiting the hormone-sensitive (and cAMP-sensitive) lipase inside adipocytes. In the liver, insulin and glucagon interact to determine the fate of FFAs that are taken up from the circulation.[210] Insulin, working indirectly through stimulation of glycolysis, promotes reesterification of FFA to triglycerides. Glucagon, working more directly on trafficking of FFAs into mitochondria, favors oxidation of FFAs to ketones. Overall, insulin's effects on ketone production are predominantly through suppression of FFA release in adipose tissue and secondarily through hepatic effects, whereas glucagon affects the liver predominantly. Insulin also appears to have important hepatic effects to stimulate synthesis of triglycerides,[292] which are elevated in pregnancy.

Insulin *promotes protein anabolism* by stimulating amino acid uptake into insulin-sensitive cells[166, 316] and by regulating protein synthesis and degradation rates.[143, 248] The effects are tissue specific and have been demonstrated in skeletal and cardiac muscle and liver. In fast-twitch skeletal muscle, insulin promotes protein synthesis through regulation of the efficiency of protein synthesis by ribosomes as well as through regulation of the synthesis and degradation of ribosomes themselves. Effects on ribosomal number predominate in slow-twitch striated and cardiac muscle. Insulin also regulates protein synthesis in the liver, but the effect is predominantly on synthesis of secretory (e.g., albumin) rather than structural proteins. Insulin appears to have lesser effects on protein degradation than on protein synthesis in the liver.[164] The mechanisms by which insulin regulates protein synthesis and degradation are unresolved but may involve regulation of gene transcription[113, 202] and prostaglandin production.[254]

Insulin in Pregnancy

Normal pregnancy is characterized by *two* major alterations in insulin physiology: a *reduction in insulin's ability to stimulate glucose uptake* and an *enhancement of B cell insulin secretion.* Between conception and delivery, the ability of insulin to stimulate glucose utilization declines 50 to 70%,[41, 263] and insulin secretory responses to nutrients such as glucose increase twofold to threefold [41, 282, 283] (Fig. 4–6). In general, the alterations in insulin physiology parallel the growth of the fetoplacental unit and circulating levels of several peptide and steroid hormones of pregnancy.[98] The parallelism suggests that the hormones of pregnancy play a role in the genesis of maternal metabolic adaptations to gestation, a suggestion supported by in vivo and in vitro studies of insulin action and islet function (see later discussion). Thus the fetoplacental unit appears capable of realigning maternal metabolism to help provide for the metabolic demands of gestation.

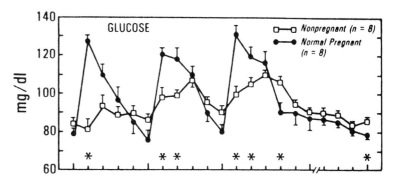

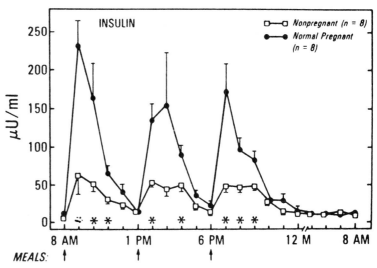

FIGURE 4–6. The effect of normal late pregnancy on the diurnal changes in plasma glucose and insulin. Note the significant increase in postprandial response. (From Phelps RL, Metzger BE, Freinkel N. Carbohydrate metabolism in pregnancy. Am J Obstet Gynecol 1981; 140:730.)

Simultaneous and interrelated changes in insulin action and B cell function make it difficult to determine whether B cell hyperfunction is a primary process leading to insulin resistance during pregnancy or whether insulin resistance occurs first and leads to a compensatory enhancement of insulin secretion. In view of the manifold actions of insulin, our use of the term *insulin resistance* in this discussion refers to cellular glucose uptake and metabolism. The fact that women with type I diabetes and no endogenous B cell function develop insulin resistance during gestation[273] provides strong evidence that insulin resistance is a primary process. In theory, the resistance could occur in any insulin-dependent tissue. In fact, most but not all available data indicate that *skeletal muscle* and *adipose tissue* from pregnant rats and humans are *resistant to insulin's effect on glucose uptake.*[4, 6, 127, 198, 262, 293, 294] Data on the response of hepatic glucose production to insulin during pregnancy are con-

flicting,[65, 126, 198] in part because of inaccuracies in tracer methods that have been used to assess insulin's effect on glucose production in vivo.[26, 212]

Mediation of insulin resistance during pregnancy may be related to the impact of several nonislet hormones on adipose tissue and skeletal muscle. Progesterone, placental lactogen, prolactin, and glucocorticoids have been shown to reduce insulin-mediated glucose transport into adipocytes and muscle tissue after exposure in vitro.[199, 231, 262] Administration of these hormones individually to nonpregnant animals and humans has also produced some alterations indicative of insulin resistance,[18, 64, 153, 155] although the resistance has generally not been of the degree seen in pregnancy. Estradiol and chorionic gonadotropin do not appear to antagonize insulin's effect on glucose utilization.[260, 262] Exposure of rat adipocytes to a combination of progesterone, human placental lactogen (hPL), prolactin, and cortisol in vitro caused a reduction in insulin action similar to that seen in cells taken from pregnant rats,[262] suggesting that the combined effects of those hormones are important for the full effects of pregnancy on insulin action.

The mechanisms by which hormones of pregnancy alter insulin action remain to be identified. Although progesterone and cortisol have been shown to reduce insulin binding to adipocytes in vitro,[231] that effect may be counterbalanced by stimulatory effects of estradiol on insulin binding.[262] Indeed, although some conflicting data exist,[21, 134] most studies have failed to detect differences in insulin binding to erythrocytes, monocytes, or adipocytes between pregnant and nonpregnant individuals.[5, 76, 115, 195, 227, 237, 293, 295] Thus *insulin resistance appears to occur at a site distal to the receptor binding step.* To date, a reduction has been reported in insulin-mediated autophosphorylation of hepatic insulin receptors from pregnant rats[206] and in the levels of key enzymes of glycolysis in adipose tissue and muscle from pregnant women.[7] Increased circulating levels and tissue content of nonesterified fatty acids, which can inhibit insulin-mediated glucose uptake,[93] also have been reported in pregnancy. Regulation of GLUT 4 transporters in pregnancy remains to be studied.

In nonpregnant controls, resistance to insulin-mediated glucose uptake causes a compensatory enhancement of the insulin secretory response to nutrients.[15, 27, 39] Thus conditions associated with insulin resistance and normal B cell function are characterized by elevated fasting and postprandial insulin levels. Much of the *hyperinsulinemia of pregnancy* may be related to this phenomenon.[39] Likewise, many of the insulinotropic effects that have been reported after in vivo administration of pregnancy hormones to nonpregnant humans and experimental animals[16, 64, 153, 269] may actually reflect B cell compensation for hormonally mediated insulin resistance, as direct exposure of islets to estradiol, progesterone, or PL causes little if any augmentation of B cell growth or insulin secretory capacity.[64, 140, 205, 228] Thus the hyperinsulinemia of pregnancy appears to result predominantly from B cell compensation for hormonally mediated insulin resistance, with perhaps a small contribution from direct stimulation of pancreatic B cells by placental hormones.

Glucagon

Synthesis, Secretion, and Clearance

Glucagon is a 29–amino acid, single-chain polypeptide synthesized predominantly in the A cells of the islets of Langerhans. Physiologic activity of glucagon depends on the three carboxy-terminal amino acids that are necessary for binding to the receptor, whereas the N-terminal portion of the glucagon molecule is involved in the activation of adenylate cyclase.[301] Similar to insulin, glucagon is synthesized as preprohormone, the synthesis of which occurs in many cells of the central nervous system and gut[23, 203] as well as in the pancreas. Depending on the cell of origin, preproglucagon may be processed to *true glucagon* or to one of six additional peptides that share variable immunoactivity and bioactivity with true glucagon.[304] In some species, significant amounts of true glucagon originate from extrapancreatic cells in the gut, but the pancreas appears to be the predominant source of true glucagon in humans. Because many of the peptide products of preproglucagon reach the circulation, only 30 to 40% of circulating immunoreactive glucagon is biologically active. The remainder represents biologically inactive but immunoreactive peptides.

Numerous factors regulate *glucagon secretion by the A cells.* Amino acids represent the predominant nutrient stimulators of release, although *amino acids differ in their relative stimulation of glucagon and insulin.* Some, such as arginine, cause release of both hormones. Others, such as alanine and glycine, stimulate glucagon release predominantly. Leucine, a good stimulant for insulin release, does not stimulate glucagon. Other branched-chain amino acids, such as isoleucine and valine, are likewise not glucagon secretogogues.[107] Physiologic concentrations of amino acids are more effective in stimulating glucagon than insulin, but the presence of glucose enhances the effect of amino acids on insulin release.[107] Thus with high-protein and low-carbohydrate meals, glucagon is released to counter the hypoglycemic effect of insulin.[301] Hormonal stimulators of glucagon release include catecholamines; the gastrointestinal hormones cholecystokinin, gastrin, and gastric inhibitory polypeptide; and glucocorticoids. Both sympathetic and parasympathetic (vagal) stimulation promote glucagon release; this is especially important in augmenting the response of the A cell to hypoglycemia. β-adrenergic stimulation augments the secretion of both insulin and glucagon.

Glucagon secretion is inhibited by glucose. The inhibition may be due in part to a paracrine effect of insulin and somatostatin, which are released in response to glucose and can inhibit the A cell directly. The demonstration, however, of A cell suppression by small increments in glucose in dogs without B cells or insulin[287] is consistent with an intrinsic glucose-sensing system in A cells. Similar to glucose, FFAs and ketones inhibit glucagon secretion,[110] as does α-adrenergic stimulation.[109] As a result of the complex regulation of glucagon secretion, *the net signal to A cells following a nutrient load* will be the summation of the opposing influences of hyperglycemic suppression and stimulation by gut hormones and amino acids.

The average fasting plasma immunoreactive glucagon level in healthy humans is approximately 75 pg/mL (25 pmol/L). The half-life of true glucagon in the circulation is 3 to 6 minutes, and it is removed largely by the kidney and liver.[157]

Actions of Glucagon

In contrast to insulin, which promotes energy storage during feeding, *glucagon promotes the release of energy substrates between meals* (see Table 4–4). The major target organ for glucagon is the liver, where glucagon stimulates glycogenolysis and gluconeogenesis. Glucagon also promotes the oxidation of FFAs to ketones in the liver. Finally, glucagon has a minor role in stimulating FFA release from adipose tissue but only in the absence or near absence of insulin. In general, the catabolic effects of glucagon occur in direct competition with the anabolic effects of insulin, and it is the *insulin: glucagon relationship* that determines the activity of regulated pathways.

Glucagon appears to have *two basic mechanisms of action on hepatocytes.* First, binding of glucagon to one population of cell surface receptors results in *generation of cAMP* through a classic guanine nucleotide-binding protein (Gs) mechanism. cAMP activates a cAMP-de-

pendent protein kinase, which phosphorylates several hepatic enzyme kinases. The kinases catalyze phosphorylation reactions that alter the activity of enzymes involved in glycogen metabolism and gluconeogenesis. Regarding glycogen metabolism, glycogen phosphorylase is activated to *promote glycogen breakdown,* and glycogen synthase is inactivated, slowing glycogen formation. Regarding gluconeogenesis, fructose 2,6-bisphosphatase is activated, resulting in lower levels of fructose 2,6-bisphosphate. Lowered fructose 2,6-bisphosphate inhibits glycolysis and *stimulates gluconeogenesis* at the level of phosphofructokinase-1.[131, 305] Fructose 2,6-bisphosphate is also an important regulator of fatty acid metabolism.[96, 210] Low levels of fructose 2,6-bisphosphate (favored by glucagon) reduce the flux through glycolysis of three-carbon fragments, which are needed for triglyceride synthesis. The reduced flux inhibits a lipogenic enzyme, malonyl CoA, and activates carnitine acyl transferase, which *allows transport of fatty acids into mitochondria for oxidation to ketones.* High levels of fructose 2,6-bisphosphate (favored by insulin) increase three-carbon flux through glycolysis, stimulating triglyceride synthesis and inhibiting ketogenesis. Thus most of the effects of glucagon on carbohydrate and lipid metabolism in the liver result from the generation of cAMP, and they occur in direct competition with the actions of insulin. The second mechanism of glucagon action involves *inositol phospholipid breakdown in hepatocytes,* presumably by binding to a separate set of cell surface receptors.[310] This mechanism generates inositol triphosphate and diacyl glycerol, which elevate cytosolic calcium and activate protein kinase C. The precise function of this second pathway is unclear, but it may explain why some compounds reproduce the actions of glucagon on hepatocytes without causing cAMP accumulation.[63]

Glucagon in Pregnancy

Fasting plasma glucagon is slightly but significantly *increased* in late normal pregnancy.[69, 150, 185, 219] Because of the relatively greater increase in insulin, the fasting molar insulin:glucagon ratio is increased.[180] *After oral glucose, glucagon suppression below fasting levels is exaggerated,* probably as a result of the higher plasma glucose levels reached because similar physiologic elevations of plasma glucose elicit an identical plasma glucagon suppression in late pregnancy and postpartum.[69, 136, 138, 180]

Oral administration of alanine is followed by a greater rise in plasma glucagon in late pregnancy than postpartum,[168] whereas most data suggest an *unchanged glucagon response to a protein-rich meal in late pregnancy*.[139, 219] This may be due to the fact that a protein-rich meal also contains glucose and lipid, modulating the glucagon secretion caused by amino acid stimulation.[168, 186] Intravenous amino acids result in an almost identical elevation of plasma glucagon levels in pregnancy and postpartum.[181, 182]

Whether the *mechanisms controlling A cell responsiveness during pregnancy* are different from the nonpregnant state is unresolved. Beck et al[19] observed that treatment of women with synthetic estrogens for 14 days reduced the glucagon secretory response to arginine.[19] The treatment had no effect on basal glucagon levels but did reduce amino acid–induced insulin secretion. Perfusion of isolated rat pancreases with hPL caused a significant but short release of glucagon, suggesting that hPL stimulates A cells. In the presence of high glucose levels, however, the islet cell stimulatory effects of hPL were absent.[189]

Data on possible changes in *hepatic responses to glucagon during pregnancy* are not available, but our review of metabolic homeostasis in pregnancy suggests that resistance to glucagon is unlikely.

Somatostatin

Secretion and Functions

The D cells at the periphery of the islets secrete somatostatin, a cyclic polypeptide containing 14 amino acids. Somatostatin is present in several tissues, including brain, the gastrointestinal tract, and the pancreas. Most stimulators of insulin secretion from pancreatic B cells also promote somatostatin release from D cells.[157] Among the stimulators are glucose, arginine, leucine, gastrointestinal hormones, and tolbutamide. Epinephrine and diazoxide inhibit both insulin and somatostatin release.[301]

Somatostatin acts in several ways to restrain the movement of nutrients from the gastrointestinal tract into the circulation. It prolongs gastric emptying, decreases gastric acid and gastrin production, diminishes pancreatic exocrine secretion, decreases splanchnic blood flow, and retards xylose absorption.[157] Low circulating somatostatin levels have been recorded in obese subjects. In some animal models of obesity associated with hyperinsulinemia, pancreatic somatostatin content is reduced, and it has been suggested that hyposomatostatinemia facilitates nutrient assimilation. Neutralization of circulating somatostatin is associated with enhanced nutrient absorption in dogs,[157] and addition of somatostatin antiserum to isolated rat islets has been shown to result in enhanced insulin secretion.[315] Thus the D cells of the pancreatic islets may exert some control over gastrointestinal function and nutrient influx.[184] Somatostatin also appears to blunt glucagon's effect on glucose release from the isolated, perfused rat liver.[10, 265]

Somatostatin in Pregnancy

The number of somatostatin-producing cells tends to diminish during normal pregnancy.[308] Further, the meal-induced rise in somatostatin is absent in late pregnancy, whereas basal somatostatin levels are unchanged.[144] Studies in pregnancy reveal an inverse correlation between birth weight and maternal somatostatin levels, and it has been suggested that low maternal somatostatin levels enhance nutrient storage in the fetoplacental unit, thereby leading to a higher birth weight.[315] Under physiologic conditions, insulin release is modulated by the inhibitory action of somatostatin,[61] and it is possible that some of the enhanced postprandial insulin response of pregnancy is facilitated by the absence of postprandial somatostatin release.

Pancreatic Polypeptide

PP is found in F cells located primarily in the islets of the posterior portion of the head of the pancreas. Circulating levels of PP increase in response to a mixed meal. Intravenous infusion of glucose or triglyceride, however, does not produce such a rise, whereas intravenous amino acids produce only a small increase. PP is released from the pancreas during antroduodenal contractions in the fasting state,[142] and the level of its release depends on vagal cholinergic tone.[274] In pregnancy, conflicting studies have reported basal plasma PP concentrations to be unchanged[143] or decreased,[138] whereas the usual postprandial rise in PP was present but significantly reduced.[143] PP responses to a protein-rich meal as well as to glucose are reduced in pregnancy, whereas the response to ingested lipids is unaffected.[137] Vagotomy abolishes the PP response to an ingested meal. A great deal remains to be elucidated about the synthesis and physiologic significance of PP, especially in pregnancy.

METABOLIC HOMEOSTASIS DURING PREGNANCY

Metabolic homeostasis during pregnancy represents an intricate interplay among metabolic fuels and hormones that facilitate maternal nutrient storage during feeding and favor utilization of stored fat as an energy source during fasting to minimize maternal protein catabolism. These metabolic realignments allow the mother to provide for the ever-increasing metabolic requirements of the fetus (Fig. 4–7) at a minimal cost to her own well-being. Insulin resistance (peripheral glucose uptake) and compensatory hyperinsulinemia appear to be the key factors favoring maternal fuel storage in the fed state. Placental hormones that stimulate lipolysis and limit hepatic glucose production, together with falling serum insulin concentrations, orchestrate the accelerated switch to fat catabolism during fasting. The net result is an accentuation of the normal interplay between fed-state anabolism and fasting catabolism that occurs during feeding and fasting in nonpregnant individuals. We describe the alterations of maternal fuel homeostasis in terms of carbohydrate, protein, and lipid metabolism in the fed compared with postabsorptive and fasted states.

Carbohydrate Metabolism

Fed State: Facilitated Anabolism

Reciprocal changes in insulin-mediated glucose disposal, which declines during gestation,[41, 263]

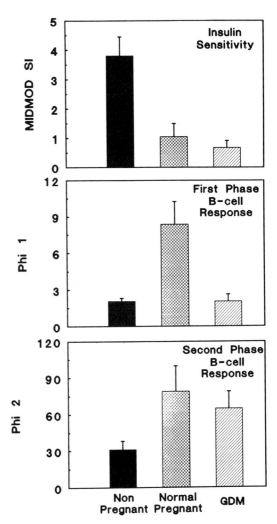

FIGURE 4–7. Insulin sensitivity and pancreatic B cell function in nonpregnant (n = 4), normal pregnant (n = 5), and gestational diabetic (n = 8) women. All women were lean, and the pregnant women were studied during the third trimester of pregnancy. S_I, Phi-1, and Phi-2 were derived from computer analysis of intravenous glucose tolerance test data using the minimal model technique. Low S_I in the two pregnant groups reflects resistance to insulin's action on glucose metabolism in late pregnancy. B cell function was increased to compensate for insulin resistance in normal pregnant women, but the compensation was incomplete in women with gestational diabetes. (From Bergman RN, Phillips LS, Cobelli C. Physiologic evaluation of factors controlling glucose disposition in man. Measurement of insulin sensitivity and beta-cell sensitivity from the response to intravenous glucose. J Clin Invest 1981; 68:1456.)

and B cell responsiveness to glucose, which increases during gestation,[41, 282, 283] maintain postprandial glucose concentrations within a fairly narrow range throughout pregnancy. There is normally, however, a *slight deterioration of glucose tolerance* during the latter half of gestation.[201] That this deterioration occurs despite twofold to threefold increases in nutrient-stimulated insulin levels reflects the insulin resistance of pregnancy described previously in this chapter. The physiologic significance of the mild postprandial hyperglycemia and marked postprandial hyperinsulinemia of pregnancy may be twofold. First, the delayed disappearance of glucose from the maternal circulation after feeding provides a greater opportunity for glucose utilization by the fetus (Fig. 4–8).[101] Second, insulin resistance in skeletal muscle may facilitate shunting of ingested carbohydrate to less resistant adipose tissue during postprandial hyperinsulinemia.[49, 101, 197] Thus hormonally mediated insulin resistance in late pregnancy *may facilitate anabolism of fetal and maternal tissues.* The clinical implications of fed state changes in carbohydrate metabolism during pregnancy relate to the diagnosis and management of maternal diabetes (see later discussion).

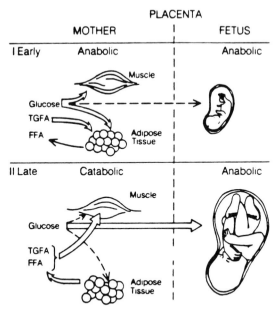

FIGURE 4–8. Fuel disposition in pregnancy of normal mothers. The upper panel represents early gestation and the lower panel late gestation. In early pregnancy, glucose represents the primary maternal metabolic fuel, while triglyceride fatty acids (TGFA) are primarily stored. Fetal glucose needs are minimal at this stage. Later in pregnancy, FFA and TGFA provide the primary maternal metabolic fuels, while glucose is diverted from maternal tissues for transport to the fetus. (From Knopp RH, Montes A, Childs M, et al. Metabolic adjustments in normal and diabetic pregnancy. Clin Obstet Gynecol 1981; 24:21.)

Postabsorptive and Fasted States: Accelerated Starvation

Plasma glucose levels after an overnight fast, when glucose production by the liver provides for all of the body's glucose requirements, normally *decline approximately 10%* over the course of pregnancy. Felig and Tyson first demonstrated the propensity toward fasting hypoglycemia in pregnancy when they compared plasma glucose concentrations during an 84-hour fast between normal nonpregnant women and pregnant women in their second trimester scheduled for elective abortion.[95] Glucose levels were lower in the pregnant group at the end of the fast. Metzger et al[218] reported hypoglycemia after a much shorter period of fasting during late pregnancy. Those authors compared women at 32 to 36 weeks' gestation with nonpregnant control women by measuring plasma glucose after 12, 14, 16, and 18 hours of fasting. They found that plasma glucose was significantly lower in the gravid patients after a 12-hour overnight fast. Continued fasting for 6 hours resulted in a significant decline of circulating glucose and alanine concentrations in the pregnant but not the nonpregnant women. In vitro studies of glucose production by livers from fasted pregnant rats[130, 214] and in vivo studies of alanine administration to pregnant women[88, 297] indicate an enhanced gluconeogenic capacity of the pregnant liver after relatively prolonged periods of fasting. Those data, combined with lowered fasting alanine and serine levels in pregnancy,[88, 101, 162] led to the characterization of fasting hypoglycemia during pregnancy as a substrate deficiency state.[216] The availability, however, of two other gluconeogenic substrates, lactate and glycerol, is adequate during pregnancy,[64] and studies by Kalhan et al[151] indicate that hepatic alanine uptake after overnight fasting in late human pregnancy is not impaired. Those findings suggest that factors other than substrate limitation of gluconeogenesis contribute to the relative hypoglycemia observed after overnight fasting in late pregnancy. *Utilization of glucose by the fetus and placenta* represents a likely contributing factor.[66, 260] Thus fasting hypoglycemia during pregnancy appears to result from a composite of maternal and fetal influences. Early on, hormonally mediated substrate limitation of gluconeogenesis leads to hypoglycemia during prolonged fasting. As pregnancy progresses, increased siphoning of maternal glucose by the fetoplacental unit contributes to fasting hypoglycemia in a progressive fashion, leading to reduced plasma glucose levels after relatively short periods of food deprivation. Fetal utilization of alanine[82] and hormonally mediated restriction of alanine release by skeletal muscle[224] may limit gluconeogenesis during prolonged fasting as well. The maternal adaptations that allow fasting hypoglycemia during pregnancy, combined with the accelerated fat catabolism of late pregnancy (see later discussion), provide a mechanism for conservation of maternal protein stores during even relatively short periods of food deprivation. Those adaptations have been termed *accelerated starvation* by Freinkel.[97]

Lipid Metabolism

Fed State: Facilitated Anabolism

After absorption from the gut, most dietary lipid exists as triglyceride in chylomicrons, which reach the blood stream via the thoracic duct lymph. Some of the triglycerides are removed from chylomicrons via lipoprotein lipase (LPL) in the capillary endothelium. Additional triglyceride is removed from chylomicron remnant particles when they reach the liver; this triglyceride is stored or secreted in very low density lipoprotein (VLDL) particles.[208] Insulin stimulates the production of triglyceride and VLDL by the liver.[292] Similar to chylomicrons, VLDL particles are stripped of triglycerides by *liproprotein lipase in the capillary endothelium* of adipose and muscle tissues. *Hydrolysis of triglycerides by LPL produces FFA and glycerol.* Most of the glycerol is released into the blood stream, whereas most of the FFAs are absorbed and either reesterified and stored as triglyceride (adipose) or B-oxidized (muscle).[208] Insulin promotes fat deposition by promoting the synthesis and activity of LPL, which increases the rate of entry into adipocytes of FFA from diet or liver-derived triglyceride.[208] Insulin also increases glucose uptake into adipose tissue by its effects on glucose transport, and it inhibits lipolysis by suppressing the hormone-sensitive lipase in fat cells.[47, 208] Thus barring additional alterations in the hormonal input into adipose tissue, the *net effect of insulin is an accumulation of triglyceride and an expansion of adipose tissue mass.*

In theory, the progressive augmentation of insulin responses to meals during pregnancy should provide a progressive stimulus to adipose tissue expansion. That theoretical effect depends on the maintenance of normal sensitivity to insulin of (1) LPL, (2) glucose transport, and (3) intracellular lipolysis during pregnancy. As already noted, data from studies in humans and experimental animals indicate some resistance to insulin-mediated glucose uptake by fat cells during late pregnancy. The resistance might be expected to limit insulin's effect on fat accumulation. The resistance, however, to insulin-mediated glucose uptake in fat is probably not as great as the resistance in skeletal muscle[197] and may be mild during the first half of gestation. Further, sensitivity to the antilipolytic effects of insulin appears to be normal in pregnancy.[60, 156] Thus meal-stimulated insulin secretion should suppress lipolysis and circulating FFA levels and, to the extent that muscle is more insulin resistant than fat, should shunt ingested glucose to adipose tissue.[49] These anabolic changes, together with increased caloric intake and perhaps increased caloric "efficiency" associated with insulin resistance,[87] appear to explain much of the *net fat accumulation of pregnancy,* especially during the first half of gestation. During later gestation, experiments in pregnant rats indicate that decreased fat synthesis in maternal adipose tissue is accompanied by (1) a decline in adipocyte conversion of glucose to fatty acids and glycerol, (2) reduction in uptake of fatty acids from plasma triglycerides caused by a decrease in LPL activity, and (3) enhanced lipolytic activity (discussed later).[130a]

In addition to changes in fat mass, pregnancy is characterized by major changes in *circulating lipid levels* (Table 4–5). Plasma triglycerides increase twofold to fourfold during gestation, and total cholesterol increases 50%.[176] VLDL levels increase 2.5-fold during gestation, and VLDL triglyceride levels increase by a similar amount. VLDL triglyceride increases linearly during the first two-thirds of gestation and exponentially thereafter.[176] Studies in experimental animals indicate that the

TABLE 4–5. Comparison of Lipoprotein and Apoprotein Concentrations (mg/dL; mean ± SD) in 36-Week Gestation versus Nonpregnant Controls

	Nonpregnant	36-Week Gestation
Total (N = 23)		
Triglyceride	59 ± 19	222 ± 60
Cholesterol	171 ± 26	251 ± 32
VLDL		
Triglyceride	33 ± 14	107 ± 41
Cholesterol		
Apo B		
LDL		
Triglyceride	14 ± 10	72 ± 21
Cholesterol	104 ± 23	161 ± 39
Apo A-I	61 ± 10	84 ± 23
HDL		
Triglyceride	2 ± 6	29 ± 9
Cholesterol	56 ± 12	64 ± 9
Apo A-I	128 ± 23	164 ± 16
HDL2 (N = 19)		
Cholesterol	22 ± 8	38 ± 12
HDL3		
Cholesterol	34 ± 5	31 ± 6

From Knopp RH, Warth MR, Charles D, et al. Lipoprotein metabolism in pregnancy, fat transport to the fetus, and the effects of diabetes. Biol Neonate 1986; 50:297. With permission.

mechanism of these VLDL changes is related to enhanced VLDL entry into the circulation and diminished adipose tissue LPL activity in late gestation, causing a rerouting of triglyceride fatty acids to other tissues, such as muscle and uterus, for oxidation rather than storage. These changes all appear to be hormonally mediated, and many are mimicked by administration of oral contraceptives or estrogens. Fasting FFA levels rise slowly during the last 10 weeks of gestation.[209] FFA levels, however, decrease after meals, consistent with a suppressive effect on lipolysis of meal-stimulated insulin release.

Postabsorptive and Fasted States: Accelerated Starvation

Fat mobilization normally occurs during fasting, resulting in *increased production of FFA and glycerol.* Most of the glycerol is released into the circulation, whereas the amount of FFA released or reesterified to triglyceride depends on two factors: the availability of glycerol-3-phosphate formed from glucose and the rate of blood flow to the adipose tissue.[208] The rate

of lipolysis is regulated by the activity of a hormone-sensitive (and cAMP-sensitive) triglyceride lipase that exists within fat cells. The rate of lipolysis is also influenced by circulating hormones, such as insulin, which is antilipolytic, and glucagon, adrenocorticotropic hormone (ACTH), and catecholamines, which stimulate lipolysis. Glucocorticoids and growth hormones promote lipolysis via permissive effects on protein synthesis that lead to inhibition of glucose metabolism by fat cells and increased sensitivity to catecholamines.[208] At rest and with moderate exercise, plasma FFAs provide the major fuel needs for skeletal and cardiac muscle (and probably uterine muscle during labor). In the fasting state, FFAs are taken up by liver cells; some are reesterified to triglycerides and released as VLDLs. A greater proportion undergo β oxidation and condensation of the acetate units to form the ketone bodies β hydroxybutyrate and acetoacetate. *Ketogenesis* then depends on the rate of lipolysis (provision of FFA) and the "set" of the liver, which favors ketogenesis when insulin levels and flux through glycolysis are low (e.g., during fasting) and glucagon levels are high.[89, 210, 211]

Lipolysis is accentuated during the second half of human pregnancy.[175] Most available data indicate that plasma FFA levels are increased after an overnight fast in pregnant women near term compared with levels measured earlier in pregnancy or in nonpregnant women.[30, 42, 86, 100, 240, 242] In vitro studies of isolated fat cells from pregnant and nonpregnant rats revealed significantly greater release of FFA and glycerol by cells from the pregnant animals.[172] Fat mobilization was enhanced without any evidence of impaired responsiveness to the antilipolytic effect of insulin.[52, 172] Basal and epinephrine-stimulated release of glycerol from human adipose tissue in vitro also has been shown to be greater during late as compared with early pregnancy.[78] Incubation of rat adipose tissue with *hPL* in concentrations of 20 to 500 μg/mL resulted in increased release of glycerol[106] and increased FFA at the higher doses,[296] implicating hPL in the enhanced lipolysis of pregnancy. hPL, however, was without a lipolytic effect on human adipose tissue incubated in vitro. Likewise, a 12-hour overnight infusion of hPL did not increase fasting

FFA levels in nonpregnant humans.[18] Thus the mediator(s) of the progressive drive to lipolysis during pregnancy has not been identified in full.

Similar to FFA, circulating ketone levels are elevated in the fasted state in late pregnancy. Felig and Tyson first demonstrated this phenomenon when they fasted women before elective abortion between 16 to 20 weeks' gestation and found enhanced ketonemia, increased urinary nitrogen excretion, and exaggerated reductions in gluconeogenic amino acids compared with nonpregnant women.[95] Metzger et al[218] measured FFA and 3-hydroxybutyrate (3-OHB) levels during a 12- to 18-hour overnight fast in the third trimester. They found that 12-hour fasted levels of both lipids were elevated in the pregnant group and that the levels of both increased markedly after only 14 to 16 hours of fasting. No change in FFA or 3-OHB levels occurred in nonpregnant women during the same interval. Thus the *enhanced lipolysis of late pregnancy results in accelerated ketosis when the fasted liver is presented with a large supply of FFA.* The acceleration of lipid catabolism during fasting is adaptive in that it allows the mother to switch rapidly to fat as a major energy source, minimizing her need for glucose production and protein breakdown during food deprivation. The drive to fat catabolism and ketosis, however, may have serious consequences for women with insulin-deficient (type I) diabetes, as discussed later.

Gestational hormones have been shown to cause effects on lipid metabolism similar to those described for pregnancy, but the effects in vivo could be related to compensatory hyperinsulinemia. Estrogens increase the plasma concentration of triglyceride and cholesterol[35] and increase glucose metabolism and fatty acid synthesis in rat adipose tissue.[111] Progesterone failed to affect these systems but has been shown in other studies to enhance fat deposition.[12, 104, 132] Low-dose tricyclic estrogen and progestin have very little effect on lipid metabolism.[170]

Protein Metabolism

The body's muscle mass is the major reservoir of amino acids. In the normal fasting state, low insulin levels signal the release of amino acids, especially alanine and glutamine.[48, 89, 258] Alanine is used primarily in the liver; 30% is used for protein synthesis, and 70% is converted to glucose.[56] Glutamine is used primarily by the gut and kidneys.[48] The branched-chain amino acids leucine, isoleucine, and valine are not glucogenic and are oxidized by muscle and adipose tissue or taken up by the placenta.

When measured in the fasting state during pregnancy, the plasma concentrations of alanine, glycine, and serine are significantly lower than concentrations in nonpregnant women.[82, 99, 162] The *rate of muscle proteolysis* seems to be somewhat *restrained* in fasting pregnant animals or women,[88, 99] despite increased catecholamine[99] and cortisol levels.[241] The reason may be the higher insulin:glucagon ratio of pregnancy in both the fasting and the fed states or the suppression of release of alanine from skeletal muscle by the rising concentration of ketones.[278] In addition, sex steroids, such as progesterone and estradiol, may restrain amino acid release from skeletal muscle.[224] The continuous active transport of amino acids across the placenta probably contributes to the relative hypoaminoacidemia of pregnancy as well.[82]

The *rise in plasma insulin after a meal containing protein stimulates the uptake of amino acids into muscle, promotes synthesis of muscle protein, and retards proteolysis.*[47] Excess amino acids are oxidized as fuel, and the nitrogen is excreted in urine.[298] The increase in plasma glucagon following a high-protein, low-carbohydrate meal increases the hepatic trapping of amino acids, so that blood levels of the glucogenic amino acids do not rise. The branched-chain amino acids leucine, isoleucine, and valine, however, represent 60 to 70% of the amino acids released by the splanchnic bed after a protein meal,[89] and their plasma concentrations increase twofold to threefold after feeding because they are not oxidized in the liver.[8] *Branched-chain amino acids* are oxidized in muscle and adipose tissue and are rapidly transported across the placenta. Leucine also serves as substrate for protein synthesis in muscle and fatty acid synthesis in adipose tissue.[48]

Women given a mixed carbohydrate-protein meal in late pregnancy demonstrate a smaller rise in the plasma concentration of amino acids than do nonpregnant women, and the amino acids disappear from the circulation more rapidly than is true 5 to 8 weeks' postpartum.[99] After a glucose load, there is a significant fall in plasma amino acid concentrations during pregnancy.[99] *The smaller incremental area for amino acids after mixed meals in pregnancy is probably related to placental uptake, to increased insulin levels, and perhaps to hepatic diversion for gluconeogenesis.*

PREGNANCY AND MATERNAL DIABETES

In general, diabetes complicates pregnancy in two situations. First, some women with diabetes become pregnant. Those women have established *pregestational* diabetes, and they may have metabolic abnormalities from the time of conception onward. The metabolic abnormalities can alter all stages of intrauterine development. During embryogenesis and organogenesis, poor maternal metabolic control is associated with an increased risk of *major congenital anomalies*[103, 116, 167, 288] and *spontaneous abortions.*[222] During the second and third trimesters, poor control is associated with accelerated fetal growth and *premature maturation of the fetal pancreatic B cells.*[238] The resultant fetal hyperinsulinemia can reduce fetal oxygenation, impair synthesis of surfactant apoprotein, and set the stage for neonatal hypoglycemia.[238] Both early and late pregnancy complications can be reduced by good maternal glycemic control, which should begin *before conception.*[103, 167, 288] The second form of diabetes complicating pregnancy occurs in women who are first found to have abnormalities of *glucose tolerance* during routine testing *in pregnancy.* Those women have gestational diabetes mellitus (GDM). Hyperglycemia in these women is usually too mild to cause overt diabetic symptoms in the mother but is sufficient to alter fetal growth and development during the second and third trimesters. Further, women with *GDM have a high risk of developing diabetes in subsequent years,* so they need special counseling and follow-up. The metabolic realignments of pregnancy described in this chapter have important implications for women with either pregestational or gestational diabetes. Those

implications are discussed in the context of changes in carbohydrate and lipid metabolism, although maternal diabetes results in increased circulating levels of carbohydrate, lipid, and protein fuels.[217]

Pregestational Diabetes

There are two types of established diabetes that may affect women of reproductive age. *Type I diabetes* (insulin-dependent diabetes mellitus [IDDM]) is an autoimmune disease[80] characterized by circulating antibodies directed against the pancreatic islets, immune cell infiltration of the islets, and selective destruction of the pancreatic B cells. The B cell destruction is generally complete, so women with type I diabetes have a severe or complete *deficiency of endogenous insulin.* As a result, hepatic glucose production, lipolysis, and ketogenesis are unchecked, and there is no postprandial utilization of glucose by insulin-sensitive tissues unless exogenous insulin is administered. Type I diabetic patients are thus dependent on exogenous insulin for survival; they develop ketoacidosis if insulin therapy is withheld. The second form of diabetes is type II diabetes (noninsulin-dependent diabetes mellitus [NIDDM]). This disease generally affects older individuals but may occur during the female reproductive years, especially in certain ethnic groups (e.g., Native and Mexican Americans). At least three metabolic defects have been identified in type II diabetes: *insulin resistance, B cell failure to compensate for the insulin resistance,* and *hepatic glucose overproduction.*[73] Although the relative importance and order of development of these abnormalities is not known with certainty, it appears that resistance to insulin's effect on glucose uptake is an early abnormality that may be inherited in patients at risk for NIDDM.[85] Inadequate B cell reserve to compensate for the insulin resistance may be a second inherited defect or may result from B cell exhaustion and the B cell toxic effects of chronic, mild hyperglycemia described earlier in this chapter.[190, 191] Hepatic glucose overproduction is generally a late finding and accounts for the development of fasting hyperglycemia in NIDDM.[28] Patients with NIDDM do not develop complete B cell failure and generally secrete sufficient insulin to suppress lipolysis and ketogenesis. They rarely develop ketoacidosis *(unless pregnant)* and have hyperglycemia as their primary metabolic manifestation.

Pregnancy has significant metabolic impact on type I and type II diabetes. Regarding carbohydrate metabolism, the alteration that has the greatest impact is the development of *progressive insulin resistance*. During the first trimester, insulin requirements generally are no different from and sometimes are slightly less than requirements of nonpregnant patients. During the latter half of pregnancy, however, there is generally a progressive increase in the amount of insulin required to maintain good glycemic regulation.[146, 259] The increase may be greatest in women with type II diabetes[188] but occurs to some extent in many women with type I (autoimmune) diabetes as well. As a result of the progressive insulin resistance, patients must be seen at frequent intervals during the second and third trimesters for review of blood glucose results and adjustment of insulin doses. Capable patients may also be taught to make minor adjustments of their own insulin doses. The insulin resistance of pregnancy abates rapidly after delivery, and many patients need very little insulin during the first few days postpartum.

Placental uptake of glucose, which is not dependent on maternal insulin, can enhance the likelihood of *severe hypoglycemia* in pregnant treated type I patients who have not recently consumed food. The risks of severe hypoglycemia are to the maternal brain and can be reduced by careful self-monitoring of capillary blood glucose and timely use of meals and snacks.

The progressive *propensity to fat catabolism* during pregnancy has two major implications for diabetic women. First, because insulin is the major hormone suppressing lipolysis and ketogenesis, pregnant women with no endogenous B cell function (type I diabetes) are at increased risk for accelerated ketone production and *ketoacidosis* whenever they omit their insulin therapy or experience an intercurrent illness. The ketoacidosis may occur rapidly and at lower plasma glucose concentrations than are typical of ketoacidosis in nonpregnant individuals. Thus physicians must maintain a high index of suspicion for ketoacidosis in pregnant

diabetic patients. The second implication of accelerated fat catabolism relates to the use of caloric restriction to treat obesity, a frequent characteristic of women with NIDDM. Because of the propensity for ketosis during caloric deprivation in pregnancy,[218] diets providing less than approximately 25 kcal/kg actual body weight should not be prescribed[173] to avoid exposure of the fetus to elevated maternal ketone levels, which have been associated with impaired intellectual development of offspring.[39, 252, 289] Milder caloric restriction may reduce hyperglycemia without ketosis in NIDDM, although monitoring for ketonuria is recommended in that setting.

Gestational Diabetes Mellitus

GDM is glucose intolerance that first occurs or is detected during gestation.[226, 290] Because pregnancy per se is associated with a slight deterioration of glucose tolerance compared with the nonpregnant condition,[201] criteria that are specific for pregnancy must be used to interpret glucose tolerance tests during gestation. The criteria currently recommended in the United States (NDDG Criteria; Table 4–6) were developed by O'Sullivan and Mahan[234] to predict maternal diabetes after pregnancy. The criteria also identify pregnancies at risk for fetal complications of macrosomia, neonatal hypoglycemia, and stillbirth.[102, 233, 252] The criteria were originally developed using venous whole blood and have been adapted to plasma values and current methodology by several groups,[50, 265] with slightly different results.

TABLE 4–6. Diagnostic Thresholds for Gestational Diabetes

	National Diabetes Data Group*	Sacks et al†
	Plasma, mg/dL (mM)	
Fasting	105 (5.8)	96 (5.3)
1-Hour	190 (10.6)	172 (9.4)
2-Hour	165 (9.2)	152 (8.3)
3-Hour	145 (8.1)	131 (7.2)

*Data from: National Diabetes Data Group. Classification and diagnosis of diabetes mellitus and other categories of glucose intolerance. Diabetes 1979; 28:1039.
†Sacks DA, Abu-Fadil S, Greenspoon JS, Fotheringham N. Do the current standards for glucose tolerance testing in pregnancy represent a valid conversion of O'Sullivan's original criteria? Am J Obstet Gynecol 1989; 161:638.

There is no widespread agreement about the correct conversion at present. *All sets of criteria, however, select the women in the upper 2 to 4% of glucose tolerance for pregnancy.*

Studies to determine the *mechanisms for glucose intolerance* in pregnant women have focused on insulin sensitivity and pancreatic B cell function (see Fig. 4–7). *Insulin sensitivity* during the third trimester in women with mild to moderate GDM (fasting glucose <130 mg/dL) is similar to that of normal pregnant women.[41] Insulin sensitivity increases after pregnancy in both groups but is lower in women with a history of GDM than in women without such a history.[312, 313] The findings suggest that women with GDM have an underlying, perhaps inherited, defect in insulin action that is masked by the physiologic insulin resistance of late pregnancy. *B cell responses to glucose* during the third trimester are less in women with GDM than in normal pregnant women, indicating a failure of B cell compensation for the marked insulin resistance of late pregnancy in women with GDM.[41] Thus as a group, women who meet current diagnostic criteria for GDM appear to have an underlying defect in insulin action that pales in the face of the great insulin resistance of late pregnancy. They also manifest reduced B cell capacity to compensate for the insulin resistance. The cellular mechanisms underlying the insulin resistance and B cell defects in women with prior GDM have not been identified. Likewise, whether either defect predominates in the eventual development of diabetes after pregnancy remains to be determined and may vary among different ethnic groups.

From a clinical standpoint, the metabolic defects that characterize GDM can be approached according to fetal risks during pregnancy and maternal risks after pregnancy. Because even mild maternal hyperglycemia during the second and third trimesters is associated with a *risk of fetal overgrowth,*[102, 147] normoglycemia should be the goal of management during pregnancy. This can be achieved with *dietary therapy* alone in many patients but requires insulin treatment if fasting (≥105 mg/dL) or postprandial (≥120 mg/dL) hyperglycemia persists despite good dietary compliance.[290] Because women with GDM have a risk of ketosis during fasting similar to normal

pregnant women,[40] the caveats about caloric restriction delivered earlier for NIDDM apply to women with GDM as well. *Exercise,* which improves carbohydrate tolerance in nonpregnant patients with diabetes, may prove a useful therapy to lower blood glucose in women with GDM.[147]

After pregnancy, women with GDM have a *50 to 70% risk of developing diabetes.*[169, 213, 215, 234] That risk dictates a special need for education about planned pregnancies, contraception, and prevention of diabetes by weight loss and exercise.[129, 170]

SUMMARY

Intermediary metabolism during pregnancy is characterized by an exaggeration of the normal daily swings between anabolism and catabolism that accompany feeding and fasting in nonpregnant people. In the *fed state,* pregnancy produces an increase in postprandial glucose, amino acid, and lipid levels despite markedly increased insulin levels. Thus by the second half of gestation, there is a relative insulin resistance, nearly compensatory hyperinsulinemia, and slightly impaired disposal of maternal glucose. The insulin resistance seems to be a postreceptor event brought on by high circulating levels of gestational hormones, and the resultant hyperinsulinemia may facilitate maternal fat storage during feeding. The elevation of circulating maternal glucose, amino acids, and lipids after eating promotes delivery of the nutrients to the fetus.

The *fasted and postabsorptive states* are characterized by lower glucose and amino acid levels and more rapid lipolysis than occurs in nonpregnant women. These changes are indicative of a progressive acceleration of fat catabolism with earlier induction of a starvation-like picture during food deprivation. Teleologically, the adaptations to fasting can be viewed as a mechanism to provide lipid substrates for maternal tissues, sparing carbohydrate and protein for the rapidly growing conceptus. During the first half to two-thirds of pregnancy, the facilitation of maternal anabolism appears to predominate to cause net accretion of fat in the mother. Later, the catabolic changes become progressively prominent and result in utilization of some of the stored nutrients.

The pancreatic islets, in particular the B cells, play a pivotal role in the orchestration of the metabolic adaptations to pregnancy. In the *absence of normal B cell reserve* (e.g., in patients with diabetes mellitus) the insulin resistance and exaggerated fat catabolism of pregnancy result in maternal metabolic derangements that can disrupt normal intrauterine development from conception onward. Dietary, behavioral, and pharmacologic therapies designed to restore normal maternal metabolism throughout pregnancy can greatly improve the metabolic environment of the developing fetus, thereby optimizing the outcome of pregnancies complicated by maternal diabetes.

REFERENCES

1. Ader M, Bergman RN. Peripheral effects of insulin dominate suppression of fasting hepatic glucose production. Am J Physiol 1990;258:E1020.
2. Ahren B, Veith RC, Taborsky GJ. Sympathetic nerve stimulation versus pancreatic norepinephrine infusion in the dog: effects on basal release of insulin and glucagon. Endocrinology 1987;121:323.
3. Andersen O. Insulin receptor binding and glucose metabolism in normal pregnancy and gestational diabetes mellitus. Dan Med Bull 1990;37:492.
4. Andersen O, Falholt K, Kuhl C. Activity of enzymes of glucose and triglyceride metabolism in adipose and muscle tissue from normal pregnant women at term. Diab Med 1989;6:131.
5. Andersen O, Kuhl C. Insulin receptor binding to monocytes and erythrocytes during normal human pregnancy. Eur J Clin Invest 1986;16:226.
6. Andersen O, Kuhl C. Adipocyte insulin receptor binding and lipogenesis at term in normal pregnancy. Eur J Clin Invest 1988;18:575.
7. Andersen O, Kuhl C, Buch I. Insulin receptors in normal pregnant women and women with gestational diabetes. Acta Endocrinol 1986;(suppl 277):27.
8. Aoki TT, Brennan MF, Muller WA, et al. Amino acid levels across normal forearm and splanchnic bed after a protein meal. Am J Clin Nutr 1976;29:340.
9. Ashby JP, Shirling D, Baird JD. Effect of progesterone on insulin secretion in the rat. J Endocrinol 1978;76:479.
10. Bailey CJ, Conlon JM, Flatt PR. Effect of ovarian hormones, pregnancy and lactation on somatostatin and substance P in the alimentary tract of mice. J Endocrinol 1989;122:645.
11. Bailey CJ, Matty AJ. Glucose tolerance and plasma insulin of the rat in relation to the oestrous cycle and sex hormones. Horm Metab Res 1972;4:266.
12. Baird JD. Some aspects of the metabolic and hormonal adaptation to pregnancy. Acta Endocrinol 1986;(suppl 277):11.
13. Bar RS, Gorden P, Roth J, et al. Fluctuations in the affinity and concentration of insulin receptors on circulating monocytes of obese patients. J Clin Invest 1976;58:1123.
14. Battaglia FC. Principal substrates of fetal metabolism:
fuel and growth requirements of the ovine fetus. In: Elliott K, O'Connor M, eds. Pregnancy metabolism, diabetes and the fetus (Ciba Foundation Symposium, new series) Amsterdam: Excerpta Medica, 1979; 63:57.
15. Beard JC, Ward WK, Halter JB, et al. Relationship of islet function to insulin action in human obesity. J Clin Endocrinol Metab 1987;65:59.
16. Beck P. Progestin enhancement of the plasma insulin response to glucose in Rhesus monkeys. Diabetes 1969;18:146.
17. Beck P. Reversal of progesterone-enhanced insulin production by human chorionic somatomammotropin. Endocrinology 1970;87:311.
18. Beck P, Daughaday WH. Human placental lactogen: studies of its acute metabolic effects and disposition in normal man. J Clin Invest 1967;46:103.
19. Beck P, Eaton RP, Arnett DM, Alsever RN. Effect of contraceptive steroids on arginine-stimulated glucagon and insulin secretion in women. I. Lipid physiology. Metabolism 1975;24:1055.
20. Beck P, Wells SA. Comparison of the mechanisms underlying carbohydrate intolerance in subclinical diabetic women during pregnancy and during postpartum oral contraceptive steroid treatment. J Clin Endocrinol 1969;29:807.
21. Beck-Nielson H, Kuhl C, Pedersen O, et al. Decreased insulin binding to monocytes from normal pregnant women. J Clin Endocrinol Metab 1979; 49:810.
22. Bell GI, Kayano T, Buse JB, et al. Molecular biology of glucose transporters. Diabetes Care 1990;13:198.
23. Bell GI, Sanchez-Pescardor R, Laybourn PJ, Najarian RC. Exon duplication and divergence in the human preproglucagon gene. Nature 1983;304:368.
24. Bellman O, Hartman E. Influence of pregnancy on the kinetics of insulin. Am J Obstet Gynecol 1975;122:829.
25. Bergman RN. Toward a physiological understanding of glucose tolerance. Diabetes 1989;38:1512.
26. Bergman RN, Finegood DT, Ader M. Assessment of insulin sensitivity in vivo. Endocr Rev 1985;6:45.
27. Bergman RN, Phillips LS, Cobelli C. Physiologic evaluation of factors controlling glucose disposition in man. J Clin Invest 1981;68:1456.
28. Best JD, Judzewitsch RG, Pfeifer MA, et al. The effect of chronic sulfonylurea therapy on hepatic glucose production in non-insulin dependent diabetes. Diabetes 1982;31:333.
29. Biezenski JJ. Maternal lipid metabolism. Obstet Gynaecol Ann 1974;3:203.
30. Bleicher SJ, O'Sullivan JB, Freinkel N. Carbohydrate metabolism in pregnancy. V. The interrelations of glucose, insulin, and free fatty acids in late pregnancy and postpartum. N Engl J Med 1964;271:866.
31. Bolaffi JL, Bruno L, Heldt A, Grodsky GM. Characteristics of desensitization of insulin secretion in fully in vitro systems. Endocrinology 1988;122:1801.
32. Bone AJ, Taylor KW. Metabolic adaptation to pregnancy shown by increased biosynthesis of insulin in islets of Langerhans isolated from pregnant rat. Nature 1976;262:501.
33. Bonner-Weir S, L Orci. New perspectives on the microvasculature of the islets of Langerhans in the rat. Diabetes 1982;31:883.
34. Bowes WA, Katta LR, Droegmemueller W, Bright T. Triphasic randomized clinical trial: comparison of effects on carbohydrate metabolism. Am J Obstet Gynecol 1989;161:1402.

35. Bradley DD, Wingerd J, Petitti DB, et al. Serum high-density-lipoprotein cholesterol in women using oral contraceptives, estrogens, and progestins. N Engl J Med 1978;299:17.

36. Brockman RP, Bergman EN, Joo PK, Mann JG. Effects of glucagon and insulin on net hepatic metabolism of glucose precursors in sheep. Am J Physiol 1975;229:1344.

37. Brunzell J, Porte D Jr, Bierman EL. Reversible abnormalities in postheparin lipolytic activity during the late phase of release in diabetes mellitus. Metabolism 1975;24:1132.

38. Brunzell JD, Robertson RP, Lerner RL, et al. Relationships between fasting plasma glucose levels and insulin secretion during intravenous glucose tolerance tests. J Clin Endocrinol Metab 1976;42:222.

39. Buchanan TA. Carbohydrate metabolism in pregnancy. Normal physiology and implications for diabetes mellitus. Isr J Med Sci 1991;27:425.

40. Buchanan TA, Metzger BE, Freinkel N. Accelerated starvation in late pregnancy: a comparison between obese women with and without gestational diabetes mellitus. Am J Obstet Gynecol 1990;162:1015.

41. Buchanan TA, Metzger BE, Freinkel N, Bergman RN. Insulin sensitivity and B-cell responsiveness to glucose during late pregnancy in lean and moderately obese women with normal glucose tolerance or mild gestational diabetes. Am J Obstet Gynecol 1990;162:1008.

42. Burt RL. Plasma nonesterified fatty acids in normal pregnancy and the puerperium. Obstet Gynecol 1960;15:460.

43. Burt RL, Davidson IW. Insulin half-life and utilization in normal pregnancy. Obstet Gynecol 1974;43:161.

44. Burt RL, Kimel CA. Peripheral utilization of glucose in pregnancy and the puerperium. Obstet Gynecol 1954;4:58.

45. Burt RL, Leake NH, Rhyne AL. Glucose tolerance during pregnancy and the puerperium. A modification with observations on serum immunoreactive insulin. Obstet Gynecol 1969;33:634.

46. Butler PC, Kryshak E, Marsh M, Rizza RA. Effect of insulin on oxidation of intracellularly and extracellularly derived glucose in patients with NIDDM. Diabetes 1990;39:1373.

47. Cahill GF Jr. The Banting Memorial Lecture 1971. Physiology of insulin in man. Diabetes 1971;20:785.

48. Cahill GF Jr, Oaki TT. The role of glucagon in amino acid homeostasis. In: Foa PP, Bajaj JS, Foa NL, eds. Glucagon: its role in physiology and clinical medicine. New York: Springer-Verlag, 1977:487.

49. Caro JF, Dohm LG, Pories WJ, Sinha MK. Cellular alterations in liver, skeletal muscle and adipose tissue responsible for insulin resistance in obesity and type II diabetes. Diab Metab Rev 1989;5:665.

50. Carpenter MW, Coustan DR. Criteria for screening tests for gestational diabetes. Am J Obstet Gynecol 1982;144:768.

51. Carpentier J-L, Gorden P, Robert A, Orci L. Internalization of polypeptide hormones and receptor recycling. Experientia 1987;53:47.

52. Chernick S, Novack M. Effect of insulin on FFA mobilization and ketosis in fasting pregnant rats. Diabetes 1970;19:563.

53. Cherrington AD, Exton BH. Studies on the role of cAMP-dependent protein kinase in the actions of glucagon and catecholamines on liver glycogen metabolism. Metabolism 1976;25(suppl):1351.

54. Chez RA, Mintz DH, Epstein MF. Fetal hormonal mechanisms for plasma glucose. In: Camerini-Davalos RA, Cole HS, eds. Early diabetes in early life. New York: Academic Press, 1975:141.

55. Chiasson JL, Liljenquist JE, Sinclair-Smith BC, Lacy WW. Gluconeogenesis from alanine in normal postabsorptive man. Intrahepatic stimulatory effect of glucagon. Diabetes 1975;24:574.

56. Chochinov RH, Perlman K, Moorhouse JA. Circulating alanine production and disposal in healthy subjects. Diabetes 1978;27:287.

57. Chou CK, Dull T, Russel D, et al. Human insulin receptors mutated at the ATP-binding site lack protein tyrosine kinase activity and fail to mediate postreceptor effects of insulin. J Biol Chem 1987; 262:1842.

58. Christensen PJ, Date JW, Schonheyder F, Volqvartz K. Amino acids in blood plasma and urine during pregnancy. Scand J Clin Lab Invest 1957;9:54.

59. Churchill JA, Berendes HW, Nemore J. Neuropsychological deficits in children of diabetic mothers: a report from the collaborative study of cerebral palsy. Am J Obstet Gynecol 1969;105:257.

60. Colart TM, Williams C. Effect of insulin on adipose tissue lipolysis in human pregnancy. Br J Obstet Gynecol 1976;83:241.

61. Colturi TJ, Unger RH, Feldman M. Role of circulating somatostatin in regulation of gastric acid secretion, gastrin release, and islet cell function. J Clin Invest 1984;74:417.

62. Cook DL, Satin LS, Ashford LJ, Hales CN. ATP-sensitive K+ channels in pancreatic B-cells. Diabetes 1988;37:495.

63. Corvera S, Huerta-Bahana J, Pelton JT, et al. Metabolic effects and cyclic AMP levels produced by glucagon, (1-N-alphatrinitrophenylhistidine, 12-homoarginine) glucagon and forskolin in isolated rat hepatocytes. Biochim Biophys Acta 1984;804:434.

64. Costrini NV, Kalkhoff RK. Relative effects of pregnancy, estradiol and progesterone on plasma insulin and pancreatic islet insulin secretion. J Clin Invest 1971;50:992.

65. Cowett RM. Hepatic and peripheral responsiveness to a glucose infusion in pregnancy. Am J Obstet Gynecol 1985;153:272.

66. Cowett RM, Susa JB, Kahn CB, et al. Glucose kinetics in nondiabetic and diabetic women during the third trimester of pregnancy. Am J Obstet Gynecol 1983;146:773.

67. Creutzfeldt W, Ebert R. New developments in the incretin concept. Diabetologia 1985;28:565.

68. Czech MP. The nature and regulation of the insulin receptor: structure and function. Ann Rev Physiol 1985;47:357.

69. Daniel RR, Metzger BE, Freinkel N, et al. Carbohydrate metabolism in pregnancy. XI. Response of plasma glucagon to overnight fast and oral glucose during normal pregnancy and in gestational diabetes. Diabetes 1974;23:771.

70. Davidson MB. Insulin resistance of late pregnancy does not include the liver. Metabolism 1984;33:532.

71. Davison JM, Hyten FE. Renal handling of glucose in pregnancy. In: Sutherland HS, Stowers JM, eds. Carbohydrate metabolism in pregnancy and the newborn. Edinburgh: Churchill-Livingstone, 1975:2.

72. Davison JS, Davison MC, Hay DM. Gastric emptying time in late pregnancy and labour. J Obstet Gynaecol Br Comm 1970;77:37.

73. DeFronzo RA. The triumvirate: B-cell, muscle and liver. A collusion responsible for NIDDM. Diabetes 1988;37:667.

74. Denton RM. Insulin signalling: search for the missing links. Nature 1990;348:286.

75. Dunning BE, Ahren B, Veith RC, et al. Galanin. A novel pancreatic neuropeptide. Am J Physiol 1975;251:E127.

76. Dwenger A, Mitzkat HJ, Holle W, et al. Insulin binding to erythrocytes from pregnant, postpartum, follicular and luteal phases. J Clin Chem Clin Biochem 1982;20:273.

77. Ebina Y, Ellis L, Jarnagin K, et al. The human insulin receptor cDNA: the structural basis of hormone activated transmembrane signalling. Cell 1985;40:747.

78. Edstrom K, Cerasi E, Luft R. Insulin response to glucose infusion during pregnancy. A prospective study of high and low insulin responders with normal carbohydrate tolerance. Acta Endocrinol 1974;75:87.

79. Efendic S, Luft R, Wajngot A. Aspects of the pathogenesis of type 2 diabetes. Endocr Rev 1984;5:395.

80. Eisenbarth GS. Type I diabetes mellitus: a chronic autoimmune disease. N Engl J Med 1986;314:1360.

81. Elliot JA. The effect of pregnancy on the control of lipolysis in fat cells isolated from human adipose tissue. Eur J Clin Invest 1975;5:159.

82. Ellis JW. Multiphasic oral contraceptives. Efficacy and metabolic impact. J Reprod Med 1987;32:28.

83. Ellis L, Clauser E, Morgan D, et al. Replacement of insulin receptor tyrosine residues 1162 and 1163 compromises insulin-stimulated kinase activity and uptake of 2-deoxyglucose. Cell 1986;45:721.

84. Ellis L, Morgan DO, Clauser E, Roth R. A membrane anchored cytoplasmic domain of the human insulin receptor mediates a constitutively elevated insulin-independent uptake of 2-deoxyglucose. Mol Endocrinol 1987;1:15.

85. Eriksson J, Franssila-Kalunki A, Ekstrand A, et al. Early metabolic defects in persons at increased risk for non-insulin-dependent diabetes mellitus. N Engl J Med 1989;321:337.

86. Fairweather DV. Changes in levels of serum nonesterified fatty acid and blood glucose in pregnancy. J Obstet Gynaecol Br Comm 1971;78:707.

87. Felig P. Insulin is the mediator of feeding-related thermogenesis: insulin resistance and/or deficiency results in a thermogenic defect which contributes to the pathogenesis of obesity. Clin Physiol 1984;4:267.

88. Felig P, Kim YJ, Lynch V, Hendler R. Amino acid metabolism during starvation in human pregnancy. J Clin Invest 1972;51:1195.

89. Felig P, Koivisto V. Body fuel metabolism. In: Freinkel N, ed. The year in metabolism 1977. New York: Plenum Press, 1978:143.

90. Felig P, Marliss E, Cahill GF Jr. Plasma amino acid levels and insulin secretion in obesity. N Engl J Med 1969;281:811.

91. Felig P, Wahren J, Hendler R. Influence of physiologic hyperglucagonemia on basal and insulin-inhibited splanchnic glucose output in normal man. J Clin Invest 1976;58:761.

92. Felig P, Wahren J, Sherwin R, Hendler R. Insulin, glucagon and somatostatin in normal physiology and diabetes mellitus. Diabetes 1976;25:1091.

93. Ferrannini E, Barrett EJ, Bevilacqua S, DeFronzo R. Effect of fatty acids on glucose production and utilization in man. J Clin Invest 1983;72:1737.

94. Field JB. Insulin extraction by the liver. In: Greep RD, Astwood EB, eds. Handbook of physiology. Endocrinology, endocrine pancreas. Vol 1. Washington, DC: American Physiology Society, 1972:505.

95. Flint DJ, Sinnett-Smith PA, Clegg RA, Vernon RG. Role of insulin receptors in the changing metabolism of adipose tissue during pregnancy and lactation in the rat. Biochem J 1979;182:421.

96. Foster DW, McGarry JD. The metabolic derangements and treatment of diabetic ketoacidosis. N Engl J Med 1983;309:159.

97. Freinkel N. Effects of the conceptus on maternal metabolism during pregnancy. In: Leibel BS, Wrenshall GA, eds. On the nature and treatment of diabetes. Amsterdam: Excerpta Medica, 1965:679.

98. Freinkel N. Of pregnancy and progeny. Banting Lecture 1980. Diabetes 1980;29:1023.

99. Freinkel N, Metzger BE, Nitzan M, et al. "Accelerated starvation" and mechanisms for the conservation of maternal nitrogen during pregnancy. Isr J Med Sci 1972;8:426.

100. Freinkel N, Metzger BE, Nitzan M, et al. Facilitated anabolism in late pregnancy: Some novel maternal compensations for accelerated starvation. In: Malaisse WJ, Pirart J, Vallance-Owen J, eds. Diabetes. Amsterdam: Excerpta Medica, 1974:474.

101. Freinkel N, Metzger BE, Nitzan M, et al. Facilitated anabolism in late pregnancy: some novel maternal compensations for accelerated starvation. In: Malaisse WJ, Pirart J, eds. Proceedings of the VIIIth Congress of the International Diabetes Federation. Amsterdam: Excerpta Medica, International Congress Series No. 312, 1974:478.

102. Freinkel N, Metzger BE, Phelps RL, et al. Gestational diabetes mellitus: heterogeneity of maternal age, weight, insulin secretion, HLA antigens, and islet cell antibodies and the impact of maternal metabolism on pancreatic B-cell function and somatic growth in the offspring. Diabetes 1985;34 (suppl 2):1.

103. Fuhrmann K, Reiher H, Semmler K, Glockner E. The effect of intensified conventional insulin therapy before and during pregnancy on the malformation rate in offspring of diabetic mothers. Exp Clin Endocrinol 1984;83:173.

104. Galleti F, Klopper A. The effect of progesterone on the quantity and distribution of body fat in the female rat. Acta Endocrinol 1964;46:379.

105. Gardner DF, Wilson HK, Podet EJ, et al. Prolonged action of regular insulin in diabetic patients: Lack of relationship to circulating insulin antibodies. J Clin Endocrinol Metab 1986;62:621.

106. Genazzani AR, Benuzzi-Badoni M, Felber JP. Human chorionic somatomammotropin (HCSM): lipolytic action of a pure preparation on isolated fat cells. Metabolism 1969;18:593.

107. Gerich JE, Charles MA, Grodsky GM. Regulation of pancreatic insulin and glucose secretion. Ann Rev Physiol 1976;38:353.

108. Gerich JE, Langlois M, Noacco C, et al. Adrenergic modulation of pancreatic glucagon secretion in man. J Clin Invest 1974;53:1441.

109. Gerich JE, Langlois M, Schneider V, et al. Effects of alternations of plasma free fatty acids levels on pancreatic glucagon secretion in man. J Clin Invest 1974;53:1284.

110. Gillmer MD, Beard RW, Brooke FM, Oakley NW. Carbohydrate metabolism in pregnancy. Part I, Diurnal plasma glucose profile in normal and diabetic women. BMJ 1975;3:399.

111. Gilmour KE, McKerns KW. Insulin and estrogen regulation of lipid synthesis in adipose tissue. Biochim Biophys Acta 1966;116:220.

112. Goldfine ID. The insulin receptor: molecular biology

and transmembrane signaling. Endocr Rev 1987; 8:235.

113. Granner DK, Andreone TL, Sasaki L, Beale E. Inhibition of transcription of the phosphoenolpyruvate carboxykinase gene by insulin. Nature 1983;305:549.

114. Grasso S, Palumbo G, Messina A, et al. Human maternal and fetal serum insulin and growth hormone (HGH) response to glucose and leucine. Diabetes 1976;25:545.

115. Gratacos JA, Neufield N, Kumar D, et al. Monocyte insulin binding studies in normal and diabetic pregnancies. Am J Obstet Gynecol 1981;141:611.

116. Greene MF, Hare JW, Cloherty JP, et al. First trimester hemoglobin A1 and risk for major malformation and spontaneous abortion in diabetic pregnancy. Teratology 1989;39:225.

117. Grillo RAI, Shima K. Insulin content and enzyme histochemistry of the human foetal pancreatic islet. J Endocrinol 1966;36:151.

118. Grodsky GM. The kinetics of insulin release. Handbk Exp Pharmacol 1975;32:1.

119. Groscurth P, Kistler G. The pancreas, embryology and anatomy. In: Labhart A, ed. Clinical endocrinology, theory and practice. New York: Springer-Verlag, 1986:750.

120. Grumbach MM, Kaplan SL, Sciarra JJ, Burr IM. Chorionic growth hormone-prolactin (CGP): secretion, disposition, biologic activity in man and postulated function as the "growth hormone" of the second half of pregnancy. Ann NY Acad Sci 1968;148:501.

121. Hadden DR. Glucose tolerance tests in pregnancy. In: Sutherland HW, Stowers JM, eds. Carbohydrate metabolism in pregnancy and the newborn. Edinburgh: Churchill-Livingstone, 1975:19.

122. Hagen A. Blood sugar findings during pregnancy in normals and possible prediabetics. Diabetes 1961; 19:438.

123. Hager D, Georg RH, Leitner JW, Beck P. Insulin secretion and content in isolated rat pancreatic islets following treatment with gestational hormones. Endocrinology 1972;91:977.

124. Hamburger AD, Kulpers AC, Van der Vies J. The effect of progesterone on plasma insulin in the rabbit. Experientia 1975;31:602.

125. Hamosh M, Clary TR, Chernick SS, Scow RO. Lipoprotein lipase activity of adipose and mammary tissue and plasma triglyceride in pregnant and lactating rats. Biochim Biophys Acta 1970;210:473.

126. Hauguel S, Gilbert M, Girard J. Pregnancy-induced insulin resistance in liver and skeletal muscles of the conscious rabbit. Am J Physiol 1987;252:E165.

127. Hauguel S, Leturque A, Gilbert M, Girard J. Effects of pregnancy and fasting on muscle glucose utilization in the rabbit. Am J Obstet Gynecol 1988; 158:1215.

128. Hellman B. The islets of Langerhans in the rat during pregnancy and lactation with special reference to the changes in the B/A cell ratio. Acta Obstet Gynecol Scand 1960;30:331.

129. Helmrich SP, Ragland DR, Leung RW, Paffenbarger RS. Physical activity and reduced occurrence of non-insulin-dependent diabetes mellitus. N Engl J Med 1991;325:147.

130. Herrera E, Knopp RH, Freinkel N. Carbohydrate metabolism in pregnancy. VI. Plasma fuels, insulin, liver composition, gluconeogenesis and nitrogen metabolism during late gestation in the fed and fasted rat. J Clin Invest 1969;48:2260.

130a. Herrera E, Lasuncion MA, Palacin M, et al. Inter-mediary metabolism in pregnancy. Diabetes 1991; 40(suppl 2):83.

131. Hers H-G, Van Schaftingen E. Fructose 2,6-bisphosphate two years after its discovery. Biochem J 1982;206:1.

132. Hervey E, Hervey GR. The effects of progesterone on body weight and composition in the rat. J Endocrinol 1967;37:361.

133. Hidaka H, Nagulesparan M, Klimes I, et al. Improvement of insulin secretion but not insulin resistance after short term control of plasma glucose in obese Type II diabetics. J Clin Endocrinol Metab 1982; 54:217.

134. Hjollund E, Pederson O, Espersen T, Klebe J. Impaired insulin receptor binding and postbinding defects of adipocytes from normal and diabetic pregnant women. Diabetes 1986;35:598.

135. Hollingsworth DR. Alterations of maternal metabolism in normal and diabetic pregnancies. Differences in insulin-dependent, non-insulin-dependent and gestational diabetes. Am J Obstet Gynecol 1983; 146:417.

136. Hornnes PJ, Kuhl C. Plasma insulin and glucagon responses to isoglycemic stimulation in normal pregnancy and postpartum. Obstet Gynecol 1980;55:425.

137. Hornnes PJ, Kuhl C. Gastrointestinal hormones and cortisol in normal pregnant women and women with gestational diabetes. Acta Endocrinol 1986;(suppl 277):24.

138. Hornnes PJ, Kuhl C, Lauritsen KB. Gastrointestinal insulinotropic hormones in normal and gestational diabetic pregnancy: response to oral glucose. Diabetes 1981;30:504.

139. Hornnes PJ, Kuhl C, Lauritsen KB. Gastroenteropancreatic hormones in normal pregnancy: response to a protein rich meal. Eur J Clin Invest 1981;11:345.

140. Howell SL, Tyhurst M, Green IC. Direct effects of progesterone on rat islets of Langerhans in vivo and in tissue culture. Diabetologia 1977;13:579.

141. Hytten FE. Weight gain in pregnancy. In: Hytten F, Chamberlain G, eds. Clinical physiology in obstetrics. Oxford: Blackwell Scientific Publications, 1980:193.

142. Janssens J, Hellemans J, Adrian TE, et al. Pancreatic polypeptide is not involved in the regulation of the migrating motor complex in man. Regul Pept 1982; 3:41.

143. Jefferson LS, Li JB, Rannels SR. Regulation by insulin of amino acid release and protein turnover in the perfused rat hemicorpus. J Biol Chem 1977;252:1476.

144. Jenssen TG, Haukland HH, Vonen B, et al. Changes in postprandial release patterns of gastrointestinal hormones in late pregnancy and the early postpartum period. Br J Obstet Gynaecol 1988;95:565.

145. Johnson JH, Ogawa A, Chen L, et al. Underexpression of B cell high Km glucose transporters in non-insulin-dependent diabetes. Science 1990;250:546.

146. Jovanovic L, Peterson CM. Optimal insulin delivery for the pregnant diabetic patient. Diabetes Care 1982;5(suppl 1):24.

147. Jovanovic-Peterson L, Durak E, Peterson CM. Randomized trial of diet versus diet plus cardiovascular conditioning on glucose levels in gestational diabetes. Am J Obstet Gynecol 1989;161:415.

148. Jovanovic-Peterson L, Peterson C, Reed GF, et al. the DIEP Study. Maternal postprandial glucose levels and infant birthweight. Am J Obstet Gynecol 1991; 164:103.

149. Kahn BB, Flier JS. Regulation of glucose transporter

gene expression in vitro and in vivo. Diab Care 1990;13:548.

150. Kahn CR. The molecular mechanism of insulin action. Ann Rev Med 1985;36:429.

151. Kalhan SC, Gilfillan CA, Tserng KY, Savin SM. Glucose-alanine relationship in normal human pregnancy. Metabolism 1988;37:152.

152. Kalhan SC, Schwartz R, Adam PA. Placental barrier to human insulin-I^{125} in insulin-dependent diabetic mothers. J Clin Endocrinol Metab 1975;40:139.

153. Kalkhoff RK, Jacobson M, Lemper D. Progesterone, pregnancy and the augmented plasma insulin response. J Clin Endocrinol 1970;31:24.

154. Kalkhoff RK, Kim HJ. Effects of pregnancy on insulin and glucagon secretion by perfused rat pancreatic islets. Endocrinology 1978;102:623.

155. Kalkhoff RK, Richardson BL, Beck P. Relative effects of pregnancy, human placental lactogen, and prednisolone on carbohydrate tolerance in normal and subclinical diabetic subjects. Diabetes 1969;18:153.

156. Kalkhoff RK, Schalch DS, Walker JL, et al. Diabetogenic factors associated with pregnancy. Trans Assoc Am Phys 1964;77:270.

157. Karam JH, Salber PR, Forsham PH. Pancreatic hormones and diabetes mellitus. In: Greenspan FS, Forsham PH, eds. Basic and clinical endocrinology. E Norwalk, CT: Appleton-Century-Crofts, 1986:523.

158. Karnieli E, Zarnowski MJ, Hissin P, et al. Insulin-stimulated translocation of glucose transport systems in the isolated rat adipose cell. J Biol Chem 1981;256:4772.

159. Kasanicki MA, Pilch PF. Regulation of glucose transporter function. Diab Care 1990;13:219.

160. Katz AI, Lindheimer MD, Mako ME, Rubenstein AH. Peripheral metabolism of insulin, proinsulin, and C-peptide in the pregnant rat. J Clin Invest 1975; 56:1608.

161. Katz AI, Rubenstein AH. Metabolism of proinsulin, insulin and C-peptide in the rat. J Clin Invest 1973;52:1113.

162. Kerr GR. The free amino acids of serum during development of Macaca mulatta. II. During pregnancy and fetal life. Pediatr Res 1968;2:493.

163. Kim H-J, Kalkhoff RR. Sex steroid influence on triglyceride metabolism. J Clin Invest 1975;56:888.

164. Kimball SR, Flaim KE, Peavy DE, Jefferson LS. Protein metabolism. In: Rifkin H, Porte D Jr, eds. Diabetes mellitus: theory and practice, ed 4. New York: Elsevier, 1990:1.

165. King KC, Butt J, Raivio K, et al. Human maternal and fetal insulin response to arginine. N Engl J Med 1971;285:607.

166. Kipnis DM, Noall MW. Stimulation of amino acid transport by insulin in the isolated rat diaphragm. Biochim Biophys Acta 1958;28:226.

167. Kitzmiller JL, Gavin LA, Gin GD, et al. Preconception care of diabetes. Glycemic control prevents congenital anomalies. JAMA 1991;265:731.

168. Kitzmiller JL, Tanenberg RJ, Aoki TT, et al. Pancreatic alpha cell response to alanine during and after normal and diabetic pregnancies. Obstet Gynecol 1980;56:440.

169. Kjos SL, Buchanan TA, Greenspoon JS, et al. Gestational diabetes mellitus: the prevalence of glucose intolerance and diabetes mellitus in the first two months postpartum. Am J Obstet Gynecol 1990; 163:93.

170. Kjos SL, Shoupe D, Douyan S, et al. Effect of low-dose oral contraceptives on carbohydrate and lipid metabolism in women with recent gestational diabetes. Am J Obstet Gynecol 1990;163:1822.

171. Kloppel G, Veld PA, Stamm B, Heitz P. The endocrine pancreas. In: Kovacs K, Asa S, eds. Functional endocrine pathology. Cambridge, MA: Blackwell Scientific, 1991:396.

172. Knopp RH, Herrara E, Freinkel N. Carbohydrate metabolism in pregnancy. 8. Metabolism of adipose tissue isolated from fed and fasted pregnant rats during late gestation. J Clin Invest 1970;49:1438.

173. Knopp RH, Magee MS, Raisys V, Benedetti T. Metabolic effects of hypocaloric diets in the management of gestational diabetes. Diabetes 1991;40(suppl 2):165.

174. Knopp RH, Saudek CD, Arky RA, O'Sullivan JB. Two phases of adipose tissue metabolism in pregnancy: maternal adaptations for fetal growth. Endocrinology 1973;92:984.

175. Knopp RH, Warth MR, Carrol CJ. Lipid metabolism in pregnancy. I. Changes in lipoprotein triglyceride and cholesterol in normal pregnancy and the effects of diabetes mellitus. J Reprod Med 1973;10:95.

176. Knopp RH, Warth MR, Charles D, et al. Lipoprotein metabolism in pregnancy, fat transport to the fetus, and the effects of diabetes. Biol Neonate 1986;50:297.

177. Kono T, Barham FW. The relationship between the insulin-binding capacity of fat cells and the cellular response to insulin. J Biol Chem 1971;246:6210.

178. Kono T, Robinson F, Blevins T, Ezaki O. Evidence that translocation of the glucose transport activity is the major mechanism of insulin action on glucose transport in fat cells. J Biol Chem 1982;257:10942.

179. Kuhl C. Glucose metabolism during and after pregnancy in normal and gestational diabetic women. I. Influence of normal pregnancy on serum glucose and insulin concentration during basal fasting conditions and after a challenge with glucose. Acta Endocrinol 1975;79:709.

180. Kuhl C, Holst JJ. Plasma glucagon and the insulin:glucagon ratio in gestational diabetes. Diabetes 1976;25:16.

181. Kuhl C, Hornnes PJ. Insulin and glucagon responses to amino acids in normal and gestational diabetic pregnancy (abstr). Diabetologia 1982;23:182.

182. Kuhl C, Hornnes PJ. Endocrine pancreatic function in women with gestational diabetes. Acta Endocrinol 1986;(suppl 277):19.

183. Kuhl C, Hornnes P, Andersen O. Aetiological factors in gestational diabetes. In: Sutherland HW, Stowers JM, eds. Carbohydrate metabolism in pregnancy and the newborn. Edinburgh: Churchill Livingstone, 1984:12.

184. Kuhl C, Hornnes P, Faber OK. Hepatic insulin extraction in human pregnancy. Horm Metab Res 1981;13:71.

185. Kuhl C, Hornnes P, Jensen SL. Effect of pregnancy on the hepatic extraction of insulin (abstr). Diabetologia 1977;13:411.

186. Kuhl C, Hornnes P, Klebe JG. Effect of pregnancy on the glucagon response to protein ingestion. Horm Metab Res 1977;9:206.

187. Lang DA, Matthews DR, Peto J, Turner RC. Cyclic oscillations of basal plasma glucose and insulin concentrations in human beings. N Engl J Med 1979;301:1023.

188. Langer O, Anyaegbunam A, Brustman L, et al. Pregestational diabetes: insulin requirements throughout pregnancy. Am J Obstet Gynecol 1988;159:616.

189. Laube H, Fussganger RD, Schroder KE, Pfeiffer EF.

Acute effect of human chorionic somatomammotropin on insulin and glucagon release in the isolated perfused pancreas. Diabetes 1972;21:1072.

190. Leahy JL, Bonner-Weir S, Weir GC. Minimal chronic hyperglycemia is a critical determinant of impaired insulin secretion after an incomplete pancreatectomy. J Clin Invest 1988;81:1407.

191. Leahy JL, Cooper HE, Deal DA, Weir GC. Chronic hyperglycemia is associated with impaired glucose influence on insulin secretion. J Clin Invest 1986;77:908.

192. Leake NH, Burt RL. Insulin-like activity in serum during pregnancy. Diabetes 1962;11:419.

193. Leake NH, Burt RL. Serum insulin-like activity after tolbutamide during pregnancy and early puerperium. Obstet Gynecol 1965;25:245.

194. Leake NH, Burt RL. Effect of HPL and pregnancy on glucose uptake in rat adipose tissue. Am J Obstet Gynecol 1969;103:39.

195. Lerario AC, Wajchenberg BL, El-Andere W, et al. Sequential studies of glucose tolerance and red blood cell insulin receptors in normal human pregnancy. Diabetes 1985;34:780.

196. Lerner RL, Porte D Jr. Relationships between intravenous glucose loads, insulin responses and glucose disappearance rates. J Clin Endocrinol 1971;33:409.

197. Leturque A, Ferre P, Burnol A-F, et al. Glucose utilization rates and insulin sensitivity in vivo in tissues of virgin and pregnant rats. Diabetes 1986;35:172.

198. Leturque A, Ferre P, Satabin P, et al. In vivo insulin resistance during pregnancy in the rat. Diabetologia 1980;19:521.

199. Leturque A, Hauguel S, Sutter DMT, et al. Effects of placental lactogen and progesterone on insulin stimulated glucose metabolism in rat muscles in vitro. Diab Metab 1989;15:176.

200. Lind T, Bell S, Gilmore E, et al. Insulin disappearance rate in pregnant and nonpregnant women and in nonpregnant women given GHRIH. Eur J Clin Invest 1977;7:47.

201. Lind T, Billewicz WZ, Brown G. A serial study of changes occurring in the oral glucose tolerance test during pregnancy. J Obstet Gynaecol Br Comm 1973;80:1033.

202. Lloyd CE, Kalinyak JE, Hutson SM, Jefferson LS. Stimulation of albumin gene transcription by insulin in primary cultures of rat hepatocytes. Am J Physiol 1987;252:C205.

203. Lund PK, Goodman RH, Montiminy MR, et al. Anglerfish islet preproglucagon II. J Biol Chem 1983; 258:3280.

204. Marshall S, Olefsky J. Characterization of insulin-induced receptor loss and evidence for internalization of the insulin receptor. Diabetes 1981;30:746.

205. Martin JM, Friesen H. Effect of human placental lactogen on the isolated islets of Langerhans in vitro. Endocrinology 1969;84:619.

206. Martinez C, Ruiz P, Andres A, et al. Tyrosine kinase activity of liver insulin receptor is inhibited in rats at term gestation. Biochem J 1989;263:267.

207. Maryama H, Hisatomi A, Orci L, et al. Insulin within the islet is a physiologic glucagon inhibitor. J Clin Invest 1984;74:2296.

208. Masoro EJ. Lipids and lipid metabolism. Ann Rev Physiol 1977;39:301.

209. McDonald-Gibson RG, Young M, Hytten FE. Changes in plasma nonesterified fatty acids and serum glycerol in pregnancy. Br J Obstet Gynaecol 1975;82:460.

210. McGarry JD. New perspectives in the regulation of ketogenesis. Diabetes 1979;28:517.

211. McGarry JD, Foster DW. Hormonal control of ketogenesis. Biochemical considerations. Arch Intern Med 1977;137:495.

212. McMahon M, Schwenk WF, Haymond MW, Rizza RA. Underestimation of glucose turnover measured with 6-[^{3}H]- and 6,6[^{2}H$_2$]- but not 6-[^{14}C]-glucose during hyperinsulinemia in humans. Diabetes 1989;38:97.

213. Mestman JH, Anderson GV, Guadalupe V. Follow-up study of 360 subjects with abnormal carbohydrate metabolism during pregnancy. Obstet Gynecol 1972; 39:421.

214. Metzger BE, Agnoli FS, Hare JW, Freinkel N. Carbohydrate metabolism in pregnancy. X. Metabolic disposition of alanine by the perfused liver of the fasting pregnant rat. Diabetes 1973;22:601.

215. Metzger BE, Bybee DE, Freinkel N, et al. Gestational diabetes mellitus. Correlations between the phenotypic and genotypic characteristics of the mother and abnormal glucose tolerance during the first year postpartum. Diabetes 1985;43(suppl 2):111.

216. Metzger BE, Hare JW, Freinkel N. Carbohydrate metabolism in pregnancy IX. Plasma levels of gluconeogenic fuels during fasting in the rat. J Clin Endocrinol 1971;33:869.

217. Metzger BE, Phelps RL, Freinkel N, Navikas I. Effects of gestational diabetes on diurnal profiles of plasma glucose, lipids and individual amino acids. Diab Care 1980;3:402.

218. Metzger BE, Ravnikar V, Vileisis RA, Freinkel N. "Accelerated starvation" and the skipped breakfast in late normal pregnancy. Lancet 1982;1:588.

219. Metzger BE, Unger RH, Freinkel N. Carbohydrate metabolism in pregnancy. XIV. Relationships between circulating glucagon, insulin, glucose and amino acids in response to a "mixed meal" in late pregnancy. Metabolism 1977;26:151.

220. Michaels RL, Sorenson RL, Parsons JA, Sheridan JD. Prolactin enhances cell-to-cell communication among B-cells in pancreatic islets. Diabetes 1987; 36:1098.

221. Miller RE. Pancreatic neuroendocrinology: peripheral neural mechanisms in the regulation of the islets of Langerhans. Endocr Rev 1981;2:471.

222. Mills JL, Simpson JL, Driscoll SG, et al. NICHD Diabetes in Early Pregnancy Study. Incidence of spontaneous abortion among diabetic women whose pregnancies were identified within 21 days of conception. N Engl J Med 1988;319:1617.

223. Moller D, Flier JS. Insulin resistance—mechanisms, syndromes and implications. N Engl J Med 1991; 325:938.

224. Morrow PG, Marshall WP, Kim H-J, Kalkhoff RK. Metabolic response to starvation. I. Relative effects of pregnancy and sex steroid administration in the rat. Metabolism 1981;30:268.

225. Naismith DJ, Morga BLG. The biphasic nature of protein metabolism during pregnancy in the rat. Br J Nutr 1976;36:563.

226. National Diabetes Data Group. Classification and diagnosis of diabetes mellitus and other categories of glucose intolerance. Diabetes 1979;28:1039.

227. Neufield N, Braustein G, Corbo LM, et al. Insulin receptors and placental proteins in normal and gestational diabetic pregnancies. Biol Res Pregnancy 1984;2:84.

228. Nielsen JH. Effects of growth hormone, prolactin and placental lactogen on insulin content and release and

DNA synthesis in cultured pancreatic islets. Endocrinology 1982;110:600.

229. Nielsen JH. Direct effects of gonadal and contraceptive steroids on insulin release from mouse pancreatic islets in organ culture. Acta Endocrinol 1984;105:245.

230. Nielsen JH, Nielsen V, Pedersen LM, Deckert T. Effects of pregnancy hormones on pancreatic islets in organ culture. Acta Endocrinol 1986;111:336.

231. Olefsky JM. Effect of dexamethasone in insulin binding, glucose transport and glucose oxidation in isolated rat adipocytes. J Clin Invest 1975;56:1499.

232. Olefsky JM. The insulin receptor: its role in insulin resistance of obesity and diabetes. Diabetes 1976; 25:1154.

233. O'Sullivan JB, Charles D, Mahan CM, Dandrow RV. Gestational diabetes and perinatal mortality rate. Am J Obstet Gynecol 1973;116:901.

234. O'Sullivan JB, Mahan CM. Criteria for the oral glucose tolerance test in pregnancy. Diabetes 1964; 13:278.

235. Pagano G, Cassader M, Massabrio M, et al. Insulin binding to human adipocytes during late pregnancy in healthy, obese and diabetic state. Horm Metab Res 1980;12:177.

236. Parker PJ, Embi N, Caudwell FB, Cohen P. Glycogen synthase from rabbit skeletal muscle. Eur J Biochem 1982;124:47.

237. Pauvilai G, Drobny EC, Domont LA, Baumann G. Insulin receptors and insulin resistance in human pregnancy: evidence for a postreceptor defect in insulin action. J Clin Endocrinol Metab 1982;54:247.

238. Pedersen J. The pregnant diabetic and her newborn infant. Baltimore: Williams & Wilkins, 1977.

239. Perlman JA, Russell-Briefel R, Ezzati T, Lieberknecht G. Oral glucose tolerance and the potency of contraceptive progestins. J Chron Dis 1985;38:857.

240. Persson B, Lunell NO. Metabolic control in diabetic pregnancy. Variations in plasma concentrations of glucose, free fatty acids, glycerol, ketone bodies, insulin, and human chorionic somatomammotropin during the last trimester. Am J Obstet Gynecol 1975;122:737.

241. Peterson RE, Imperato-McGinley J. Cortisol metabolism in the perinatal period. In: New MI, Fiser RH Jr, eds. Diabetes and other endocrine disorders during pregnancy and in the newborn. New York: Alan R Liss, 1976:141.

242. Picard C, Ooms HA, Balassse E, Conard V. Effect of normal pregnancy on glucose assimilation, insulin, and nonesterified fatty acid levels. Diabetologia 1968;4:16.

243. Pipe NGJ, Smith T, Halliday D, et al. Changes in fat, fat-free mass and body water in human normal pregnancy. Br J Obstet Gynaecol 1979;86:929.

244. Porte D Jr, Graber AL, Kuzuya T, Williams RH. The effect of epinephrine on immunoreactive insulin levels in man. J Clin Invest 1966;45:228.

245. Porte D Jr, Williams R. Inhibition of insulin release by norepinephrine in man. Science 1966;152:1248.

246. Posner BI. Insulin receptors in human and animal placental tissue. Diabetes 1974;23:209.

247. Rajan AS, Aguilar-Bryan L, Nelson DA, et al. Ion channels and insulin secretion. Diab Care 1990; 13:340.

248. Rannels DE, Kao R, Morgan GE. Effect of insulin on protein turnover in heart muscle. J Biol Chem 1975;250:1694.

249. Ravnikar V, Metzger BE, Freinkel N. Is there a risk of "accelerated starvation" in normal human pregnancy? (abstr). Diabetes 1978;27:463.

250. Rehfeld JF, Larsson LI, Goltermann NR, et al. Neural regulation of pancreatic hormone secretion by C-terminal tetrapeptide of CCK. Nature 1980;284:33.

251. Rehfeld JF, Lindkaer JS. The effect of gastrin and cholecystokinin on the endocrine pancreas. Front Horm Res 1980;7:108.

252. Rizzo T, Metzger BE, Burns WJ, Burns K. Correlations between antepartum maternal metabolism and intelligence of offspring. N Engl J Med 1991;325:911.

253. Roach PJ, Rosell-Perez M, Larner J. Muscle glycogen synthase in vivo state: effects of insulin administration on the chemical and kinetic properties of the purified enzyme. FEBS Lett 1977;80:95.

254. Rodeman-Granner HP, Goldberg AL. Arachidonic acid, prostaglandin E_2 and F_{2a} influence rates of protein turnover in skeletal and cardiac muscle. J Biol Chem 1982;257:1632.

255. Rosen OM. After insulin binds. Science 1987; 237:1452.

256. Rosen OM. Structure and function of insulin receptors. Diabetes 1989;38:1508.

257. Rosetti L, Giaccari A, DeFronzo RA. Glucose toxicity. Diab Care 1990;13:610.

258. Ruderman NB. Muscle amino acid metabolism and gluconeogenesis. Ann Rev Med 1975;26:245.

259. Rudolph MCJ, Coustan DR, Sherwin RS, et al. Efficacy of the insulin pump in the home treatment of pregnant diabetics. Diabetes 1981;30:891.

260. Rushakoff RJ, Kalkhoff RK. Effects of pregnancy and sex steroid administration on skeletal muscle metabolism in the rat. Diabetes 1981;30:545.

261. Rushakoff RJ, Kalkhoff RK. Relative effects of pregnancy and corticosterone administration on skeletal muscle metabolism in the rat. Endocrinology 1983;113:43.

262. Ryan EA, Enns L. Role of gestational hormones in the induction of insulin resistance. J Clin Endocrinol Metab 1988;67:341.

263. Ryan EA, O'Sullivan MJ, Skyler JS. Insulin action during pregnancy. Diabetes 1985;34:380.

264. Sacks DA, Abu-Fadil S, Greenspoon JS, Fotheringham, N. Do the current standards for glucose tolerance testing in pregnancy represent a valid conversion of O'Sullivan's original criteria? Am J Obstet Gynecol 1989;161:638.

265. Sacks H, Waligora K, Matthews J, Pimstone B. Inhibition by somatostatin of glucagon induced glucose release from the isolated perfused rat liver. Endocrinology 1977;101:1751.

266. Saltiel AR. Second messengers of insulin action. Diab Care 1990;13:244.

267. Saltiel AR, Fox A, Sherline P, Cuatrecasas P. Insulin stimulated hydrolysis of a novel glycolipid generates modulators of cAMP phosphodiesterase. Science 1986;233:967.

268. Samaan NA, Goplerud CP, Bradbury JT. Effect of arginine infusion on plasma levels of growth hormone, insulin, and glucose during pregnancy and the puerperium. Am J Obstet Gynecol 1970;107:1002.

269. Samaan N, Yen SCC, Gonzalez D. Metabolic effects of placental lactogen in man. J Clin Endocrinol Metab 1968;28:485.

270. Sando H, Grodsky GM. Dynamic synthesis and release of insulin and proinsulin from perfused islets. Diabetes 1973;22:354.

271. Sasaki K, Cripe T, Kochs S, et al. Multihormonal regulation of phosphoenolpyruvate carboxykinase gene

transcription: the dominant role of insulin. J Biol Chem 1984;259:15242.

272. Schalch DS, Kipnis DM. Abnormalities in carbohydrate tolerance associated with elevated plasma non-esterified fatty acids. J Clin Invest 1965;44:2010.

273. Schmitz O, Klebe J, Moller J, et al. In vivo insulin action in type I (insulin dependent) diabetic pregnant women as assessed by the insulin clamp technique. J Clin Endocrinol Metab 1985;61:877.

274. Schwartz TW. Pancreatic polypeptide: A hormone under vagal control. Gastroenterology 1983;85:1411.

275. Seifter S, England S. Carbohydrate metabolism. In: Rifkin H, Porte D Jr, eds. Diabetes mellitus: theory and practice, ed 4. New York: Elsevier, 1990:1.

276. Seyffert WA, Madison LL. Physiologic effects of metabolic fuels on carbohydrate metabolism. Diabetes 1967;16:765.

277. Sheridan JD, Anaya PA, Parsons JA, Sorenson RL. Increased dye coupling in pancreatic islets from rats in late-term pregnancy. Diabetes 1988;37:908.

278. Sherwin RS, Hendler RG, Felig P. Effect of ketone infusions on amino acid and nitrogen metabolism in man. J Clin Invest 1975;55:1382.

279. Shirling D, Ashby JP, Baird JD. A direct anabolic effect of progesterone in the intact female rat. J Endocrinol 1983;99:47.

280. Spellacy WN. Insulin and growth hormone measurements in normal and high risk pregnancies. In: Crosignani PG, Pardi G, eds. Fetal evaluation during pregnancy and labor. New York: Academic Press, 1971:110.

281. Spellacy WN, Ellingson AB, Keith G, et al. Plasma glucose and insulin levels during the menstrual cycle of normal women and premenstrual syndrome patients. J Reprod Med 1990;35:508.

282. Spellacy WN, Goetz FC. Plasma insulin in normal late pregnancy. N Engl J Med 1963;268:988.

283. Spellacy WN, Goetz FC, Greenberg BZ, Ellis J. Plasma insulin in normal mid-pregnancy. Am J Obstet Gynecol 1965;92:11.

284. Srivastava MC, Oakley NW, Tompkins CV, et al. Insulin metabolism, insulin sensitivity and hormonal responses to insulin infusion in patients taking oral contraceptive steroid. Eur J Clin Invest 1975;5:425.

285. Stagner JI, Samols E. Modulation of insulin secretion by pancreatic ganglionic nicotinic receptors. Diabetes 1986;35:849.

286. Stagner JI, Samols E, Weir GC. Sustained oscillations of insulin glucagon and somatostatin from the isolated canine pancreas during exposure to a constant glucose concentration. J Clin Invest 1980;65:939.

287. Starke A, Grundy S, McGarry JD, Unger RH. Correction of hyperglycemia by inducing renal malabsorption of glucose restores the glucagon response to glucose in insulin-deficient dogs: implications for human diabetes. Proc Natl Acad Sci USA 1985;82:1544.

288. Steele JM, Johnstone FD, Hepburn DA, Smith AF. Can prepregnancy care of diabetic women reduce the risk of abnormal babies? BMJ 1990;301:1070.

289. Stehbens JA, Baker GL, Kitchel M. Outcome at ages 1, 3, and 5 years of children born to diabetic women. Am J Obstet Gynecol 1977;127:408.

290. Summary and Recommendations of the Third International Workshop-Conference on Gestational Diabetes Mellitus. Diabetes 1991;40(suppl 2):197.

291. Thorens B, Charron MJ, Lodish HF. Molecular physiology of glucose transporters. Diab Care 1990;13:209.

292. Topping DL, Mayes PA. The immediate effects of insulin and fructose on the metabolism of the perfused liver. Biochem J 1972;126:295.

293. Toyoda N, Deguchi T, Murata K, et al. Postbinding insulin resistance around parturition in the isolated rat epitrochlearis muscle. Am J Obstet Gynecol 1991;165:1475.

294. Toyoda N, Murata K, Sugiyama Y. Insulin binding, glucose oxidation, and methylglucose transport in isolated adipocytes from pregnant rats near term. Endocrinology 1985;116:998.

295. Tsibris JCM, Raynor LO, Buhi WC, et al. Insulin receptors in circulating erythrocytes and monocytes from women on oral contraceptives or pregnant women near term. J Clin Endocrinol Metab 1980;51:711.

296. Turtle JR, Kipnis DM. The lypolytic action of human placental lactogen on isolated fat cells. Biochim Biophys Acta 1967;144:583.

297. Tyson JE, Austin K, Thomas G. Prolonged nutritional deprivation in pregnancy: factors contributing to hypoglycemia. Am J Obstet Gynecol 1971;109:1080.

298. Tyson JE, Jones GS, Huth J, Thomas P. Patterns of insulin, growth hormone, and placental lactogen release after protein and glucose-protein ingestion in pregnancy. Am J Obstet Gynecol 1971;110:934.

299. Tyson JE, Rabinowitz D, Merimee TJ, Friesen H. Response of plasma insulin and human growth hormone to arginine in pregnant and postpartum females. Am J Obstet Gynecol 1969;103:313.

300. Ullrich A, Bell JR, Chen EY, et al. Human insulin receptor and its relationship to the tyrosine kinase family of oncogenes. Nature 1985;313:756.

301. Unger RH. Glucagon and somatostatin. In: Freinkel NF, ed. The year in metabolism 1977. New York: Plenum, 1978:101.

302. Unger RH, Dobbs RE, Orci L. Insulin, glucagon, and somatostatin secretion in the regulation of metabolism. Ann Rev Physiol 1978;40:307.

303. Unger RH, Orci L. Glucagon secretion and metabolism in man. In: DeGroot LJ, ed. Endocrinology. Philadelphia: WB Saunders, 1989:1318.

304. Unger RH, Orci L. Glucagon. In: Rifkin H, Porte D Jr, eds. Diabetes mellitus: theory and practice, ed 4. New York: Elsevier, 1990:104.

305. Uyeda K, Furuya E, Luby LJ. The effect of natural and synthetic D-fructose-2,6-bisphosphate on the regulatory kinetic properties of liver and muscle phosphofructokinases. J Biol Chem 1981;256:8394.

306. Vague P, Moulin J-P. Defective glucose sensitivity of the B-cell in non insulin dependent diabetes. Improvement after twenty hours of normoglycemia. Metabolism 1982;31:139.

307. Van Assche FA. Quantitative morphologic and histoenzymatic study of the endocrine pancreas in nonpregnant and pregnant rats. Am J Obstet Gynecol 1974;118:39.

308. Van Assche FA, Aerts L, Gepts W. Immunocytochemical study of the endocrine pancreas in the rat during normal pregnancy and during experimental diabetic pregnancy. Diabetologia 1980;18:487.

309. Van Assche FA, Hoet JJ, Jack P. The endocrine pancreas of the pregnant mother, fetus, and newborn. In: Beard RW, Nathanielsz PW, eds. Fetal physiology and medicine. Philadelphia: WB Saunders, 1982:127.

310. Wakelam MJ, Murphy GJ, Hruby VJ, Housley ND. Activation of two signal transduction systems hepatocytes by glucagon. Nature 1986;323:68.

311. Walker AP, Flint DJ. Absence of down-regulation of

the insulin receptor by insulin. Biochem J 1983; 210:373.

312. Ward WK, Johnston CLW, Beard JC, et al. Abnormalities of islet B-cell function, insulin action and fat distribution in women with a history of gestational diabetes: relation to obesity. J Clin Endocrinol Metab 1985;61:1039.

313. Ward WK, Johnston CLW, Beard JC, et al. Insulin resistance and impaired insulin secretion in subjects with a history of gestational diabetes mellitus. Diabetes 1985;34:861.

314. Wheeler TJ, Hinkle PC. The glucose transporter of mammalian cells. Ann Rev Physiol 1985;47:503.

315. Widstrom AM, Matthiesen AS, Winberg J, Uvnas-Moberg K. Maternal somatostatin levels and their correlation with infant birth weight. Early Hum Dev 1989;20:165.

316. Wool IG, Krahl ME. Incorporation of C14-amino acids into protein of isolated diaphragms: an effect of insulin independent of glucose entry. Am J Physiol 1959;196:961.

317. Yang YJ, Hope ID, Ader M, Bergman RN. Insulin transport across capillaries is rate limiting for insulin action in dogs. J Clin Invest 1989;84:1620.

318. Yen SS. Metabolic homeostasis during pregnancy. In: Yen SS, Samman N, Jaffe RB, eds. Reproductive endocrinology. Philadelphia: WB Saunders, 1978:537.

319. Yen SS, Tsai CC, Vela P. Gestational diabetogenesis: quantitative analysis of glucose interrelationship between normal pregnancy and pregnancy with gestational diabetes. Am J Obstet Gynecol 1971;111:792.

320. Yen SS, Vela P, Tsai CC. Impairment of growth hormone secondary in response to hypoglycemia during early and late pregnancy. J Clin Endocrinol 1970;31:29.

321. Young M, Prenton MA. Maternal and fetal plasma amino acid concentrations during gestation and in retarded fetal growth. J Obstet Gynaecol Br Comm 1969;76:333.

Hypertension in Pregnancy

Bahij S. Nuwayhid

Edmond W. Quillen

Hypertension affects 10 to 15% of pregnancies and remains the leading cause of maternal and fetal mortality and morbidity. The 1980s saw the introduction of new diagnostic tools, such as ultrasound, Doppler technology, and Swan-Ganz catheterization. New management strategies were also introduced, with prophylactic low-dose aspirin among the most promising. In the area of pathogenesis, the maternal immune response to the fetal allograft and the role of the prostaglandins, superoxides, and endothelium-derived factors are being actively investigated as factors involved in the pathogenesis of pregnancy-induced hypertension. Together these exciting new approaches may increase our understanding of the subject, but it may be another decade before their cumulative effect on maternal and fetal mortality and morbidity can be assessed.

CLASSIFICATION

Numerous classifications of hypertension in pregnancy have been suggested,[25, 68] but the most commonly used is that of the Committee on Terminology of the American College of Obstetricians and Gynecologists:[56, 80]

I. Preeclampsia-eclampsia.
II. Chronic hypertension.
III. Preeclampsia-eclampsia superimposed on chronic hypertension.
IV. Transient or late hypertension.

Preeclampsia-eclampsia is unique to pregnancy and affects 5 to 10% of pregnancies, more frequently primigravid women. Although most commonly diagnosed during the third trimester, preeclampsia might occur as early as 20 weeks' gestation. The term *eclampsia* is applied when tonic-clonic seizures develop in a preeclamptic woman. Preeclampsia is characterized by hypertension, proteinuria, and edema, although edema by itself is not a reliable sign. Hypertension is defined as blood pressure (BP) >140/90 after 20 weeks' gestation if earlier readings of BP are not available or a rise of 30 mmHg in systolic pressure and 15 mmHg in diastolic pressure when BP is known. Proteinuria is defined as >300 mg/L per 24-hour urine specimen.

Severe preeclampsia is characterized by

1. Arterial pressures >160/110 mmHg.
2. Proteinuria >5 g per 24-hour specimen.
3. Oliguria <400 mL per 24-hour specimen.
4. Platelet count <100,000.
5. An increase in bilirubin level or liver enzymes.
6. Symptoms such as epigastric pain, scatomata, severe headache.

A variant of severe preeclampsia is the *HELLP* syndrome, which is characterized by *h*emolysis, *e*levated *l*iver enzymes, and *l*ow *p*latelet count. Gestational hypertension or nonproteinuric preeclampsia is defined as an increase in arterial pressure during pregnancy but no proteinuria. The difficulty with this category is that it includes a large proportion of primigravid women who do not develop hypertension or preeclampsia. Chesley[14] in a large study of white American primigravidas showed that 5% of the women had a diastolic BP >90 mmHg during the first half of pregnancy, and this percentage rose to 20% at term. Other studies[67, 92] also suggest that an increase in diastolic BP of 20 mmHg between 24 and 40 weeks occurred in more than 20% of primigravidas (range 19 to 57%).

Chronic hypertension affects 5 to 6% of all pregnancies. It is more common in multiparas and black women. A history of mild to moderate hypertension preceding pregnancy might be obtained from the patient, although more often none is available. Secondary causes of hypertension must be looked for. A BP of 140/90 mmHg before 20 weeks' gestation is presumptive evidence of chronic hypertension. Failure of BP to decrease at midgestation might suggest a more complicated course.[83]

Chronic hypertension with superimposed preeclampsia usually carries the worse prognosis for both mother and fetus. Most frequently, the diagnosis is in error because it is difficult to ascertain whether the hypertension is getting worse or there is superimposition of preeclampsia. Most clinicians rely on development of massive proteinuria, changes in liver enzymes, or changes in coagulation profile to assign patients to this category.

Late or transient hypertension includes those patients who develop hypertension but no proteinuria during the latter part of gestation, during labor, and during the early postpartum period. Usually BP returns to normal within 1 week after delivery. This category is significant for two reasons: (1) It includes some patients with mild preeclampsia or chronic hypertension who never develop proteinuria, and as such the prognosis for their pregnancy is much better than either preeclampsia or hypertension alone. (2) Women in this category are at a greater risk of developing chronic hypertension later in life.[15]

Despite these definitions, clinical diagnosis of preeclampsia remains difficult. Fisher et al[39] reported that in 60% of multiparous women the clinical diagnosis of preeclampsia was erroneous. Likewise, Katz et al[59] using renal biopsies failed to show evidence of preeclampsia in 40% of patients with chronic renal disease who were clinically diagnosed as having superimposed preeclampsia.

SURVEILLANCE

Obstetric, Family, and Medical Histories

The association between parity and preeclampsia is well documented. MacGillivray[66] reported that preeclampsia was present in approximately 6% of nulliparous women but only in 0.3% of women in their second pregnancy. Similarly, Chesley and Cooper[16] reported that transient hypertension was diagnosed in 25% of first pregnancies and 2 to 3% of subsequent pregnancies.

A familial tendency to preeclampsia has been shown, and several studies provided evidence that preeclampsia is inherited in a manner consistent with a recessive single gene hypothesis,[16, 21, 60] with a calculated gene frequency of 0.20 to 0.25%. The overall risk for development of preeclampsia increases fourfold for nulliparous pregnancies if there is a documented history of preeclampsia in the mother and sixfold if in a biologic sister.[81]

The medical history is also important because patients with multiple gestation, extremes of ages, diabetes mellitus, chronic hypertension, and a variety of autoimmune diseases are at an increased risk for developing superimposed preeclampsia.

Arterial Pressure at Midgestation

Several investigators have used noninvasive determination of arterial pressure to predict the development of preeclampsia.[3, 76, 83, 113] The cutoff point for normal diastolic BP during midgestation was set at 90 mmHg. The largest study, done by Page and Christianson,[83] included more than 10,000 patients, who were studied during the first pregnancy. Only 2.7% of their patients with diastolic pressure >90 mmHg developed preeclampsia. The specificity of the method averaged 88% and the sensitivity 41%. The predictive value of a positive test result was low (8%) and that for a negative value was quite high (98%), suggesting that a negative test result is very assuring. More recent studies by Moutquin et al,[76] Villar and Sibai,[113] and Ales et al[3] show qualitatively similar results.

The introduction of 24-hour ambulatory monitoring devices[18] has permitted determination of arterial pressure levels during the subject's routine activities. Villar et al[112] reported that bed rest, positional changes, and home environment all contributed to lower readings at home. An ongoing study by Moutquin and colleagues[73–75] suggests that failure of mean arterial pressure to decrease during sleep period (night time) is associated with higher rates of preeclampsia. The day to night variability in arterial pressure was maintained in chronic hypertension patients, suggesting a different disease entity.

Doppler Flow Velocimetry

In the last few years, Doppler flow velocimetry of the umbilical and uterine circulations has been used to predict the development of hypertension in pregnancy. The basic concepts underlying this technique are simple: Doppler technology is capable of detecting flow velocity wave forms in the uterine and umbilical arteries; during normal pregnancy, there is an increase in the uteroplacental and umbilicoplacental circulations secondary to reduced vascular resistance, which is reflected by a qualitative change in the wave form velocities. Using the uterine or umbilical artery wave forms, a systolic to diastolic (S/D) ratio or a pulsatility index (PI) or resistance index (RI) can be calculated.[35] These indices have been termed frequently as *resistance indices,* although they are qualitative indices and do not measure or calculate the vascular resistances. Regardless of the terminology, it seems there is positive correlation between abnormal indices and poor maternal, fetal, and neonatal outcomes.

One of the largest studies assessing the routine use of early Doppler velocimetry for predicting development of hypertension later in pregnancy was done by Steel et al.[104] A total of 1014 nulliparous women were screened at 16 to 22 weeks' gestation and again at 24 week's gestation if abnormally high uterine resistance was detected. The group with abnormal results had a greater incidence of preeclampsia. Farmakides et al[37] reviewed the literature and included their own data on the utility of uterine and umbilical flow velocimetry in predicting maternal and fetal outcome in a high-risk population. They reported little change in the flow velocimetry of the uterine arteries until the end of the second trimester. An S/D ratio <2.6 at 26 weeks and absence of a diastolic notch suggested normal uteroplacental development. For the umbilical artery, a cut-off point of 3.0 for the S/D ratio after 30 weeks was suggestive of normal umbilicoplacental development. Their conclusions can be summarized as follows:

1. Pregnancies with abnormal uterine flow velocimetry resulted in a higher incidence of stillbirth, premature births, intrauterine growth retardation (IUGR), maternal preeclampsia, and increased rate of cesarean sections for fetal distress. The sensitivity and specificity for predicting maternal and fetal morbidity was high (>80%). Further, abnormal velocimetry preceded clinical disease in most cases and was more specific and sensitive than mean arterial pressure, uric acid, and creatinine clearance in predicting maternal, fetal, and neonatal morbidity.

2. Pregnancies with abnormal umbilical flow velocimetry resulted in a higher rate of fetal growth retardation and secondarily higher rates of fetal distress in labor, cesarean sections, and neonatal intensive care unit admissions.

3. When both uterine and umbilical vascular patterns were abnormal, both mother and fetus were affected. There were higher rates of preeclampsia in mother and severe IUGR in the fetus.

Based on these findings, Farmakides et al[37] suggested the use of flow velocimetry for surveillance purposes in high-risk pregnancies, with the first examination done at about 24 weeks' gestation and a repeat measurement at 32 to 34 week's gestation. These recommendations were not supported by Jacobson et al,[57] who studied 93 women at risk for preeclampsia or IUGR and analyzed the uterine flow velocity wave forms at 20 and 24 weeks' gestation. They found that although higher resistance indices were more common in women who developed preeclampsia or IUGR, the correlation was not close enough to be useful as a clinical test.

Pressor Tests

It is well known that there is increased vascular sensitivity to vasoactive compounds during preeclampsia. The classic study of Gant et al[47] extended these findings and for the first time suggested that pressor tests could be used to predict development of preeclampsia later in pregnancy. Using the interval between 28 and 32 weeks of gestation, they found that 87% of subsequently normotensive women required >8 ng/kg per minute of angiotensin II to elevate diastolic pressure by 20 mmHg. Among those women who later developed preeclampsia, 90% required an angiotensin II dose <8 ng/kg per minute to achieve the same increase in diastolic pressure.

The drawbacks to this study are that (1) it was done in a predominantly poor black population, where the incidence of pregnancy-induced hypertension is high; (2) only one positive test was used to classify patients as having a positive or negative test result, although serial testing was done; and (3) a cuff sphygmomanometer was used. Morris et al[72] reported high false-positive results when they included all serial tests in the calculation and replaced the cuff sphygmomanometer with a Doppler device. Öney and Kauhausen[82] using a primigravid white population found the pressor test to have less predictive value. Presently the pressor test is rarely used because of the difficulty and risk of administration and low predictability value for development of preeclampsia.

Gant et al,[46] aware of the difficulties of routine administration of angiotensin II sensitivity test, developed a new noninvasive test termed the *rollover test*. Briefly stated, the test is performed by placing the gravida (28 to 32 weeks' gestation) on her side and recording the BP and then turning her to the back position and recording the BP immediately and after 5 minutes. An increase in the diastolic pressure of 20 mmHg or more is sufficient to term this test as positive. The authors reported a strong positive correlation between the rollover test and angiotensin II sensitivity test and later development of pregnancy-induced hypertension. Several investigators[58, 86] attempted to duplicate the findings with various degrees of success: Reported sensitivity ranged from as low as 10% to a high of 88%, and predictive value for a positive test ranged from 39 to 94%. The highest agreement among all the studies was in a predictive value for a negative test.[81] These observations suggest that a negative test result is highly indicative that the nulligravida will not develop pregnancy-induced hypertension. As with the angiotensin II sensitivity test, the high false-positive results and low predictability values for this test discouraged clinicians from using it routinely for surveillance purposes.

Calcium Metabolism

Taufield et al[108] in a well-planned study showed that total and fractional 24-hour urinary calcium excretion of preeclamptic women is significantly lower than that of normotensive controls. Independent confirmation of these findings was provided by other groups.[44, 96] Sanchez-Ramos et al[96] reported on a prospective study in which 103 consecutive nulliparous women at risk for preeclampsia were studied. Twenty-four–hour urinary calcium excretions were collected serially at 10 to 24 weeks, 25 to 32 weeks, and 33 weeks to term. Results showed that patients who later developed preeclampsia had lower rates of calcium excretion during the three collection periods. Using a

predictive threshold for calcium excretion of 195 mg per 24 hours, the authors found a higher incidence of preeclampsia in hypocalciuric women (87 versus 2%). In addition, the relationship between hypocalciuria and parathyroid hormone (PTH) levels in preeclamptic women was studied by Frenkel et al.[44] Fourteen preeclamptic women were compared with 12 women with chronic hypertension and 11 normotensive women all in the third trimester. Compared with normotensive controls, preeclamptic women had the lowest 24-hour urinary calcium excretion (62.1 ± 32.8 mg per 24 hours versus 225.6 ± 146.9 mg per 24 hours) and the lowest serum PTH levels (9.8 ± 5.5 pg/mL versus 16.4 ± 3.2 pg/mL). The ionized calcium, phosphorus, albumin, and calcitriol serum levels were not significantly different among the various groups. The authors suggested that the hypocalciuria of preeclampsia is independent of the PTH-calcitriol axis, and the hypocalciuria of preeclampsia may be due to intrinsic renal tubular dysfunction.

Increased intracellular calcium has been implicated in the pathogenesis of hypertension.[64, 102, 105] The level of free intracellular calcium is a major determinant of vascular smooth muscle tone and consequently of peripheral vascular resistance. Sowers et al[101] in a study of 47 primigravid black women at ≥35 weeks' gestation showed an increase in erythrocyte calcium levels without any change in sodium, potassium, or magnesium cellular levels. In a follow-up study, the same authors investigated platelet calcium metabolism as an early predictor of increased peripheral vascular resistance and preeclampsia.[118] A total of 48 nulliparous black women were studied during each trimester of pregnancy. The arterial pressure, forearm vascular resistance, and basal and arginine vasopressin (AVP) stimulated intracellular platelet calcium concentration were measured. Data on the 14 women (29%) who developed preeclampsia were compared with the other 34 women who remained normotensive. Pertinent results were as follows:

1. Although basal levels of platelet intracellular calcium did not differ among the women who developed preeclampsia or remained normotensive, there was a striking increase in the sensitivity of platelet intracellular calcium lev-

els to AVP stimulation in the group with pre-eclampsia.

2. The decrease in peripheral vascular resistance seen in normal pregnancy was not accompanied by a change in the level of platelet intracellular calcium.

The significance of this study, if confirmed, is that an alteration in platelet calcium metabolism is predictive of preeclampsia as early as the first trimester of pregnancy and that this altered metabolism precedes any vascular changes. Redmen[91] and others[6, 81] in reviewing the work of Sowers and colleagues[101, 118] commented that it is important to ascertain that these changes in platelet metabolism are induced by pregnancy and not inherent in the individuals studied and that follow-up studies to document return to normal platelet metabolism during the puerperium are also needed. Questions about the criteria used to diagnose preeclampsia and use of selected population were raised.

ARTERIAL PRESSURE REGULATION DURING NORMAL PREGNANCY

The long-term steady-state level of mean arterial pressure (MAP) is known to be determined by the equilibrium between the intake and output of fluid and electrolytes as governed by the renal body fluid feedback system.[53] Accordingly any imbalance in the net rate of input and output is reflected over time, as a change in the total extracellular fluid and blood volumes. The volume and tone of the vascular system govern the average peripheral driving force and resistance for blood to return to the heart. The input pressure to the heart and the contractile state of the heart govern the level of cardiac output. Based on this level of blood flow, the peripheral tissues exert an autoregulatory modulation of total peripheral resistance. The product of any given level of cardiac output and total peripheral resistance is the arterial pressure, which is the main factor in the control of urinary output.

According to this renal body fluid feedback system, a sustained increase in the blood volume and cardiac output with no change in the total peripheral resistance leads to a volume loading type of hypertension. The increase in blood pressure produces pressure diuresis and natriuresis and returns the cardiac output and blood volume to near normal levels, but this is accomplished at the expense of further increases in total peripheral resistance. As a new steady state is established, volume homeostasis is maintained by shifting the equilibrium point for the relationship between arterial pressure and sodium excretion to a higher pressure level.[19, 69]

The *renal function curve,* which describes the relationship between arterial pressure and sodium and water excretion, is very steep in the normal, nonpregnant state. This relationship has not previously been determined during pregnancy. In nonpregnant animals, a fourfold to fivefold increase in sodium intake is excreted by the kidneys, with only a 2 to 3 mmHg change in the arterial pressure. The set-point, or equilibrium point, of this curve occurs at the arterial pressure level, which is required to excrete the exact amount of salt and water coming into the system, i.e., to maintain fluid and electrolyte balance. Alterations of this set-point are therefore the only means by which the long-term average level of arterial pressure can be changed. For example, a shift in the renal function curve to the right may be brought about by higher circulating levels of angiotensin II or aldosterone or decreased renal mass. Conversely, a shift of the renal function curve to the left might be brought about by decreasing the renal vascular resistance or tubular reabsorption.[27, 79]

Changes in sympathetic nervous system activity may also raise the set-point of the renal function curve and consequently increase the level of arterial blood pressure. Indeed, chronic stimulation of the renal nerves[63] and intrarenal arterial infusion of norepinephrine[23] result in hypertension. Autonomic activity is thought to increase during pregnancy because high spinal anesthesia or ganglionic blocking agents produce dramatic decreases in MAP, whereas MAP in nongravid women does not change.[110] Similarly, nonpregnant sheep treated with 6-hydroxydopamine do not exhibit significant hemodynamic perturbations, but MAP is chronically reduced by 15 to 20 mmHg in the gravid ewe.[107]

Over the last 5 years, we have investigated a variety of mechanisms that influence arterial pressure regulation during pregnancy. These investigations have confirmed earlier observations that cardiac output, renal blood flow, and glomerular filtration rate (GFR) are increased and MAP is reduced during normal pregnancy. More importantly, these investigations have provided considerable new information with regard to cardiovascular homeostasis during pregnancy.

Initially the mechanisms responsible for the increase in cardiac output were studied in anesthetized guinea pigs, as illustrated in Figure 5–1.[11] The mean systemic filling pressure was increased from 7.1 ± 0.2 to 8.0 ± 0.5 mmHg, but the resistance to venous return was unchanged. The cardiac function curves, i.e., the instantaneous relationship between right atrial pressure and cardiac output, were determined to be shifted so that a greater cardiac output was obtained for any given level of right atrial pressure. These data indicate that the vascular system of pregnant guinea pigs is slightly overfilled. The data also demonstrate that the increase in cardiac output results primarily from an increase in the cardiac pumping ability and to a lesser extent from a slight increase in the pressure gradient for venous return to the heart.

Subsequent studies have employed conscious instrumented sheep. Working on the hypothesis that there was a primary change in proximal tubular function that was responsible for the increased level of GFR during pregnancy, pregnant ewes were subjected to saline loads. Proximal tubular reabsorption was determined to be elevated, but when the increase in GFR was taken into account, fractional proximal tubular reabsorption was demonstrated to be similar in nonpregnant and pregnant sheep. The degree, however, of suppression of proximal and distal tubular reabsorption by saline loading was less in pregnant ewes than in nonpregnant ewes. It results in a reduced cumulative excretion of sodium and water in response to saline loading (Fig. 5–2) and may predispose to excess volume expansion during pregnancy.[12]

Another vulnerability of renal function was demonstrated by the determination of the capacity to autoregulate renal blood flow. The breakpoint below which reductions of renal perfusion pressure result in reduction of renal blood flow is increased during pregnancy, as shown in Figure 5–3.[13] This reduced renal blood flow autoregulatory capacity combined with the reduced average level of arterial pressure contributes to a reduced safety margin within which renal perfusion pressure can fall without compromising renal blood flow during pregnancy.

Regardless of these possible deficiencies in renal function, the steady-state capacity for a

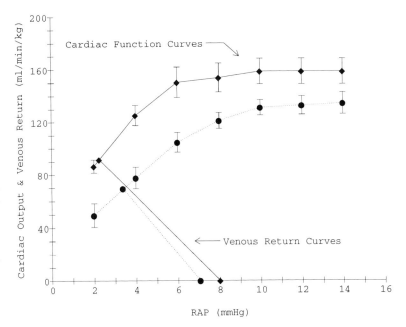

FIGURE 5–1. Cardiac function and venous return curves for nonpregnant (dotted lines) and pregnant (solid lines) guinea pigs. The resistance to venous return is illustrated by the slope of the venous return curves. The mean systemic filling pressure is indicated by the intercept of the venous return curve with the x axis at zero cardiac output. (From Cha SC, Aberdeen GW, Nuwayhid BS, Quillen EW Jr. Influence of pregnancy on mean systemic filling pressure and the cardiac function curve in guinea pigs. Can J Physiol Pharmacol 1992; 70:669.)

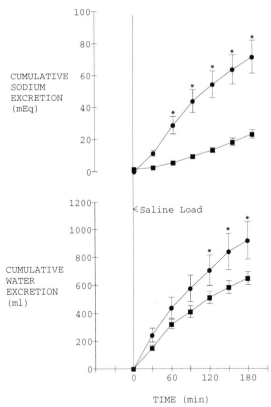

FIGURE 5–2. Cumulative sodium and water excretions for pregnant (solid square) and nonpregnant (solid circle) animals after saline load. Values are mean ± SEM. (From Cha SC, Mukaddam-Daher S, Quillen EW Jr, Nuwayhid BS. Tubular handling of fluid and electrolytes during ovine pregnancy. Am J Physiol in press, 1993.)

given change in arterial pressure to alter the urinary excretion of salt and water is maintained during pregnancy.[89] Indeed, the steady-state relationship between arterial pressure and urinary sodium excretion, i.e., the renal function curve, was shifted in a parallel fashion to the left during pregnancy (Fig. 5–4). Given the reduction in the average level of arterial pressure that is known to occur during pregnancy, this left shift of the renal function curve at moderate levels of sodium intake is not surprising. The parallel nature of this shift, however, was sustained over the extreme range of 5 to 1200 mmol per day total sodium intake.

This parallel left shift of the renal function curve was nevertheless unexpected because plasma levels of angiotensin II were suppressed by increases in sodium intake to a lesser extent in pregnant as compared with nonpregnant sheep. Acting alone, this type of

angiotensin II profile should have reduced the slope of the renal function curve or, stated differently, resulted in a salt-sensitive form of hypertension during pregnancy. These findings illustrate the importance of vasodilatory and natriuretic factors that have yet to be identified in the modulation of the arterial pressure–urinary output relationships during pregnancy.

Additional studies conducted in our laboratory have pointed to the role of the reduced renal perfusion pressure (decreased arterial pressure) and increased renal sympathetic nerve activity as factors that are at least partly responsible for the elevation of renin secretion and consequently plasma angiotensin II during pregnancy.[1, 36]

Although these elevated levels of angiotensin II have generally been judged inconsequential based on the demonstrations of reduced direct vasoconstrictor actions, it is becoming increasingly clear that the renin-angiotensin system is an important factor in arterial pressure regulation during pregnancy. By studying totally sinoaortic baroreceptor denervated sheep with and without ganglionic blockade, we have shown that circulating angiotensin II acts within the brain to produce approximately 20% of the total systemic pressor responses. During pregnancy, this indirect, autonomically mediated component of the angiotensin II pressor response is increased to about 65% of the overall response (Fig. 5–5).[88]

Circulating angiotensin II can also influence urinary sodium reabsorption by actions on the brain.[77] Long-term selective stimulation of this action of angiotensin II on the central nervous system, by continuous intracarotid infusion of the hormone, resulted in a sustained hypertension in association with a urinary sodium and water retention (Fig. 5–6). This effect was more readily exhibited (3 to 4 days) in pregnant sheep as compared with nonpregnant sheep (3 to 10 days). Because the peripheral plasma levels of angiotensin II and other hormones, including AVP and atrial natriuretic peptide, were not altered, the results of these studies suggest that this central nervous system action of angiotensin II is mediated by the renal nerve.

Finally, data from our laboratory[1, 36, 77, 78] and elsewhere[7, 70] are increasingly pointing to an enhanced role for the autonomic nervous system in arterial pressure regulation during

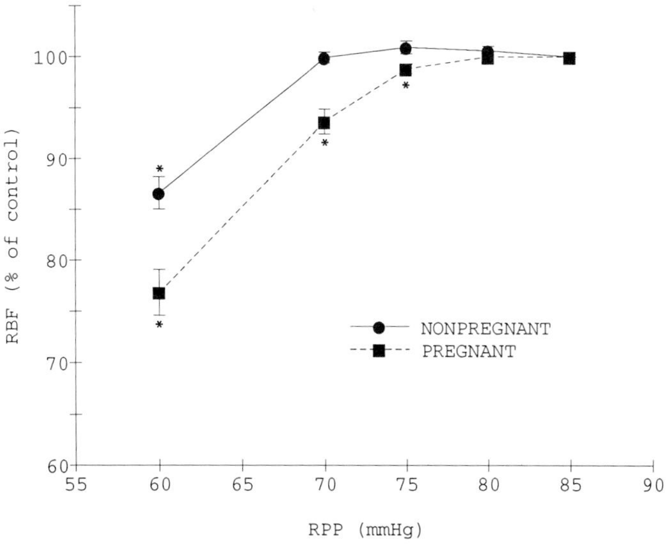

FIGURE 5–3. Renal blood flow (RBF) during reduction of renal perfusion pressure (RPP) in nonpregnant and pregnant sheep. *Indicates a difference (p <0.05) from control condition. (From Cha SC, Mukaddam-Daher S, Quillen EW Jr, Nuwayhid BS. Autoregulation of renal blood flow during ovine pregnancy. Hypertension in Pregnancy. 1993; 12:71.)

pregnancy. We have already cited studies that suggest (1) an increased role of the autonomic nervous system in the systemic pressor response to angiotensin II, (2) the role of the renal nerve in mediating the effect of central nervous system action of angiotensin II on urinary sodium excretion, and (3) the role of the renal nerve in promoting renin secretion. In addition, our observations of sheep prepared with one inner-

vated and one denervated kidney have suggested that the renal nerves have an enhanced influence on the conservation of sodium during the transition from high to low sodium intake states.[1] Also, the renal nerves may be an important component in the maintenance of sodium balance during ovine pregnancy.

PATHOPHYSIOLOGY OF PREECLAMPSIA

The cause and pathophysiology of preeclampsia are still unclear; over the last decade, however, it became apparent that hypertension as the major pathologic feature of preeclampsia is less credible, as up to 20% of preeclamptic women do not have BPs exceeding 140/90 mmHg. Further, as described earlier, the changes in vascular sensitivity to pressor agents, changes in umbilical and uterine wave form velocities, and changes in calcium metabolism all antedate development of hypertension by several weeks to several months. No doubt preeclamptic women are a heterogeneous group, and at least in one subset, hypertension is the major pathologic feature. It has been suggested that preeclampsia is a trophoblastic disease, in which an abnormal maternal immune response might lead to platelet and endothelial cell dysfunction.[91, 95] Secondary manifestations of this dysfunction include hypertension, coagulation abnormalities, and multisystem failure.

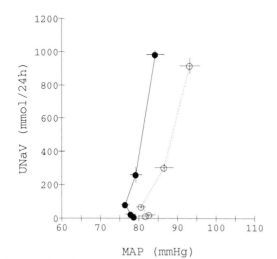

FIGURE 5–4. Renal function curve illustrating steady-state relationship of mean arterial pressure (MAP) and 24-hour urinary sodium excretion (UNaV) in pregnant (open circles and interrupted line), and nonpregnant (closed circles and continuous line) sheep. (From Quillen EW Jr, Nuwayhid BS. Steady-state arterial pressure–urinary output relationships during ovine pregnancy. Am J Physiol 1992; 263:R1141.)

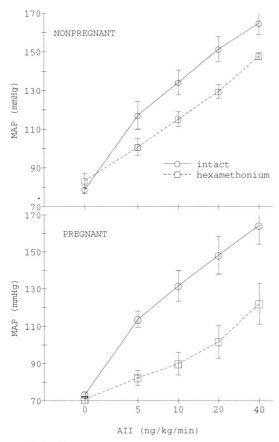

FIGURE 5–5. Relationship between dose of infused angiotensin II (AII) and mean arterial pressure (MAP) in totally sinoaortic denervated nonpregnant (top) and pregnant (bottom) sheep. The difference between the intact and hexamethonium-treated groups represents the centrally mediated component of the total AII pressor response. (From Quillen EW Jr, Aljabari AW, Nuwayhid BS. Central nervous system contributions to the pressor action of angiotensin II in sinoaortic denervated pregnant sheep, in preparation, 1993.)

Hyperdynamic Model of Hypertension

Traditionally preeclampsia has been characterized by elevated BP, normal or reduced cardiac output, reduced blood volume, and high systemic vascular resistance. Over the last decade, the increased utility of Swan-Ganz catheters in the management of women with severe preeclampsia has permitted the construction of left ventricular pressure–volume curves for assessment of cardiac performance and calculation of systemic vascular resistances.

Compilation of data from several studies showed that for the same level of MAP, cardiac output ranged from a low of 4 L per minute

to a high of 12 L, and the systemic vascular resistance (determined as the MAP divided by cardiac output) showed similar variations.[9, 17, 22] Many investigators attributed the heterogeneity of the data to the fact that therapeutic interventions, gestational age, severity, and underlying cause of the disease process were not controlled for. Groenendijk and Wallenburg[51] reported on a small series of nulliparous preeclamptic women in whom measurements of MAP and cardiac output were taken before fluid loading and antihypertensive treatment. Uniformly the patients were found to be vasoconstricted, and when the patients were hydrated or treated with antihypertensive medications, the systemic vascular resistance decreased. These latter findings suggested that preeclampsia is characterized by high systemic vascular resistance.

Using noninvasive Doppler techniques for measuring cardiac output, Easterling et al[32] conducted a cross-sectional study of 36 preeclamptic women before treatment. Preeclamptic women had higher systemic vascular resistances than normotensive women; however, cardiac outputs and systemic vascular resistances varied widely, suggesting heterogeneity among the study population. The same authors conducted a prospective longitudinal study in which 179 women were enroled before 22 weeks' gestation.[31] Doppler studies were repeated at the time of the routine prenatal clinical visits and at 6 to 8 weeks' postpartum, and the results were blinded from the clinicians. Of the total study population, 45% developed gestational hypertension and 5% preeclampsia (hypertension plus proteinuria). When the cardiac outputs and systemic vascular resistances were plotted against the gestational age for both the hypertensive and normotensive women, the former group had higher cardiac outputs and lower systemic vascular resistances throughout pregnancy. Even at 6 to 8 weeks' postpartum, when all the clinical signs and symptoms of preeclampsia disappeared and BP returned to normal, cardiac output remained higher and systemic vascular resistance lower in the hypertensive group.

In a follow-up retrospective study,[30] these investigators reviewed the charts of 76 patients who were diagnosed with pregnancy-induced hypertension before 28 weeks' gestation and in whom cardiac output was measured during

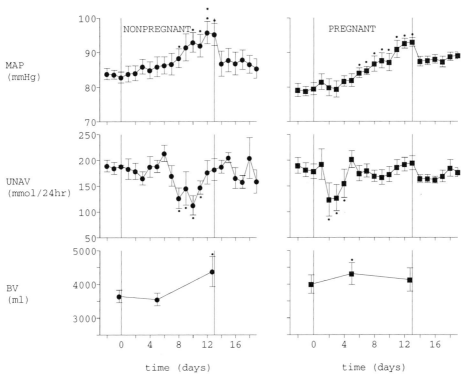

FIGURE 5–6. Effect of chronic intracarotid angiotensin II infusion (0.7 ng/kg/min) on mean arterial pressure (MAP), 24-hour sodium excretion (UNaV), and blood volume (BV) in nonpregnant (circles) and pregnant (squares) sheep. (From Mukaddam-Daher S, Cha SC, Nuwayhid BS, Quillen EW Jr. Indirect hypertensive actions of long-term intracarotid angiotensin II infusion during ovine pregnancy. Can J Physiol Pharmacol, submitted for publication, 1993.)

the pregnancy. They used a cut-off value of 1150 dynes.cm.sec^{-5} for total peripheral resistance and identified 36 low-resistance patients, 32 high-resistance patients, and 8 patients who exhibited crossover from low to high resistance. Aside from the hemodynamic data, there were no significant differences in the maternal parameters between the two groups. Comparison of the neonatal outcome showed that neonates of the high-resistance group were delivered earlier and were smaller in size (lower percentile rank) than neonates of the low-resistance group. The crossover group was too small for statistical analysis; however, it included a high number of intrauterine fetal demises and poor neonatal outcome, suggesting that a crossover from low to high maternal total peripheral resistance is ominous for the fetus.

Based on these findings, Easterling[29] suggested a hemodynamic model for pregnancy-induced hypertension based in part on the volume-loading hypertension model of Guyton.[53] Guyton showed that an increase in blood volume secondarily increases cardiac output and, in the absence of significant changes in the systemic vascular resistance, increases arterial pressure. Because an increase in cardiac output is costly in terms of energy requirements and might lead to tissue hyperperfusion, systemic vascular resistance gradually increases. The further increase in arterial pressure brought about by the increase in resistance leads to pressure diuresis and a return of the cardiac output and blood volume to near normal values. Although initial increases in arterial pressure were reached at the expense of higher blood volume and cardiac output, long-term maintenance of the arterial pressure is supported by high total systemic vascular resistance. This scenario has the effect that small changes in blood volume could lead to profound increases or decreases in arterial pressure.

Although this hypothesis for development of hypertension in pregnancy is ingenious, the documented evidence is not compelling. First, most of the studies reported in the literature[99] using invasive and noninvasive methods have documented a normal to low cardiac index and normal to high systemic vascular resistance in preeclamptic women. Second, the longitudinal prospective study by the authors showed that women who developed hypertension during pregnancy had higher cardiac outputs and lower total peripheral resistances than normotensive women during the whole pregnancy and at 6 to 8 weeks' postpartum. Because 45% of these patients developed hypertension with no proteinuria, a high percentage of them might fit the essential hypertension category. The hyperdynamic type of hypertension described by Guyton includes this group of patients. Third, the categorization of hypertensive pregnant women as *low or high resistance* might be of help for predicting neonatal outcome but not maternal prognosis. Here again the near equal division of hypertensive pregnant women between the low-resistance and high-resistance groups suggests a bimodel distribution for the population studied. Fourth, the authors emphasized the crossover from the low-resistance to the high-resistance category as support for the hyperdynamic hypertension model. There is no doubt that such a phenomenon occurs as documented by different experimental models; however, the small numbers of women who crossed over argues against this phenomenon being a natural progression of the disease process.

The aforementioned data document the heterogeneity of patients who develop hypertension in pregnancy and show that in the low-resistance group fetal and neonatal unit outcome is fairly good. More studies are needed to define this hyperdynamic model for development of hypertension in pregnancy.

Multistage Hypothesis for Development of Pregnancy Hypertension

Abnormal Maternal Immune Response

The concept that preeclampsia is an immunologic disorder has been proposed for several decades; however, only more recently and mainly owing to technical advancements in the field of immunology, interest in this area resurfaced.[33]

Accumulated evidence supporting the concept of an immune component in preeclamp-sia arose from the findings that women affected by this disorder are mainly primigravid, have pregnancies with different partners or in inconsanguineous marriages, or have a history of previous use of barrier methods for contraception. In situations in which there is increased trophoblastic mass, such as hydatidiform mole, the incidence of preeclampsia is also higher. In contrast, previous abortion, multiparity, pregnancies after previous blood transfusions, consanguineous marriages and frequent exposure to seminal fluid seem to have a protective effect.[98] MacGillivray[66] studied the incidence of preeclampsia in women who were followed during two consecutive pregnancies. He found a higher incidence of preeclampsia in the first as compared with the second pregnancy. Also, he found that a history of previous abortion had a protective effect in the development of preeclampsia. These findings were not confirmed by Campbell and Moore and colleagues,[10, 71] who found that neither a previous abortion nor a previous pregnancy delivered before term reduced the incidence of preeclampsia in the subsequent pregnancy. Further, Campbell et al reported that the outcome of a second pregnancy as it relates to preeclampsia was dependent on the outcome of the first pregnancy. If the first pregnancy was complicated by proteinuric preeclampsia, the incidence of this condition in the second pregnancy was similar to that in the first pregnancy. For women who were normotensive in the first pregnancy and delivered at term, however, the incidence of preeclampsia in a second pregnancy was reduced. As to the effect of changing partners between the first and second pregnancy, the same authors studied a subset of patients and showed that the incidence of preeclampsia in a second pregnancy is dependent on the development of preeclampsia in the first pregnancy but not on a change of partners.

The association between barrier contraception and preeclampsia was investigated by Klonoff-Cohen et al[62] in a case-control study of 110 primiparous women with preeclampsia and 115 pregnant women without preeclampsia. They found that women who used barrier contraceptives were more than twice as likely to develop preeclampsia. Further, women who were exposed to smaller amounts of sperm were at a greater risk of developing preeclampsia.

The role of various lymphocyte subsets, complement, circulating antibodies, and human leukocyte antigen (HLA) in the pathogenesis of preeclampsia has been investigated.[33] Although most studies found no changes in the serum levels of immunoglobulins, the serum concentrations of various complement components were altered in cases of severe preeclampsia. This latter finding could be the result of an acute phase reaction. The role of various lymphocyte subsets in development of preeclampsia was investigated,[4, 71, 103] and Moore et al[71] showed a slight increase in the T helper cells; this slight increase, however, did not support a major role for these cells in the pathogenesis of preeclampsia.

The association between autoantibodies and preeclampsia has been investigated.[42, 50] Foidart et al[42] reported that sera of preeclamptic women contained higher titer of antilaminin and suggested that these antibodies might play a role in the pathogenesis of preeclampsia. Gregorini et al[50] hypothesized that lupus-like anticoagulant antibodies, present in both preeclampsia and recurrent abortions, impaired synthesis of prostaglandin I_2 (PGI_2) and interfered with normal placentation.

The role of different HLA types in development of preeclampsia has also been studied.[60, 94] Redman et al[94] found an increased incidence of double homozygosity for HLA-A and HLA-B antigens in preeclamptic women, whereas Kilpatrick et al[60] reported an increased incidence of preeclampsia in the presence of $HLA-DR_4$. These findings were not confirmed by others, suggesting that HLA typing might be of limited value in surveillance for preeclampsia.

Greer et al[49] reported that neutrophil activation in the placental vascular bed occurs in preeclampsia. They suggested that activated neutrophils release various substances, such as elastases and proteases, that destroy the integrity of the vessel wall. Oxygen free radicals also released by activated neutrophils cause membrane lipid peroxidation, disruption of endothelial integrity, and secondarily increased vascular permeability. Leukotriene, especially leukotriene B_4 production levels are reported to be higher in preeclampsia,[85] and these in-creased levels might contribute to increased arteriopathy. Although it is not known what pathogenic factors are involved, it is thought that the activation of neutrophils is most probably secondary to some immunologic mechanisms implicated in preeclampsia.

Endothelial Cell Dysfunction

Endothelial cell injury or altered cell function is thought to play a role in the pathogenesis of preeclampsia. The increased levels of factor VIII–related antigens, fibronectin and fibronectin ED_1, and the disturbance of tissue plasminogen activator/plasminogen activator inhibitor (tPA/PAI) and PGI_2/thromboxane A_2 (TXA_2) balances suggests that endothelial cell damage may be involved in the pathogenesis of preeclampsia.[95]

Plasma fibronectin is derived primarily from liver and endothelial cells and has been used as a marker of endothelial cell damage. During the course of a normal pregnancy, plasma fibronectin concentration rises by about 20% during the third trimester (average 200 to 395 $\mu g/mL$).[54] Several studies have shown that with mild to severe preeclampsia, there is a twofold to threefold increase in plasma fibronectin levels.[34, 106]

The predictive value of fibronectin levels in normotensive gravid women destined to become preeclamptic was assessed by Lazarchick et al.[65] In 16 of 17 normotensive women who subsequently developed preeclampsia, plasma fibronectin levels were abnormally high (>400 $\mu g/mL$). Further, 13 of the women (76%) had elevated levels detectable more than 4 weeks before the onset of hypertension.

With regard to preeclampsia, PGI_2 and TXA_2 are the most relevant eicosanoids. TXA_2 is a potent vasoconstrictor and a stimulus to platelet aggregation, whereas PGI_2 has the opposite effect on platelet function and vascular tone. Preeclampsia is thought to be a state of relative PGI_2 deficiency and TXA_2 dominance.[115] Fitzgerald and colleagues[40, 41] reported that urinary excretion of TXA_2 metabolites correlated with some of the indices for severity of preeclampsia. Further, they showed that a decrease in the PGI_2 excretion precedes clinical disease. For the decrease in vasodilator prostaglandins to produce hypertension, the intrarenal production of PGI_2 and PGE_2 should decrease[38, 84] and the renal action of angiotensin II become unopposed. The arterial pressure–sodium excretion curve, which normally shifts to the left during pregnancy (see Fig. 5-4), would then shift to the right with a decrease in its slope, and the arterial pressure would increase to maintain sodium and fluid balance. Although the imbalance between PGI_2/TXA_2 explains many of the clinical findings of preeclampsia, so far it has not been shown that this disturbed balance is the principal pathogenic mechanism.

Several studies suggest that PGI_2 deficiency is not the primary change in the pathogenesis of preeclampsia. Further, vasodilator prostaglandins do not appear to be the major vasodepressor agents of pregnancy.[20] For example, Sorensen et al[100] determined BP and cardiac output before and after an 18-hour interval during which 23 pregnant women were given 75 mg indomethacin. Those authors found that the increase in vascular resistance was minimal and concluded that other vasodilators were largely responsible for the decreased peripheral vascular resistance of normal pregnancy. In addition, we have determined the influence of continuous indomethacin infusion on the steady-state relationships between arterial pressure and urinary sodium excretion in nonpregnant and pregnant sheep.[78] Over a wide range of sodium intakes, the urinary excretions of PGE_2 and the prostacyclin metabolite, 6 keto-$PGF_1\alpha$, were reduced to approximately 50% of these control levels by indomethacin. Nevertheless, the arterial pressure–urinary sodium excretion relationships were not altered in either nonpregnant or pregnant sheep. These data are in agreement with the conclusion that vasodilator prostaglandins are not the principal depressor agents of pregnancy. In addition, these findings suggest that prostaglandins have a minimal role in the maintenance of pressure and volume homeostasis during pregnancy.

The physiologic vasodilation during pregnancy and the pathologic vasoconstriction in preeclampsia might be mediated by endothelial-derived relaxing or constricting factors (EDRF and EDCF). Evidence supporting a physiologic role for EDRF includes the following: EDRF released from uterine vascular endothelium is increased during pregnancy, treatment of rabbits with 17-β estradiol increased endothelium-dependent relaxation to acetylcholine; and decrease in arterial pressure in pregnancy in spontaneously hypertensive rats was completely dependent on EDRF release.[2, 48, 116] In preeclampsia, EDRF production by the umbilical vessels secondary to bradykinin stimulation is reduced,[87] and sera of antepartum patients with preeclampsia show elevated levels of endothelial cytotoxic activity[95] and antivascular endothelial cell antibodies.[90] More recently, endothelin, an endothelium-derived circulating peptide with potent vasoactive properties, was found to be significantly increased in preeclamptic pregnant women. Plasma concentrations returned to normal within 48 hours after delivery.[109] Present data are highly suggestive that the endothelium plays a major role in normal pregnancy and preeclampsia; however, it is not known to what extent EDRF is involved with the physiologic vasodilatation of pregnancy nor to what extent endothelial injury might be a major pathologic factor in preeclampsia.

Platelet Dysfunction and Coagulation Abnormalities

Redman[91] suggested that preeclampsia is "a trophoblast-dependent process mediated by platelet dysfunction." In the absence of adequate production of PGI_2 and EDRF in the uteroplacental circulation, surface-mediated activation of platelets occurs. Both TXA_2 and serotonin are generated locally, seconday to platelet activation. TXA_2 is a known vasoconstrictor and enhances platelet aggregation. Serotonin released by platelets is partially destroyed by endothelial enzymes; however, its circulatory effects might depend on the intactness of the vascular endothelium. Van-Houtte[111] argued that in a vessel with intact endothelium, serotonin interacts with the S_1 serotoninergic receptors located on the endothelial cells. A positive feedback signal is generated, which increases the local synthesis of PGE_2 and EDRF. This mechanism is thought to provide protection against excess accumulation of platelets and thrombi formation. Alternatively, the response of diseased or denuded vascular wall to serotonin differs in that serotonin interacts with the S_2 serotoninergic receptors on the vascular smooth muscle cells to cause direct contraction. Additionally, the S_2 receptor stimulation amplifies the vasoconstrictor action of catecholamines and angiotensin II. Stimulation of the S_2-serotoninergic receptors on the platelets amplifies the aggregation process, with the release of more serotonin, thus leading to a positive feedback loop.

The pivotal function of platelets in preeclampsia is suggested by the results of several low-dose aspirin studies.[8, 97, 114] Administration of 60 to 100 mg per day of aspirin, a dose adequate to blunt platelet aggregation, prevents the clinical symptoms of preeclampsia in women with increased responsiveness to angiotensin II.

Preeclampsia is associated with enhanced activation of blood coagulation and increased risk of thrombosis and thromboembolism.[26] The increased factor VIII–related antigen to VIII coagulant ratio in preeclampsia may reflect enhanced thrombin generation. Antithrombin III activity is also reduced in preeclampsia, probably as a secondary response to its increased consumption because there is a progressive increase in thrombin–antithrombin III complexes in pregnancy-induced hypertension.

The increased blood coagulability that is associated with preeclampsia may also be explained, in part, by elevated fibrin levels. There is a decreased fibrinolytic activity in patients with preeclampsia that is attributed to increased plasma levels of PAI-1 and PAI-2.[5] In addition, an imbalance between tPA and PAI activities appears to contribute to the persistence of fibrin in the uteroplacental and renal microcirculation.

Oxygen Free Radicals

Oxygen free radical formation and increased lipid peroxidation have been suggested to be among the main factors responsible for endothelial cell injury. Free radicals are produced during normal physiologic processes, ischemia, ischemia-reperfusion, and immune reactions.[61] The superoxide anion shifts the PGI_2/TXA_2 ratio in favor of TXA_2, which in turn enhances vasoconstriction and platelet aggregation. Superoxide can also be cytotoxic to the cells by enhancing lipid peroxidation of the cellular membranes. The peroxides in turn damage the endothelium, break down EDRF, and activate the coagulation system.[52]

The contribution of oxygen free radicals to the pathogenesis of preeclampsia has been studied by several investigators.[28, 55] Hubel et al[55] hypothesized that a "placental oxidant-antioxidant imbalance intensifies the release of placental lipid peroxidation products into the circulation." The lipid peroxidation products in turn damage the endothelial lining and selectively reduce PGI_2 synthesis.

Multistage Hypothesis for Development of Preeclampsia

Zeeman and Dekker[117] proposed a unifying hypothesis for development of pregnancy-induced hypertension. It states that pregnancy is a state of immunologic tolerance between the fetus (paternal allograft) and maternal tissue. Adaptation of the immune system leads to endovascular trophoblast invasion of the uteroplacental circulation with loss of autonomic innervation and muscular layer of the spinal arteries.[43] Simultaneously the endovascular trophoblasts and the endothelium increase synthesis of vasodilating substances, such as EDRF and PGI_2 and consequently the uteroplacental circulation becomes a high-flow, low-resistance system.

In preeclampsia, immunologic maladaptation results in insufficient ingrowth of trophoblast and activation of neutrophils, macrophages, and T cells. Tissue ischemia and neutrophil activation produce oxygen free radicals, which in turn might cause vascular endothelial cell damage. EDRF activity and PGI_2 synthesis are decreased, and platelet-derived TXA_2 production is increased. Further, in the absence of adequate production of PGI_2 and disruption of the vascular endothelium, platelet activation and activation of coagulation system might occur. In addition, serotonin and TXA_2 levels are increased and result in further vasoconstriction. As mentioned earlier,[111] serotonin in the presence of intact endothelium might stimulate the S_1 serotoninergic receptors and through a positive feedback mechanism increase production of vasodilators such as PGI_2 and EDRF. In situations in which the endothelium is disrupted, the S_2 serotoninergic receptors on vascular smooth muscle cells are stimulated and vasoconstriction occurs. The combination of vasoconstriction, microangiopathy, and thrombosis leads to decreased uteroplacental perfusion as seen in severe preeclampsia.

Roberts et al[95] suggested that preeclampsia is an endothelial cell disorder. They speculated that decreased placental perfusion, be it secondary to maternal vasculitis, inadequate trophoblast invasion, or increased trophoblast mass, leads to production of endothelial cytotoxins and generalized endothelial cell injury. Endothelial cell injury in turn leads to development of generalized vasospasm, activation of intravasular coagulation mechanisms, and fibrin deposition.[45]

Redman[91] suggested that preeclampsia is a trophoblastic disease "mediated by platelet dysfunction." The rationale being (1) platelets contribute to the pathogenesis of preeclampsia,[93] (2) the disturbances in the platelets occur earlier than that in the smooth muscle,[118] and (3) the disease can be prevented or ameliorated by low-dose aspirin.[24]

SUMMARY

Regardless of minor differences among the various hypotheses, there is general agreement that abnormal maternal immune responses, endothelial cell injury, and platelet dysfunction play an important role in the pathogenesis of preeclampsia. Still the major question to be answered relates to the primary immunologic or biochemical mechanisms leading to the development of preeclampsia.

REFERENCES

1. Aberdeen GW, Cha SC, Mukaddam-Daher S, et al. Renal nerve effects on renal adaptation to changes in sodium intake during ovine pregnancy. Am J Physiol 1992;262:F823.
2. Ahokas RA, Mercer BM, Sibia BM. Enhanced endothelium-derived relaxing factor activity in pregnant spontaneously hypertensive rats (abstr). Am J Obstet Gynecol 1991;164(suppl):242.
3. Ales KL, Norton ME, Dryzen ML. Early prediction of antepartum hypertension. Obstet Gynecol 1989;73:928.
4. Bailey K, Herrod HL, Younger R, et al. Functional aspects of T-lymphocyte subsets in pregnancy. Obstet Gynecol 1985;66:211.
5. Ballegeer V, Spitz B, Kieckens L, et al. Predictive value of increased plasma levels of fibronectin in gestational hypertension. Am J Obstet Gynecol 1989;161:432.
6. Barr SM, Lees KR, Butters L, et al. Platelet intracellular free calcium concentration in normotensive and hypertensive pregnancies in the human. Clin Sci 1989;76:67.
7. Barron WM, Mujais SK, Zinamann M, et al. Plasma catecholamine responses to physiologic stimuli in normal human pregnancy. Am J Obstet Gynecol 1986;154:80.
8. Beaufils M, Vzan S, Donsimoni R, et al. Prevention of preeclampsia by early antiplatelet therapy. Lancet 1985;1:840.
9. Bendetti TJ, Cotton DB, Read JC, Miller FC. Hemodynamic observations in severe pre-eclampsia with a flow-directed pulmonary artery catheter. Am J Obstet Gynecol 1980;136:465.
10. Campbell D, MacGillivray I, Carr-Hill P. Preeclampsia in second pregnancy. Br J Obstet Gynaecol 1985;92:131.
11. Cha SC, Aberdeen GW, Nuwayhid BS, Quillen EW Jr. Influence of pregnancy on mean systemic filling pressure and the cardiac function curve in guinea pigs. Can J Physiol Pharmacol 1992;70:669.
12. Cha SC, Mukaddam-Daher S, Quillen EW Jr, Nuwayhid BS. Tubular handling of fluid and electrolytes during ovine pregnancy. Am J Physiol 1993, 265: (in press).
13. Cha SC, Mukaddam-Daher S, Quillen EW Jr, Nuwayhid BS. Autoregulation of renal blood flow during ovine pregnancy. Hypertension in Pregnancy 1993;12:71.
14. Chesley LC. Proposal for classification. In: Friedman EA, ed. Blood pressure, edema and proteinuria in pregnancy. New York: Alan R. Liss, 1976:251.
15. Chesley LC. Hypertension in pregnancy: definitions, familial factor and remote prognosis. Kidney Int 1980;18:234.
16. Chesley LC, Cooper DW. Genetics of hypertension in pregnancy: possible single gene control of preeclampsia on the descendants of eclamptic women. Br J Obstet Gynaecol 1986;93:898.
17. Clark SL, Greenspoon JS, Aldahl D, Phelan JP. Severe preeclampsia with persistent oliguria: management of hemodynamic subsets. Am J Obstet Gynecol 1986;154:490.
18. Clark S, Hofmeyer G, Coats A, et al. Ambulatory blood pressure monitoring during pregnancy: evaluation of the TM-2420 monitor. Obstet Gynecol 1991;77:152.
19. Coleman GT, Guyton AC. Hypertension caused by salt loading in the dog. III. Onset transients of cardiac output and other circulatory variables. Circ Res 1969;25:153.
20. Conrad KP, Colpays ML. Evidence against the hypothesis that prostaglandins are the vasodepressor agents of pregnancy. J Clin Invest 1986;77:236.
21. Cooper DW, Hill JA, Chesley LC, et al. Genetic control of susceptibility to eclampsia and miscarriage. Br J Obstet Gynaecol 1988;95:644.
22. Cotton DB, Lee W, Huhta JC, Dorman KF. Hemody-

namic profile of severe pregnancy-induced hypertension. Am J Obstet Gynecol 1988;158:523.

23. Cowley AW, Lohmeier TE. Changes in renal vascular sensitivity and arterial pressure associated with sodium intake during long-term intrarenal norepinephrine infusion in dogs. Hypertension 1979;1:549.

24. Cunningham FG, Gant NF. Prevention of preeclampsia—a reality? N Engl J Med 1989;321:606.

25. Davey DA, MacGillivray I. The classification and definition of the hypertensive disorders of pregnancy. Am J Obstet Gynecol 1988;158:892.

26. deBoer K, tenCate JW, Sturk A, et al. Enhanced thrombin generation in normal and hypertensive pregnancy. Am J Obstet Gynecol 1989;160:95.

27. DeClue JW, Guyton AC, Cowley AW Jr, et al. Subpressor angiotensin infusion, renal sodium handling, and salt-induced hypertension in the dog. Circ Res 1978; 43:503.

28. Dekker GA, Kraayenbrink AA. Oxygen free radicals in preeclampsia (abstr). Am J Obstet Gynecol 1991; 164(suppl):273.

29. Easterling TR. The maternal hemadynamics of preeclampsia. Clin Obstet Gynecol 1992;35:375.

30. Easterling TR, Benedetti TJ, Carlson KC, et al. The effect of maternal hemodynamics on fetal growth in hypertensive pregnancies. Am J Obstet Gynecol 1991;165:902.

31. Easterling TR, Benedetti TJ, Schmucker BL, et al. Maternal hemodynamics in normal and preeclamptic pregnancies: a longitudinal study. Obstet Gynecol 1990;76:1061.

32. Easterling TR, Watts DH, Schmucher BC, et al. Measurement of cardiac output during pregnancy: a validation of Doppler technique and clinical observations in preeclampsia. Obstet Gynecol 1987;69:845.

33. El-Raeiy A, Gleicher N. The immunologic concept of preeclampsia. In: Rubin PC, ed. Handbook of hypertension: hypertension in pregnancy. Vol 10. New York: Elsevier Science, 1988:257.

34. Erikson HO, Hansen PK, Brocks V, et al. Plasma fibronectin concentration in preeclampsia. Acta Obstet Gynecol Scand 1987;66:25.

35. Fairlie FM. Doppler flow velocimetry in hypertension in pregnancy: hypertension and pregnancy. Clin Perinatol 1991;18:749.

36. Fan L, Archambault D, Chavez S, et al. Influences of renal nerves on renin secretion during ovine pregnancy. Am J Physiol 1993, In press.

37. Farmakides G, Schulman H, Schneider E. Surveillance of the pregnant hypertensive patient with doppler flow velocimetry. Clin Obstet Gynecol 1992; 35:387.

38. Ferris TF. Prostanoids in normal and hypertensive pregnancy. In: Rubin PC, ed. Handbook of hypertension: hypertension in pregnancy. Vol 10. New York: Elsevier, 1988:102.

39. Fisher KA, Luger A, Sporgo BH, et al. Hypertension in pregnancy: clinical-pathological correlations and remote prognosis. Medicine 1981;60:267.

40. Fitzgerald DJ, Entman SS, Mullay K, et al. Decreased prostacyclin biosynthesis preceding the clinical manifestations of pregnancy induced hypertension. Circulation 1987;75:956.

41. Fitzgerald DJ, Rocki W, Murray R, et al. Thromboxane-A2 synthesis in pregnancy induced hypertension. Lancet 1990; 1:335:751.

42. Foidart JM, Hunt J, Lopiere LM, et al. Antibodies to laminin in preeclampsia. Kidney Int 1986;29:1050.

43. Fox H. The placenta in pregnancy hypertension. In: Rubin PC, ed. Handbook of hypertension: hypertension in pregnancy. Vol 10. New York: Elsevier Science Publishers, 1988:16.

44. Frenkel Y, Barkai G, Mashiach S, et al. Hypocalciuria of preeclampsia is independent of parathyroid hormone level. Obstet Gynecol 1991;77:689.

45. Friedman SA, Taylor RN, Roberts JM. Pathophysiology of preeclampsia: hypertension in pregnancy. Clin Perinatol 1991;18:661.

46. Gant NF, Chand S, Worley RJ, et al. A clinical test useful for predicting the development of acute hypertension in pregnancy. Am J Obstet Gynecol 1974; 120:1.

47. Gant WF, Daley GL, Chand S, et al. A study of angiotensin II pressor response throughout primigravid pregnancy. J Clin Invest 1973;52:2682.

48. Gischard V, Miller VM, Vanhoulte PM. Effect of 17-β estradiol on endothelium-dependent responses in the rabbit. J Pharmacol Exp Ther 1988;244:19.

49. Greer IA, Butterworth B, Liston WA, et al. Neutrophil activation in PIH: localization to the placental bed (abstr). Proceedings of the VII World Congress of Hypertension in Pregnancy, Perugia, Italy, 1990:276.

50. Gregorini G, Setti G, Remuzzi G. Recurrent abortion with lupus anticoagulant, and preeclampsia: a common final pathway for two different diseases? Case Report. Br J Obstet Gynaecol 1986;93:194.

51. Groenendijk R, Trimbos JBMJ, Wallenburg HCS. Hemodynamic measurements in preeclampsia: preliminary observations. Am J Obstet Gynecol 1984; 150:232.

52. Gryglewski RJ, Palmer RMJ, Moncada S. Superoxide anion is involved in the breakdown of endothelium-derived vascular relaxing factor. Nature 1989; 320:454.

53. Guyton AC. Arterial pressure and hypertension. Philadelphia: WB Saunders, 1980.

54. Hess LW, O'Brien WF, Holmberg JA, et al. Plasma and amniotic fluid concentrations of fibronectin during normal pregnancy. Obstet Gynecol 1986;68:25.

55. Hubel CA, Roberts JM, Taylor RN, et al. Lipid peroxidation in pregnancy: New perspectives on preeclampsia. Am J Obstet Gynecol 1989;161:1025.

56. Hughes EL. Obstetric gynecology terminology. Philadelphia: FA Davis, 1972.

57. Jacobson SL, Imhof R, Manning N, et al. The value of Doppler assessment of the uteroplacental circulation in predicting preeclampsia or intrauterine growth retardation. Am J Obstet Gynecol 1990; 162:110.

58. Karbhari D, Harrigan JT, LaMagra R. The supine hypertensive test as a predictor of incipient preeclampsia. Am J Obstet Gynecol 1977;127:620.

59. Katz AI, Davison JM, Hayslett JP, et al. Pregnancy in women with kidney disease. Kidney Int 1980;18:192.

60. Kilpatrick DL, Gibson F, Liston WA, et al. Association between susceptibility to preeclampsia within families and HLA DR4. Lancet 1989;1:1063.

61. Kloner RA, Przyklenk K, Whittaker P. Deleterious effects of oxygen radicals in ischemia/reperfusion, resolved and unresolved issues. Circulation 1989; 80:1115.

62. Klonoff-Cohen HS, Savitz DA, Cefalo RC, et al. An epidemiological study of contraception and preeclampsia. JAMA 1989;262:3143.

63. Kottke FJ, Kubilek WG, Visscher MB. The production of arterial hypertension by chronic renal artery-nerve stimulation. Am J Physiol 1945;145:38.

64. Kwan CY. Dysfunction of calcium handling by smooth

muscle in hypertension. Can J Physiol Pharmacol 1985;63:366.

65. Lazarchick J, Stubbs TM, Romein L, et al. Predictive value of fibronectin levels in normotensive gravid women destined to become preeclamptic. Am J Obstet Gynecol 1986;154:1050.

66. MacGillivray I. Some observations on the incidence of preeclampsia. Br J Obstet Gynaecol 1958;65:536.

67. MacGillivray I, Rose GA, Rowe B. Blood pressure survey in pregnancy. Clin Sci 1969;37:395.

68. Management of preeclampsia. ACOG Technical Bulletin 1986;91:1.

69. Manning RD Jr, Coleman TG, Guyton AC, et al. Essential role of mean circulatory filling pressure in salt-induced hypertension. Am J Physiol 1979;236:H314.

70. McLaughlin MK, Mathews T, Cooke R. Vascular catecholamine sensitivity during pregnancy in the ewe. Am J Obstet Gynecol 1989;160:47.

71. Moore MP, Carter NP, Redman CWG. Lymphocyte subsets in normal and preeclamptic pregnancies. Br J Obstet Gynaecol 1983;90:326.

72. Morris JA, O'Grady JP, Hamilton CJ, Davidson EC. Vascular reactivity to angiotensin II infusion during gestation. Am J Obstet Gynecol 1978;130:379.

73. Moutquin JM, Desmarais L. Circadian recording of ambulatory blood pressure in normotensive and hypertensive pregnancies (abstr #280). Presented at the Society for Gynecologic Investigation, San Diego, CA 1989.

74. Moutquin JM, Desmarais L, Bastide A, et al. Prédiction de la prééclampsie: la tension artérielle ambulatoire. J Obstet Gynecol Biol Reprod 1992;21:313.

75. Moutquin JM, Desmarais L, Marie V, et al. Diagnostic value of circadian ambulatory blood pressure monitoring in pregnancy hypertension (abstr #305). Presented at the Society for Gynecologic Investigation, San Antonio, Texas, 1992.

76. Montquin JM, Rainville C, Giroux L, et al. A prospective study of blood pressure in pregnancy: prediction of preeclampsia. Am J Obstet Gynecol 1985;151:191.

77. Mukaddam-Daher S, Cha SC, Nuwayhid BS, Quillen EW Jr. Indirect hypertensive actions of long-term intracarotid angiotensin II infusion during ovine pregnancy. Can J Physiol Pharmacol 1992; submitted.

78. Mukaddam-Daher S, Moutquin J-M, Nuwayhid B, Quillen EW. Effects of prostaglandin inhibition on the renal function curve during ovine pregnancy. Am J Obstet Gynecol 1993. Submitted.

79. Murray RH, Luft FC, Black R, et al. Blood pressure responses to extremes of sodium intake in normal man. Proc Soc Exp Biol Med 1978;159:432.

80. National High Blood Pressure Education Program Working Group. Report on high blood pressure in pregnancy. Bethesda MD: Department of Health and Human Services, National Heart, Lung and Blood Institutes, 1990.

81. O'Brien WF. The prediction of preeclampsia. Clin Obstet Gynecol 1992;35:351.

82. Öney T, Kauhausen H. The value of the angiotensin sensitivity test in the early diagnosis of hypertensive disorders in pregnancy. Am J Obstet Gynecol 1982;142:17.

83. Page EW, Christianson R. The impact of mean arterial pressure in the middle trimester upon the outcome of pregnancy. Am J Obstet Gynecol 1976;125:740.

84. Pedersen EB, Aakjaer C, Christensen AJ, et al. Renin, angiotensin II, aldosterone, catecholamines, prosta-

glandins and vasopressin: the importance of pressor and depressor factors for hypertension in pregnancy. Scand J Clin Lab Invest 1984;44(suppl 169):48.

85. Pelusi G, Scagliarini G, Biagi G, et al. Neutrophil production of leukotriene-B4 is increased in gestational hypertension (abstr). Proceedings VII World Congress of Hypertension in Pregnancy, Perugia, Italy, 1990:199.

86. Phelan JP, Everidge GJ, Wilder TL, Newman C. Is the supine pressor test an adequate means of predicting acute hypertension in pregnancy? Am J Obstet Gynecol 1977;128:173.

87. Pinto A, Sorrentino R, Sorrentino P, et al. Endothelial-derived relaxing factor released by endothelial cells of human umbilical vessels and its impairment in pregnancy-induced hypertension. Am J Obstet Gynecol 1991;164:507.

88. Quillen EW Jr, Aljabari AW, Nuwayhid BS. Central nervous system contributions to the pressor action of angiotensin II in sinoaortic denervated pregnant sheep, in preparation.

89. Quillen EW Jr, Nuwayhid BS. Steady-state arterial pressure–urinary output relationships during ovine pregnancy. Am J Physiol 1992; 263:R1141.

90. Rappaport VJ, Hirata G, Yap HK, Jordan SC. Antivascular endothelial cell antibodies in severe preeclampsia. Am J Obstet Gynecol 1990;162:138.

91. Redman CWG. Platelets and the beginning of preeclampsia (edit). N Engl J Med 1990;323:478.

92. Redman CWG, Beilin LJ, Bonnar J. Variability of blood pressure in normal and abnormal pregnancy. In: Lindheimer MD, Katz AI, Zuspan FP, eds. Hypertension in pregnancy. New York: John Wiley, 1976:53.

93. Redman CWG, Bonnar J, Beilin L. Early platelet consumption in preeclampsia. BMJ 1978;1:467.

94. Redman CWG, Bodmer WF, Bodmer JH, et al. HLA antigens in severe preeclampsia. Lancet 1978;2:397.

95. Roberts JM, Taylor RN, Musci TJ, et al. Preeclampsia: an endothelial cell disorder. Am J Obstet Gynecol 1989;161:1200.

96. Sanchez-Ramos L, Jones DC, Cullen MT. Urinary calcium as an early marker for preeclampsia. Obstet Gynecol 1991;77:685.

97. Schiff E, Pelez E, Goldenberg M, et al. The use of aspirin to prevent pregnancy-induced hypertension and lower the ratio of the thromboxane A2 to prostacyclin in relatively high risk pregnancies. N Engl J Med 1989;321:351.

98. Sibai BM. Immunologic aspects of preeclampsia. Clin Obstet Gynecol 1991;34:27.

99. Sibai BM, Mabie WC. Hemodynamics of preeclampsia: hypertension and pregnancy. Clin Perinatol 1991;18:727.

100. Sorensen TK, Easterling TR, Carbon KL, et al. The maternal hemodynamic effect of indomethacin in normal pregnancy. Obstet Gynecol 1992;79:661.

101. Sowers JR, Zemel MB, Bronsteen RA, et al. Erythrocyte cation metabolism in preeclampsia. Am J Obstet Gynecol 1989;161:441.

102. Sowers JR, Zemel MB, Standley PR, et al. Calcium and hypertension. J Lab Clin Med 1989;114:338.

103. Sridama V, Yang S-L, Moawad A, DeGroot LJ. T-cell subsets in patients with preeclampsia. Am J Obstet Gynecol 1983;147:566.

104. Steel SA, Pearce JM, McParkland P, Chamberlin GVP. Early doppler ultrasound screening in prediction of hypertensive disorders of pregnancy. Lancet 1990; 1:335:1548.

105. Strazzullo P, Nunziata V, Cirillo M, et al. Abnormali-

ties of calcium metabolism in essential hypertension. Clin Sci 1983;65:137.

106. Stubbs TM, Lazarchick J, Horger EO. Plasma fibronectin levels in preeclampsia: a possible biochemical marker for vascular endothelial damage. Am J Obstet Gynecol 1984;150:885.

107. Tabsh K, Rudelstrofer R, Nuwayhid B, et al. Circulatory responses to hypovolemia in the pregnant and nonpregnant sheep after pharmacologic sympathectomy. Am J Obstet Gynecol 1986;154:411.

108. Taufield PA, Ales KL, Resnick LM, et al. Hypocalciuria in preeclampsia. N Engl J Med 1987;316:715.

109. Taylor RN, Varma M, Teng NNH, et al. Women with preeclampsia have higher plasma endothelin levels than women with normal pregnancies. J Clin Endocrinol Metab 1990;71:1675.

110. Ushioda E, Nuwayhid B, Kleinman G, et al. The contribution of the β-adrenergic system to the cardiovascular response to hypovolemia. Am J Obstet Gynecol 1983;147:423.

111. VanHoutte PM. Serotonergic antagonists and vascular disease. Cardiovasc Drugs Ther 1990;4:7.

112. Villar J, Repke J, Markush L, et al. The measuring of blood pressure during pregnancy. Am J Obstet Gynecol 1989;161:1019.

113. Villar MA, Sibai BM. Clinical significance of elevated mean arterial blood pressure in second trimester and threshold increase in systolic or diastolic blood pressure during third trimester. Am J Obstet Gynecol 1989;160:419.

114. Wallenburg HCS, Dekker GA, Makovitz JW, et al. Low dose aspirin prevents pregnancy-induced hypertension and preeclampsia in angiotensin sensitive primigravidae. Lancet 1986;1:1.

115. Walsh SW. Preeclampsia: an imbalance in placental prostacyclin and thromboxane production. Am J Obstet Gynecol 1985;152:335.

116. Weiner CE, Martinez E, Zhu LK, et al. In vitro release of endothelium-derived relaxing factor by acetylcholine is increased during the guinea pig pregnancy. Am J Obstet Gynecol 1989;161:1599.

117. Zeeman GG, Dekker GA. Pathogenesis of preeclampsia: a hypothesis. Clin Obstet Gynecol 1922; 35:317.

118. Zemel MB, Zemel PC, Berry S, et al. Altered platelet calcium metabolism as an early predictor of increased peripheral vascular resistance and preeclampsia in urban black women. N Engl J Med 1990;32:434.

The Renin-Angiotensin-Aldosterone System and Vasopressin

Ellen W. Seely

Thomas J. Moore

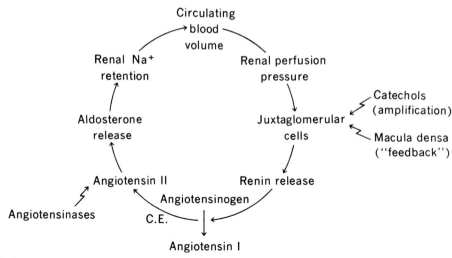

FIGURE 6–1. Renin release is controlled by a number of factors, with a major one being a volume-mediated negative feedback loop. (Adapted from Williams GH, Dluhy RG, Thorn GW. In: Thorn GW, et al, eds. Harrison's Principles of Internal Medicine, ed 8. New York: McGraw-Hill, 1977:520. With permission.)

Pregnancy is characterized by important changes in fluid and electrolyte balance, which are largely dictated by pregnancy-induced changes in the *renin-angiotensin-aldosterone (RAS) axis* and in *vasopressin*.

RENIN-ANGIOTENSIN-ALDOSTERONE SYSTEM

Since 1954, when aldosterone, the principal salt-retaining hormone of the adrenal, was identified by Simpson et al,[84] an extensive body of literature on the potential role of this hormone in diseases associated with sodium retention has accumulated. Because the renin-angiotensin system is a major regulator of aldosterone secretion (angiotensin also being the most potent vasoconstrictor agent endogenously produced), a critical role for the RAS axis has been advocated in edema disorders and hypertension. Considerable changes occur in sodium and water balance during pregnancy. Thus it is not surprising that the RAS axis has been implicated both in the edema accompanying normal pregnancy and in the hypertensive states (preeclampsia and eclampsia) associated with pregnancy. This chapter reviews the regulation of the RAS system and potential alterations in its control in the nonpregnant state, during pregnancy, and in the developing fetus.

Renin and Angiotensin

Research has suggested that renin-angiotensin system plays a much broader role in physiologic processes than has traditionally been appreciated. In addition to the renin and angiotensin present in the circulating plasma, it is now known that renin and angiotensin are synthesized and stored in a variety of peripheral tissues.[10, 42] These "local" renin-angiotensin systems may, in fact, affect some of the functions previously attributed to the circulating system. In addition, these local systems also provide the potential for renin and angiotensin to play a role in several novel physiologic functions. In describing our current understanding of the renin-angiotensin system, we discuss both the classic, circulating system and local systems.

Circulating Renin-Angiotensin System

Renin is a proteolytic enzyme produced and stored in the granules of the renal juxtaglomerular cells that surround the afferent arterioles of the cortical glomeruli. After release, renin splits a decapeptide, angiotensin I, from its circulating substrate, the α_2 globulin angiotensinogen (Fig. 6–1). Angiotensin I is then enzymatically converted by angiotensin-converting enzyme located in the lung and elsewhere to the octapeptide, angiotensin II. Angiotensin II is a potent pressor compound, exerting its pressor action by a direct effect on arterial smooth muscle.[47] In addition, angiotensin II is a potent direct stimulus for the production of aldosterone. Angiotensinases in plasma, erthyrocytes, and vascular endothelium rapidly destroy angiotensin II, which has a half-life of approximately 1 minute.

Renin release by the kidney is controlled by several factors.[18] These are interdependent, and the amount of renin released is a composite of the input of all factors. The juxtaglomerular cells, which are specialized myoephithelial cells of the afferent arteriole, act as miniature pressor transducers that sense renal perfusion pressure. The changes in pressure are perceived as distortions in the stretch on the arterial wall. Thus for example, with reduction in circulating blood volume, a corresponding reduction of renal perfusion pressure and in afferent arteriolar pressure occurs. This is perceived by the juxtaglomerular cells, which then release more renin to normalize blood volume and blood pressure via the effect of angiotensin II on aldosterone and vascular tone. So the RAS system subserves volume control by appropriate modification of renal tubular sodium transport.

A second control mechanism for renin release is centered in the macula densa cells of the distal convoluted tubule. It has been suggested that these cells may function as chemoreceptors, monitoring the sodium load present in distal tubules, and that such information is directly fed back to the juxtaglomerular cells, where appropriate modifications of renin release take place. The evidence for this hypothesis, however, is conflicting. Third, the sympathetic nervous system is the predominant factor regulating renin release in response to assuming the upright posture. The mechanism by which sympathetic activity alters renin release is largely via a direct effect on the juxtaglomerular cells.

Finally, a number of circulating factors may alter renin release, such as potassium[22] (increasing dietary potassium directly decreases renin release) and angiotensin II[107] (increasing angiotensin II concentration reduces renin release via a direct *short feedback loop*). The control of renin release is certainly complex, consisting of both intrarenal (pressor receptor and macula densa) and extrarenal (sympathetic nervous system, potassium, angiotensin) mechanisms.[18]

Local Tissue Renin-Angiotensin Systems

In addition to the circulating renin-angiotensin system, it is now well established that many tissues in addition to the kidney synthesize renin and angiotensins. These tissues include the pituitary gland, vascular smooth muscle, adrenal cortex, ovarian follicles, and uterus.[10, 42, 55, 56, 63] The specific functions of these local systems have not been entirely elucidated. Some local specific function, however, seems likely in view of the fact that, in several of the tissues, the local production of renin and angiotensin II appears to be regulated by appropriate physiologic stimuli. For example, in the adrenal zona glomerulosa (where aldosterone is made), the cellular content of angiotensin II increases during sodium restriction and decreases during oral salt loading in the rat[55] (Fig. 6–2). Because these same variations in salt intake also increase and decrease aldosterone production, it seems likely that local angiotensin II formation plays a role in aldosterone production. In the ovary, follicular fluid contains a high concentration of the renin precursor, prorenin.[37] Some of this prorenin enters the circulation: Plasma prorenin levels increase twofold at the time of ovulation[80] (Fig. 6–3). In addition, the plasma prorenin level increases ten-fold in pregnancy. The specific function, however, of ovarian renin in reproductive function is unclear.

Aldosterone

Biochemistry and Metabolism of Aldosterone

Aldosterone is the most potent mineralocorticoid produced in humans and is secreted exclusively by the outer (glomerulosa) cells of the adrenal cortex.[70, 104, 105] Other mineralocorticoids secreted by the adrenal cortex include 11-deoxycorticosterone (DOC), 18-hydroxy 11-deoxycorticosterone, and 18-hydroxycorticosterone. These other steroids can be secreted

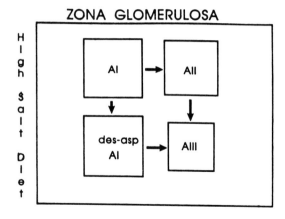

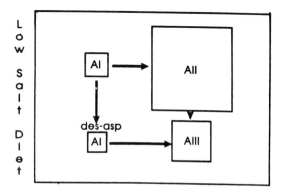

FIGURE 6–2. Relative contents of angiotensin peptides in the adrenal zona glomerulosa of rats ingesting high-salt diets (top panel) and low-salt diets (bottom panel). The area of each square reflects peptide content. On the low-salt intake, there is a preferential shift to angiotensin II. (From Kifor I, Moore TJ, Fallo F, et al. The effect of sodium intake on angiotensin content of the rat adrenal gland. Endocrinology 1991;128:1277. With permission.)

both by the glomerulosa and by the reticularis/fasciculata layers of the adrenal cortex. Except for DOC, the other steroids secreted by the adrenal cortex have so little mineralocor-

ticoid activity that it is unlikely they contribute significantly to the control of sodium and potassium homeostasis.[70]

After secretion, aldosterone, similar to other

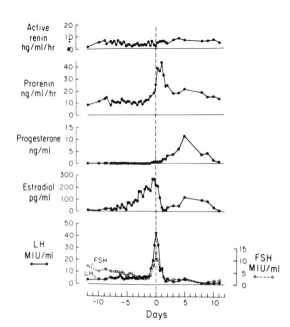

FIGURE 6–3. Hormonal changes occurring throughout the normal menstrual cycle in one normal woman. *Day O* indicates day of ovulation. Note the increase in plasma prorenin levels (with no changes in active renin) at the time of ovulation. (From Sealey JE, Cholst I, Glorioso N, et al. Sequential changes in plasma LH and plasma prorenin during the menstrual cycle. J Clin Endocrinol Metab 1987;65:1. With permission.)

steroid hormones, is bound to circulating proteins. The extent of aldosterone's binding to proteins, however, is much smaller than that of either testosterone or cortisol. In plasma, only 50% of aldosterone is protein bound.

The average daily secretion rate of aldosterone varies from 50 to 250 μg in normal subjects on a normal sodium intake, with the plasma concentration ranging between 5 and 15 ng/dL. More than 75% of the circulating aldosterone is normally inactivated during a single passage through the liver. Under certain circumstances, however, such as congestive heart failure, this percentage may be reduced. Approximately 10% of aldosterone appears in the urine as a glucuronide conjugate from which free aldosterone is released when the pH is lowered to 1. This *acid-labile conjugate* is formed both in the liver and in the kidney, and the amount in the urine is often used as an index of aldosterone secretion. On an average salt intake, the 24-hour urinary excretion of this conjugate ranges from 2 to 20 μg.[106]

Aldosterone Physiology

Under normal circumstances, aldosterone has two important mineralocorticoid activities: (1) It is a major regulator of extracellular fluid balance, as noted, and (2) it is a major determinant of potassium metabolism.[70, 105, 106] It regulates volume through a direct effect on the renal distal tubular transport of sodium. Aldosterone enhances the active reabsorption of sodium ion, which causes a fall in transmembrane potential, thus producing an environment favorable for the flow of positive ions out of the cell into the tubular lumen. Because the major, intracellular monovalent cation is potassium, potassium is lost in the urine in exchange for the active reabsorption of sodium.

Aldosterone and other mineralocorticoids also act on the epithelium of the salivary ducts and sweat glands and the epithelial cells of the gastrointestinal tract to promote reabsorption of sodium in "exchange" for potassium ions. The subcellular mechanism of action of aldosterone, similar to other steroids, involves aldosterone binding to its receptor in the cell cytoplasm, transport into the nucleus, and subsequent alteration in protein synthesis as a critical intermediary step in its action.

To protect against the untoward consequences of inappropriately increased levels of aldosterone or other mineralocorticoids, humans and other animals have the ability to "escape" from the sodium-retaining effects of these compounds. Thus when a normal individual is given aldosterone, sodium retention occurs only for 2 to 3 days. The individual then "escapes" from the sodium-retaining effect, thereby preventing the formation of clinical edema. Renal potassium loss persists.[106]

Three well-defined control mechanisms for aldosterone release exist: the renin-angiotensin system, potassium, and adrenocorticotrophic hormone (ACTH).[44, 70, 105] The renin-angiotensin system is primarily focused on regulating extracellular fluid volume and blood pressure. Potassium ions regulate aldosterone, which in turn maintains appropriate potassium balance.[46] ACTH also stimulates aldosterone secretion; however, its effect is transient unless ACTH is given in pulsatile fashion.[82] Thus although physiologic levels of ACTH under certain circumstances may stimulate aldosterone secretion, ACTH seems to be less important than potassium and the renin-angiotensin system in the normal control of aldosterone production,[108] whereas the renin-angiotensin system and potassium are roughly of equal importance.

Laboratory Assessment of the Activity of the Renin-Angiotensin-Aldosterone System

A variety of laboratory tests have been developed to assess the various components of the renin-aldosterone axis, including plasma renin activity (PRA), plasma renin substrate concentration, plasma angiotensin II, and plasma or urine aldosterone levels.[106] The appropriate use of these tests requires an understanding of their limitations.

Plasma Renin Activity

PRA is a measurement of renin's *enzymatic activity*. The assay involves measuring the amount of angiotensin I generated in vitro under controlled conditions. In most laboratories, endogenous renin substrate is added to the plasma sample, and the angiotensin I that is then generated is measured by radioimmunoassay (RIA). Two modifications may be used in the assay that may affect the results. First, some studies have suggested that collecting the samples on ice may increase the apparent renin activity owing to cryoactivation of prorenin in plasma. Prorenin is a renin precursor that is normally inactive. It can be activated, however, by cold temperature (6 to 10°C) or acidification (to pH 3.0).[68, 81] This cryoactivation, however, may not be a problem in an operational sense because several hours on ice may be required before activation occurs.[34] The pH at which the plasma sample is incubated may modify the results. The pH optimum for the reaction is 5.5 to 5.6.[33] Some laboratories use this pH, whereas others use pH 7.4[85] The amounts of angiotensin I generated under these circumstances are significantly different. Thus the same concentration of enzyme may produce varying levels of calculated renin *activity*, depending on how the sample was collected, the pH, temperature, and the time of the incubation reaction.

Plasma Renin Substrate

The concentration of angiotensinogen (renin substrate) in a plasma sample is assessed by adding an excess amount of renin and measuring the amount of angiotensin I generated after the angiotensinogen is exhausted.

Plasma Angiotensin II and Aldosterone Levels

Plasma angiotensin II and aldosterone are assessed directly by RIA, most often after some form of purification procedure to separate closely related contaminants that may cross react in the RIA system.[33] Although aldosterone assays are widely available, angiotensin II assays are limited to a few academic centers.

Clinical Evaluation

Because of wide fluctuations in the plasma levels of the components of this axis, random measurement of any of them provides an inadequate index of the functional state of the axis. Thus as with most endocrine diseases, the levels should be measured only after appropriate suppression (if hyperfunction is suggested) or stimulation (if hypofunction is being assessed). Stimulation of the entire axis is produced by volume depletion. A simple, potent stimulus consists of sodium restriction and upright posture. After 3 to 5 days on a 10-mEq sodium intake, aldosterone excretion rates range from 17 to 44 µg per day, whereas supine morning plasma aldosterone levels range from 12 to 40 ng/dL. In addition, plasma levels increase twofold to fourfold in response to upright posture (25 to 80 ng/dL). Following sodium restriction, recumbent plasma renin activity ranges between 2 and 8ng/mL per hour, rising to 2.5 to 15 ng/mL per hour following 2 to 3 hours of ambulation.[33] Likewise, suppression of the axis is accomplished by volume expansion. This is produced with the administration of salt intravenously or orally. A convenient suppression test is the intravenous infusion of 500 mL of normal saline per hour for 4 hours, which normally suppresses plasma aldosterone levels to <8 ng/dL if the subject is on a low sodium intake or <5 ng/dL if the subject is on a normal sodium intake.[54, 93]

Alterations in the Renin-Angiotensin System in Normal Pregnancy and with Estrogen Therapy

Pregnancy induces a number of significant alterations in fluid and sodium balance and modifies the activity of the RAS axis. It is still unclear, however, whether the RAS modifications are in response to or are the cause of the changes in fluid and sodium balance.

Hemodynamic Changes in Pregnancy

The normal pregnant woman demonstrates a reduction in systolic, diastolic, and mean blood pressure during the first half of pregnancy[15] (Fig. 6–4). In the latter half of preg-

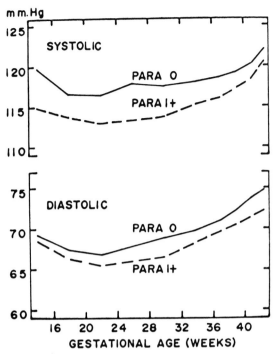

FIGURE 6–4. Changes in mean arterial pressure of 1046 primigravidas and 2227 multigravidas during the course of pregnancy. All patients were white between the ages of 25 and 34 years and delivered live infants. (From Christiansen RE. Studies on blood pressure during pregnancy. I. Influence of parity and age. Am J Obstet Gynecol 1976;125:509. With permission.)

nancy, blood pressure gradually rises until the mean blood pressure in most near-term pregnant subjects is approximately equal to that in the nonpregnant state. The fall in blood pressure is accompanied by an increase in plasma volume and cardiac output and a reduction in peripheral resistance.[75, 96] The increase in plasma volume is secondary to the activation of the normal homeostatic mechanisms responding to the fall in arterial pressure. Thus there is a change in hormonal factors that promotes sodium retention—the net result is an enhancement of sodium retention, fluid retention, and volume expansion. Renal blood flow and glomerular filtration rates are thus increased by 50% in early pregnancy, with a return of prepregnancy levels at the time of gestation.[24, 96] This increased glomerular filtration rate, along with the fall in renal vascular resistance and the natriuretic effect of the increased levels of progesterone, should produce increased renal sodium loss. The increases in estrogen and aldosterone, however,

promote sodium retention. The net effect is the observed increase in plasma volume. As a result of these factors, many women demonstrate some peripheral edema during the course of their pregnancy.[92]

Changes in the Renin-Angiotensin-Aldosterone System During Pregnancy

Renin and Angiotensin

PRA increases substantially during normal pregnancy.[11, 12, 16, 43, 66, 98, 103] Levels increase early in pregnancy, reaching a peak at 12 weeks (approximately twice the normal level) and remain elevated thereafter (Fig. 6–5). There is also an increase in the amount of renin observed in early pregnancy, which may be largely an inactive form of renin that is activated in vitro.[86] This inactive form of renin (prorenin) has been intensively investigated,

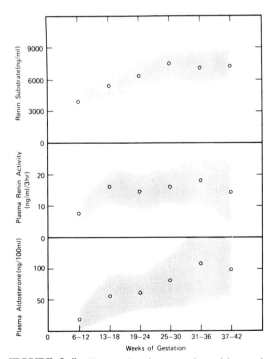

FIGURE 6–5. Changes in plasma renin activity, renin substrate, and aldosterone levels during normal pregnancy. The mean level is represented by the open circle, and ± 1 SD is represented by the hatch area. (From Weinberger MH, Kramer NJ, Petersen LP, et al, eds. Hypertension in Pregnancy. New York: John Wiley & Sons, 1976:263. With permission.)

but it is unclear whether it is derived from the kidney, the uterus, or the chorion.[38, 90, 91]

Angiotensin II levels also increase to nearly twice normal within 2 to 3 weeks of conception.[102] These levels rise to a peak of 3 to 4 times the nonpregnant state at about 30 weeks' gestation. Whether angiotensin II levels fall during the latter stages of pregnancy is still uncertain. All studies have documented a gradual increase in renin substrate concentration[45] during the course of pregnancy, which reaches a peak at 30 weeks' gestation at a level twofold to threefold greater than in the nonpregnant state. Because estrogen administration to nonpregnant women also increases renin substrate, it is likely that estrogen is the major stimulus for the renin substrate increase in pregnancy.

Even though the angiotensin II concentration is significantly elevated during the course of the pregnancy, the elevated levels in normal pregnancy do not produce an increase in blood pressure. Indeed, when directly challenged with angiotensin II infusion, both the renal and the systemic vasculatures have a *reduced* responsiveness to angiotensin II.[1, 14, 41, 67] The mechanism underlying this reduced responsiveness is not clear. In normal subjects, modification of the circulating levels of angiotensin II produces changes in the responsiveness of the vasculature to infused angiotensin II.[47] Thus, increasing basal angiotensin II concentration reduces vascular responses to infused angiotensin II and vice versa. Because circulating angiotensin II levels are elevated in pregnancy, this may explain the reduced responsiveness. Inhibitors of prostaglandin synthesis have been shown to restore normal vascular responsiveness to angiotensin II when given to pregnant individuals.[36] Thus an increase in prostaglandin production by the uterus or placenta may potentially contribute to the reduced vascular responsiveness.

Aldosterone

In 1957, Venning et al[95] documented an increased excretion rate of *aldosterone* during pregnancy. Since then, it has been documented that aldosterone's plasma levels and secretory rates are increased.[5, 7, 28, 30, 32, 51, 97, 99, 102] Indeed, studies suggest that as early as 2 weeks

after conception plasma aldosterone concentration is already significantly above the normal range. By the 24th week, it has usually reached a plateau at 3 to 5 times greater than in the nonpregnant state, reaching a peak at about the 36th week at a level some eightfold to tenfold higher than in nonpregnant women (see Fig. 6–5).

Even though plasma aldosterone levels are markedly increased during pregnancy, the regulation of aldosterone secretion appears to be normal. For example, when pregnant women are given either DOC acetate or 9-α-fluorohydrocortisone (both mineralocorticoids) to promote sodium retention, aldosterone secretion is suppressed significantly.[31] Likewise, aldosterone responsiveness to ACTH administration is normal.[29, 31] Some studies suggest that the elevated aldosterone levels are necessary to maintain normal sodium balance and that pregnancy is indeed a chronic sodium-losing state. Thus aldosterone secretion is increased to compensate for this salt-losing tendency. When its secretion is inhibited, salt wasting occurs, with significant reduction in weight and postural hypotension.[28]

An interesting feature of the increased levels of mineralocorticoids in pregnancy is that the expected potassium wasting does not occur. Thus even though pregnant women have eightfold to tenfold increases in aldosterone secretion rates, their serum potassium levels are normal. This apparent paradox can probably best be explained by the elevated *progesterone* levels observed in pregnancy.[94] Progesterone acts as an antagonist to aldosterone at the renal tubule and inhibits both its sodium-retaining and potassium-losing tendencies.[59] Support for this thesis comes from experimental studies as well as clinical experience: e.g., the documented amelioration of hypokalemia in women with either primary aldosteronism or Bartter's syndrome when they become pregnant[5, 57] and the parallel increases in aldosterone and progesterone levels during pregnancy.[30, 62]

Changes in the Renin-Angiotensin-Aldosterone Axis at Delivery

It has now been clearly documented that the levels of plasma aldosterone in the maternal circulation are significantly lower than in venous or arterial cord blood at the time of delivery.[52] Further, the level of aldosterone at delivery, as indicated earlier, can be modified by the level of volume depletion occurring before delivery. Thus the increase in plasma aldosterone observed with volume depletion in the mother is also observed in cord blood and the plasma of the neonate during the first 3 days postpartum.

The increased aldosterone concentration is probably a reflection of an increased angiotensin II level. The level of angiotensin II, however, seems in part related to the method of delivery[72] (Fig. 6–6). Patients with elective cesarean sections show concentrations of angiotensin II in cord, venous, and arterial blood similar to that in maternal venous blood. Vaginal delivery significantly increases both venous and arterial cord angiotensin II concentrations. Further, the level achieved is directly related to the duration of the second stage of labor, which suggests that changes in cord angiotensin II concentration are a consequence of changes in fetal or placental angiotensin II production. Renin activity is not consistently elevated in cord blood compared with the maternal circulation, whereas renin substrate is considerably lower in cord blood than in the maternal circulation.

Effects of Estrogen on the Renin-Angiotensin-Aldosterone Axis

Many of the responses of pregnancy so far described are reproduced in normal subjects given estrogen, with certain important exceptions. The most significant exception is the difference in hemodynamic responses. In general, blood pressure tends to *increase* in individuals given estrogen, with increases into the hypertensive range in a minority of patients.[71, 101, 109] The renal circulation is particularly sensitive to this, with significant reductions in renal blood flow compared with normal subjects matched in age and diet[48] (Fig. 6–7). As would be anticipated, there are significant increases in the plasma levels of aldosterone, renin activity, renin substrate, and angiotensin II when estrogen-containing oral contraceptives are administered—the initial event is an increase in renin substrate.[11, 16, 61, 87] Further, these changes may persist for 1 to 3 months after the oral contraceptive is stopped, and the hypertension may last indefinitely in some patients. Whether the increased activity of the RAS axis can be accounted for by the increase in renin substrate is unclear. Some data suggest that progestational compounds in the oral contraceptive may also contribute to the absolute level by blocking the effect of aldosterone on the distal renal tubule.[48] The progestational compounds in the oral contraceptive agents probably also explain why the increased aldosterone levels do not result in potassium loss and hypokalemia.

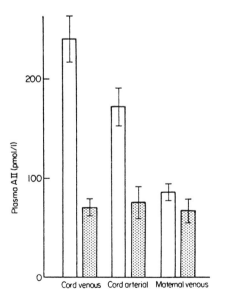

FIGURE 6–6. Mean ± SEM plasma angiotensin II concentration in cord and maternal blood obtained after either cesarean section (stippled columns) or vaginal delivery (open columns). The levels from infants delivered vaginally were significantly higher. (From Pipkin FB, Symonds EM. Factors affecting angiotensin II concentrations in the human infant at birth. Clin Sci Mol Med 1977;52:449. With permission.)

VASOPRESSIN

Vasopressin was synthesized by du Vigneaud[27] in 1954 and, with the earlier synthesis of oxytocin, provided the first evidence that the hypothalamus has endocrine function. In humans, vasopressin plays a role in volume homeostasis together with the RAS system and has a primary role in the control of osmolality.

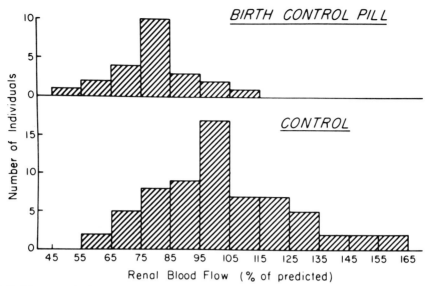

FIGURE 6–7. Histogram display of renal blood flow; expressed as percent of predicted for age and diet in women taking (above) or not taking (below) oral contraceptives. The predicted values were derived from regression relationships relating renal blood flow to age and sodium intake in healthy individuals. (From Hollenberg NK, Williams GH, Burger B, et al. Reciprocal influence of salt intake on adrenal glomerulosa and renal vascular responses to angiotensin II in normal man. Circ Res 1976;38:35. With permission.)

Biochemistry and Metabolism of Vasopressin

Arginine vasopressin (AVP) contains nine amino acid residues and has a molecular weight of approximately 1100 daltons.[17] Its structure is similar to oxytocin, the other major hormone produced in the hypothalamus (Fig. 6–8). Vasopressin is the hormone that plays the role of antidiuretic hormone (ADH) in most mammals. Lower vertebrates have a peptide hormone, vasotocin, that subserves this function. Vasotocin differs from vasopressin via a single-base substitution of isoleucine for phenylalanine at position 3, which disrupts the ring structure. Of interest, vasotocin is also present in the human fetal hypothalamus, which is discussed later in this section. Vasopressin is synthesized in the paraventricular and supraoptic nuclei. There it is packaged with neurophysin (which is its carrier protein), and together they make an insoluble complex.[6] The complex is transported down the axons to the median eminence and posterior pituitary, where it is stored until its release.[78]

The binding of vasopressin to its neurophysin is optimal at pH 5.2 to 5.8 and has a Kd of 2×10^5M. As a result, almost all of the vasopressin that circulates in human plasma is free

from its neurophysin because the complex dissociates in plasma. Vasopressin is cleared from the circulation by two main routes: degradation and renal excretion. Many tissues are capable of inactivating vasopressin, with the two most important organs being liver and kidney. The vasopressin that is not metabolized is cleared by the kidney (approximately 25% of the total clearance).[3] The total clearance of plasma vasopressin via both of these mechanisms is approximately 2 to 4 mL per minute per kg body weight and results in a biological half-life of 30 to 40 minutes.[3]

Mechanisms of Vasopressin Actions

Vasopressin exerts its effects by binding to tissue receptors of two types. V1 receptors are located on smooth muscle and liver cells and are responsible for the vasoconstrictor properties of vasopressin. V2 receptors are located on the renal epithelial cells, activate adenyl cyclase, and are responsible for the antidiuretic properties of vasopressin.[17]

Regulation of Vasopressin Secretion

The two major stimuli for vasopressin release are osmolality and blood volume. Other stim-

POSITION

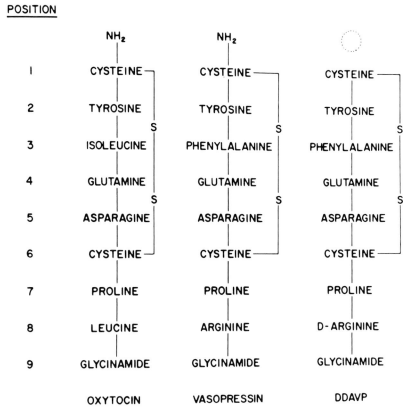

FIGURE 6–8. Structures of oxytocin, vasopressin, and DDAVP. Physiology of vasopressin, oxytocin and thirst. In: Becker H, ed. (From Robertson GL. Principles and Practice of Endocrinology and Metabolism. Philadelphia: JB Lippincott, 1990:223. With permission.)

uli include nausea,[74] hypoglycemia,[4] angiotensin,[69] and stress.[83]

Osmolality

Osmolality is the major regulator for vasopressin under normal situations. Osmolality is sensed by osmoreceptors, which are located in the anterior hypothalamus. Changes in osmolality as small as 1% result in a change in vasopressin levels of about 1 pg/mL, which is sufficient to change urine concentration.[73] When plasma osmolality falls, vasopressin levels fall to low or undetectable levels. As plasma osmolality rises, there is a sharp rise in vasopressin levels (Fig. 6–9), once a threshold for release is reached at approximately 285 mOs/kg in normal nonpregnant subjects.

Blood Pressure and Volume

Vasopressin response to changes in blood pressure is mediated by baroreceptors located in the heart and large arteries. Changes in blood volume are sensed by receptors in the cardiac atria and pulmonary veins. Impulses from these receptors travel via the vagus and the glossopharyngeal nerves to the brain stem, where pathways continue on to the supraoptic and paraventricular nuclei. In contrast to the extremely tight link between osmolality and vasopressin release, the relation between vasopressin and blood pressure or blood volume is exponential: A change in blood pressure of 5 to 10% may result in no change in vasopressin levels, whereas a larger change of 20 to 30% can result in very high vasopressin levels, greater than those required to achieve maximal antidiuresis.[73]

Biologic Actions of Vasopressin

The major effect of vasopressin is to inhibit water loss by the kidney. Vasopressin acts on

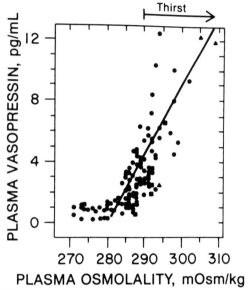

FIGURE 6–9. The relationship of plasma vasopressin levels and thirst to plasma osmolality in healthy nonpregnant individuals. (From Robertson GL. Thirst and vasopressin function in normal and disordered states of water balance. J Lab Clin Med 1983;101:351. With permission.)

the distal and collecting tubules in the kidney, allowing increased reabsorption of free water by making the tubules permeable to water. Water then passes from the tubular lumen into the hyperosmolar interstitium of the renal medulla. In the absence of vasopressin, the tubules are impermeable to water, and the hypotonic fluid from the proximal nephron passes through the distal segments, resulting in a urine flow of 20 to 30 L per day.[73]

Other effects of vasopressin include a role in potentiating anterior pituitary responsiveness to corticotropin.[73] It remains unclear whether vasopressin plays a role in the regulation of blood pressure in humans.

DISORDERS OF VASOPRESSIN

Syndrome of Inappropriate Antidiuretic Hormone

As already described, vasopressin is released in response to an increase in plasma osmolality or decrease in pressure or volume. When vasopressin is released owing to *nonosmotic* factors (resulting in a decrease in osmolality), the re-

lease is considered inappropriate and termed the *syndrome of inappropriate ADH secretion* (SIADH). A diagnosis of SIADH therefore is made when simultaneous measurements of plasma and urine show plasma hypo-osmolality with inappropriately hypertonic urine in a patient who is euvolemic. It must be determined that thyroid and adrenal function (both necessary for appropriate free water clearance) are normal. Clinically, patients may be asymptomatic when the onset is less rapid or the degree of hyponatremia less severe or may present within the spectrum of confusion to seizures to coma. Laboratory analysis reveals hyponatremia with decreased plasma osmolality and an inappropriately concentrated urine (>100 mOs/kg). Once a diagnosis is made, a search for underlying causes of SIADH must be undertaken. Acute treatment involves free water restriction (approximately 800 mL per day) if the patient is asymptomatic. If a patient has confusion, seizures, or coma, the hyponatremia should be reversed more rapidly by administering normal saline and furosemide or even hypertonic (3%) saline. Chronic treatment involves free water restriction. Oral demeclocycline, which inhibits vasopressin action, is an alternative if free water restriction fails.

Diabetes Insipidus

Both vasopressin deficiency and resistance to vasopressin's effect result in diabetes insipidus (DI), which manifests clinically as polyuria and polydipsia. DI can be either central (i.e., hypothalamic pituitary) or nephrogenic in origin. In central DI, there are low levels of vasopressin. Deficiency results from insufficient vasopressin release from the posterior pituitary. Most commonly central DI results following pituitary surgery but can also result from hypothalamic or pituitary tumors (primary or metastatic) or head trauma. In nephrogenic DI, vasopressin levels are high, but the kidney is unable to respond to vasopressin. Most commonly renal resistance to AVP is acquired and results from medication use, with the leading cause being lithium carbonate. Rarely nephrogenic DI is inherited in an X-linked mode with full penetrance in males and partial in females.

A diagnosis of DI can be made in a patient with hypernatremia and high plasma osmolality, who is excreting large volumes of inappropriately dilute urine. If the thirst mechanism is intact and free access to water available, however, these patients often have normal serum sodium and plasma osmolality at the expense of a large fluid intake. In this situation, a water deprivation test is useful in making a diagnosis and distinguishing between primary polydipsia and central or nephrogenic DI.

Water Deprivation Test

This test is performed by restricting fluid intake while measuring plasma and urine osmolality. The goal is to stimulate AVP release by a rise in plasma osmolality. Usually 6 hours of fluid deprivation is sufficient to make a diagnosis. The test should be performed in a carefully monitored situation because the major risk is dehydration if the patient has the diagnosis. Fluids should be withheld starting in the morning and urine osmolality measured hourly until there is a plateau of osmolality on three specimens. Plasma osmolality and weight should be determined before the test and every 2 hours during the test. The test should be terminated for hypotension, an increase in serum osmolality to greater than 300 mOsm/kg, or a loss in body weight of more than 3%. At termination of the test, serum osmolality and urine osmolality should be determined. If the patient remains clinically stable throughout the test, a dose of either 5 units aqueous vasopressin or 1 μg 1-deamino-8-D-arginine vasopressin (DDAVP) subcutaneously or 10 μg DDAVP intranasally should be given. Urinary osmolality should be remeasured 30 to 60 minutes later.

A failure to raise urinary osmolality to >800 mOsm/kg during the test with a rise of serum osmolality to >288 mOsm/kg is compatible with a diagnosis of DI. The subsequent administration of vasopressin in a normal person does not increase urinary osmolality more than 9% beyond that achieved during water deprivation alone. In patients with central DI, administration of vasopressin increases urine osmolality more than 9%. Patients with nephrogenic DI fail to concentrate the urine with dehydration and do not respond to vasopressin administration.

A plasma vasopressin level drawn at the end of the water deprivation test in a patient who fails to concentrate urine can be helpful distinguishing central from nephrogenic DI, being low in the former and elevated in the latter.

Special considerations must be undertaken when performing this test during pregnancy. (see next section).

VASOPRESSIN IN PREGNANCY

Plasma osmolality is usually maintained in a tight range in nonpregnant humans, averaging 285 mOsm/kg. Changes from these levels in the nonpregnant state are usually the result of an underlying disease or medication. In contrast, normal healthy pregnancy is a state in which a decrease in osmolality of 7 to 10 mOsm/kg characteristically occurs along with a decrease in the osmotic threshold for thirst. This section describes the hypo-osmolality of pregnancy, offers possible mechanisms for its occurrence, reviews dysregulation of osmolality (DI of pregnancy), and discusses the role of vasopressin in the fetus.

Plasma osmolality and plasma sodium begin to decrease within days after conception and are significantly lower than nonpregnant levels by 5 weeks' gestation.[21] A nadir is reached at approximately 10 weeks' gestation, which is then maintained until term (Fig. 6–10). Of note, because only 1.5 mOsm/kg of this decrease is due to lower levels of plasma urea, the majority of the decrease in osmolality is due to a decrease in plasma sodium and its associated anions and therefore indicates a true decrease in "effective" osmolality.

Associated and contributing to this decrease in osmolality is an increase in the total body water of 7 to 8 L which is distributed approximately 50/50 between the maternal and fetal placental compartments. The majority of fluid in the mother is in the interstitial and intravascular compartment. The increase in total body water begins in the first trimester, increasing more rapidly in the second trimester and peaking around 32 weeks' gestation.[65]

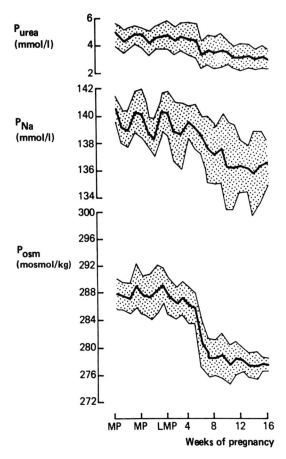

FIGURE 6–10. Changes in plasma urea (P_{urea}), sodium (P_{Na}), and osmolality (P_{osm}) before conception and through the first trimester of pregnancy. MP = Menstrual period; LMP = last menstrual period. (From Davison JM, Vallottan MB, Lindheimer MD. Plasma osmolality and urinary concentration during and after pregnancy: Evidence that lateral recumbency inhibits maximal urinary concentrating ability. Br J Ob Gyn 1981;88:474. With permission.)

Regulation of Osmolality and Vasopressin Secretion

Despite the lower plasma osmolality in pregnancy, there is no increase in urine volume or water diuresis as would occur if a similar osmolality were reached in the nonpregnant state. This observation suggests that the osmolality set-point is reset to a lower level in pregnancy that is maintained in the face of osmotic challenges.

For example, studies of pregnant women by Davison et al[19, 20] have demonstrated that, despite lower basal plasma osmolality, the response of vasopressin to water loading, fluid restriction, and infusion of 5% saline is well maintained. Basally in the face of a lower plasma osmolality, plasma vasopressin levels are similar to those in the nonpregnant state. Fluid deprivation results in a similar magnitude of rise of plasma and urine osmolality and plasma vasopressin levels as compared with postgestation. Similarly with water loading, there is lowering of plasma osmolality with a suppression of vasopressin to nondetectable levels. In response to infusion of 5% saline, there is a steady rise in vasopressin in pregnancy in response to the rise in osmolality. A comparison of the response of vasopressin to change in osmolality before and after pregnancy allows an estimation of the threshold for vasopressin release in the pregnant and nonpregnant state. These manipulations of osmolality support a resetting of the osmotic threshold for vasopressin release (Fig. 6–11).

Concomitant with the decrease in osmotic threshold for vasopressin release in pregnancy is a resetting of the osmotic threshold for thirst (Fig. 6–11). The women who received infusion of hypertonic saline noted a desire to drink at an osmolality approximately 10 mOsm/kg lower than postpartum.

It is thought that this combination of a lower osmotic threshold for both vasopressin release and thirst works in parallel to maintain the decrease in osmolality seen in pregnancy. With a decrease in the osmotic threshold for thirst, there is increased free water intake, leading to hemodilution. This hemodilution and lowering of plasma osmolality would usually result in a lowering of vasopressin and free water diuresis. Because of the concomitant lowering of the osmotic threshold for vasopressin release, however, AVP secretion is not suppressed, and a new steady-state osmolality is reached.

Arginine Vasopressin Metabolism in Pregnancy

The metabolic clearance rate (MCR) of vasopressin increases greatly between 8 and 22 weeks' gestation, reaching a peak in midpregnancy (threefold to fourfold the rate of nonpregnant women) that is maintained through the third trimester.[20] The mechanisms for the

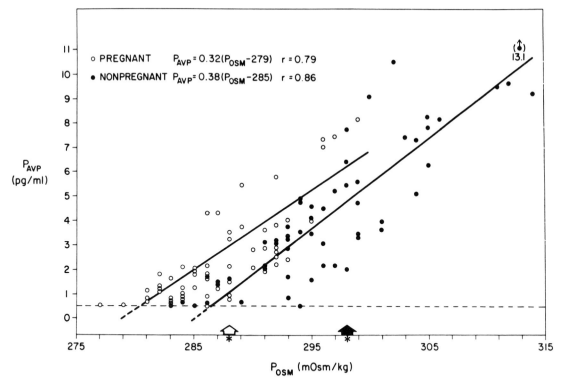

FIGURE 6–11. The relationship between plasma osmolality (P_{osm}) and vasopressin (P_{avp}) during infusion of 5% saline over 2 hours in pregnant women. Open symbols represent third-trimester values and closed symbols represent values 6 to 8 weeks postpartum. The arrows represent thirst thresholds. (From Davison JM, Gilmore EA, Durr J, et al. Altered osmotic thresholds for vasopressin secretion and thirst in human pregnancy. Am J Physiol 1984;246:F105. With permission.)

increased MCR are unclear. Possibilities include increased renal and hepatic degradation secondary to increased blood flow to these organs or placental degradation via production of vasopressinase.[60] Vasopressinase is produced in the placenta and is present in large amounts in the blood of pregnant women and in vitro has been demonstrated to inactivate large quantities of vasopressin.[76] This enzyme not only increases the clearance of vasopressin, but also complicates the study of vasopressin in pregnancy. Measuring vasopressin during pregnancy requires the addition of inhibitors of vasopressinase to the sample at the time of blood drawing.[19] Despite this increase in MCR, plasma levels of vasopressin remain similar in a given woman throughout pregnancy, suggesting a concomitant increase in vasopressin production.[64]

Vasopressinase (cysteine aminopeptidase) cleaves the ring structure of vasopressin between cysteine and tyrosine (Fig. 6–12). The cleaved peptide no longer has antidiuretic ac-

tivity[25] but may retain pressor activity.[39] DDAVP, owing to its amino terminus modification, is not affected by this enzyme.

Potential Causes for the Altered Osmoregulation in Pregnancy

Several hormones that are elevated in pregnancy have been investigated in animal studies for their effect on vasopressin release. These include estradiol, progesterone, and prolactin. Levels of these hormones seen in pregnancy, however, do not have a significant effect on plasma osmolality or the osmotic threshold for vasopressin release in animal studies.[26] Human chorionic gonodotropin (hCG) is another possible candidate. Women receiving hCG in the luteal phase demonstrate a lowering of osmotic threshold and thirst threshold.[20] In addition, a woman with hydatidiform disease demonstrated a decrease in plasma osmolality

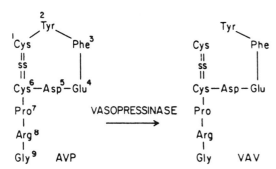

FIGURE 6–12. Vasopressinase cleaves the cysteine-tyrosine bond and changes vasopressin (AVP) to vasopressin-altered vasopressinase (VAV), which does not retain antidiuretic activity. (From Krege JH, Katz VL. A proposed relationship between vasopressinase altered vasopressin and preeclampsia. Medical Hypothesis 1990;31:284. With permission.)

and a lowering of the osmotic threshold for vasopressin release and thirst.[20]

DISORDERS OF VASOPRESSIN REGULATION IN PREGNANCY

DI of pregnancy, although at first thought to be rare, is being recognized with increasing frequency. In the most classic presentation, the DI is transient, manifestating itself in the third trimester and resolving within several weeks postpartum. The DI may recur with subsequent pregnancies.[43] A potential association with acute fatty liver of pregnancy[9] and hypertension[2, 25, 40, 50] has been noted. There is also a striking predominance of male infants born to women with transient DI of pregnancy.[2, 9, 40, 43, 50]

Original reports of DI in pregnancy proposed it to be a vasopressin-resistant state because of a lack of response to exogenously administered vasopressin.[2] It was then appreciated, however, that increased levels of endogenous vasopressinase seen in pregnancy could degrade the exogenously administered aqueous vasopressin, giving the appearance of resistance.[25] In support of this, reports indicate that DDAVP (see Fig. 6–8), which is resistant to vasopressinase, is effective in DI of pregnancy.[25, 49]

DDAVP is, however, not universally successful in the treatment of DI in pregnancy.[40] More recently, it has been recognized that many of the reported cases may have had an underlying partial central or nephrogenic DI, which was not manifested until pregnancy but which was detected by a diagnostic workup postpartum.[50] Prior partial central DI could become clinically manifest because of the presence of increased vasopressinase in maternal serum, which may reduce maternal vasopressin levels in women with limited vasopressin secretory reserve. The cause for an exacerbation of nephrogenic DI during pregnancy is less clear. It may be that in partial nephrogenic DI, high levels of AVP are able to compensate partially for the defect and that during pregnancy placental vasopressinase prevents maintenance of these high levels. The realization that the pregnant state may make either central or nephrogenic DI manifest may explain the discrepancy between reports of whether DDAVP is effective[49] or not effective.[40] At present, the most likely explanation for DI of pregnancy has two components: a reduction in vasopressin secretory capacity or in the response to vasopressin (present beforehand) plus accelerated vasopressin degradation.

DI in pregnancy can be suspected in a woman with polyuria and polydipsia. A diagnosis can be made when the simultaneous measurement of plasma and urine osmolality reveal plasma hyperosmolality (normal osmolality in pregnancy being in the range of 275 to 278 mOsm/kg) with inappropriately dilute urine. Most women with transient central or nephrogenic DI in pregnancy do not require treatment and are able to maintain their plasma osmolality with increased oral fluid intake. If the amount of water needed each day is so excessive that the woman is not able to prevent hyperosmolality, medical therapy may be indicated. If the diagnosis is suspected but not confirmed by basal blood and urine measurements, a diagnosis of DI should be confirmed via a water deprivation test. A water deprivation test has not been standardized for pregnancy as it has for the nonpregnant state. Given that osmolality is approximately 7 to 8 mOsm/kg lower in pregnancy, it is reasonable to adjust the water deprivation test accordingly. In our institution, we make the following modifications during pregnancy: Plasma osmolality is not allowed to rise to more than 290 mOsm/kg or body weight to fall by more than 1 kg. Because the osmotic threshold for AVP release is lower in pregnancy, these modifications should allow manifestation of the AVP effect. AVP levels (drawn with vasopressinase inhibitor) at the end of the test can help distinguish central from nephrogenic DI. Alternately, DDAVP can be given if the test is compatible with DI to distinguish central and nephrogenic DI. If central DI is present, DDAVP can be continued through delivery with careful monitoring of serum sodium and osmolality. If nephrogenic DI is present, hydrochlorothiazide has been reported to be successful,[40] but given the lack of any series of patients treated in this manner and risk of dehydration, caution must be exercised. Because transient DI of pregnancy may represent an unmasking of partial preexistent DI, women should be retested postpartum.

Pregnancy can also occur in a woman with documented preexisting DI. A 1978 review of 67 reported cases of pregnancy in women with preexisting DI indicated a deterioration of the DI in 58%, no change in 15%, and an improvement in 20%. The cause of DI in these 67 cases, however, is not well defined. Women with previously diagnosed central DI preceding pregnancy can be managed with DDAVP, usually requiring an increased dose. Little information exists as to the course of nephrogenic DI during pregnancy. As discussed earlier, idiopathic nephrogenic DI is a rare disorder with X-linked inheritance and partial expression in affected women.[46a] In addition, DI can be a manifestation of Sheehan's syndrome (postpartum hypopituitarism), usually in conjunction with other hormone deficiencies (see Chapter 7).

VASOPRESSIN AND OSMOREGULATION IN THE FETUS

Vasopressin is usually detectable in the human fetal neurohypophysis at 11 to 12 weeks' gestation[88] and increases 1000-fold over the next 12 to 16 weeks.[8] Also present in the neurohypophysis is arginine vasotocin, a naturally occurring vasopressin analog[89] whose physiologic function is unknown in the fetus but experimentally can decrease renal free water clear-

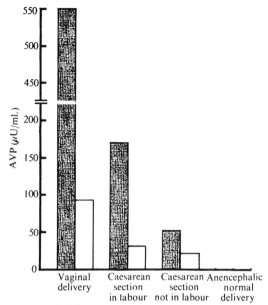

FIGURE 6–13. Vasopressin (AVP) levels determined on umbilical plasma (stippled = arterial; open = venous) at delivery. (From Chard T, Hudson CN, Edwards CRW, Boyd NRH. Release of oxytocin and vasopressin by the human foetus during labour. Nature 1971;234:353. With permission.)

ance and increase blood pressure.[35] An anencephalic neonate with no morphologic evidence of neurohypophyseal tissue had no detectable vasopressin in cord blood, indicating that vasopressin in fetal plasma is of fetal origin. Further support comes from the observation that levels are higher in umbilical arterial blood compared with venous blood[13] (Fig. 6–13).

The role of fetal vasopressin is unclear. Circulating levels are measurable by midgestation, are lower in fetuses with severe anemia, and increase in response to intravascular transfusion without a stimulus of a change in osmolality[100] for unclear reasons.

Animal studies have documented a rise in fetal plasma vasopressin in response to hypotension.[23, 53, 77] Labor appears to be a stimulus for vasopressin release by the fetus, with higher levels being found in neonates whose mothers had been in labor than in those whose mothers were delivered by cesarean section without labor[13] (see Fig. 6–13).

REFERENCES

1. Abdul-Karim R, Assali NS. Pressor response to angiotensin in pregnant and nonpregnant women. Am J Obstet Gynecol 1961;82:246.

2. Barron WM, Cohen LH, Ulland LA, et al. Transient vasopressin resistant diabetes insipidus of pregnancy. N Engl J Med 1984;310:442.

3. Bauman G, Dingham JF. Distribution, blood transport, and degradation of antidiuretic hormone in man. J Clin Invest 1976;57:1109.

4. Baylis PH, Zerbe RL, Robertson GL. Arginine vasopressin responses to insulin induced hypoglycemia in man. J Clin Endocrinol Metab 1981;53:935.

5. Biglieri EG, Slaton PE Jr. Pregnancy and primary aldosteronism. J Clin Endocrinol 1967;27:1628.

6. Breslow E. The neurophysins. Adv Enzyme 1974; 40:271.

7. Brown RD, Strott CA, Liddle GW. Plasma deoxycorticosterone in normal and abnormal human pregnancy. J Clin Endocrinol 1972;35:736.

8. Burford GD, Robinson IC. Oxytocin, vasopressin and neurophysins in the hypothalamo-neurohypophysial system of the human fetus. J Endocrinol 1982;95:403.

9. Cammu H, Velkeniers B, Charels K, et al. Idiopathic acute fatty liver of pregnancy associated with transient diabetes insipidus. Case report. Br J Obstet Gynaecol 1987;94:173.

10. Campbell DJ. Circulating and tissue angiotensin systems. J Clin Invest 1987;79:1.

11. Catt KJ, Baukal A, Ashburn M. The renin-angiotensin system during oral contraceptive therapy and pregnancy. In: Fregly MJ, Fregly MS, eds. Oral contraceptives and high blood pressure. Gainesville, FL: Dolphin Press, 1974:211.

12. Cession G. Plasma renin in the menstrual cycle, normal pregnancy and late gestational hypertension. Bull Soc Roy Belg Gynaecol Obstet 1967;37:287.

13. Chard T, Hudson CN, Edwards CRW, Boyd NRH. Release of oxytocin and vasopressin by the human foetus during labour. Nature 1971;234:352.

14. Chesley LC, Wynn RM, Silverman NI. Renal effects of angiotensin II infusions in normotensive pregnant and nonpregnant women. Circ Res 1963;13:232.

15. Christiansen RE. Studies on blood pressure during pregnancy. 1. Influence of parity and age. Am J Obstet Gynecol 1976;125:509.

16. Crane MG, Harris JJ. Effects of estrogens and gestagens on the renin-aldosterone system. In: Fregly MJ, Fregly MS, eds. Oral contraceptives and high blood pressure. Gainesville, FL: Dolphin Press, 1974:100.

17. Culpepper RM, Hebert SC, Andreoli TE. The posterior pituitary and water metabolism. In: Wilson JD, Foster DW, eds. Williams textbook of endocrinology, ed 7. Philadelphia: WB Saunders, 1985:619.

18. Davis JO, Freeman RH. Mechanisms regulating renin release. Physiol Rev 1976;56:2.

19. Davison JM, Gilmor EA, Durr J, et al. Altered osmotic thresholds for vasopressin secretion and thirst in human pregnancy. Am J Physiol 1984;246:F105.

20. Davison JM, Shiells EA, Philips PR, Lindheimer MD. Serial evaluation of vasopressin release and thirst in human pregnancy. J Clin Invest 1988;81:798.

21. Davison JM, Vallottan MB, Lindheimer MD. Plasma osmolality and urinary concentration during and after pregnancy: evidence that lateral recumbency inhibits maximal urinary concentrating ability. Br J Obstet Gynaecol 1981;88:472.

22. Dluhy RG, Underwood RH, Williams GH. Influence of dietary potassium on plasma renin activity in normal man. J Appl Physiol 1970;28:299.

23. Drummand WH, Rudolph AM, Keil LC, et al. Arginine vasopressin and prolactin after hemorrhage in the fetal lamb. Am J Physiol 1980;238:E214.

24. Dunlop W. Investigations into the influence of posture on renal plasma flow and glomerular filtration rate during late pregnancy. Br J Obstet Gynaecol 1976;83:17.

25. Durr JA, Hoggard JG, Hunt JM, Schrier RW. Diabetes insipidus in pregnancy associated with abnormally high circulating vasopressinase activity. N Engl J Med 1987;316:1070.

26. Durr JA, Stamoutsos B, Lindheimer MD. Osmoregulation during pregnancy in the rat. Evidence for resetting of the threshold for vasopressin secretion during gestation. J Clin Invest 1981;68:337.

27. Du Vigneaud V. Hormones of the posterior pituitary: oxytocin and vasopressin. In: Harvey Lectures 1954–1955. New York: Academic Press, 1956:1.

28. Ehrlich EN. Heparinoid-induced inhibition of aldosterone secretion in pregnant women. The role of augmented aldosterone secretion in sodium conservation during normal pregnancy. Am J Obstet Gynecol 1971;109:963.

29. Ehrlich EN, Biglieri EG, Lindheimer MD. ACTH-induced sodium retention in pregnancy. Role of desoxycorticosterone and corticosterone. J Clin Endocrinol 1974;38:7601.

30. Ehrlich EN, Laves M, Lugibihl K, et al. Progesterone-aldosterone interrelationships in pregnancy. J Lab Clin Med 1962;59:588.

31. Ehrlich EN, Lindheimer MD. Effect of administered mineralocorticoid or ACTH in pregnant women: attenuation of kaliuretic influence of mineralocorticoids during pregnancy. J Clin Invest 1972;51:1301.

32. Ehrlich EN, Nolten WE, Oparil S, Lindheimer MD. Mineralocorticoids in normal pregnancy. In: Lindheimer MD, Katz AI, Zuspan FP, eds. Hypertension in pregnancy. New York: John Wiley & Sons, 1976:189.

33. Emanuel RL, Cain JP, Williams GH. Double antibody RIA of renin activity and angiotensin II in human peripheral plasma. J Lab Clin Med 1973;81:632.

34. Emanuel RL, Williams GH. Should blood samples for assay of plasma renin activity be chilled? Clin Chem 1978;24:2042.

35. Ervin MG, Ross MG, Leake RD, et al. Changes in steady state plasma arginine vasotocin levels affect ovine fetal renal and cardiovascular function. Endocrinology 1986;118:759.

36. Everett RB, Worley RJ, MacDonald PC, Gant NF. Effect of prostaglandin synthetase inhibitors on pressor response to angiotensin II in human pregnancy. J Clin Endocrinol Metab 1978;46:1007.

37. Fernandez LA, Tarlatzis BC, Rzasa PJ, et al. Renin-like activity in ovarian follicular fluid. Fertil Steril 1985;44:219.

38. Ferris TF, Stein JH, Kauffman J. Uterine blood flow and uterine renin secretion. J Clin Invest 1972; 51:2827.

39. Fong CT, Silver L, Louie DD. Necessity of the disulfide bond of vasopressin for antidiuretic activity. Biochem Biophys Res Commun 1964;14:302.

40. Ford SM. Transient vasopressin-resistant diabetes insipidus of pregnancy. Obstet Gynecol 1986;68:288.

41. Gant NF, Daley GL, Chand S, et al. A study on AII pressor response throughout primigravid pregnancy. J Clin Invest 1973;52:2682.

42. Ganten D, Hermann K, Unger TH, Lang RE. The tissue renin-angiotensin system: focus on brain angiotensin adrenal gland, and arterial wall. Clin Exp Hypertens Theor Pract 1983;A5:1099.

43. Goodman H, Sachs BP, Phillipe M, Moore T. Tran-

sient recurrent nephrogenic diabetes insipidus. Am J Obstet Gynecol 1984;149:910.

44. Gross F. The regulation of aldosterone secretion by the renin-angiotensin system under various conditions. Acta Endocrinol 1967;124:41.

45. Helmer OM, Judson WE. Influence of high renin substrate levels on renin-angiotensin system in pregnancy. Am J Obstet Gynecol 1967;99:9.

46. Himathongkam T, Dluhy RG, Williams GH. Potassium-aldosterone-renin interrelationships. J Clin Endocrinol Metab 1975;41:153.

46a. Hime MC, Richardson JA. Diabetes insipidus and pregnancy. Obstet Gynecol Surv 1978;33:375.

47. Hollenberg NK, Chenitz WR, Adams DF, Williams GH. Reciprocal influence of salt intake on adrenal glomerulosa and renal vascular responses to angiotensin II in normal man. J Clin Invest 1974;54:34.

48. Hollenberg NK, Williams GH, Burger B, et al. Renal blood flow and its response to AII: an interaction between oral contraceptive agents, sodium intake and the renin-angiotensin system in healthy young women. Circ Res 1976;38:35.

49. Hughes JM, Barron WM, Vance ML. Recurrent diabetes insipidus associated with pregnancy: Pathophysiology and therapy. Obstet Gynecol 1989;73:462.

50. Iwasaki Y, Oiso Y, Kondo K, et al. Aggravation of subclinical diabetes insipidus during pregnancy. N Engl J Med 1991;324:522.

51. Jones KM, Lloyd-Jones Roindel A. Aldosterone secretion and metabolism in normal men and women and in pregnancy. Acta Endocrinol 1959;30:321.

52. Katz FH, Beck P, Makowski EL. The renin-aldosterone system in mother and fetus at term. Am J Obstet Gynecol 1974;118:51.

53. Kelly RT, Rose JC, Meis PJ, et al. Vasopressin is important for restoring cadiovascular homeostasis in fetal and adult sheep. Am J Obstet Gynecol 1983;146:807.

54. Kem DC, Weinberger MH, Mayes DM, Nugent CA. Saline suppression of plasma aldosterone in hypertension. Arch Intern Med 1971;128:380.

55. Kifor I, Moore TJ, Fallo F, et al. The effect of sodium intake on angiotensin content of the rat adrenal gland. Endocrinology 1991;128:1277.

56. Kifor I, Moore TJ, Fallo F, et al. Potassium-stimulated angiotensin release from superfused adrenal capsules and enzymatically dispersed cells of the zona glomerulosa. Endocrinology 1991;129:823.

57. Klaus D, Klumpp F, Rossler R. Einfluss der Schwangerschaft auf das Bartter Syndrome. Klin Wochenschr 1971;49:1280.

58. Krege JH, Katz VL. A proposed relationship between vasopressinase altered vasopressin and preeclampsia. Med Hypoth 1990;31:283.

59. Landau RL, Lugibihl K. Inhibition of the sodium-retaining influence of aldosterone by progesterone. J Clin Endocrinol 1958;18:1237.

60. Landon MJ, Copas DK, Shiells EA, Davison JM. Degradation of radiolabelled arginine vasopressin (^{125}I-AVP) by the human placenta perfused in vitro. Br J Obstet Gynaecol 1988;95:488.

61. Laragh JH, Sealey JE, Ledingham JG, Newton MA. Oral contraceptives, renin, aldosterone, and high blood pressure. JAMA 1967;201:918.

62. Ledoux F, Genest J, Nowaczynski W, et al. Plasma progesterone and aldosterone in pregnancy. J Can Med Assoc 1975;112:943.

63. Lightman A, Palumbo A, DeCherney AH, Naftolin F. The ovarian renin-angiotensin system. Sem Reprod Endocrinol 1989;7:79.

64. Lindheimer MD, Barron WM, Davison JM. Osmoregulation of thirst and vasopressin release in pregnancy. Am J Physiol 1989;257:F159.

65. Lindheimer MD, Barron WM, Durr J, Davison JM. Water homeostasis and vasopressin secretion during gestation. Adv Nephrol 1986;15:1–24.

66. Lindheimer MD, del Greco F, Ehrlich EN. Postural effects on Na and steroid excretion, and serum renin activity during pregnancy. J Appl Physiol 1973;35:343.

67. Lumbers ER. Peripheral vascular reactivity to angiotensin and noradrenalin in pregnant and non-pregnant women. Aust J Exp Biol Med Sci 1970;48:493.

68. Lumbers ER. Activation of renin in human amniotic fluid by low pH. Enzymologia 1971;40:329.

69. Mauw D, Bonjour JD, Malvin RL, Vander A. Central action of angiotensin in stimulating ADH release. Am J Physiol 1971;220:239.

70. Muller J. Regulation of aldosterone biosynthesis. New York: Springer-Verlag, 1971.

71. Pfefter RI, Van den Noort S. Estrogen use and stroke risk in post menopausal women. Am J Epidemiol 1976;103:445.

72. Pipkin FB, Symonds EM. Factors affecting angiotensin II concentrations in the human infant at birth. Clin Sci Mol Med 1977;52:449.

73. Robertson GL. Physiology of vasopressin, oxytocin and thirst. In: Becker KL, ed. Principles and practice of endocrinology and metabolism. Philadelphia: JB Lippincott, 1990:223.

74. Robertson GL, Athar S, Shelton RL. Osmotic control of vasopressin function. In: Andreoli TE, Granthan JJ, Rector FC, eds. Disturbances in body fluid osmolality. Bethesda, MD: American Physiological Society 1977:125.

75. Rose DJ, Badre ME, Bader RA, Braunwald E. Catheterization studies of cardiac hemodynamic in normal pregnant women with reference to left ventricular work. Am J Obstet Gynecol 1956;72:233.

76. Rosenbloom AA, Sack J, Fisher DA. The circulating vasopressinase of pregnancy: species comparison with radioimmunoassay. Am J Obstet Gynecol 1975; 121:316.

77. Ross MG, Ervin MG, Leake RD, et al. Isovolemic hypotension in the ovine fetus: plasma vasopressin response and urinary effects. Am J Physiol 1986; 250:E564.

78. Scharrer E, Scharrer B. Hormones produced by neurosecretory cells. Rec Prog Horm Res 1954;10:183.

79. Schrier RW. Pregnancy: an overfill or underfill state? Am J Kid Dis 1987;10:284.

80. Sealey JE, Cholst I, Glorioso N, et al. Sequential changes in plasma luteinizing hormone and plasma prorenin during the menstrual cycle. J Clin Endocrinol Metab 1987;63:1.

81. Sealey JE, Laragh JH. Prorenin in human plasma? Methodological and physiological implications. Circ Res 1975;36 & 37(suppl 1):1.

82. Seely EW, Conlin PR, Brent GA, Dluhy RD. Adrenocorticotropin stimulation of aldosterone: prolonged continuous versus pulsatile infusion. J Clin Endocrinol Metab 1989;69:1028.

83. Segar WE, Moor WW. The regulation of antidiuretic hormone release in man. J Clin Invest 1968;47:2143.

84. Simpson SA, Tait JF, Wettstein A, et al. Isolierung eines neuen kristallisierten Hormons aus nebennieren mit besonders hoher Weiksamkeit aus den Meneralstofswechsel. Experientia (Basel) 1953;9:33.

85. Skinner SL. Improved assay methods for renin concentration and activity in human plasma. Circ Res 1967;20:391.

86. Skinner SL, Cran EJ, Gibson R, et al. Angiotensin I and II, active and inactive renin, renin substrate, renin activity and angiotensinase in human liquor amnii and plasma. Am J Obstet Gynecol 1975; 121:626.

87. Skinner SL, Lumbers ER, Symonds EM. Alterations by oral contraceptives of normal menstrual changes in plasma renin activity, concentration and substrate. Clin Sci 1969;36:67.

88. Skowsky WR, Fisher DA. Fetal neurohypophysical arginine vasopressin and arginine vasotocin in man and sheep. Pediatr Res 1977;11:627.

89. Smith A, McIntosh N. Neurohypophysial peptides in the human fetus: presence in pituitary extracts of immunoreactive arginine-vasotocin. J Endocrinol 1983;99:441.

90. Symonds EM, Skinner SL, Stanley MA, et al. An investigation of the cellular sources of renin in human chorion. J Obstet Gynaecol Br Comm 1970;77:885.

91. Symonds EM, Stanley MA, Skinner SL. Production of renin by in vitro cultures of human chorion and uterine muscle. Nature 1968;217:1152.

92. Thomson AM, Hytten FE, Billewicz WZJ. The epidemiology of edema during pregnancy. J Obstet Gynaecol Br Comm 1967;74:1.

93. Tuck ML, Dluhy RG, Williams GH. A specific role for saline or the sodium ion in the regulation of renin and aldosterone secretion. J Clin Invest 1974;53:988.

94. Tulchinsky D, Okada DM. Hormones in human pregnancy. IV. Plasma progesterone. Am J Obstet Gynecol 1975;121:293.

95. Venning EH, Primrose T, Caligaris LCS, et al. Aldosterone excretion in pregnancy. J Clin Endocrinol 1957;17:473.

96. Walters WAW, Lim YL. Changes in the maternal cardiovascular system in human pregnancy. Surg Gynecol Obstet 1970;131:765.

97. Watanabe M, Meeker CI, Gray MJ, et al. Secretion of aldosterone in normal pregnancy. J Clin Invest 1963;42:1619.

98. Weinberger MH, Kramer NJ, Petersen LP, et al. Sequential changes in the renin-aldosterone system and plasma progesterone concentration in normal and abnormal human pregnancy. In: Lindheimer MD, Katz AK, Zuspan FP, eds. Hypertension in pregnancy. New York: John Wiley & Sons, 1976:263.

99. Weinberger MH, Petersen LP, Herr MJ, et al. Observations of the renin-angiotensin-aldosterone system in pregnancy. In: Fregly MJ, Fregly MS, eds. Oral contraceptives and high blood pressure. Gainesville, FL: Dolphin Press, 1974:237.

100. Weiner CP, Smith F, Robillard JE. Arginine vasopressin and acute intravascular volume expansion in the human fetus. Fetal Ther 1989;4:69.

101. Weir RJ, Briggs E, Mack A, et al. Blood pressure in women taking oral contraceptives. BMJ 1974;1:533.

102. Weir RJ, Brown JJ, Fraser R, et al. Relationship between plasma renin substrate, angiotensin II, aldosterone and electrolytes in normal pregnancy. J Clin Endocrinol 1975;40:108.

103. Weir RJ, Paintin DB, Brown JJ, et al. A serial study in pregnancy of the plasma concentrations of renin, corticosteroids, electrolyte and proteins and of haematocrit and plasma volume. J Obstet Gynaecol Br Comm 1971;78:590.

104. Williams GH, Cain JP, Dluhy RG, Underwood RH. Studies of the control of plasma aldosterone concentration in normal man. I. Response to posture, acute and chronic volume depletion and sodium loading. J Clin Invest 1972;51:1731.

105. Williams GH, Dluhy RG. Aldosterone biosynthesis. Interrelationship of regulatory factors. Am J Med 1972;53:595.

106. Williams GH, Dluhy RG. Diseases of the adrenal cortex. In: Wilson JD, Braunwald E, Isselbacher KJ, eds. Harrison's principles of internal medicine, ed 12. New York: McGraw-Hill, 1991:1713.

107. Williams GH, Hollenberg NK, Moore TJ, et al. Failure of renin suppression by angiotensin II in hypertension. Circ Res 1978;42:46.

108. Williams GH, Rose LI, Dluhy RG, et al. Aldosterone response to sodium restriction and ACTH stimulation in panhypopituitarism. J Clin Endocrinol 1971; 32:27.

109. Woods JW. Oral contraceptives and hypertension. Lancet 1967;2:653.

CHAPTER 7

The Maternal Adenohypophysis

Robert L. Barbieri

The structure and function of the anterior lobe of the pituitary gland (adenohypophysis) are significantly altered by pregnancy. In this chapter, the structural and functional changes of the adenohypophysis during pregnancy are reviewed. This review is followed by a discussion of diseases of the adenohypophysis that can occur during pregnancy and the puerperium.

PITUITARY STRUCTURE THROUGHOUT PREGNANCY

The pituitary gland is composed of three major parts: an anterior lobe (adenohypophysis), an intermediate lobe (prominent in the fetus but atrophic in adult life), and a posterior lobe (the neurohypophysis). The anterior and posterior lobes have distinct embryologic origins. The anterior lobe is formed from an upward extension of ectoderm from the primitive oral cavity (Rathke's pouch). The posterior pituitary lobe arises from a downgrowth of the hypothalamus and fuses with Rathke's pouch. The roof of the sella turcica is formed from dura (diaphragm sellae). The posterior wall of the sella is formed by dorsum sellae (bone), and the lateral walls are formed by fibrous tissue proximate to the medial walls of the cavernous sinus.

The pituitary lies near cranial nerves II (superiorly) and III, IV, V, and VI (laterally). In the nonpregnant state, the pituitary gland is approximately 15 mm across, 10 mm long, and 5 mm deep and weighs approximately 0.5 to 1 g. During pregnancy, the volume of the pituitary gland increases significantly, and the shape of the gland changes. An autopsy study of 118 pregnant women demonstrated a 30% increase in the weight of the gland (term, 1070 mg; nonpregnant, 820 mg).[22] Using magnetic resonance imaging, a continuous increase in gland volume has been demonstrated throughout gestation[34] (Table 7–1). The total increase in pituitary volume from the nonpregnant state to the third trimester was 136%. This increase in pituitary volume results in a change in the shape of the gland with the development of a convex, domed appearance of the diaphragm sellae.[41] This upward bulging of the pituitary and compression of the optic chiasm

TABLE 7–1. Volume of the Pituitary Gland Throughout Pregnancy as Determined by Magnetic Resonance Imaging

Gestational Age (weeks)	Subject Number	Pituitary Volume (mm³)
Nonpregnant	20	300 ± 60
9	10	437 ± 90
21	11	534 ± 124
37	11	708 ± 123

Data from Gonzalez JG, Elizondo G, Saldivar D, et al. Pituitary gland growth during normal pregnancy: an in vivo study using magnetic resonance imaging. Am J Med 1988;85:217.

may account, in part, for the bitemporal hemianopsia observed in some pregnant women.[16, 24] Of interest, at term the posterior pituitary is difficult to image.[24] This is in contrast to the nonpregnant state, in which the posterior pituitary can be imaged using a T1-weighted signal.[24]

The adenohypophysis is composed of six distinct cell types: thyrotrope, gonadotrope, corticotrope, somatotrope, lactotrope, and "other." During pregnancy, the number, structure, and function of four of these six cell types change significantly. The greatest changes occur in the lactotropes. Before pregnancy, approximately 20% of pituitary cells are lactotropes. In the third trimester, as many as 60% of the pituitary cells are lactotropes.[5, 75] The increase in the number of prolactin-producing cells is most striking in the lateral aspects of the gland. By 1 month postpartum, the number of lactotropes decreased in nonlactating women.[75] Postpartum resolution of lactotrope hyperplasia is not complete, and nonpregnant multiparae have more lactotropes than nulligravidae.[5, 75] The number of gonadotropes and α-secreting cells decreases markedly during pregnancy. The number of somatotropes decreases throughout pregnancy.[75] Little change occurs in the number of thyrotrope cells.[75]

ANTERIOR PITUITARY FUNCTION THROUGHOUT PREGNANCY

The structural changes in the pituitary throughout pregnancy (Table 7–2) are paral-

Table 7–2. Cross-Sectional Area (Anteroposterior by Transverse Diameter) of the Pituitary Gland at Autopsy Throughout Gestation

Group	Subject Number	Cross-Sectional Area (mm^2)
Nonpregnant	10	60
First trimester	1	45
Second trimester	2	68
Third trimester	9	104
Postpartum (days)		
<30	2	122
30–59	3	96
60–120	3	73

Data from Scheithauer BW, Sano T, Kovacs ST, et al. The pituitary gland in pregnancy: a clinicopathologic and immunohistochemical study of 69 cases. Mayo Clin Proc 1990;65:461.

leled by important functional changes. During pregnancy, pituitary production of prolactin and adrenocorticotropic hormone (ACTH) increase. Pituitary production of gonadotropins and growth hormone (GH) decreases. Little change occurs in pituitary production of thyrotropin, vasopressin, or oxytocin except during labor, when oxytocin levels increase significantly.

PROLACTIN

During pregnancy, there are three major sources of prolactin production: maternal pituitary, fetal pituitary, and uterine decidua. Most prolactin in the maternal circulation is derived from the maternal pituitary. Throughout pregnancy, prolactin levels rise from <20 ng/mL in the nonpregnant state to 60 ng/mL at 14 weeks' gestation, 100 ng/mL at 24 weeks' gestation, and 140 ng/mL at term[71] (Fig. 7–1). The factors that account for this rise have not been definitively defined, but estradiol is thought to play an important role in causing the hyperprolactinemia of pregnancy. In laboratory animals, estradiol increases the concentration of prolactin mRNA and increases prolactin secretion. Estradiol may produce these effects by a direct effect on the lactotrope and by an indirect effect on the hypothalamus and median eminence. As an example of this possible indirect effect, estradiol increased the median eminence concentration of vasoactive intestinal peptide, and vasoactive intestinal peptide is known to stimulate lactotrope

growth in vitro and is a secretagogue from prolactin.[65, 66]

As already noted, the decidua is a major site of prolactin production during pregnancy, and amniotic fluid prolactin concentrations peak at 6000 ng/mL near the end of the second trimester.[23] Evidence to support the contention that significant quantities of decidual prolactin do not enter the maternal circulation is provided by observations that in pregnant women with preexisting hypopituitarism, prolactin in the maternal circulation is low throughout pregnancy.[50, 70]

The control of pituitary prolactin secretion during pregnancy appears to be preserved except for the presence of a higher set-point to basal secretion. For example, in pregnant women, prolactin secretion is stimulated by thyrotropin-releasing hormone,[39] arginine, meals,[67] and sleep[13] in a manner similar to that observed in nonpregnant women. Following delivery, prolactin concentrations decrease to nonpregnant levels within 3 months in nonnursing mothers.[12] In nursing women, baseline serum prolactin concentrations slowly decrease to nonpregnant levels, and intermittent episodic pulses of prolactin secretion in conjunction with nursing are observed.

During pregnancy, there is a major change in the biochemistry of circulating prolactin. In the nonpregnant state, most circulating prolactin is an N-linked glycosylated form (G-PRL). As pregnancy progresses, increasing amounts of nonglycosylated prolactin as compared with G-PRL appear in the circulation.[56] In the third trimester, the concentration of circulating nonglycosylated prolactin exceeds that of G-PRL. After parturition in nonnursing mothers, the proportion of nonglycosylated prolactin in the circulation decreases markedly.[56] G-PRL and nonglycosylated prolactin may serve different physiologic roles. In some systems, nonglycosylated prolactin is more biologically active than G-PRL.[64] In pregnancy and lactation, more of the nonglycosylated prolactin may be produced to prepare the breast for lactation.[56]

ADRENOCORTICOTROPIN

Pregnancy is marked by an increase in the concentration of ACTH, similar to that of prolac-

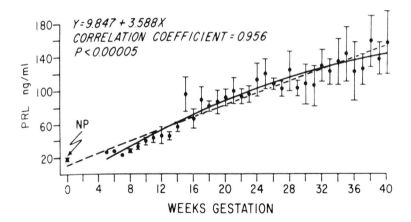

$Y = 9.847 + 3.588X$
CORRELATION COEFFICIENT = 0.956
$P < 0.00005$

FIGURE 7–1. Circulating prolactin throughout gestation. (From Rigg LA, Lein A, Yen SSC. Pattern of increase in circulating prolactin levels during human gestation. Am J Obstet Gynecol 1977; 129:454. With permission.)

tin, in the maternal circulation. For example, Carr et al[15] reported an increase in ACTH in the maternal circulation from 10 pg/mL in the nonpregnant state to 50 pg/mL at term (Fig. 7–2). Further increases in ACTH in the maternal circulation (300 pg/mL) were observed in labor.[15] Although the placenta can produce ACTH,[29] the majority of the ACTH in the maternal circulation is probably derived from the maternal pituitary.[28]

The increase in ACTH is associated with an increase in serum free cortisol,[62, 63] salivary free cortisol,[76] and urinary free cortisol.[18, 62, 63] Maternal hypercortisolemia is also observed in complete molar pregnancy, suggesting that the excess cortisol is derived exclusively from the maternal adrenal. The parallel increase in ACTH and cortisol during pregnancy suggests that the elevated ACTH is causing the increase in adrenal cortisol production and that there is an abnormal set-point in the negative feedback control between ACTH and cortisol. Further evidence to suggest that there is an abnormal set-point in ACTH-cortisol feedback is provided by the observation that in pregnancy short-term and long-term dexamethasone suppression fails to suppress total serum cortisol and urinary free cortisol normally.[62, 63, 68]

Evidence is accumulating that corticotropin-releasing hormone (CRH) produced by the placenta may be the cause of the abnormal ACTH-cortisol set-point observed in pregnancy.[31–33] In nonpregnant women, circulating CRH is in the range of 10 to 100 pg/mL. In the third trimester of pregnancy, maternal CRH concentrations are 500 to 3000 pg/mL, and these levels decline rapidly after delivery.[33]

Elevated placental CRH may play a role in altering the maternal ACTH-cortisol set-point. Goland et al[31] have reported a series of experiments in baboons that indicate that pituitary response to CRH and vasopressin is abnormal during pregnancy. In nonpregnant baboons, low doses (0.5 μg/kg) and high doses (5 μg/kg) of exogenous CRH produce significant increases in circulating ACTH and cortisol.[31] In pregnant baboons near term, low doses (0.5 μg/kg) of CRH fail to stimulate increases in circulating ACTH and cortisol. High doses (5 μg/kg) of CRH, however, fail to stimulate rises in ACTH and cortisol in the pregnant animals.[31] In sharp contrast to the resistance of the pregnant pituitary to CRH is the sensitivity of the pregnant pituitary to vasopressin.[32] In pregnant baboons near term, vasopressin (0.3 unit, 3.0 units) produced larger increases in ACTH and cortisol than those observed in nonpregnant controls. These investigators conclude that chronic placental CRH stimulation of the maternal pituitary-adrenal axis during pregnancy leads to an enhanced response to vasopressin and a down-regulation of the response to CRH.[31, 32]

GROWTH HORMONE

During pregnancy, secretion of GH (somatotropin) by the maternal pituitary is markedly suppressed. This discovery is in sharp contrast to the previously accepted belief that the maternal concentration of pituitary GH is normal.[49] The discovery of two forms of human GH has significantly advanced our understand-

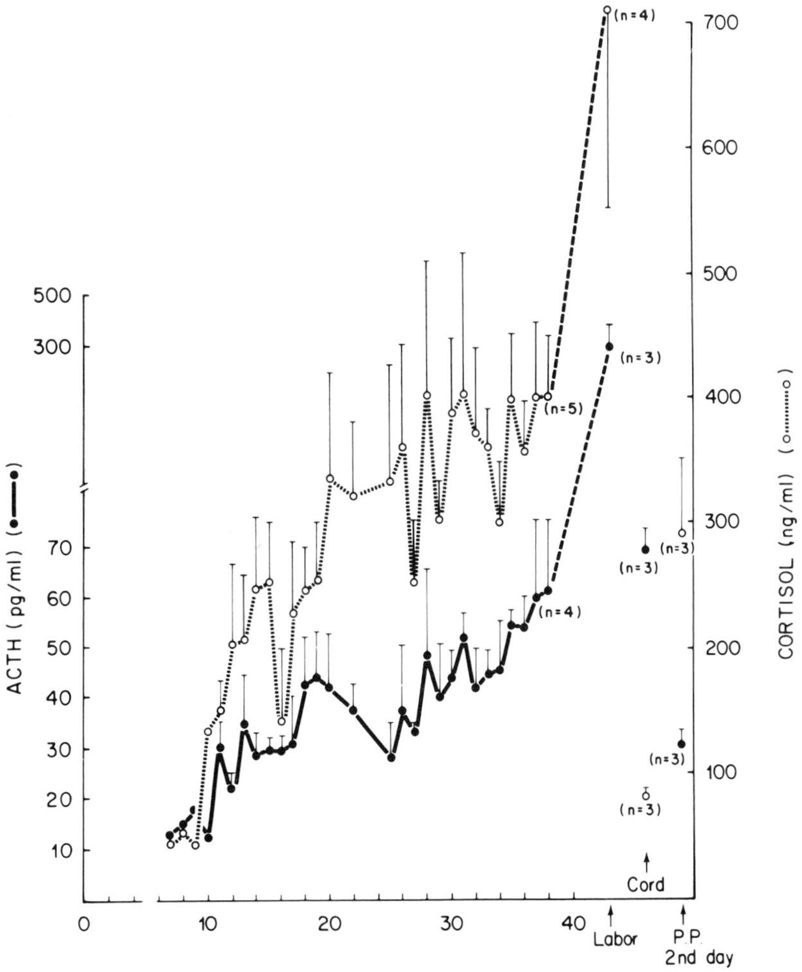

FIGURE 7–2. Circulating ACTH throughout gestation. (From Carr BR, Parker CR Jr, Madden JD, et al. Maternal plasma adrenocorticotropin and cortisol relationships throughout human pregnancy. Am J Obstet Gynecol 1981; 139:416. With permission.)

ing of GH economics in pregnancy. During pregnancy, the placenta produces a variant of GH (GH-V) that is encoded by its own gene and differs by 13 amino acids from pituitary GH.[25, 26] GH-V is secreted in a nonpulsatile manner, with minimal diurnal variation, and appears to be biologically active[20, 25, 26] (Fig. 7–3). Near term only 3% of circulating GH bioactivity is derived from maternal pituitary secretion, 85% is derived from placental secretion of GH-V, and 12% is derived from the actions of chorionic somatomammotropin.[20] The circulating GH-V probably stimulates insulin-like growth factor-I (IGF-I) secretion, resulting in negative feedback suppression of maternal GH secretion.[20] Blunted GH response to insulin[84] (Fig. 7–4) and arginine[73] (Fig. 7–5) during pregnancy may be accounted for, in part, by suppression of maternal GH secretion. The elevated GH-V and IGF-I concentrations and the decreased insulin-like growth factor binding protein concentrations in pregnancy may make the third trimester of pregnancy an "acromegalic-like" state.

GONADOTROPINS

During pregnancy, maternal serum luteinizing hormone (LH) and follicle-stimulating hor-

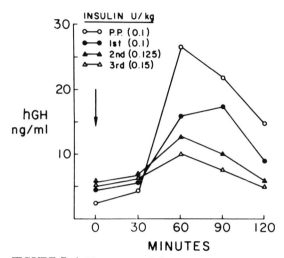

FIGURE 7–4. Human growth hormone response to insulin throughout pregnancy. (From Yen SSC, Vela P, Tsai CC. Impairment of growth hormone secretion in response to hypoglycemia during early and late pregnancy. J Clin Endocrinol Metab 1970; 31:29. With permission.)

mone (FSH) concentrations are decreased by 6 to 7 weeks of pregnancy and are near or below the detection limits of most assays in the second and third trimesters[59, 69, 72] (Fig. 7–6). Immunohistochemical and immunochemical analysis of pituitary glands from pregnant women demonstrate a decrease in pituitary LH and FSH concentration.[21, 75] During pregnancy, LH and FSH response to exogenous GnRH is diminished[59, 69, 72] (see Fig. 7–6). It is likely that the markedly elevated concentrations of estradiol and progesterone during pregnancy are causally involved in the suppression of maternal LH and FSH secretion. Inhibin, secreted by the corpus luteum and placenta, may act in concert with estradiol to suppress FSH secretion.[1, 57] After delivery, maternal concentrations of estradiol, progesterone, and inhibin decrease rapidly, and circulating LH and FSH concentrations slowly return to normal.[59, 69, 72]

THYROTROPIN

Maternal concentrations of thyrotropin, or thyroid-stimulating hormone (TSH), are within the normal range, and TSH response to thyrotropin-releasing hormone (TRH) is normal throughout pregnancy.[40, 48] At 9 to 13 weeks' gestation, there appears to be a modest

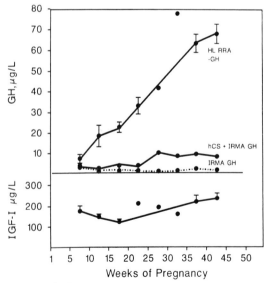

FIGURE 7–3. Circulating growth hormone throughout gestation. (From Daughaday WH, Trivedi B, Winn HN, Yan H. Hypersomatotropism in pregnant women, as measured by a human liver radioreceptor assay. J Clin Endocrinol Metab 1990; 70:215. With permission.)

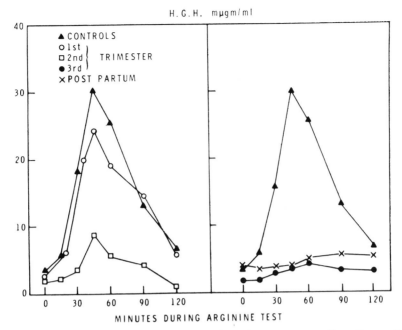

FIGURE 7–5. Human growth hormone response to arginine throughout pregnancy. (From Samaan NA, Goplerud CP, Bradbury JT. Effect of arginine infusion on plasma levels of growth hormone, insulin and glucose during pregnancy and the puerperium. Am J Obstet Gynecol 1970; 107:1002. With permission.)

decline in maternal circulating TSH concentrations[30, 37] (Fig. 7–7). This change coincides with peak placental production of human chorionic gonadotropin (hCG). The decrease in TSH may be due to the weak thyrotropic properties of hCG.[61, 80] An alternative hypothesis is that the placenta secretes a chorionic TSH or TRH, but more recent findings do not support this concept.[36, 37]

IMPRINTING OF THE PITUITARY DURING PREGNANCY

Pregnancy may produce changes in pituitary function that persist long after delivery. Imprinting of the pituitary is best documented with respect to prolactin secretion. Musey et al[60] studied serum LH, FSH, and prolactin secretion in 24 women both before and after pregnancy and in 40 nulliparous controls. Basal serum LH and FSH concentrations and LH and FSH response to GnRH were identical before and after pregnancy in the 24 experimental subjects. In contrast, basal serum prolactin concentrations and prolactin response to per-

phenazine were lower after pregnancy.[60] To expand on these results, basal prolactin levels were measured in a cross-sectional study of 19 nulliparous women and 29 parous women.[60] Serum prolactin was lower in the parous women (4.8 ± 0.4 ng/mL) than in the nulliparous women (8.9 ± 1.4 ng/mL, $P < 0.01$). These investigators conclude that pregnancy may decrease the risk of developing breast cancer by permanently lowering prolactin secretion. Similar results have been reported by Yu et al[85] and Kwa et al.[53]

PITUITARY TUMORS DURING PREGNANCY

Laboratory findings demonstrate that many pituitary tumors are monoclonal, i.e., derived from a single stem cell. For example, in one study clonality was demonstrated in 100% of GH-producing tumors, 100% of prolactin-producing tumors, and 75% of ACTH-producing tumors.[38] Somatic mutations that alter the gene for the Gs protein may play a role in tumorigenesis of many pituitary tumors, especially GH-secreting tumors. G proteins regulate adenylate cyclase activity and are com-

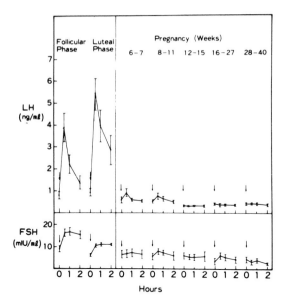

FIGURE 7–6. Serum levels of LH and FSH before and after a 100-μg bolus of GnRH in pregnant women and normal menstruating women. (Miyake A, Tanizawa O, Aono T, Kurachi K. Pituitary responses in LH secretion to LHRH during pregnancy. Obstet Gynecol 1977; 49:549. With permission.)

posed of proteins that transfer stimulatory (Gs) or inhibitory (Gi) signals from cell surface receptors to enzyme catalytic units. In one report, of 25 GH-secreting tumors studied, 10 had mutations in the Gs gene, resulting in the production of a mutant Gs protein that is chronically activated.[55] Genetic mutations may be the primary cause of pituitary tumor growth. Factors that may change during pregnancy (e.g., estrogen, progesterone, dopamine) may play a secondary role in controlling tumor growth.

PROLACTINOMAS DURING PREGNANCY

In general, women with significant hyperprolactinemia are anovulatory and require endocrine treatment (bromocriptine) to ovulate and achieve a pregnancy. The effects of pregnancy on a preexisting prolactinoma have been evaluated in a large number of cases.[27, 35, 45, 51, 79, 81] In general, bromocriptine was discontinued when the pregnancy was first diagnosed. Neurologic outcomes differed among

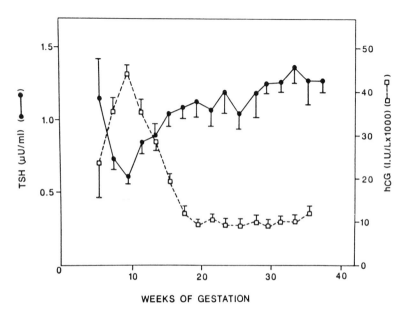

FIGURE 7–7. Serum TSH and hCG as a function of gestational age. (From Glinoer D, De Nayer P, Bourdoux P, et al. Regulation of maternal thyroid during pregnancy. J Clin Endocrinol Metab 1990; 71:276. With permission.)

patients with microprolactinomas and macro-prolactinomas. Therefore these results are discussed separately. Of the 215 patients with microprolactinomas,[27, 35, 45, 51, 79, 81] fewer than 1% had changes in their visual fields, polytomograms, or neurologic signs. Approximately 5% developed headaches. Of the 60 patients with macroadenomas,[29, 35, 54] approximately 20% developed changes in their visual fields, polytomograms, or neurologic signs. Some of these patients required reinstitution of bromocriptine, addition of glucocorticoids, or neurosurgical intervention owing to an expanding tumor mass.

Pregnancy can be induced with bromocriptine in a patient with a microprolactinoma with the expectation that few serious neurosurgical complications will occur. For the patient with a macroprolactinoma, mild neurosurgical complications occur frequently. In general, these can be treated by the reinstitution of bromocriptine.[14] Some authorities recommend surgical treatment or radiotherapy before induction of ovulation and pregnancy with bromocriptine in women with macroprolactinomas to decrease the incidence of intrapartum neurologic complications. Surgical intervention or radiotherapy, however, can often result in a loss of gonadotropin reserve and produce a need for ovulation induction with gonadotropins. Loss of gonadotropin reserve owing to bromocriptine has not been observed. Therefore women with macroprolactinomas might best be treated by using bromocriptine throughout their pregnancy.

Cushing's disease is typically associated with depressed gonadotropin secretion, and consequently pregnancy rarely occurs in women with Cushing's disease.[3] In pregnant women with Cushing's disease, premature labor, pregnancy-induced hypertension, and gestational diabetes are unusually common.[3] Most cases of Cushing's disease are due to microadenomas, and consequently neurosurgical problems caused by a pituitary mass effect are unlikely to occur during pregnancy. In most cases, definitive treatment of Cushing's disease can be delayed until after delivery.

Acromegaly is often associated with anovulation, but pregnancy sometimes occurs. In general, except for possible complications of pituitary enlargement, acromegaly does not appear to have a marked detrimental effect on pregnancy outcome.[2] In most cases, definitive treatment for acromegaly can be deferred until after delivery. Bromocriptine therapy[19, 83] and transsphenoidal surgery have been successfully used to treat acromegaly during pregnancy.

SHEEHAN'S SYNDROME

Sheehan's syndrome is the development of hypothalamic and pituitary dysfunction following severe obstetric hemorrhage near term. As already noted, the pituitary increases in volume by approximately 100% during pregnancy. This increase in size and the low-flow, low-pressure nature of the pituitary (portal) capillary circulation may make the pituitary, and parts of the hypothalamus, vulnerable to ischemia caused by obstetric hemorrhage and shock. In developed countries, the availability of sophisticated blood banks, high-quality anesthesia services, and well-equipped and well-staffed obstetric operating rooms has significantly decreased the incidence of postpartum pituitary necrosis. In contrast, in developing countries, obstetric hemorrhage and shock remain major problems. In these countries, Sheehan's syndrome is a major cause of hypopituitarism.[47]

In Sheehan's syndrome, virtually any pattern of pituitary hormone deficiency can be observed. GH and prolactin deficiency, however, are the most common abnormalities in Sheehan's syndrome. Jialal et al[47] studied 10 African women with Sheehan's syndrome using a combined intravenous insulin (0.1 unit/kg), TRH (200 μg), and GnRH (100 μg) challenge test. The pattern of pituitary dysfunction observed among the women was as follows: 100% had prolactin deficiency, 100% had GH deficiency, 90% had cortisol deficiency, 80% had TSH deficiency, 70% had LH deficiency, and 40% had FSH deficiency.[47]

These pituitary abnormalities can cause failure of lactation, failure of hair growth over areas shaved for delivery, poor wound healing after cesarean section, and weakness. Organic psychosis is also a common problem in women with Sheehan's syndrome.[6, 52] Probably the safest, most simple test for Sheehan's syndrome would be to perform an intravenous TRH (100 μg) stimulation test with prolactin measurements at time 0 minutes and 30 minutes. The ratio of prolactin at time 30 minutes to prolactin at time 0 should be ≥3.[10, 47] If the ratio of prolactin response to TRH is subnormal, the patient should undergo a complete evaluation for possible panhypopituitarism.

Disorders of anterior pituitary function are the most common presentation for Sheehan's syndrome. Mild posterior pituitary dysfunction, however, occurred frequently in women with Sheehan's syndrome. A pathologic study by Sheehan and Whitehead[78] indicated that 90% of patients with postpartum hypopituitarism demonstrated ''atrophy and scarring'' of the neurohypophysis. None of these patients, however, displayed symptoms of diabetes insipidus. Whitehead[82] performed detailed pathologic studies on the hypothalamus of 13 patients previously studied with Sheehan[78] and found that atrophy of the supraoptic, nucleus, and to a lesser extent the paraventricular nucleus was directly correlated with the degree of neurohypophyseal atrophy present but not with that of the adenohypophysis. The site of the primary lesion leading to the atrophic changes in the hypothalamic nuclei and the posterior pituitary could not be determined. These studies emphasize that although clinical diabetes insipidus is seldom associated with Sheehan's syndrome, pathologic abnormalities in the hypothalamus and posterior pituitary are common in this syndrome.[77]

Clinical studies demonstrate that most women with Sheehan's syndrome have mild defects in vasopressin secretion and maximal urinary concentrating ability.[8, 9, 11, 43, 46] The hypothyroidism and hypocortisolemia present in Sheehan's syndrome can produce hyperlipidemia[42] and blunted responses of renin and aldosterone to volume depletion.[7]

LYMPHOCYTIC HYPOPHYSITIS

Lymphocytic hypophysitis is a rare disorder involving infiltration of the adenohypophysis by lymphocytes and plasma cells, which, in some cases, results in hypopituitarism. Most cases of lymphocytic hypophysitis occur in women in the third trimester of pregnancy or immediately postpartum. In cases in which hypopituitarism is present, ACTH deficiency is extremely common. Circulating antipituitary antibodies, antinuclear antibodies, and antimitochondria antibodies can be detected in some cases. Pituitary enlargement can occur and cause neurologic complications requiring transsphenoidal surgery. Bromocriptine and high-dose glucocorticoids can sometimes be effective in managing the neurologic sequelae (headache, visual field defects, cranial nerve palsies) of severe lymphocytic hypophysitis.[4, 17, 58]

REFERENCES

1. Abe Y, Hasegawa Y, Miyamoto K, et al. High concentrations of plasma immunoreactive inhibin during normal pregnancy in women. J Clin Endocrinol Metab 1990;71:133–137.
2. Abelove WA, Rupp JJ, Paschkis KE. Acromegaly and pregnancy. J Clin Endocrinol Metab 1954;14:32–44.
3. Aron DC, Schnall AM, Sheeler LR. Cushing's syndrome and pregnancy. Am J Obstet Gynecol 1990;162:244–252.
4. Asa SL, Bilbao JM, Kovacs K, Josse RG, Kreines L. Lymphocytic hypophysitis of pregnancy resulting in hypopituitarism: a distinct clinicopathologic entity. Ann Intern Med 1981;95:166–171.
5. Asa SL, Penz G, Kovacs K, Ezrin C. Prolactin cells in the human pituitary: a quantitative immunocytochemical analysis. Arch Pathol Lab Med 1982;106:360–363.
6. Bahemkura M, Rees PH. Sheehan's syndrome presenting with psychosis. E Afr Med J 1981;58:324–329.
7. Bakiri F, Benmiloud M, Vallotton MB. The renin-angiotensin system in panhypopituitarism: Dynamic studies and therapeutic effects in Sheehan's syndrome. J Clin Endocrinol Metab 1983;56:1042–1047.
8. Bakiri F, Benmiloud M, Vallotton MB. Arginine-vasopressin in postpartum panhypopituitarism: urinary excretion and kidney response to osmolar lead. J Clin Endocrinol Metab 1984;58:511–515.
9. Bakiri F, Benmiloud M. Antidiuretic function in Sheehan's syndrome. Br Med J 1984;289:579–580.
10. Barbieri RL, Cooper DS, Daniels GH, et al. Prolactin responses to thyrotropin releasing hormone in patients with hypothalamic-pituitary disease. Fertil Steril 1985;43:66.
11. Barbieri RL, Randall RW, Saltzman DH. Diabetes insipidus occurring in a patient with Sheehan's syndrome during a gonadotropin-induced pregnancy. Fertil Steril 1985;44:529.
12. Bonnar J, Franklin M, Nott PN, McNeilly AS. Effect of breast-feeding on pituitary-ovarian function after childbirth. BMJ 1975;4:82.
13. Boyar RM, Finkelstein JW, Kapen S, Hellman L. Twenty-four hour prolactin (PRL) secretory patterns during pregnancy. J Clin Endocrinol Metab 1975; 40:1117.
14. Canales ES, Garcia IC, Ruiz JE, Zarate A. Bromocriptine as prophylactic therapy in prolactinoma during pregnancy. Fertil Steril 1981;36:524.
15. Carr BR, Parker CR Jr, Madden JD, et al. Maternal plasma adrenocorticotropin and cortisol relationships

throughout human pregnancy. Am J Obstet Gynecol 1981;139:416.

16. Carvill M. Bitemporal contractions of the visual fields during pregnancy. Am J Ophthalmol 1923;6:885.

17. Castle D, DeVilliers JC, Melvill R. Lymphocytic adenohypophysitis. Report of a case with demonstration of spontaneous tumour regression and a review of the literature. J Neurosurg 1988;2:401.

18. Cousins L, Rigg L, Hollingsworth D, et al. Qualitative and quantitative assessment of the circadian rhythm of cortisol in pregnancy. Am J Obstet Gynecol 1983; 145:411.

19. Cundy R, Grundy EN, Melville H, Sheldon J. Bromocriptine treatment of acromegaly following spontaneous conception. Fertil Steril 1984;42:134.

20. Daughaday WH, Trivedi B, Winn HN, Yan H. Hypersomatotropism in pregnant women, as measured by a human liver radioreceptor assay. J Clin Endocrinol Metab 1990;70:215.

21. De la Lastra M, Llados C. Luteinizing hormone content of the pituitary gland in pregnant and non-pregnant women. J Clin Endocrinol Metab 1977;44:921.

22. Erdheim J, Stumme E. Uber die schwangerschaftsveranderung der hypophyse. Beitr Z Pathol Anat 1909; 46:1.

23. Fang VS, Kim MH. Study on maternal, fetal, and amniotic human prolactin at term. J Clin Endocrinol Metab 1975;41:1030.

24. Finlay CE. Visual field defects in pregnancy. Arch Ophthalmol 1934;12:207.

25. Frankenne F, Closset J, Gomez F, et al. The physiology of growth hormones (GHs) in pregnant women and partial characterization of the placental GH variant. J Clin Endocrinol Metab 1988;66:1171.

26. Frankenne F, Rentier-Delrue F, Scippo ML, et al. Expression of the growth hormone variant gene in human placenta. J Clin Endocrinol Metab 1991; 64:635.

27. Gemzell C, Wang CF. Outcome of pregnancy in women with pituitary adenoma. Fertil Steril 1979; 31:363.

28. Genazzani AR, Felber JP, Fioretti P. Immunoreactive ACTH, immunoreactive human chorionic somatomammotropin (HCS) and 11-OH steroid plasma levels in normal and pathological pregnancies. Acta Endocrinol 1977;83:800.

29. Genazzani AR, Fraioli F, Hurlimann J, et al. Immunoreactive ACTH and cortisol plasma levels during pregnancy. Detection and partial purification of corticotropin-like placental hormone: the human chorionic corticotropin (HCC). Clin Endocrinol 1975;4:1.

30. Glinoer D, De Nayer P, Bourdoux P, et al. Regulation of maternal thyroid during pregnancy. J Clin Endocrinol Metab 1990;71:276.

31. Goland RS, Stark RI, Wardlaw SL. Response to corticotropin-releasing hormone during pregnancy in the baboon. J Clin Endocrinol Metab 1990;70:925.

32. Goland RS, Wardlaw SL, MacCarter G, et al. Adenocortistropin and cortisol response to vasopressin during pregnancy. J Clin Endocrinol Metab 1991;73:257.

33. Goland RS, Wardlaw SL, Stark RI, et al. High levels of corticotropin-releasing hormone immunoreactivity in maternal and fetal plasma during pregnancy. J Clin Endocrinol Metab 1986;63:1199.

34. Gonzalez JG, Elizondo G, Saldivar D, et al. Pituitary gland growth during normal pregnancy: an in vivo study using magnetic resonance imaging. Am J Med 1988;85:217.

35. Griffith RW, Turkalj I, Braun P. Pituitary tumors dur-

ing the pregnancy in mothers treated with bromocriptine. Br J Clin Pharmacol 1979;1:393.

36. Harada A, Hershman JM. Extraction of human chorionic thyrotropin (hCT) from term placentas: failure to recover thyrotropic activity. J Clin Endocrinol Metab 1978;47:681.

37. Harada A, Hersham JM, Reed AW, et al. Comparison of thyroid stimulators and thyroid hormone concentrations in the sera of pregnant women. J Clin Endocrinol Metab 1979;48:793.

38. Herman V, Fagin J, Melmed S. Clonal origin of pituitary tumors. J Clin Endocrinol Metab 1990;71:1427.

39. Hersham JM, Burrow GN. Lack of release of human chorionic gonadotropin by thyrotropin-releasing hormone. J Clin Endocrinol Metab 1976;42:970.

40. Hershman JM, Kojima A, Friesen HG. Effect of thyrotropin-releasing hormone on human pituitary thyrotropin, prolactin, placental lactogen and chorionic thyrotropin. J Clin Endocrinol Metab 1973;36:497.

41. Hinshaw DB, Hasso AN, Thompson JR, Davidson BJ. High resolution computed tomography of the post partum pituitary gland. Neuroradiology 1984;26:299.

42. Ishibashi S, Murase T, Yamada N, et al. Hyperlipidemia in patients with hypopituitarism. Acta Endocrinol 1985;110:456.

43. Iwasaki Y, Oiso Y, Yamaguchi K, et al. Neurohypophyseal function in postpartum hypopituitarism: impaired plasma vasopressin response to osmotic stimuli. J Clin Endocrinol Metab 1989;68:560.

44. Jeppsson S, Rannevik G, Kullander S. Studies on the decreased gonadotropin response after administration of LH/FSH-releasing hormone during pregnancy and the puerewicz. Am J Obstet Gynecol 1974;120:1029.

45. Jewelewicz R, Vande Wiele RL. Clinical course and outcome of pregnancy in twenty-five patients with pituitary microadenomas. Am J Obstet Gynecol 1980; 136:339.

46. Jialal I, Desai RK, Rajput MC. An assessment of posterior pituitary function in patients with Sheehan's syndrome. Clin Endocrinol 1987;27:91.

47. Jialal I, Naidoo C, Norman RJ, et al. Pituitary function in Sheehan's syndrome. Obstet Gynecol 1984;63:15.

48. Kannan V, Sinha MK, Devi PK, Rastogi GK. Plasma thyrotropin and its response to thyrotropin releasing hormone in normal pregnancy. Obstet Gynecol 1973;42:547.

49. Kaplan SL, Grumbach MM. Serum chorionic growth hormone-prolactin and serum pituitary growth hormone in mother and fetus at term. J Clin Endocrinol Metab 1965;21:1370.

50. Kauppila A, Chatelain P, Kirkinen P, et al. Isolated prolactin deficiency in a woman with puerperal lactogenesis. J Clin Endocrinol Metab 1987;64:309.

51. Kelly WF, Doyle FH, Mashiter K, et al. Pregnancies in women with hyperprolactinemia: clinical course of 41 pregnancies in 27 women. Br J Obstet Gynaecol 1979; 86:698.

52. Khanna S, Ammini A, Saxena S, Mohan D. Hypopituitarism presenting as delirium. Int J Psychiat Med 1988;18:89.

53. Kwa HG, Cleton F, Bulbrook RD, et al. Plasma prolactin levels and breast cancer: relation to parity, weight and height and age at first birth. Int J Cancer 1981; 28:31.

54. Lamberts SWJ, Klijn JGM, deLange SA, et al. The incidence of complications during pregnancy after treatment of hyperprolactinemia with bromocriptine in patients with radiologically evident pituitary tumors. Fertil Steril 1979;31:614.

55. Landis CA, Harsh G. Clinical characteristics of acromegalic patients whose pituitary tumors contain mutant Gs protein. J Clin Endocrinol Metab 1990; 71:1416.

56. Markoff E, Lee DW, Hollingsworth DR. Glycosylated and nonglycosylated prolactin in serum during pregnancy. J Clin Endocrinol Metab 1988;67:519.

57. McLachlan RI, Healy DL, Robertson DM, et al. The human placenta: a novel source of inhibin. Biochem Biophys Res Commun 1986;140:485.

58. Meichner RH, Riggio S, Manz HJ, Earll JM. Lymphocytic adenohypophysitis causing pituitary mass. Neurology 1987;37:158.

59. Miyake A, Tanizawa O, Aono T, Kurachi K. Pituitary responses in LH secretion to LHRH during pregnancy. Obstet Gynecol 1977;49:549.

60. Musey VC, Collins DC, Musey PI, et al. Long-term effect of a first pregnancy on the secretion of prolactin. N Engl J Med 1987;316:229.

61. Nisula BC, Ketelslegers JM. Thyroid-stimulating activity and chorionic gonadotropin. J Clin Invest 1974; 54:494.

62. Nolten WE, Lindheimer MD, Ruekert PA, et al. Diurnal patterns and regulation of cortisol secretion in pregnancy. J Clin Endocrinol Metab 1980;51:466.

63. Nolten WE, Ruekert PA. Elevated free cortisol index in pregnancy: possible regulatory mechanisms. Am J Obstet Gynecol 1981;139:492.

64. Pellegrini I, Gunz G, Ronin C, et al. Polymorphism of prolactin secreted by human prolactinoma cells: immunological, receptor binding, and biological properties of the glycosylated and non-glycosylated forms. Endocrinology 1988;122:2667.

65. Prysor-Jones RA, Silverlight JJ, Kennedy SJ, Jenkins JS. Vasoactive intestinal peptide and the stimulation of lactotroph growth by oestradiol in situ. J Endocrinol 1988;116:259.

66. Prysor-Jones RA, Silverlight JJ, Jenkins JS. Oestradiol, vasoactive intestinal peptide and fibroblast growth factor in the growth of human pituitary tumor cells in vitro. J Endocrinol 1989;120:171.

67. Quigley ME, Ishizuka B, Ropert JF, Yen SSC. The food-entrained prolactin and cortisol release in late pregnancy and prolactinemia patients. J Clin Endocrinol Metab 1982;54:1109.

68. Rees LH, Burke CW, Chard T, et al. Possible placental origin of ACTH in normal human pregnancy. Nature 1975;254:620.

69. Reyes FI, Winter JSD, Faiman C. Pituitary gonadotropin function during human pregnancy: serum FSH and LH levels before and after LHRH administration. J Clin Endocrinol Metab 1976;42:590.

70. Riddick DH, Luciano AA, Kusmick WF, Maslar IA. Evidence for a nonpituitary source of amniotic fluid prolactin. Fertil Steril 1979;31:35.

71. Rigg LA, Lein A, Yen SSC. Pattern of increase in circulating prolactin levels during human gestation. Am J Obstet Gynecol 1977;129:454.

72. Rubinstein LM, Parlow AF, Derzko C, Hershman JM. Pituitary gonadotropin response to LHRH in human pregnancy. Obstet Gynecol 1978;52:172.

73. Samaan NA, Goplerud CP, Bradbury JT. Effect of arginine infusion on plasma levels of growth hormone, insulin and glucose during pregnancy and the puerperium. Am J Obstet Gynecol 1970;107:1002.

74. Sasaki A, Liotta AS, Luckey MM, et al. Immunoreactive corticotropin releasing factor is present in human maternal plasma during the third trimester of pregnancy. J Clin Endocrinol Metab 1984;59:812.

75. Scheithauer BW, Sano T, Kovacs ST, et al. The pituitary gland in pregnancy: a clinicopathologic and immunohistochemical study of 69 cases. Mayo Clin Proc 1990;65:461.

76. Schulte HM, Weisner D, Allolio B. The corticotropin releasing hormone test in late pregnancy: lack of adrenocorticotropin and cortisol response. Clin Endocrinol 1990;33:99.

77. Schwartz AR, Leddy AL. Recognition of diabetes insipidus in postpartum hypopituitarism. Obstet Gynecol 1982;59:394.

78. Sheehan HL, Whitehead R. The neurohypophysis in postpartum hypopituitarism. J Pathol 1965;85:145.

79. Shewchuk AB, Adamson GD, Lessard P, Ezrin C. The effect of pregnancy on suspected pituitary adenomas after conservative management of ovulation defects associated with galactorrhea. Am J Obstet Gynecol 1980;136:659.

80. Silverberg J, O'Donnell J, Sugenoya A, et al. Effect of human chorionic gonadotropin on human thyroid tissue in vitro. J Clin Endocrinol Metab 1978;46:420.

81. Thorner MO, Edwards CRW, Charlesworth M, et al. Pregnancy in patients presenting with hyperprolactinemia. BMJ 1979;2:771.

82. Whitehead R. The hypothalamus in post-partum hypopituitarism. J Pathol 1965;86:55.

83. Yap AS, Clouston WM, Mortimer RH, Drake RF. Acromegaly first diagnosed in pregnancy: the role of bromocriptine therapy. Am J Obstet Gynecol 1990; 163:477.

84. Yen SSC, Vela P, Tsai CC. Impairment of growth hormone secretion in response to hypoglycemia during early and late pregnancy. J Clin Endocrinol Metab 1970;31:29.

85. Yu MC, Gerkins VR, Henderson BE, et al. Elevated levels of prolactin in nulliparous women. Br J Cancer 1981;43:826.

86. Zarate A, Canales ES, Alger M, Forsbach G. The effect of pregnancy and lactation on pituitary prolactin-secreting tumors. Acta Endocrinol (Copenh) 1979; 92:407.

The Maternal Thyroid and Parathyroid Glands

Michael M. Kaplan

THYROID HORMONE PHYSIOLOGY

Thyroid Hormone Action

The biologically active thyroid hormones are L-thyroxine (T_4 or 3,5,3',5'-tetraiodo-L-thyronine), and 3,5,3'-triiodo-L-thyronine (T_3). The predominant mode of thyroid hormone action is a nuclear receptor mechanism that requires several processes (Table 8–1). Entry of circulating T_4 and T_3 into cells occurs via active transport from plasma and perhaps by passive diffusion as well. T_3 is the main active thyroid hormone within target cells at normal intracellular T_4 and T_3 concentrations. T_4 is mainly a prohormone, activated to T_3 in many organs. T_4 can also function directly as a thyroid hormone by binding to the T_3 receptor; intracellular T_4, however, accounts for only a small fraction of thyroid hormone effects except in unusual conditions of selective elevation of intracellular T_4 levels.

The nuclear T_3 receptors belong to the steroid hormone receptor superfamily. Two T_3 receptor genes each direct synthesis of more than one receptor isoform. There is differential expression of the T_3 receptor isoforms in various organs, but the precise role of each isoform is not yet clear. After T_3 or T_4 binds to a receptor, the occupied receptor binds to regulatory regions, termed T_3 *response elements*, of thyroid hormone–responsive genes. The DNA nucleotide sequences of T_3 response elements vary among different genes. Tissue-specific factors may also be important in modulating T_3 effects on gene transcription rates, which are stimulated in some cases and inhibited in others. The mRNAs produced by gene transcription then direct synthesis of thyroid hormone–dependent proteins. A few thyroid hormone actions appear to involve nonnuclear mechanisms, which are less well understood.

Thyroid Hormone Biosynthesis and Metabolism

The steps in T_4 and T_3 biosynthesis are listed in Table 8–2. Trapping of iodide from plasma is followed by organification of the iodide, i.e. iodination of tyrosine residues of the thyroglobulin molecule. Next, a small number of specific iodotyrosine residues are coupled by an ether linkage of the phenolic carbons to form iodothyronines, still part of thyroglobulin. Thyroglobulin is stored within the lumen of the thyroid follicle as the colloid protein. When needed, the stored thyroglobulin is subjected to proteolysis by lysosomal enzymes. The resulting T_4 and T_3 are secreted. Some T_4 is deiodinated to T_3 during the secretory process. Most of the iodinated tyrosines in thyroglobulin never become T_3 and T_4 but are liberated from thyroglobulin along with T_4 and T_3 and deiodinated within the thyrocytes, and the iodine is salvaged for re-use.

All of these biosynthetic processes as well as thyroid cell growth are stimulated by thyrotropin (thyroid-stimulating hormone) [TSH]. TSH acts through a cell surface receptor, which is homologous to the common receptor for luteinizing hormone (LH) and human chorionic gonadotropin (hCG) and is coupled to adenylate cyclase. Cyclic adenosine monophosphate (cAMP) is the most important intracellular second messenger for TSH action,

---

TABLE 8–1. Steps in Thyroid Hormone Action via the Nuclear T_3 Receptor

1. Entry of thyroid hormones into target cells
2. For T_4 deiodination to T_3
3. Binding of T_3 to its nuclear receptor(s)
4. Binding of the T_3-receptor complex to regulatory elements of thyroid hormone–responsive genes, stimulating or inhibiting gene transcription
5. Possible additional modulation of gene transcription rates by tissue-specific factors
6. mRNA translation into peptide gene products

TABLE 8–2. Steps in Thyroid Hormone Biosynthesis

1. Iodide trapping: active transport of iodide via a thyrocyte anion channel
2. Organification: iodination into tyrosine residues of thyroglobulin by the action of the enzyme thyroperoxidase
3. Coupling of iodotyrosine residues into iodothyronines, also catalyzed by thyroperoxidase
4. Storage of iodinated thyroglobulin as colloid in thyroid follicles
5. Proteolysis of thyroglobulin, releasing iodothyronines and iodotyrosines
6. Deiodination of iodotyrosines and salvage of iodide
7. Deiodination of some T_4 into T_3
8. Secretion of T_4 and T_3

but some TSH effects may be mediated by other second messenger systems, e.g., that involving phospholipase C and inositol phosphates.

The other important regulatory factor for thyroid hormone biosynthesis is intracellular iodide. Acutely a raised intracellular iodide concentration inhibits iodide organification (the Wolff-Chaikoff effect) and also inhibits thyroglobulin proteolysis and T_4 and T_3 secretion. Normally the thyroid gland escapes from these inhibitory actions after a short time, but thyroid glands that have been damaged, e.g., by thyroiditis or radiation, may not adapt. Exposure of such damaged thyroid glands to large amounts of iodide may cause hypothyroidism.

In the plasma, T_4 and T_3 circulate almost entirely bound to proteins, mainly thyroxine-binding globulin (TBG) and secondarily to transthyretin (formerly called prealbumin), albumin, and lipoproteins. Less than 0.05% of plasma T_4 and less than 0.5% of plasma T_3 are free, i.e., not protein bound, yet only the free T_4 and free T_3 enter cells of target organs.

Thyroidal secretion is the only source of T_4. About 20% of the T_3 in the circulation is secreted by the thyroid gland. The rest is produced by extrathyroidal T_4 5'-deiodination. T_4 is deiodinated to T_3 in many organs, including liver, kidney, pituitary, and brain. Much of the resulting T_3 returns to the circulation, but some remains within the organ of production. Thus there are two potential sources of intracellular T_3: plasma T_3 and T_3 produced locally. In some organs, such as heart and skeletal muscle, plasma T_3 is by far the main source of intracellular T_3. In others, such as liver and kidney, both sources are important. In yet other target organs, including pituitary and brain, locally produced T_3 predominates.

Deiodination of T_4 to T_3 is inhibited by fasting; by several drugs, including glucocorticoids; during and after surgery; and in virtually any serious nonthyroid illness. This reduction in T_3 production results in a selective reduction in serum total and free T_3 concentrations, sometimes termed the *low-T_3 syndrome*, which may have a beneficial, protein-sparing effect in hypocaloric or catabolic states. Pregnant women who have toxemia or preeclampsia have a low T_3 state similar to that seen in other nonthyroidal illnesses.

T_4 is also deiodinated to a biologically inactive T_3 isomer called *reverse-T_3*. T_3 and reverse-T_3 are deiodinated to diiodothyronines and monoiodothyronines. This cascade of deiodinations is the main pathway of T_4 and T_3 disposal. Sulfation and glucuronidation of T_4 and T_3 are minor disposal pathways. None of the other iodothyronines besides T_4 and T_3, and none of the esters, have any known hormonal effects at physiologic concentrations.

Hypothalamic-Pituitary-Thyroid Regulatory Axis

Secretion of TSH by the pituitary gland is inhibited by thyroid hormones, in a classic negative feedback loop. Thus serum TSH concentrations rise in hypothyroidism and fall in hyperthyroidism. Several hypothalamic factors also regulate TSH secretion. Most importantly, thyrotropin-releasing hormone (TRH) stimulates TSH secretion. There is also direct inhibition by T_3 of TRH production, a process termed *long loop negative feedback*. Somatostatin and dopamine, released from the hypothalamus into the pituitary portal system, appear to be inhibitory modulators of TSH secretion but are less important than TRH. High plasma levels of endogenous or exogenous glucocorticoids inhibit TSH secretion.

Changes in Thyroid Hormone Economy During Normal Pregnancy

Changes in the thyroid hormone economy of the normal pregnant woman are listed in Table 8–3. The hypothalamic-pituitary-thyroid axis functions normally during pregnancy. In the first trimester, there is a slight, transient decrease in the mean serum TSH concentration,[30, 35] in compensation for the mild thyrotropic actions of high plasma levels of hCG, as discussed further subsequently. The response of maternal TSH to stimulation by exogenous TRH is generally within the normal range, although the mean TSH increment may be slightly increased.[15]

The renal clearance of iodide increases during pregnancy,[1] in parallel with the rise in glomerular filtration rate. In geographic areas of iodine deficiency or borderline iodine sufficiency, the resulting urinary iodide loss can cause goiter[30] and an increased thyroidal iodine uptake. Because iodine deficiency is nonexistent in North America, it is not surprising that echographic estimates of thyroid size in American women show a mean increase of only 10% during pregnancy,[47, 58] not enough to be of clinical importance.

Circulating levels of TBG, the main thyroid hormone–binding protein in the plasma, double during pregnancy.[30] The increase in TBG level is roughly linear in the first 20 weeks of pregnancy, with no significant change thereafter. The TBG increase is due to a change in its pattern of glycosylation induced by the high circulating estrogen levels of pregnancy, leading to a longer plasma half-life. The consequence of the TBG increase is that total serum T_4 and total serum T_3 concentrations also rise substantially, by an average of about 30% in the first trimester and 50 to 65% in the second and third trimesters. These increases require normal pituitary and thyroid function. Even slight decreases in serum free T_4 or free T_3 levels due to increased binding to TBG should trigger an increase in TSH production. Higher TSH levels ought, in turn, to increase secretion of T_4 and T_3 from the thyroid gland until normal serum free T_4 and free T_3 concentrations are restored. In seven women in whom daily T_4 turnover rates were measured during pregnancy, results were normal, implying normal thyroidal secretory rates.[22] A study in an area of borderline-low iodine supply, however, suggested an increase in thyroidal secretory activity in early pregnancy.[30] Moreover, many hypothyroid women taking T_4 need increased doses during pregnancy,[52] again suggesting the possibility of an increase in T_4 secretion during gestation.

The great majority of pregnant women with normal thyroid function have serum free T_4 and free T_3 levels within ranges that are normal for nonpregnant individuals. The average serum free T_4 and free T_3 concentrations during pregnancy are reported to be unchanged, slightly increased, and slightly decreased,[7, 8, 30, 35, 62] and there are occasional women who have values outside of the normal range in either direction without other evidence of thyroid disease. The reasons for these discrepant results reported for mean serum free hormone concentrations are not clear.

Placenta and Thyroid Hormone Economy

The impact of the placenta on thyroid hormone economy is summarized in Table 8–4. hCG, because of its structural resemblance to TSH, can bind to the TSH receptor and has intrinsic thyrotropic activity.[56] Accumulating evidence suggests that hCG accounts for a substantial minority of the total serum thyrotropic activity in early pregnancy and contributes to

---

TABLE 8–3. Changes in Thyroid Hormone Economy in Normal Pregnancy

No major change in hypothalamic-pituitary-thyroid axis. Slight TSH suppression at the time of peak serum chorionic gonadotropin levels in the first trimester. Slight increase in mean serum TSH increment after exogenous TRH administration
Increased renal iodide clearance
Increased thyroid size: minimal (about 10%) in areas of dietary iodine sufficiency, about 30% in areas of borderline dietary iodine deficiency
Increased serum levels of TBG
Increased total serum T_4 and total serum T_3 levels secondary to increased TBG binding. No major change in serum free T_4 and free T_3 concentrations
Placental aspects (see Table 8–4)

TABLE 8–4. The Placenta in Thyroid Hormone Economy

hCG has intrinsic thyroid-stimulating activity. It causes hyperthyroidism in trophoblastic diseases and, probably, in hyperemesis gravidarum
Placenta expresses pro-TRH mRNA and contains TRH-like immunoreactivity
A placental barrier limits transfer of maternal T_4 and T_3 to the fetus, although athyrotic fetuses receive some maternal thyroid hormone at term
Placental enzymes inactivate T_4 and T_3 by 5-deiodination. This process appears to be a major component of the barrier between maternal and fetal thyroid hormone economies
Placental cells can activate T_4 by 5′-deiodination to T_3, suggesting the placenta as a thyroid hormone target organ. The human placental lactogen gene is thyroid hormone–responsive in model systems
Women with autoimmune thyroid diseases have antibodies to the TSH receptor that rarely cross the placenta in sufficient amounts to stimulate or inhibit fetal thyroid function
Some drugs that affect the fetal thyroid gland cross the placenta readily: thionamides, TRH, inorganic iodide (radioactive or nonradioactive)

the increase in maternal thyroid size.[30] The very high serum hCG levels in trophoblastic diseases can cause hyperthyroidism. In this setting, the abnormal glycosylation of hCG may increase its thyrotropic potency. There is no convincing evidence of any placental thyrotropic factor besides hCG. Rat placenta expresses the mRNA for pro-TRH and the TRH precursor peptide.[46] Human placenta contains TRH-like immunoreactivity, but it is not known whether this TRH-like material in the placenta has physiologic significance.

The placenta is a barrier between the maternal hypothalamic-pituitary-thyroid axis and that of the fetus.[67] T_4, T_3, and TSH cross the placenta poorly. In infants with complete congenital thyroid deficiency, the quantity of maternal T_4 that crosses the placenta at term is enough only to maintain a mean cord serum T_4 concentration of half the normal level.[78] When exogenous T_4 and T_3 have been given to pregnant women, the doses needed to deliver biologically significant amounts of these hormones to the fetuses were equal to 4 to 10 times the normal daily production rates.[25, 65] The placenta has an enzyme, iodothyronine deiodinase type III, that inactivates T_4 by conversion to reverse-T_3 and inactivates T_3 by conversion to diiodothyronine.[67] This enzyme is probably the major component of the barrier to transplacental passage of T_4 and T_3, but other physicochemical barriers may also exist.

There are two clinical implications of the relative separation of maternal and fetal thyroid hormone economies. First, maternal thyroid hormone excess or deficiency should have little or no significant effect on the thyroid status of the fetus. Second, fetal thyroid hormone deficiency cannot be corrected by administration of thyroid hormone to the mother without inducing maternal thyrotoxicosis.

Human placental cells have another iodothyronine deiodinase, designated type II, which activates T_4 by converting it to T_3.[38] The presence of this enzyme suggests that the placenta itself may be a thyroid hormone target organ. If so, one conceivable reason for the increased incidence of spontaneous abortion in pregnancies complicated by either hyperthyroidism or hypothyroidism might be placental dysfunction induced by thyroid hormone excess or deficiency. One possible placental thyroid hormone action is the regulation of human placental lactogen (hPL). The hPL gene has a thyroid hormone response element, and hPL gene expression is stimulated by thyroid hormone in model systems.[77] To date, however, there has not been direct proof that hPL production is thyroid hormone dependent in actual pregnancies.

Women with autoimmune thyroid diseases sometimes have circulating autoantibodies against the TSH receptor that can either stimulate thyroid function, as in Graves' disease, or inhibit thyroid function, as in Hashimoto's thyroiditis. There are rare cases in which high enough levels of maternal TSH receptor antibodies cross the placenta to stimulate or inhibit hormone secretion by the fetal thyroid. Some drugs used in the diagnosis and treatment of maternal thyroid diseases can cross the placenta in high enough amounts to cause biologic effects on the fetus.

Laboratory Assessment of Maternal Thyroid Function

Thyroid diseases are common in young women. Further, hyperthyroidism and hypothyroidism each have potentially adverse effects on pregnancy outcome. Therefore many women need their thyroid function evaluated during pregnancy. Efficient and accurate tests to establish or rule out thyroid abnormalities are important. Intuitively the most direct approach would be measurement of serum thyroid hormone concentrations. Although this has been the traditional approach, the use of a high-sensitivity serum TSH assay as the first-line test of thyroid function has become a better strategy, as is discussed subsequently.

Serum Thyroid Hormone Measurements During Pregnancy

Accurate measurement of serum total T_4 and T_3 concentrations by radioimmunoassay are readily available. The major increase, however, in the serum TBG concentration during pregnancy means that the normal ranges for serum T_4 and T_3 values in the nonpregnant individual do not apply to the pregnant woman. Further,

TABLE 8–5. Alterations in Serum Thyroid Hormone Measurements in Normal Pregnancy and Pregnancy Complicated by Abnormal Thyroid Function*

Pregnancy Category	Serum T$_4$	Serum T$_3$	Free T$_4$ Index	Free T$_3$ Index	Serum Free T$_4$	Serum Free T$_3$
Normal	nl–high	nl–high	nl–high	nl–high	nl	nl
Hyperthyroid	high	high	high	high	high	high
Hypothyroid, mild	nl–high	nl–high	nl–low	nl	nl–low	nl
Hypothyroid, moderate	nl	nl	nl–low	nl	nl–low	nl
Hypothyroid, severe	nl–low	nl–low	low	nl–low	low	nl–low

*Normal (nl), high, and low indicate the relationship of expected values to the normal range for adults who have no thyroid disease and are not pregnant or taking estrogens.

the percent increase in serum TBG level varies among pregnant women, resulting in normal serum T$_4$ and T$_3$ ranges that are unacceptably wide. Thus the diagnostic sensitivities of the tests deteriorate.

Estimates of serum free T$_4$ and free T$_3$ concentrations[41, 45] are therefore more useful than total T$_4$ and T$_3$ measurements during pregnancy. Equilibrium dialysis is the reference method for measuring free T$_4$ and free T$_3$ concentrations but so far has been too laborious and expensive for routine use. The oldest alternative method, still in wide use owing to its low cost, is the free thyroxine index, obtained by multiplying the serum total T$_4$ level by the result of the T$_3$ (or T$_4$) uptake test. The latter is an indirect estimate of the percent free T$_4$. At extremes of high or low binding of T$_4$ to TBG, the relationship of the T$_3$ uptake value to the percent free T$_4$ becomes nonlinear, as the uptake test is usually performed. Consequently, in some normal pregnant women, the T$_3$ uptake test underestimates the amount of T$_4$ bound to TBG and gives an erroneously high free T$_4$ index. A similar free T$_3$ index can be calculated as the product of the T$_3$ uptake value and the total serum T$_3$ concentration. This index can be useful during pregnancy, but few laboratories establish a normal range for it.

Kinetic immunoextraction (two-step) free T$_4$ radioimmunoassays, which are available commercially in kit form, give reliable results during pregnancy. They are relatively expensive to perform. *Unbound analog* free T$_4$ and free T$_3$ radioimmunoassays use as tracers labeled T$_4$ and T$_3$ analogs that are not bound to TBG. Some unbound analog assays give more accurate results during pregnancy than many free hormone index methods do, but some un-

bound analog free hormone assays give inaccurate results owing to the decrease in serum albumin levels during pregnancy.

There are biologic limitations to the use of free thyroid hormone serum measurements, besides these technical considerations. First, all methods have broad normal ranges, in which the upper limits of normal for both free T$_4$ and free T$_3$ levels are about 2.5 times the lower limits of normal. Thus a woman whose normal serum free T$_4$ level is near the upper limit of normal can have a 50% decrease in T$_4$ supply and be hypothyroid but have a low-normal serum free T$_4$ value. Second, many patients with mild to moderate hypothyroidism maintain normal serum free T$_3$ levels. Therefore the serum free T$_3$ test is not useful in the diagnosis of hypothyroidism, whether or not the patient is pregnant, because of low sensitivity. Third, nonthyroid illnesses and medications can cause euthyroid patients to have abnormal serum free T$_4$ levels (high or low) and low serum free T$_3$ levels. Toxemia of pregnancy is just such a nonthyroid illness.[62] In these conditions, the diagnostic accuracy of abnormal serum free T$_4$ or free T$_3$ values is suboptimal because of false-positive values. The results of serum thyroid hormone measurements in normal pregnancy and in pregnancy complicated by abnormal thyroid function are summarized in Table 8–5.

Serum Thyroid-Stimulating Hormone Measurements During Pregnancy

Since the mid-1980s, serum TSH assays have become available that are 20 to 100 times more sensitive than the conventional radioimmunoassays available previously. The increased sensitivity is achieved by the use of monoclonal antibodies directed at specific parts of the TSH molecule, combined with chemiluminescent, rather than radioactive, labeling; hence they are called *immunochemiluminescent assays*. These newer assays can measure serum TSH concentrations below 0.1 µU/mL, some as low as 0.01 µU/mL, compared with the lower limit of normal of about 0.3 to 0.5 µU/mL. TSH methods that fulfill established criteria[36] for a high-sensitivity assay avoid the limitations of serum thyroid hormone measurements. It is presently necessary, however, to determine specifically that a proper TSH assay will be used for pregnant patients because many laboratories do not routinely use high-sensitivity TSH methods. In even mild hypothyroidism, serum TSH levels are uniformly elevated except in patients with hypopituitarism or hypothalamic diseases (who are unlikely to be pregnant). In even mild hyperthyroidism, when true high-sensitivity assays are used, serum TSH levels are uniformly below 0.1 µU/mL, i.e., well below normal. Other than hypothyroidism and hyperthyroidism, the clinical situations causing abnormal serum TSH levels, listed in Table 8–6, are uncommon.

THYROID DISEASES

Hyperthyroidism

Hyperthyroidism complicates about 0.2% of pregnancies.[20, 60] Graves' disease (toxic diffuse goiter) is the cause in the great majority of cases (Table 8–7). Toxic multinodular goiter, the next most common in the general population, usually occurs after age 50. Toxic multimodular goiter and single toxic adenomas together probably account for fewer than 10% of cases of hyperthyroidism during pregnancy. Other causes are rare during pregnancy.

Graves' disease is an autoimmune disease, in which autoantibodies against the TSH receptor act as TSH agonists. The precipitating factors that initiate production of these TSH receptor antibodies are not known. Genetic factors are suggested by familial clusters of autoimmune thyroid diseases, both Graves' disease and Hashimoto's thyroiditis, and by linkage of Graves' disease to the histocompatibility

TABLE 8–6. Causes of Abnormal Serum Thyroid-Stimulating Hormone Concentrations

Clinical Setting	Expected TSH Values (µU/mL)
Normal for nonpregnant adults	0.3–5.0
Severe nonthyroid illness	0.1–7.0
TSH levels above normal	
Hypothyroidism	any >5
Recovery phase of severe nonthyroid illness	>5 up to 20
Pituitary or hypothalamic hyperthyroidism	any >5
Serum antibodies against mouse immunoglobulins*	any >5
TSH levels below normal	
Hyperthyroidism	<0.05
First trimester of pregnancy	0.2–5.0
Hyperemesis gravidarum	<0.1–5.0
Exogenous T_4 in suppressive or excessive doses	any <0.3
Glucocorticoid or dopamine therapy	0.1–5.0

Patients with antibodies against mouse immunoglobulins can have artifactually elevated serum TSH values in assays based on mouse monoclonal anti-TSH antibodies. In the other settings listed, the abnormal TSH values are true serum TSH concentrations.

antigens HLA-B8, DR5, and DR3. It is thought by some, but is not proved, that severe emotional stress can trigger Graves' disease.

Many of the symptoms and signs of hyperthyroidism also occur in euthyroid pregnant women: fatigue, increased appetite, amenorrhea, vomiting, palpitation, tachycardia, heat intolerance, increased warmth and perspiration, dyspnea, increased urinary frequency, insomnia, and emotional lability. Therefore those other findings of hyperthyroidism, which are not also typical of pregnancy, are of more help in suggesting the presence of coexistent hyperthyroidism: tremor, brisk reflexes, and weight loss. The most specific symptoms and

TABLE 8–7. Causes of Hyperthyroidism

Graves' disease (toxic diffuse goiter)
Toxic multinodular goiter
Toxic autonomously functioning adenoma
Hyperemesis gravidarum
Trophoblastic diseases (molar pregnancy, choriocarcinoma)
Subacute thyroiditis
Excessive doses of exogenous thyroid hormone
Iodide-induced thyrotoxicosis
Hypersecretion of TSH
Follicular thyroid cancer (widespread disease)
Hashimoto's thyroiditis (transient, early in the disease)
Struma ovarii

signs are those of Graves' ophthalmopathy, including stare, lid lag, eye irritation and chemosis, exophthalmos, periorbital swelling, and diplopia. About 95% of patients with Graves' disease have thyroid enlargement, although the degree of enlargement is sometimes slight. The activity of Graves' disease often fluctuates spontaneously during pregnancy, presumably because of the changes in immune function that accompany the pregnant state. Graves' disease tends to worsen in the first trimester but to become less severe in the second and third trimesters.[4]

Untreated, persistent hyperthyroidism during pregnancy increases risks to both the mother and the fetus (Table 8–8). Maternal problems include increased incidences of preeclampsia, heart failure, low weight gain, and, possibly, infection and anemia.[20] The most dangerous complication of hyperthyroidism is thyroid storm, in which there is cardiovascular compromise (often high output failure), hyperpyrexia, and delirium. This rare but potentially fatal condition occurs most often in patients with preexisting hyperthyroidism who sustain another major physiologic stress. Toxemia of pregnancy or parturition can be the precipitating factor in thyroid storm.[20] For the fetus, there are increased risks of first-trimester spontaneous abortion, premature labor and delivery, stillbirth, and low birth weight.[20, 60]

Fetal and neonatal thyrotoxicosis is another potentially dangerous concomitant of maternal Graves' disease, estimated to occur in about 1% of pregnancies in women who have Graves' disease.[24] The cause is stimulation of the fetal thyroid gland by maternal stimulatory TSH receptor antibodies transferred across the placenta. Hyperthyroidism can occur in fetuses of women whose thyroid glands have been ablated and who are euthyroid on T_4 treatment during pregnancy but who still have high serum titers of the TSH receptor antibody. The activity of maternal serum TSH receptor stimulatory antibodies, determined by bioassay measuring cAMP production in vitro by thyroid cells, can be used to predict the risk of intrauterine or neonatal hyperthyroidism. In most affected cases, the maternal stimulatory antibody activity is reported to be more than 500% of the activity of control serum, although I have seen a case in which the activity was 380% of control. For women at risk, it seems prudent to measure maternal serum TSH receptor stimulatory antibodies in the second trimester. Levels that suggest an increased risk of fetal hyperthyroidism can then be followed up by clinical and ultrasound evaluation of the fetus. If the condition is present, control can be attempted by giving the pregnant woman antithyroid drugs that cross the placenta.[48]

Unique to pregnancy are those cases of hyperthyroidism that are due to thyroid stimulation by high levels of hCG. This phenomenon occurs in trophoblastic diseases (both molar pregnancy and choriocarcinoma), hyperemesis gravidarum, and other unusual situations accompanied by unusually high serum hCG levels. In patients with hyperthyroidism due to trophoblastic diseases,[9, 40, 57, 61] weight loss and fatigue are prominent symptoms. Other typical manifestations of hyperthyroidism, including goiter, are uncommon, presumably owing to the short duration of thyroid stimulation. The elevated serum thyroid hormone levels and symptoms and signs of hyperthyroidism normalize rapidly after removal of the molar tissue or effective therapy of the choriocarcinoma.

Hyperthyroidism, with high serum free T_4 and free T_3 levels and suppressed serum TSH values, accompanies hyperemesis gravidarum about 20% of the time.[11, 13, 75] Occasional patients with less severe nausea and vomiting in early pregnancy show the same thyroid abnormalities.[56] In these groups of patients, there is

TABLE 8–8. Complications of Abnormal Maternal Thyroid Function During Pregnancy

Hyperthyroidism	Hypothyroidism
Increased Fetal Risks	
Spontaneous abortion	Spontaneous abortion
Premature labor and delivery	Low birth weight
Stillbirth	Fetal death
Low birth weight	
Fetal/neonatal thyrotoxicosis	
Increased Maternal Risks	
Preeclampsia	Preeclampsia
Maternal heart failure	Placental abruption
Low maternal weight gain	Postpartum hemorrhage
Infection	Cardiac ventricular dysfunction
Anemia	Anemia

an inverse correlation between serum TSH and hCG concentrations, implicating hCG as the causative factor. Some patients with hyperemesis have isolated elevations of serum free T_4 levels, with normal serum free T_3 and TSH levels.[11] These latter cases appear to be instances of the high serum free T_4 levels due to malnutrition or nonthyroid illness. Antithyroid treatment is not known to be helpful. Once the nausea and vomiting abate, thyroid function and thyroid function test results return to normal.

Hyperthyroidism has been reported in a case of hyperplacentosis with a high serum hCG value[32] and in three pregnancies in one woman who had hyperemesis once and had two other pregnancies without nausea or vomiting but in which she had very high serum hCG levels.[39] I have treated a patient with a multinodular goiter having three areas of functional autonomy but normal preconception free T_4 and free T_3 values, whose serum free T_3 levels were slightly above normal throughout a pregnancy during which she had symptoms of mild hyperthyroidism. Antithyroid treatment was not necessary. After parturition, her serum free T_3 values returned to their mid-normal preconception levels. TSH concentrations were suppressed and free T_4 levels were normal before, during, and after pregnancy. There was no evidence of thyroid autoimmunity. hCG was not measured but would seem to be the most likely thyroid stimulator.

For the laboratory diagnosis of hyperthyroidism, serum TSH (by high-sensitivity assay), free T_4, and free T_3 levels are obtained. Table 8–6 lists the expected findings from the various methods currently used to estimate the serum free T_4 and free T_3 concentrations. The minimum findings needed to establish the diagnosis are clearly elevated values for either the serum free T_4 or free T_3, combined with a suppressed TSH. If the serum TSH level is normal, hyperthyroidism is ruled out with a high degree of confidence. The use of a high-sensitivity TSH assay makes a TRH stimulation test unnecessary. In uncertain cases, the presence of elevated antithyroid antibody titers, goiter, or eye signs are helpful confirmatory findings.

If hyperthyroidism is initially diagnosed during pregnancy, the presumptive cause is Graves' disease. The radioactive iodine uptake test and thyroid scintiscanning, ordinarily useful to determine the cause of hyperthyroidism, are contraindicated during pregnancy. In a hyperthyroid patient, the presence of a single palpable thyroid nodule, especially one 3 cm in diameter or larger, suggests a toxic thyroid adenoma rather than Graves' disease. The causes of hyperthyroidism unique to pregnancy are suggested by the clinical setting and the absence of findings characteristic of Graves' disease.

Because therapy for hyperthyroidism during pregnancy requires frequent patient monitoring, and all treatment strategies have the potential for adverse effects on the pregnancy, prevention of hyperthyroidism during pregnancy is desirable. Hyperthyroid women diagnosed when not pregnant should be informed of the implications of the disease during pregnancy. Radioactive iodine (^{131}I) treatment can be offered for definitive therapy. Patients thus treated are usually euthyroid on T_4 treatment within 6 months. Pregnancies after that are almost always straightforward to manage. There is no evidence of adverse effects of ^{131}I treatment on the outcome of a subsequent pregnancy,[48] even in the ^{131}I doses used for thyroid cancer treatment, which are 5 to 20 times higher than those typically used to treat hyperthyroidism.[70]

The choices for management of hyperthyroidism during pregnancy include observation alone, antithyroid drugs, β-adrenergic blocking drugs, and thyroid surgery. ^{131}I treatment is contraindicated during pregnancy. Helpful supportive measures include an adequate dietary caloric intake and multiple vitamins because both pregnancy and hyperthyroidism increase caloric needs, and vitamin deficiency may accompany hyperthyroidism. Bed rest and reduction of physical and emotional stress can improve symptoms but are often not practical.

Both pharmacologic and surgical therapy for hyperthyroidism have the potential for causing an adverse outcome of a pregnancy. Therefore observation alone may be acceptable for patients who have clinically mild hyperthyroidism, with no evidence of cardiovascular compromise, and whose serum free T_4 and free T_3 levels are only mildly elevated. Clinical judgment is the only available criterion for the selection of such patients, who must be willing to have evaluations about every 3 to 4 weeks during the pregnancy. Therapeutic intervention may become necessary if the severity of hyperthyroidism increases or other complications of the pregnancy arise.

Antithyroid drug treatment is the preferred therapy for almost all pregnant hyperthyroid women who are not candidates for observation alone. The two thionamide antithyroid drugs available in the United States, propylthiouracil (PTU) and methimazole (Tapazole), have similar effects within the thyroid gland.[17] Methimazole is about 15 times more potent than PTU on a weight basis. Both drugs reduce T_4 and T_3 biosynthesis by inhibition of iodide organification and of coupling of the iodinated tyrosines. PTU also inhibits conversion of T_4 to T_3 outside of the thyroid gland, a potentially advantageous property in the early phase of treatment. Both PTU and methimazole cross the placenta and can inhibit fetal thyroid function. PTU crosses the placenta less efficiently than methimazole, but even so cord serum PTU levels exceed paired maternal serum levels.[26]

Side effects of the two drugs are similar.[17] The most common is a skin rash, often intensely pruritic, occurring in 2 to 8% of patients. A lupus-like syndrome and arthralgias can also occur. About 50% of patients who have an allergic reaction to one of the thionamides are also allergic to the other. The most dangerous side effects, occurring in about 0.5% of patients, are agranulocytosis and hepatic necrosis. Rare deaths have occurred from these complications. A congenital skin defect, aplasia cutis, has been reported in about a dozen infants exposed to methimazole in utero. The lesion, consisting of circumscribed areas of undeveloped skin, has not been reported in infants of mothers treated with PTU, nor have other teratogenic effects been reported for PTU.[17]

PTU is the preferred thionamide during pregnancy because it is less likely to cause fetal thyroid suppression and has not been associated with aplasia cutis. If a mild allergic reaction occurs to PTU, methimazole may be tried. High doses of either drug, 800 to 1200 mg daily of PTU or 60 to 80 mg daily of methimzole, completely block thyroid hormone biosynthesis. Lower doses, however, e.g., 450

mg daily of PTU or 30 mg daily of methimazole, are usually sufficient to control hyperthyroidism within 4 to 8 weeks. The drugs can often be given in a single daily dose, but because some patients require two or three divided doses, it seems advisable to start with divided doses in the pregnant patient. After initial control of thyroid function is achieved, doses can almost always be reduced to maintain a euthyroid state.

The aim of thionamide treatment is to use the lowest dose necessary to maintain maternal serum free T_4 and free T_3 levels at, or just above, the upper limit of normal. This strategy minimizes the chances of fetal goiter and thyroid suppression. When more than 300 mg daily of PTU or 30 mg daily of methimazole is taken chronically, fetal goiter and hypothyroidism occur, but there is no predictable dose-response relationship. When long-term doses are kept to no more than 300 mg daily for PTU, or 20 mg daily for methimazole, fetal goiter is uncommon, effects on fetal thyroid function are minimal,[16] and the outcome of the pregnancy is usually satisfactory.

It is important to anticipate probable changes in the patient's responses to the thionamides. She should be evaluated clinically and with serum free T_4 and free T_3 assessments every 3 to 4 weeks. A rapid improvement in the values means that the drug dose should be decreased; otherwise the free T_4 and free T_3 levels usually fall too low. The typical amelioration of the activity of Graves' disease in the second trimester should also be anticipated.[56] As many as 40% of patients can discontinue thionamide treatment entirely in mid to late pregnancy and remain euthyroid.[54] Even if not, PTU doses as low as 25 to 50 mg once daily are often sufficient. The rare woman with Graves' disease who has had successful thyroid ablation but who still has high enough stimulatory TSH receptor activity to cause fetal hyperthyroidism can be treated with a combination of T_4, which will keep her euthyroid, and PTU to control the fetal thyroid.

At the start of thionamide treatment, baseline granulocyte counts and liver function tests should be obtained because there may be mild granulocytopenia or elevated liver enzymes caused by the hyperthyroidism itself. If so, only a worsening of the results necessitates discontinuation of the medication. These tests should also be monitored at the same time as thyroid hormone levels because some patients, although not all, who develop serious reactions do so gradually. Patients should be instructed to stop taking the thionamide at the first sign of a possible reaction and to call the physician for instructions. A granulocyte count and liver enzyme activities should then be determined.

In the first few months postpartum, the activity of Graves' disease often increases.[56] Women who can discontinue treatment during pregnancy may need to resume it if they are nursing or consider ^{131}I treatment if they are not breast-feeding. During lactation, PTU and methimazole appear in breast milk. PTU is transported into milk less efficiently than methimazole and is present in sufficiently low concentrations that inhibition of the infant's thyroid function is unlikely.[17] The nursing mother taking PTU can be informed that the American Academy of Pediatrics considers maternal PTU treatment "usually compatible with breast-feeding,"[2] but the infant should be monitored for goiter. Checking the breast-fed infant's serum TSH level at age 3 to 4 weeks seems prudent, but the frequency of abnormal results is not known.

B-adrenergic blockers can be useful adjuncts in the treatment of hyperthyroidism during pregnancy, especially to relieve sympathetic-like manifestations, such as tremor, tachycardia, and palpitations. Propranolol and atenolol weakly inhibit extrathyroidal conversion of T_4 to T_3 and thus are preferable to other β blockers. The usual contraindications to β blockade apply: obstructive lung disease, heart block, heart failure, and insulin use. There may be adverse fetal effects of long-term maternal use of β blockers, such as cardiac dysfunction, intrauterine growth retardation, and neonatal bradycardia and hypoglycemia. The incidence of these problems is probably low,[50] but it would seem best to keep the duration of β blocker treatment as short as possible and reserve it for the pregnant thyrotoxic woman whose tremor, palpitations, or tachycardia is debilitating.

Surgical treatment of hyperthyroidism, i.e., subtotal thyroidectomy, is effective and reasonably safe. When performed by a skilled surgeon, the procedure is complicated by permanent hypoparathyroidism or recurrent laryngeal nerve damage in fewer than 1% of cases. The potential adverse effects, however, of general anesthesia and surgical stress on the outcome of pregnancy must also be considered. General anesthesia during organogenesis may have teratogenic effects, and there can be pregnancy loss or premature labor shortly after surgery. Therefore medical treatment is preferred to surgery, unless that mother is allergic to both PTU and methimazole, or her hyperthyroidism cannot be controlled except by PTU doses greater than 300 mg daily. When surgery is necessary, the hyperthyroid state should be controlled as well as possible before operation, to minimize the risks of complications. Treatment for 7 to 10 days preoperatively by a combination of bed rest, a thionamide drug if tolerated, a β adrenergic blocker, and inorganic iodide (e.g., Lugol's solution, 3 drops daily) usually produces considerable improvement.

Hypothyroidism

The causes of hypothyroidism are given in Table 8–9. The great majority of cases are due either to chronic lymphocytic (Hashimoto's) thyroiditis or to prior ablative treatment with ^{131}I or thyroid surgery. In 2000 consecutive pregnant women in Maine, 2.5% had elevated TSH concentrations at 15 to 18 weeks' gestation, and 0.3% had both an elevated serum TSH level and an estimated serum free T_4 level

TABLE 8–9. Causes of Hypothyroidism

Common
Chronic lymphocytic (Hashimoto's) thyroiditis
Thyroid ablation by radioactive iodine or surgery
Uncommon
Subacute granulomatous (DeQuervain's) thyroiditis
Subacute lymphocytic ("painless") thyroiditis
Congenital
External radiation exposure to the upper body
Hypopituitarism or hypothalamic disease
Antithyroid drug overdosage
Goitrogenic drugs, e.g., lithium, sulfonylureas, iodine-
    containing agents
Infiltrative diseases, e.g., cystinosis, amyloidosis
Iodine deficiency (variable geographic prevalence;
    nonexistent in U.S.)
Thyroid hormone resistance

below normal.[43] This systematic survey confirms previous prevalence estimates, which depended on less accurate methods to assess thyroid function.[60] The diagnosis of Hashimoto's thyroiditis is confirmed by the presence of goiter and by elevated serum levels of antithyroid antibodies. The majority of the women in the Maine survey had elevated antithyroperoxidase antibody levels.

The symptoms of hypothyroidism are nonspecific. Knowing when to suspect the disease is particularly difficult during pregnancy because normal pregnancy can be accompanied by several of the symptoms of mild to moderate hypothyroidism: fatigue, constipation, muscle cramps, fluid retention, and carpal tunnel syndrome. Other findings of thyroid hormone deficiency include cold intolerance and dry or thickened skin and hair. In most cases of mild to moderate disease, the only abnormal physical finding is thyroid gland enlargement, present in about 95% of cases of Hashimoto's thyroiditis but often absent after thyroidectomy and usually absent after ^{131}I treatment. In more severe hypothyroidism, mentation and speech may be slow, and physical findings include a low-pitched voice, thick tongue, serous effusions, and slow tendon reflexes. The extreme of hypothyroidism is myxedema coma, with hypothermia, bradycardia, hypoventilation, and a depressed sensorium.

Moderate to severe hypothyroidism during pregnancy is associated with increased risks of complications and adverse outcomes[19, 60] (see Table 8–8). Mild hypothyroidism is associated with a far lower frequency of these problems;[19] systematic data are lacking to determine whether the level of risk associated with mild disease is above normal. In two studies, the presence of maternal thyroid autoimmunity was associated with a doubling of the rate of spontaneous abortion, independent of whether the affected women were hypothyroid.[31, 73] An unsettled issue is possible deleterious effects of maternal hypothyroidism on fetal central nervous system development. Animal studies suggest this possibility. Human data are inconclusive. Data suggesting neural developmental abnormalities in offspring of hypothyroid women[51] are flawed by imprecise estimates of the severity of maternal hypothyroidism and a failure to separate effects of maternal thyroid

hormone deficiency from those of environmental factors and of possible concomitant fetal hypothyroidism.

Because of the known and suspected adverse effects of hypothyroidism on pregnancy outcome, it seems prudent to correct even mild maternal hypothyroidism during pregnancy. Oral T_4 treatment restores a euthyroid state and carries no known risks in appropriate replacement doses. It was previously thought that replacement doses of T_4 were similar in pregnant and nonpregnant women. Studies show, however, that a high percentage of hypothyroid women need increased T_4 doses during pregnancy to remain euthyroid.[42, 64, 76]

To develop practical guidelines for monitoring and adjusting T_4 doses during pregnancy, data were analyzed from 77 pregnancies in 65 T_4-treated, hypothyroid women in my practice.[40a] High serum TSH levels were found during pregnancy in 76% of women with prior thyroid ablation by radioiodine or surgery and in 47% of those with Hashimoto's thyroiditis, all of whom continued to take T_4 doses that maintained normal serum free T_4 and TSH levels before pregnancy. Serum TSH elevations were seen as early as 4 weeks' postconception. Serum free T_4 concentrations fell below normal in 13% of the 65 women, who all had high serum TSH levels. Major TSH elevations, >20 $\mu U/mL$, were observed in another 9%, who had serum free T_4 levels at the lower limit of normal. In women tested after an initially normal serum TSH value during pregnancy, 30% had an elevated serum TSH level later in the pregnancy. Thus it seems reasonable to advise pregnant hypothyroid women treated with T_4 to have serum TSH tests at least at 6 to 8 weeks' and at 6 months' gestation, to determine if the T_4 dose needs to be increased.

The increment in T_4 dose needed to correct an elevated serum TSH level can be estimated from the abnormal TSH value. In my patients, the mean ($\pm$ SD) T_4 dose increments needed to normalize the TSH were 41 ± 24 μg per day for women with serum TSH values that were elevated but less than 10 $\mu U/mL$, 65 ± 19 μg per day for TSH elevations between 10 and 20 $\mu U/mL$, and 105 ± 32 μg per day for serum TSH elevations above 20 $\mu U/mL$. Patients should be reassessed 4 weeks after raising the T_4 dose to determine if a further dose adjustment is needed. The average T_4 dose needed to keep pregnant hypothyroid women euthyroid was about 150 µg/day. In 12 women followed through two successive pregnancies, 10 required increased T_4 doses in both pregnancies, 1 needed no change in dose in either pregnancy, and 1 needed an increase in one of two pregnancies. After delivery, the T_4 dose should be reduced back to the amount that produced a normal serum TSH level before conception and the woman's thyroid status reassessed 6 weeks postpartum to verify that this dose is correct.

Thyroid Nodules and Cancer

Thyroid nodules are occasionally discovered during pregnancy. Most are harmless, but some can have adverse health effects. About 10% of thyroid nodules are malignant. About 5 to 10% of nodules are autonomously functioning adenomas, a few of which secrete enough T_4 and T_3 to cause thyrotoxicosis. Some thyroid nodules are due to Hashimoto's thyroiditis; these may be the first clue to hypothyroidism. Thus thyroid nodules discovered during pregnancy warrant investigation.

Evaluation includes a serum TSH level by high-sensitivity assay, antithyroid antibody levels, and fine-needle aspiration cytology. An abnormal serum TSH value, suggesting hyperthyroidism or hypothyroidism, is followed up by an estimate of the serum free T_4 concentration if hypothyroidism is suggested or by estimates of serum free T_4 and free T_3 levels if hyperthyroidism is suspected. Antithyroid antibody titers give an indication of the likelihood of Hashimoto's thyroiditis as the cause of the nodule; this information is most useful in cases in which needle aspiration cytology proves uninformative. Thyroid ultrasound is often performed to evaluate nodules but is unnecessary; it is often inaccurate as performed and interpreted in the community setting and does not eliminate the need for needle aspiration. Scintigraphy, which is ordinarily useful to identify autonomously functioning nodules, for which malignancy can be reliably ruled out, is contraindicated during pregnancy because of the attendant x-ray exposure.

Needle aspiration cytology is the most important element of the evaluation because it provides the most specific information about the probability of malignancy. An adequate cytology specimen with benign findings is greatly reassuring to the patient. A finding of a high probability of malignancy allows advance planning of therapy. Pregnancy does not alter the natural course of well-differentiated (papillary or follicular) thyroid carcinoma. Thus suspicious or malignant cytology is not a reason to recommend termination of pregnancy. Moreover, the chances of a papillary or follicular thyroid cancer progressing from a curable to an incurable stage during the course of a pregnancy are low. Accordingly the patient can be offered the option of thyroid surgery during the same hospitalization as delivery. Such a strategy would minimize disruption of breastfeeding and maternal care of the newborn infant. If a cancer is discovered in the first or second trimester and the patient or physician does not wish to delay surgery until delivery, surgery can be planned for the second trimester, when the risk of affecting the outcome of pregnancy is lowest.

Postpartum Thyroid Dysfunction Due to Painless Subacute Thyroiditis

Thyroid abnormalities develop in the postpartum period in about 5% of white and Asian women and 1 to 2% of black American women. The most common cause in this clinical setting is painless postpartum subacute thyroiditis,[3, 28, 33, 37, 59, 63] an autoimmune, lymphocytic thyroiditis that differs histologically from both Hashimoto's thyroiditis and painful subacute granulomatous thyroiditis. The thyroid abnormalities usually start between 1 and 4 months' postpartum, and include asymptomatic goiter, hyperthyroidism, or hypothyroidism, alone or in combination. Patients often have a preexisting goiter or preexisting elevated serum levels of antithyroid antibodies. Two-thirds of euthyroid pregnant women with elevated serum antithyroperoxidase (microsomal) antibody titers develop at least biochemical evidence of postpartum thyroid dysfunction.[37]

In the full-blown subacute postpartum thyroiditis syndrome, there is an initial hyperthyroid phase, followed by a subsequent hypothyroid phase, and goiter is present in the majority of cases.[3, 59] The hyperthyroid phase usually has its onset in the first 3 months after delivery and lasts for several weeks up to 3 months. In this phase, widespread damage to the thyroid parenchyma results in release into the circulation of T_4 and T_3 that were previously synthesized and stored in the thyroid gland. Serum free T_4 and free T_3 levels are usually both elevated, but the serum T_3 to T_4 ratio is not usually increased, in distinction to Graves' disease, in which this ratio is typically above normal. Serum TSH levels are suppressed. Thyroidal ^{131}I uptake is low, as would be expected in the absence of TSH or a stimulatory antibody. The low ^{131}I uptake in the presence of elevated serum free T_4 and free T_3 levels is a characteristic finding, useful in distinguishing the hyperthyroid phase of postpartum thyroiditis from Graves' disease. In the latter, the thyroidal ^{131}I uptake is almost never low. If the patient is breast-feeding, it is best, and almost always possible, to defer radioactive tracer studies. Serum antithyroglobulin and antithyroperoxidase antibody levels are often present but may be negative or present in low titers.

The hyperthyroid phase of postpartum thyroiditis is self-limited. Antithyroid drug treatment is not effective because there is no ongoing thyroid hormone biosynthesis. Symptomatic treatment with β-adrenergic blockers can be useful, if symptoms are severe. Reassurance is often sufficient.

The hypothyroid phase of postpartum subacute thyroiditis, when it occurs, may or may not be preceded by a hypothyroid phase. There are no laboratory test results that specifically indicate postpartum subacute thyroiditis. The diagnosis is suggested by the timing of hypothyroidism in relation to pregnancy and sometimes by symptoms or test results suggesting recent hyperthyroidism. Women with postpartum hypothyroidism have a higher than normal incidence of impaired mental concentration and emotional depression.[37] Therefore if a patient is diagnosed in the early phase of this condition and is having such symptoms or is having other symptoms of hypothyroidism, T_4 treatment is advisable.

Postpartum subacute thyroiditis resolves completely in about 70% of cases.[59, 63] In these patients, the hypothyroid phase usually ends by 9 months' postpartum. Therefore patients treated with T_4 should have treatment withdrawn 9 to 12 months' postpartum to determine if healing has occurred. Up to 30% may have persistent hypothyroidism or goiter. This incidence of permanent thyroid dysfunction appears to be greater than the corresponding incidence of less than 10% in patients who have subacute thyroiditis at other times of life. I have seen patients with persistent euthyroid goiter after postpartum subacute thyroiditis who developed hypothyroidism years later. These patients have also had persistently elevated levels of the antithyroid antibodies. Accordingly periodic reevaluation of the thyroid function in such patients is appropriate.

PARATHYROID DISEASES

Calcium Economy in Pregnancy

Normal fetal skeletal mineralization requires that 30 g of calcium be supplied to the fetus by the pregnant woman. To meet this demand, daily intestinal absorption of dietary calcium increases during pregnancy from about 150 mg before pregnancy up to 400 mg by the second trimester.[6] Vitamin D is a crucial calcitropic factor, via its action to stimulate intestinal calcium absorption. The active form of vitamin D, 1,25-dihydroxyvitamin D or calcitriol, is normally produced from precursors by the kidney. The placenta can also synthesize calcitriol; placental calcitriol may help maintain normal serum calcitriol levels in women with kidney diseases.[14] During pregnancy, the total serum calcitriol concentration doubles. Some of this increase is due to raised levels of the serum protein that binds calcitriol, but the unbound calcitriol also increases significantly[10] and is probably the main factor responsible for the increase in dietary calcium absorption.

Intracellular calcium is an important second messenger in many organs. The main determinant of the intracellular calcium concentration is the serum ionized calcium concentration, which amounts to 45 to 50% of the total serum calcium level. Another 40 to 45% of the calcium in the circulation is bound to albumin, and 5 to 10% is complexed to anions; these nonionized forms do not affect intracellular functions. During pregnancy, the serum albumin concentration falls, by about 20% at term. Correspondingly the total serum calcium level falls during pregnancy, by about 10% on average, but there is no significant change in the mean serum ionized calcium concentration.[21]

The serum ionized calcium concentration is tightly regulated, mainly by parathyroid hormone (PTH), made by parathyroid glands. The intact 84–amino acid PTH molecule is thought to be the biologically active form. PTH stimulates bone resorption, renal tubular calcium reabsorption, and renal synthesis of calcitriol. Raised levels of serum ionized calcium inhibit PTH secretion, and low serum ionized calcium levels stimulate PTH secretion. Calcitriol also inhibits PTH secretion. During pregnancy, serum intact PTH levels fall by an average of about 50%,[21] possibly in response to the increases in vitamin D levels and the increased intestinal calcium absorption.

Other hormones that may influence calcium economy are calcitonin and PTH-related protein (PTH-RP). The functions of the latter two peptides during pregnancy are uncertain. The placenta has calcitonin receptors, but no specific placental effects of calcitonin have been described. There is evidence that the placenta secretes PTH-RP, which may regulate placental calcium transport from mother to fetus.[72]

Hyperparathyroidism

Fewer than 100 cases of hyperparathyroidism diagnosed during pregnancy have been reported, but there have been no systematic surveys to determine disease prevalence during gestation. It seems likely that some mild cases are not identified, and cases managed without complication may not be reported. Hyperparathyroidism is caused by a single parathyroid adenoma 80 to 90% of the time, multiglandular disease (usually hyperplasia) 10 to 20% of the time, and carcinoma 1% of the time or less.[6] In many cases, multiglandular parathyroid hyperfunction is due to one of several familial syndromes: multiple endocrine neoplasia type 1 and 2a, familial hyperparathyroidism, and familial hypocalciuric hypercalcemia.[6] Thus family members of patients found to have multiglandular parathyroid hyperfunction should be screened for parathyroid disease.

Hyperparathyroidism is mild and asymptomatic in half of the cases diagnosed in nonpregnant individuals. An abnormal serum calcium is the only significant finding in these cases. When symptoms are present, the most common ones are fatigue, muscle weakness, renal stones, emotional changes, headache, gastrointestinal symptoms, and bone disease. The most specific symptoms are renal stones and bone disease. Fewer than 10% of patients with renal stones, however, have hyperparathyroidism as the cause. The most mild form of bone disease is demineralization. As bone involvement advances, subperiosteal bone resorption develops, most characteristically in the middle phalanges of the fingers. The most severe form of hyperparathyroid bone disease is osteitis fibrosa cystica, consisting of bone pain, pathologic fractures, and localized bone swelling, which appears radiologically as lucent cystic lesions, termed *brown tumors* of bone.[6]

Hyperparathyroidism can cause additional problems during pregnancy.[18, 27, 44, 49, 55, 71] About 6% of reported patients with hyperparathyroidism during pregnancy have had pancreatitis.[18, 44, 66] This is a higher incidence figure than that for pancreatitis in hyperparathyroidism outside of pregnancy, but some reported pregnant patients also had other risk factors for pancreatitis. Patients with hyperparathyroidism sometimes have *parathyroid crisis*, with severe hypercalcemia leading to weakness, mental obtundation, coma, and renal failure. Dehydration is often a contributory factor in parathyroid crisis. For that reason, its incidence may be increased in the immediate postpartum period.[23] Maternal hyperparathyroidism during pregnancy can have adverse effects on the outcome of pregnancy (Table 8–10). In the reported untreated cases, spontaneous abortion or fetal death occurred in about 15% and neonatal hypocalcemic tetany in about 30%.[18, 27, 44, 49, 55, 66, 71] The latter condition is usually transient but is sometimes so severe as to be fatal. There are two factors that probably contribute to neonatal tetany.

TABLE 8–10. Complications of Abnormal Maternal Parathyroid Function During Pregnancy

Hyperparathyroidism	Hypoparathyroidism
Increased Fetal/Neonatal Risks	
Fetal death	Low birth weight
Spontaneous abortion	Skeletal demineralization
Neonatal hypocalcemic tetany	Subperiosteal bone resorption
Neonatal hypomagnesemia	
Increased Maternal Risks	
Pancreatitis	Usual symptoms*
Postpartum parathyroid crisis	
Usual symptoms*	

*Usual symptoms *indicates symptoms of the diseases when they occur in nonpregnant individuals.*

First, there may be sustained fetal hypercalcemia due to maternal hypercalcemia, leading to prolonged suppression of PTH secretion in the neonate.[5] Second, the maternal hypomagnesemia of hypoparathyroidism may cause neonatal hypomagnesemia, which in turn can impair PTH secretion and inhibit PTH action.[5]

The diagnosis of hyperparathyroidism is established by demonstrating an inappropriately elevated serum PTH level at a time of hypercalcemia. Several forms of PTH are present in the circulation: intact PTH and several fragments. Assays are available that measure various fragments as well as intact PTH. The most recently developed assays, which measure only intact PTH, are the most accurate for the diagnosis of hyperparathyroidism.[21] Because of the normal decrease in the total serum calcium concentration during pregnancy, it may be helpful in cases of borderline elevations of total serum calcium values to obtain measurements of ionized calcium. For accurate ionized calcium values, care must be taken to draw and process the blood sample according to the stated requirements of the method. Measurement of urinary calcium excretion and the ratio of urinary calcium and creatinine clearances distinguish familial hypocalciuric hypercalcemia from hyperparathyroidism. The former condition is almost always asymptomatic and does not require treatment.[6]

The standard treatment of hyperparathyroidism during pregnancy is surgery. Because so few cases of hyperparathyroidism during pregnancy have been reported, published cases are conceivably biased toward severe disease or cases with complications. Nevertheless, the frequency of reported complications in untreated cases is so high that observation without treatment seems hazardous. A small number of patients have had successful medical treatment with oral phosphate,[55] but not enough patients have been treated by this medication to formulate guidelines for its use.

Surgical treatment appears to lessen the risk of complications of hyperparathyroidism in pregnancy. Of 28 reported cases treated surgically, 3 operations were unsuccessful in correcting the hyperparathyroidism, 3 patients had spontaneous abortion or premature labor within a few hours of surgery, 3 infants had neonatal tetany despite correction of the maternal hypercalcemia, and the rest of the infants were healthy. Surgery during the second trimester minimizes the chances of teratogenic effects of anesthetics and early spontaneous abortion, which are potential problems in the first trimester, and premature labor in the third trimester.

Hypoparathyroidism

Hypoparathyroidism is an uncommon disease in which hypocalcemia is caused by low serum PTH levels. The most common cause is permanent parathyroid gland damage, or removal of all parathyroid tissue, during thyroid or parathyroid surgery. Spontaneous hypoparathyroidism is rare. It is usually sporadic but sometimes occurs in the familial syndrome of multiple endocrine deficiencies associated with mucocutaneous candidiasis.[6] Another rare familial syndrome causing hypocalcemia is pseudohypoparathyroidism, in which serum PTH levels are normal or high but in which there is a defective guanine nucleotide binding subunit in the PTH receptor–adenylate cyclase complex.[6] Severe magnesium depletion interferes with PTH secretion and PTH action, thus causing a secondary form of hypoparathyroidism. Vitamin D deficiency or resistance causes hypocalcemia owing to low intestinal calcium absorption, but serum PTH levels are high in these conditions.[6]

The hypocalcemia of hypoparathyroidism causes neuromuscular irritability, with paresthesias, positive Chvostek's and Trousseau's signs, carpopedal spasm, and, in the most severe cases, laryngospasm and seizures. There may be mental changes, ocular cataracts, and calcifications of the cerebral falx and basal ganglia. The basal ganglion calcifications are sometimes associated with extrapyramidal neurologic signs. During pregnancy, untreated maternal hypoparathyroidism causes fetal hypocalcemia and, in response, fetal parathyroid hyperplasia.[5] High fetal serum PTH levels in turn cause generalized skeletal demineralization and subperiosteal bone resorption[74] (see Table 8–10). Low birth weight is common. The affected infants who survive have a spontaneous return of normal parathyroid function over several months. Children of women with pseudohypoparathyroidism also sometimes exhibit transient neonatal hyperparathyroidism.[29]

The diagnosis of hypoparathyroidism is established by the findings of low serum total and ionized calcium concentrations along with an inappropriately low serum intact PTH level. The serum phosphate level is elevated owing to increased renal tubular phosphate reabsorption. In pseudohypoparathyroidism, there are characteristic phenotypic abnormalities, normal or high serum PTH levels, and a deficient response of urinary cAMP and phosphate excretion to exogenous PTH administration.[6] In patients with hypocalcemia due to nonparathyroid causes, serum magnesium and 25-hydroxyvitamin D measurements reveal magnesium deficiency, in which the serum PTH level is inappropriately low, and vitamin D deficiency, in which the serum PTH level is high.[6]

The goal of therapy in the pregnant hypoparathyroid woman is to keep the serum ionized calcium level, or the total calcium level corrected for the serum albumin, in the lower part of the normal range. Serum calcium levels higher than that, even if within the normal range, can increase the risk of kidney stone formation because fractional excretion of filtered urinary calcium is increased in PTH deficiency.[6] In addition, higher serum calcium levels increase the risk of an overshoot into the hypercalemic range because serum calcium levels can fluctuate unpredictably in some patients.

Therapy of hypoparathyroidism consists of oral calcium and vitamin D.[12, 34, 53, 68, 69] PTH is not available for replacement therapy. Typical oral calcium doses are 2 to 3 g of elemental calcium daily, taken as the carbonate (pure or as "oyster shell calcium"), lactate, phosphate, or other salts. For best absorption of calcium from carbonate preparations, products that meet USP solubility standards should be used. Vitamin D can be given orally as vitamin D_2 in high doses; as dihydrotachysterol, a synthetic analog that does not require PTH-dependent renal activation; or as calcitriol. The vitamin D dose requirement of hypoparathyroid women sometimes increases substantially during pregnancy and decreases dramatically after parturition.[12, 68, 69] Average daily doses during pregnancy are 100,000 units of vitamin D_2, 0.5 to 1.0 mg of dihydrotachysterol, and 0.25 to 1.0 µg of calcitriol. Patients need careful and frequent monitoring of their serum calcium levels and adjustments of the vitamin D and calcium doses.

The lactating breast makes PTH-RP, high concentrations of which are found in milk.[72] It is likely that this peptide appears in the blood of the postpartum patient and acts as a PTH surrogate, contributing to the decrease in vitamin D requirement after parturition. The hypoparathyroid woman can breast-feed successfully. Her serum calcium levels must be monitored carefully and therapy adjusted as necessary.

REFERENCES

1. Aboul-Khair SA, Crooks J, Turnbull AC, Hytten FE. The physiological changes in thyroid function during pregnancy. Clin Sci 1964;27:195.
2. American Academy of Pediatrics Committee on Drugs. The transfer of drugs and other chemicals into breast milk. Pediatrics 1983;375.
3. Amino N, Mori H, Iwatani Y, et al. High prevalence of transient post-partum thyrotoxicosis and hypothyroidism. N Engl J Med 1982;306:849.
4. Amino N, Tanizawa O, Mori H, et al. Aggravation of thyrotoxicosis in early pregnancy and after delivery in Graves' disease. J Clin Endocrinol Metab 1982;55:108.
5. Anast C. Disorders of mineral and bone metabolism. In: Avery ME, Taeusch HW, eds. Schaffer's diseases of the newborn, ed 5. Philadelphia: WB Saunders, 1984:464.
6. Aurbach GD, Marx SJ, Spiegel AM. Parathyroid hormone, calcitonin and the calciferols. In: Wilson JD, Foster DW, eds. Williams' textbook of endocrinology, ed 7. Philadelphia: WB Saunders, 1985:1137.
7. Avruskin TW, Mitsuma T, Shenkman L, et al. Measure-

ment of free and total serum T3 and T4 in pregnant subjects and neonates. Am J Med Sci 1976;271:309.

8. Ballabio M, Poshyachinda M, Ekins RP. Pregnancy-induced changes in thyroid function: role of human chorionic gonadotropin as putative regulator of maternal thyroid. J Clin Endocrinol Metab 1991;73:824.

9. Berghout A, Endert E, Wiersinga WM, Touber JL. The application of an immunoradiometric assay of plasma thyrotropin (TSH-IRMA) in molar pregnancy. J Endocrinol Invest 1988;11:15.

10. Bikle DD, Gee E, Halloran B, Haddad JG. Free 1,25-dihydroxyvitamin D levels in serum from normal subjects, pregnant subjects, and subjects with liver disease. J Clin Invest 1984;74:1966.

11. Bober SA, McGill AC, Tunbridge WMG. Thyroid function in hyperemesis gravidarum. Acta Endocrinol 1986;111:404.

12. Bouillon R. Vitamin D metabolites in human pregnancy. In: Holick MF, Gray TK, Anast CS, eds. Perinatal calcium and phosphorus metabolism. New York: Elsevier Science Publishers, 1983:291.

13. Bouillon R, Naesens M, Van Assche FA, et al. Thyroid function in patients with hyperemesis gravidarum. Am J Obstet Gynecol 1982;143:922.

14. Breslau N, Zerwekh JE. Relationship of estrogen and pregnancy to calcium homeostasis in pseudohypoparathyroidism. J Clin Endocrinol Metab 1986;62:45.

15. Burrow GN, Polackwich R, Donabedian R. The hypothalamic-pituitary-thyroid axis in normal pregnancy. In: Fisher DA, Burrow GN, eds. Perinatal thyroid physiology and disease. New York: Raven Press, 1975:1.

16. Cheron RG, Kaplan MM, Larsen PR, et al. Neonatal thyroid function after propylthiouracil therapy for maternal Graves' disease. N Engl J Med 1981;304:525.

17. Cooper DS. Antithyroid drugs. N Engl J Med 1984;311:1353.

18. Croom RD III, Thomas CG Jr. Primary hyperparathyroidism during surgery. Surgery 1984;96:1109.

19. Davis LE, Leveno KJ, Cunningham FG. Hypothyroidism complicating pregnancy. Obstet Gynecol 1988;72:108.

20. Davis LE, Lucas MJ, Hankins GDV, et al. Thyrotoxicosis complicating pregnancy. Am J Obstet Gynecol 1989;160:63.

21. Davis OK, Hawkins DS, Rubin LP, et al. Serum parathyroid hormone (PTH) in pregnant women determined by an immunoradiometric assay for intact PTH. J Clin Endocrinol Metab 1988;67:850.

22. Dowling JT, Appleton WG, Nicoloff JT. Thyroxine turnover during human pregnancy. J Clin Endocrinol Metab 1967;27:1749.

23. Fischinger W, Haufe S. Hyperkalzamische Krise bei primarem Hyperparathyreoidismus in der Schwangerschaft mit medullarer Nephrokalzinose. Med Klin 1988;83:195.

24. Fisher DA. Pathogenesis and therapy of neonatal Graves' disease. Am J Dis Child 1976;130:133.

25. Fisher DA, Lehman H, Lackey C. Placental transfer of thyroxine. J Clin Endocrinol Metab 1964;24:393.

26. Gardner DF, Cruikshank DP, Hays PM, Cooper DS. Pharmacology of propylthiouracil (PTU) in pregnant hyperthyroid women: correlation of maternal PTU concentrations with cord serum thyroid function tests. J Clin Endocrinol Metab 1986;62:217.

27. Gelister JSK, Sanderson JD, Chapple CR, et al. Management of hyperparathyroidism in pregnancy. Br J Surg 1989;76:1207.

28. Gerstein HC. How common is postpartum thyroiditis?

A methodologic overview of the literature. Arch Intern Med 1990;150:1397.

29. Glass EJ, Barr DG. Transient neonatal hyperparathyroidism secondary to maternal pseudohypoparathyroidism. Arch Dis Child 1981;56:565.

30. Glinoer D, De Nayer P, Bourdoux P, et al. Regulation of maternal thyroid during pregnancy. J Clin Endocrinol Metab 1990;71:276.

31. Glinoer D, Fernandez Soto M, Bourdoux P, et al. Pregnancy in patients with mild thyroid abnormalities: maternal and neonatal repercussions. J Clin Endocrinol Metab 1991;73:421.

32. Ginsberg J, Lewanczuk, RZ, Honore RLH, et al. Hyperplacentosis: a new cause of hyperthyroidism. Program of the 65th Meeting of the American Thyroid Association. Thyroid 1991;1(suppl 1):S-10.

33. Ginsberg J, Walfish PG. Post-partum transient thyrotoxicosis with painless thyroiditis. Lancet 1977;1:1125.

34. Goodenday LS, Gordan GS. No rise from vitamin D in pregnancy. Ann Intern Med 1971;75:807.

35. Harada A, Hershman JM, Reed AW, et al. Comparison of thyroid stimulators and thyroid hormone concentrations in sera of pregnant women. J Clin Endocrinol Metab 1979;48:793.

36. Hay ID, Bayer MF, Kaplan MM, et al. American Thyroid Association assessment of current free thyroid hormone and thyrotropin measurements and guidelines for future clinical assays. Clin Chem; 1991; 37:2002.

37. Hayslip CC, Fein HG, O'Donnell VM. The value of serum antimicrosomal antibody testing in screening for symptomatic postpartum thyroid dysfunction. Am J Obstet Gynecol 1988;159:203.

38. Hidal JT, Kaplan MM. Characteristics of thyroxine 5'-deiodination in cultured human placental cells. Regulation by iodothyronines. J Clin Invest 1985;76:947.

39. Higgins HP. Clinical hyperthyroidism caused by normal pregnancy. Program of the 65th Meeting of the American Thyroid Association. Thyroid 1991;1(suppl 1):S-17.

40. Higgins HP, Hershman JM, Kenimer JG, et al. The thyrotoxicosis of hydatidiform mole. Ann Intern Med 1975;83:307.

40a. Kaplan MM. Monitoring thyroxine treatment during pregnancy. Thyroid 1992;2:147.

41. Kaplan MM, Hamburger JI. Nonthyroidal causes of abnormal thyroid function test results. J Clin Immunoassay 1989;12:90.

42. Kimura M, Amino N, Tamaki H, et al. Physiologic thyroid activation in normal early pregnancy is induced by circulating hCG. Obstet Gynecol 1990; 75:775.

43. Klein RZ, Haddow JE, Faix JD, et al. Prevalence of thyroid deficiency in pregnant women. Clin Endocrinol 1991;35:41.

44. Kristoffersson A, Dahlgren S, Lithner F, Järhult J. Primary hyperparathyroidism in pregnancy. Surgery 1985;97:326.

45. Larsen PR, Alexander NM, Chopra IJ, et al. Revised nomenclature for tests of thyroid hormones and thyroid-related proteins in serum. J Clin Endocrinol Metab 1987;64:1089.

46. Lee SL, Megazzini KM, Yang IM. Ontogeny of thyrotropin releasing hormone gene expression in rat placenta. Presented at the 73rd Annual Meeting of the Endocrine Society, Washington, DC, 1991:247.

47. Levy RP, Newman DM, Rejali LS, Barford DAG. The myth of goiter in pregnancy. Am J Obstet Gynecol 1980;137:701.

48. Levy WJ, Schumacher OP, Gupta M. Treatment of childhood Graves' disease. A review with emphasis on radioiodine treatment. Cleve Clin J Med 1988;55:373.

49. Lowe DK, Orwoll ES, McClung MR, et al. Hyperparathyroidism and pregnancy. Am J Surg 1983;145:611.

50. Mabie WC, Sibai B. Chronic hypertension and antihypertensive drugs. In: Gleicher N, ed. Principles and practice of medical therapy in pregnancy, ed 2. Norwalk, CT: Appleton & Lange, 1992:888.

51. Man EB, Jones WS, Holden RH, Mellits ED. Thyroid function in human pregnancy. VIII. Retardation of progeny aged 7 years: relationships to maternal age and maternal thyroid function. Am J Obstet Gynecol 1971;111:905.

52. Mandel SJ, Larsen PR, Seely EW, Brent GA. Increased need for thyroxine during pregnancy in women with primary hypothyroidism. N Engl J Med 1990;323:91.

53. Marx SJ, Swart EG Jr, Hamstra AJ, DeLuca HF. Normal intrauterine development of the fetus of a woman receiving extraordinarily high doses of 1,25-dihydroxyvitamin D_3. J Clin Endocrinol Metab 1980;51:1138.

54. Momotani N, Noh J, Oyanagi H, et al. Antithyroid drug therapy for Graves' disease during pregnancy. Optimal therapy for fetal thyroid status. N Engl J Med 1986;315:24.

55. Montoro MN, Collea JV, Mestman JH. Management of hyperparathyroidism in pregnancy with oral phosphate therapy. Obstet Gynecol 1980;55:431.

56. Mori M, Amino N, Tamaki H, et al. Morning sickness and thyroid function in normal pregnancy. Obstet Gynecol 1988;72:355.

57. Nagataki S, Mizune M, Sakamoto S, et al. Thyroid function in molar pregnancy. J Clin Endocrinol Metab 1977;44:254.

58. Nelson M, Wickus GG, Caplan RH, Beguin EA. Thyroid gland size in pregnancy: an ultrasound and clinical study. J Reprod Med 1987;32:888.

59. Nikolai TF, Turney SL, Roberts RC. Postpartum lymphocytic thyroiditis. Prevalence, clinical course. Arch Intern Med 1987;147:221.

60. Niswander KR, Gordon M, eds. The Collaborative Perinatal Study of the National Institute of Neurological Disease and Stroke: The Women and Their Pregnancies. Washington, DC: U.S. Department of Health, Education and Welfare, 1972:246.

61. Norman RJ, Green-Thompson RJ, Jialal I, et al. Hyperthyroidism in gestational trophoblastic neoplasia. Clin Endocrinol 1981;15:395.

62. Osathanondh R, Tulchinsky D, Chopra IJ. Total and free thyroxine and triiodothyronine in normal and complicated pregnancy. J Clin Endocrinol Metab 1976;42:98.

63. Othman S, Philips DIW, Parkes AB, et al. A long-term follow-up of postpartum thyroiditis. Clin Endocrinol 1990;32:559.

64. Pekonen F, Teramo K, Ikonen E, et al. Women on thyroid hormone therapy: pregnancy course, fetal outcome, and amniotic fluid thyroid hormone level. Obstet Gynecol 1984;63:635.

65. Raiti S, Holsman GB, Scott RL, Blizzard RM. Evidence for the placental transfer of triiodothyronine in human beings. N Engl J Med 1967;277:456.

66. Rajala B, Abbasi RA, Hutchinson HT, Taylor T. Acute pancreatitis and primary hyperparathyroidism in pregnancy: treatment of hypercalcemia with magnesium sulfate. Obstet Gynecol 1987;70:460.

67. Roti E, Gnudi A, Braverman LE. The placental transport, synthesis and metabolism of hormones and drugs which affect thyroid function. Endocr Rev 1983;4:131.

68. Sadeghi-Nejad A, Wolfsdorf, Senior B. Hypoparathyroidism and pregnancy. Treatment with calcitriol. JAMA 1980;243:254.

69. Salle BL, Barthezene F, Glorieux FH, et al. Hypoparathyroidism during pregnancy: treatment with calcitriol. J Clin Endocrinol Metab 1981;52:810.

70. Sarkar SD, Beierwaltes WH, Gill SP, Cowley BJ. Subsequent fertility and birth histories of children and adolescents treated with ^{131}I for thyroid cancer. J Nucl Med 1976;17:460.

71. Shangold MM, Dor N, Welt SI, et al. Hyperparathyroidism and pregnancy: a review. Obstet Gynecol Survey 1982;37:217.

72. Singer FR. Parathyroid hormone-related protein. Mayo Clin Proc 1990;65:1502.

73. Stagnaro-Green A, Roman SH, Cobin RH, et al. Detection of at-risk pregnancy by means of highly sensitive assays for thyroid autoantibodies. JAMA 1990; 264:1422.

74. Stuart C, Aceto T Jr, Kuhn JP, Terplan K. Intrauterine hyperparathyroidism. Postmortem findings in two cases. Am J Dis Child 1979;133:67.

75. Swaminathan R, Chin RK, Lao TTH, et al. Thyroid function in hyperemesis gravidarum. Acta Endocrinol 1989;120:155.

76. Tamaki H, Amino N, Takeoka K, et al. Thyroxine requirements during pregnancy for replacement therapy of hypothyroidism. Obstet Gynecol 1990;76:230.

77. Voz ML, Peers B, Belayew A, Martial JA. Characteristics of an unusual thyroid response unit in the promoter of the human placental lactogen gene. J Biol Chem 1991;266:13397.

78. Vulsma T, Gons MH, deVijlder JJM. Maternal-fetal transfer of thyroxine in congenital hypothyroidism due to a total organification defect or thyroid agenesis. N Engl J Med 1989;321:13.

The Maternal Adrenal Cortex

George T. Griffing

James C. Melby

The achievement, maintenance, and successful outcome of pregnancy depend on a normal maternal endocrine system. Many endocrine adaptations are central to maintaining a healthy metabolic relationship between the mother and the fetus. Throughout pregnancy, every endocrine gland in the mother's body is apparently or actually affected. These changes are mainly adaptive, enabling the mother to nurture the developing fetus. Perhaps the most complex and fascinating endocrine changes are those involving the maternal adrenal cortex. This chapter reviews these changes in context with normal adrenal cortex function.

MORPHOLOGY

Adrenal morphology does not change substantially during pregnancy. Normally the adrenal glands are paired, triangular-shaped tissues lying superior and sometimes anterior to each kidney. The adrenal gland weighs 5 g, and the outer portion or the cortex makes up 80% of the adrenal weight. The adrenal gland is functionally and morphologically two separate glands: the adrenal cortex, which is embryologically derived from coelomic mesoderm, and the adrenal medulla, from the neural crest ectoderm. The adrenal cortex synthesizes corticosteroids, and the adrenal medulla synthesizes catecholamines.

The adrenal cortex is composed of three morphologically distinct zones: the zona glomerulosa, the zona fasciculata, and the zona reticularis. Each zone is responsible for synthesizing a predominant class of corticosteroids. The outermost zone, the zona glomerulosa, exclusively elaborates the major mineralocor-

ticoid, aldosterone. The zona fasciculata is the principal source of the prevailing glucocorticoid, cortisol. The innermost zone, the zona reticularis, produces the C-19 androgens, androstenedione and its precursor, dehydroepiandrosterone (DHEA) (Table 9–1).

ZONA FASCICULATA GLUCOCORTICOID SYNTHESIS

Corticosteroid biosynthesis qualitatively follows the nonpregnant pattern, even though quantitative synthesis is increased during pregnancy. Many different types of corticosteroid are secreted by the adrenal cortex, but only cortisol (glucocorticoid) and aldosterone (mineralocorticoid) are essential to sustain human life. All corticosteroids are derived from cholesterol and have a similar cyclic nucleus resembling phenanthrene (rings A, B, and C) to which a cyclopentane is attached (ring D). This structure has been designated the *cyclopentenoperhydrophenanthrene nucleus* (Fig. 9–1).

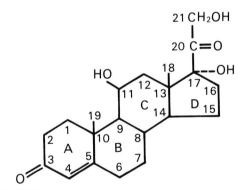

FIGURE 9–1. The chemical structure of cortisol and the nomenclature of the basic steroid nucleus.

TABLE 9–1. Corticoid Classification, Biologic Control, and Effects

Hormone	Class	Stimuli	Biologic Effects
Cortisol	Glucocorticoid	ACTH	Gluconeogenesis Protein catabolism Lipolysis
Aldosterone	Mineralocorticoid	A-II* K+† ACTH	Sodium reabsorption Potassium secretion
DHEA	Sex steroid precursor	ACTH ?other	Secondary sexual characteristics

*A-II = Angiotensin II.
†K⁺ = Local concentration of potassium.

Adrenal cholesterol is found in abundance in the adrenal cortex and may be either synthesized endogenously from acetate or extracted from circulating lipoproteins. In the formation of corticosteroids, the cholesterol side chain is cleaved, removing a six-carbon fragment, which results in a delta-5-pregnenolone (PREG), a precursor to all further steroidogenesis. Four additional enzymatic steps are required for the synthesis of cortisol (Fig. 9–2). In this sequence of steps, pregnenolone is hydroxylated to a 17α-hydroxyprogesterone, which is then sequentially hydroxylated at the 21 and 11a positions to form 11-deoxycortisol (compound S) and eventually cortisol.

REGULATION

In normal nonpregnant individuals, cortisol secretion is regulated by the central nervous system. Several centers within the central nervous system control the elaboration and secretion of a hypothalamic compound, corticotropin-releasing hormone (CRH). CRH is carried in the hypothalamic hypophyseal portal system to the anterior pituitary, where it directly stimulates the release of adrenocorticotropin (ACTH).

ACTH is a 39–amino acid polypeptide that is the major secretogogue for cortisol. After release into the circulation, ACTH attaches to a specific receptor on the adrenal cell wall, which activates adenyl cyclase. This activation generates the second messenger, adenosine-3′,5′-monophosphate (cAMP) and triggers the secretion of cortisol.

During pregnancy, the placenta secretes large amounts of CRH into the maternal and fetal circulation. Placental CRH production probably explains the high maternal plasma CRH levels along with the high ACTH concentrations and urinary free cortisol levels. ACTH and cortisol responses to exogenous CRH,

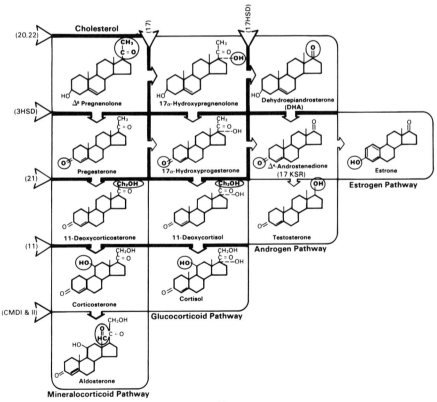

FIGURE 9–2. The biochemical pathways for the synthesis of corticosteroid hormones. Abbreviations for the steroidogenic enzymes are given in parentheses. (20,22) = cholesterol side-chain cleavage; (3HSD) = 3β-hydroxysteroid dehydrogenase; (17) = 17α-hydroxylase; (17-HSD) = 17-hydroxysteroid dehydrogenase; (21) = 21α-hydroxylase; (11) = 11β-hydroxylase; and (CMO I & II) = aldosterone synthetase.

however, are blunted during pregnancy. The decreased ACTH and cortisol responses are probably due to down-regulation of the pituitary CRH receptors because the response to another ACTH-releasing factor, vasopressin, actually increased rather than decreased.

DIURNAL RHYTHM

The large majority (70%) of the daily cortisol secretion (15 to 25mg) is released between 5:00 and 9:00 AM. Throughout the rest of the day, the cortisol secretion rate remains low, reaching a nadir at 9:00 PM. The regulation of this rhythm is a function of one's sleep-wake habits. The timing and duration of the pituitary adrenal secretory cycle can be altered by consistent revision of the timing and duration of the sleep-wake schedule. The diurnal variation of plasma cortisol is maintained during pregnancy, but cortisol secretion is increased.

FEEDBACK REGULATION

In nonpregnant individuals, ACTH secretion is subject to negative feedback regulation by cortisol at both the hypothalamic and the pituitary levels. This is a classic example of a negative feedback or *servomechanism,* which is important in maintaining homeostasis. Thus low circulating glucocorticoid levels result in a marked elevation of ACTH, and administration of exogenous cortisol suppresses pituitary secretion of ACTH. This negative feedback inhibition is subservient, however, to the diurnal rhythm because no rise in ACTH occurs during the nocturnal nadir of plasma cortisol levels (9:00 PM).

In pregnancy, the diurnal rhythm and cortisol response to stress are maintained. Normal feedback regulation, however, is lost in pregnancy. Cortisol suppression by dexamethasone is lessened, probably as a result of the autonomous placental contribution of CRH and ACTH.

STRESS

Stress can override both the diurnal rhythm and the negative feedback inhibition of ACTH. Almost any significant stress leads to increased release of ACTH and stimulation of cortisol secretion. Among the stresses that have been shown to increase adrenocortical activity are severe trauma, pyrogens, acute hypoglycemia, acute anxiety, severe depression, acute and chronic alcoholism, serious infections, convulsive treatments, and injections of histamine. Cortisol levels also increase greatly during pregnancy. These stimuli work through the central nervous system, and an intact hypothalamic-pituitary axis is critical for the mediation of the stress response (Fig. 9–3).

PLASMA BINDING

Once secreted from the adrenal cortex, the majority of plasma cortisol (90%) is bound to a specific carrier protein, cortisol-binding globulin (CBG). CBG levels can vary in indi-

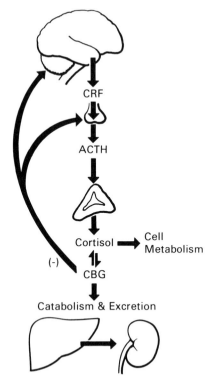

FIGURE 9–3. The regulation and metabolism of cortisol. Neural stimuli trigger release of CRH, which discharges pituitary ACTH, leading to adrenal cortisol secretion. The secreted cortisol has one of several fates: (1) becomes bound to CBG, (2) binds to cortisol receptors at target tissues, (3) is catabolized by the liver or kidney, or (4) induces feedback inhibition at the pituitary or central nervous system.

viduals and may increase twofold to threefold during pregnancy. Hepatic CBG synthesis increases owing to the effects of high levels of estrogen. CBG is usually saturated at plasma level concentrations of approximately 20 μg/dL. In pregnancy, despite the large increase in CBG, plasma cortisol exceeds this level, resulting in an increase in the unbound free plasma cortisol level.

Plasma free cortisol is the metabolically active component and is able to enter target tissues or become filtered and excreted in the urine. This is the basis for the measurement of urinary free cortisol, the best index of the level of biologically active cortisol. In pregnancy, despite the fact that total and bound plasma cortisol is increased twofold, plasma and urinary free cortisol is also increased. Therefore pregnancy is a state of hypercortisolism similar to Cushing's syndrome.

MECHANISM OF ACTION

Corticosteroids in general modify the phenotypic expression of genetic information. They appear to be freely diffusible across the cell membrane of the target tissue and interact with a specific cytosolic receptor protein. The steroid hormone–receptor complex is then transferred to the nucleus, where it binds with a specific nuclear receptor protein. This interaction influences RNA transcription of the DNA template, resulting ultimately in alterations in the rate of protein synthesis. The time course of these events is relatively slow, requiring minutes to hours for their full expression.

Glucocorticoids exert widespread effects on the metabolism of most tissues. The term *glucocorticoid* has been applied to steroids that have distinct effects on the promotion of gluconeogenesis by the liver and subsequent elevation of blood glucose concentration. These hormones also have significant catabolic effects on muscle and fat, resulting in protein catabolism and lipolysis, reflected in increased nitrogen excretion and elevated circulating free fatty acids. The elevated free cortisol in pregnancy may have some important biologic effects. Hypercortisolism probably contributes to insulin resistance, and this may be especially true in the third trimester—a time when both free cortisol and insulin resistance are maximal. Hypercortisolism may also contribute to the abnormal striae during pregnancy, but most full-blown signs of Cushing's syndrome do not appear. The high progesterone levels may act as a glucocorticoid antagonist and prevent some cortisol effects during pregnancy.

METABOLISM

Cortisol is metabolized almost entirely by the liver. Its biologic half-life is from 6 to 12 hours, and its plasma half-life is approximately 80 minutes. More than 90% of cortisol is excreted in the urine within 48 hours, and the remaining 10% appears in the feces. Cortisol metabolism is decreased in pregnancy owing to the increase of plasma binding CBG. This results in a prolongation of the plasma half-life of cortisol.

In general, it can be said that corticosteroid catabolism leads to an increase in water solubility, usually by the introduction of more hydrophilic groups (i.e., *oxo* groups are reduced to hydroxyls, and double bonds are saturated). Corticosteroid catabolism is increased during pregnancy, as reflected by increased urinary metabolites (e.g., 17-hydroxycorticosteroids). The major hepatic catabolic reactions are summarized next (Fig. 9–4).

Oxidoreduction of the C11 Group on the Molecule (Cortisol $ Cortisone)

The 11β-hydroxysteroid dehydrogenase (11β-HSD) catalyzes this reaction. In the case of cortisol, the biologically inactive compound *cortisone* is formed. Because this reaction is reversible, administration of cortisone can be converted to the biologically active cortisol. The equilibrium of this reaction is markedly affected by thyroxine: Hyperthyroidism increases the conversion of cortisol to cortisone, whereas hypothyroidism does the opposite.

The presence of 11β-HSD in the human placenta has been known for more than 20 years. This enzyme is present in the placenta at the seventh week of gestation, and it is believed to protect the fetus from high maternal cortisol levels.

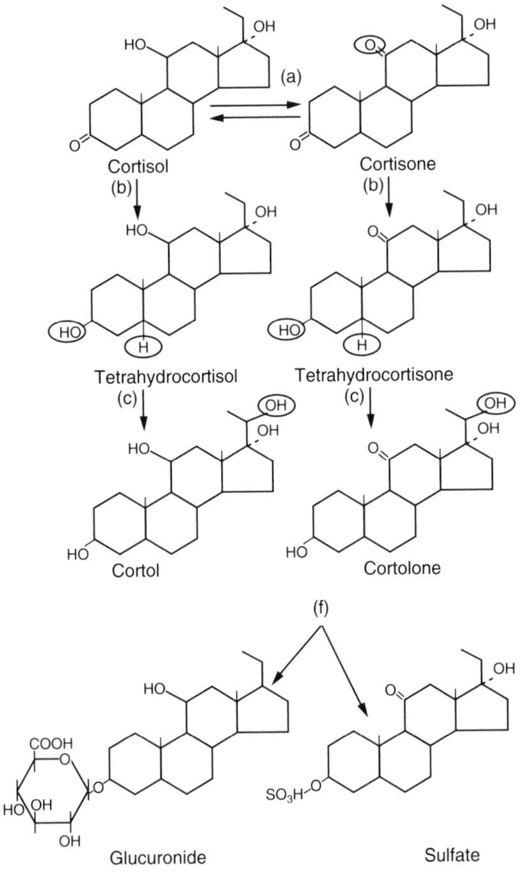

FIGURE 9–4. Major catabolic pathways of cortisol: (a) reversible oxido-reduction of the 11-group by 11β-hydroxysteroid dehydrogenase, (b) tetrahydroreduction at the 3α,5β-position, (c) 20-oxo-reduction by 20-hydroxysteroid dehydrogenases, (d) C-3 glucuronide (major) or sulfate (minor) conjugation of either cortol or cortolone.

Tetrahydroreduction of the A Ring (Cortisol [F], Cortisone [E] ⇆ THF, THE)

Reduction of a four to five double bond in ring A results in a *dihydro* intermediate that is quickly converted to the *tetrahydro* derivative by subsequent reductions at the 3-oxo group.

20-Oxoreduction (Cortisol [F], Cortisone [E] ⇆ Cortols, Cortolones)

Cortisols, cortisone, and other corticosteroids with 20-oxo groups can be acted on by enzymes that convert the 20-oxo to 20-hydroxyl groups. The enzyme 20-hydroxysteroid dehy-

drogenase carries out this reaction, which converts tetrahydrocortisol to the cortols or tetrahydrocortisone to the cortolones.

C-21 Side-Chain Cleavage (Cortisol ⇆ 17-Ketosteroid)

This reaction involves cleavage of the 17 to 20 carbon linkage by a desmolase enzyme resulting in a 17-ketosteroid. This reaction is limited to corticosteroids with a 17α-hydroxyl and 20-oxo group, such as cortisol. This enzyme is also primarily responsible for the conversion of 17-hydroxyprogesterone to androstenedione in the androgen pathway.

6β-Hydroxylation (Cortisol ⇆ 6β-Hydroxycortisol)

The 6β-hydroxylation pathway results in formation of the product, 6β-hydroxycortisol. This is a minor pathway under normal conditions, but 6β-hydroxycortisol may be excreted in relatively large amounts in newborn infants, during late pregnancy, and following drug administration. These drugs include estrogens, phenytoin, phenobarbital, and o'p'-DDD (3,3 bis[p-aminophenyl] butanone).

Other minor pathways of cortisol catabolism are known to exist but are relatively unimportant in normal adrenal physiology. The major hepatic metabolites of the aforementioned pathways include tetrahydrocortisol, tetrahydrocortisone, cortols, and cortolones and are measured as 17α-hydroxycorticosteroids (17-OHCS) in the urine.

C-3 Conjugation

The aforementioned reduced corticosteroid metabolites are conjugated in the liver via the oxygen at the C-3 position to form the corresponding water-soluble glucuronide or less soluble sulfate. These conjugated products form the predominant urinary metabolites measured in most clinical laboratories. Hepatic conjugation is increased during pregnancy, as are all of the aforementioned catabolic pathways.

ZONA GLOMERULOSA

In both pregnant and nonpregnant individuals, the zona glomerulosa is responsible for the synthesis and secretion of the major mineralocorticoid, aldosterone. The synthesis of aldosterone, similar to cortisol, proceeds through progesterone, but no 17α-hydroxylation takes place in the zona glomerulosa (see Fig. 9–2). Instead, three hydroxylations occur at the C21-position (deoxycorticosterone), C11-position (corticosterone), and the C18-position (18-hydroxycorticosterone). The final step in aldosterone synthesis is dehydrogenization of the 18-hydroxyl group, resulting in an 18-aldehyde, which then forms a hemiacetal ring. This is the biologically active mineralocorticoid, aldosterone (Fig. 9–5).

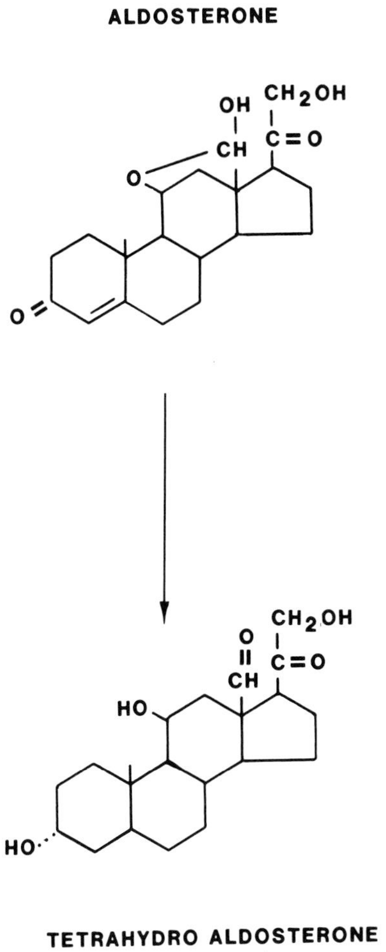

FIGURE 9–5. Aldosterone and its major hepatic metabolite, tetrahydroaldosterone.

SECRETION

Plasma aldosterone is markedly elevated during pregnancy. This increase is due to increased secretion of aldosterone and not to increased binding or decreased clearance. The peak in aldosterone production is reached by midpregnancy and is maintained until delivery. The augmented aldosterone secretion in pregnancy is due to increased zona glomerulosa stimulation by regulatory factors.

The three major regulators of aldosterone secretion that have been elucidated are (1) angiotensin II, (2) extracellular potassium, and (3) ACTH. Although ACTH in pharmacologic doses is an extremely potent stimulator of aldosterone release, at physiologic levels, ACTH appears to play a minor role in the control of aldosterone secretion. A diurnal variation of aldosterone secretion in supine humans is probably related to nyctohemeral changes in ACTH secretion. Besides ACTH, other related proopiomelanocortin (POMC) peptides have been proposed as important aldosterone secretogogues, the leading candidate being γ-melanocyte-stimulating hormone. POMC peptides are usually produced by the pituitary, but placental synthesis has also been documented. The role of POMC peptides in aldosterone physiology is under investigation and will have to await further elucidation.

Extracellular fluid potassium has a direct and potent effect on aldosterone secretion. This is especially important in anephric individuals who have no source of angiotensin II generation. An increase in extracellular potassium results in a marked rise in aldosterone secretion, whereas potassium depletion markedly suppresses aldosterone release even in aldosterone-producing adrenal adenomas. It is unknown whether potassium has an important aldosterone secretory role during pregnancy.

Angiotensin II is the predominant factor controlling aldosterone secretion in the normal state and is the end product of a series of reactions initiated by renin. Renin is an enzyme that is released from the renal juxtaglomerular apparatus. The juxtaglomerular apparatus elaborates and secretes renin in response to several physiologic stimuli: (1) reduced renal blood flow monitored by the renal afferent arteriolar baroreceptor, (2) sodium depletion detected by the macula densa in the distal nephron, and (3) β_2-adrenergic stimuli.

Renin may be released in either the active or inactive form, depending on factors that have not been elucidated at present. It is possible that renal kallikrein may be important for the activation of renin, but as yet this mechanism remains speculative. Renin acts on renin substrate (angiotensinogen), an α_2 globulin synthesized in the liver. Renin cleaves a decapeptide from angiotensinogen, which is converted to angiotensin II (octapeptide), by an enzyme, angiotensin-converting enzyme (ACE).

ACE is found predominantly in the lung. It is a metallocarboxydipeptidase, a zinc-containing enzyme that cleaves a dipeptide (histidine-9-leucine-10) from the carboxyterminal end of angiotensin I. The product of this reaction, angiotensin II, is a potent octapeptide that produces vasoconstriction and stimulates synthesis of aldosterone (Fig. 9–6).

During pregnancy, estrogen increases the hepatic synthesis of angiotensinogen as well as renin. This leads to increased angiotensin II and stimulation of aldosterone production. The renin-angiotensin system responds normally to physiologic stimuli during pregnancy but at a higher baseline level. For example, low and high dietary sodium intake modulate plasma renin activity (PRA) normally in pregnancy, but the levels for PRA and plasma aldosterone are severalfold higher in pregnant compared with nonpregnant women.[3] Angiotensin II is a potent vasoconstrictor, and normally high levels produce hypertension. During pregnancy, however, vascular sensitivity to angiotensin II is diminished, and even in the first trimester, exogenous angiotensin II blood

pressure rise is less than in the nonpregnant state.[7]

MECHANISM OF ACTION

The major effect of aldosterone is to stimulate transepithelial sodium transport across a number of tissues, including kidney, sweat glands, salivary glands, and the gastrointestinal tract. Aldosterone binds to specific mineralocorticoid cytosol receptors (type 2) present in these tissues. The aldosterone receptor complex then crosses into the nucleus and interacts with nuclear receptors to alter DNA-dependent synthesis of RNA and translation of specific transport proteins. This ultimately results in the stimulation of active sodium transport and a loosely coupled potassium secretion by the target cell.

Pregnant women, despite marked hyperaldosteronism, show few signs of aldosterone excess. There is no tendency for hypokalemia as hypernatremia, and blood pressure is usually lower than in the nonpregnant state. It has been suggested that the edema of late pregnancy is due to these changes, but hyperaldosteronism in nonpregnant women leads to hypertension and not edema. One of the explanations for the lack of mineralocorticoid signs in pregnancy is the high levels of progesterone.

Progesterone is a competitive inhibitor of aldosterone. Exogenous progesterone (but not synthetic progestins) are natriuretic and potassium sparing in humans, whereas it has no effect in adrenalectomized humans not receiving exogenous mineralocorticoids. Because progesterone blunts the kidney's response to aldosterone, the pregnancy increase in renin and aldosterone may simply be an appropriate response to the high levels of progesterone that occur in pregnancy.

Patients with pregnancy-induced hypertension (PIH) have reduced PRA and aldosterone levels compared with normal pregnancy. Overall mineralocorticoid status in PIH, however, is increased rather than decreased. Evidence for this is that mineralocorticoid receptors on circulating mononuclear leukocytes in PIH are down-regulated and a mineralocorticoid bioassay (rectal-oral subtraction potential differ-

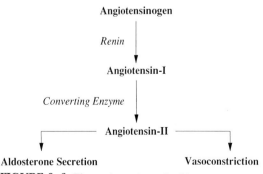

FIGURE 9–6. The renin-angiotensin-aldosterone system (see text for details).

ence) in PIH is increased.[2, 20] This suggests a nonaldosterone mineralocorticoid mechanism for this disease. One possibility is deoxycorticosterone (DOC). DOC levels increase during pregnancy, but the DOC levels in PRH are not different from normal pregnancy. Regulation of DOC during pregnancy is altered because it does not respond to ACTH or glucocorticoids. The source of DOC appears to be conversion of progesterone to DOC in peripheral tissues, especially the kidney.

METABOLISM

The aldosterone secretion rate in normal subjects is 0.05 to 0.15 mg per day. In pregnancy, aldosterone secretion increases progressively with gestation, and at the end of the third trimester, it may be increased eightfold to tenfold. In contrast to cortisol, aldosterone is poorly bound to CBG and, as a result, has a relatively short plasma half-life (20 to 30 minutes). Therefore the effect of increasing CBG during pregnancy would be expected to have little effect on plasma aldosterone, but this has not been well studied.

Aldosterone is excreted predominantly in the urine as tetrahydroaldosterone, 18-monoglucuronide aldosterone, and free aldosterone. Tetrahydroaldosterone is the major urinary metabolite that is formed by A-ring reduction in the liver. The 18-monoglucuronide is formed by conjugation of glucuronide at the 18-oxo position. This is formed both in the liver and in the kidney. It can be cleaved readily by acid and is sometimes designated as *acidlabile aldosterone*. The ratio of the three major aldosterone metabolites is unchanged with pregnancy.

ZONA RETICULARIS

The zona reticularis is relatively less important physiologically than the zona fasciculata or zona glomerulosa. Functionally the cells of the zona reticularis appear to produce predominantly steroids of the androgen and estrogen series. In normal pregnancy, adrenal androgen is only slightly increased. The predominant pathway for corticosteroid synthesis in

this zone is the Δ5 pathway, resulting in steroids of the androst-5-ene structure. Corticosteroids in this pathway undergo 17α-hydroxylation similar to what occurs with cortisol, resulting in 17α-hydroxy-pregnenolone (see Fig. 9–2).

This compound then undergoes a 17,20-desmolase reaction to form DHEA. DHEA is classified as an adrenal androgen but is without biologic activity. DHEA is subsequently converted by 3β-hydroxysteroid dehydrogenase to Δ4-androstenedione. Some androstenedione is converted to a potent androgen, testosterone, by the action of 17β-hydroxysteroid dehydrogenase. When ranked with testosterone, the androgenicity of adrenal steroids is as follows: *dihydrotestosterone > testosterone > androstenedione > dehydroepiandrosterone.*

Some androstenedione may be converted to the predominant adrenal estrogen, estrone, by aromatization of the A-ring. Estrone is a weak estrogen but can be peripherally converted to the most biologically active estrogen, estradiol, by the action of 17β-hydroxysteroid dehydrogenase. Also, some androstenedione may be converted to the predominant adrenal estrogen, estrone, by aromatization of the A-ring. The major estrogen of pregnancy is estriol, which is synthesized in the placenta from fetal 16α-hydroxy-DHEA. The potency of the estrogens is *estradiol > estrone > estriol.*

The most important determinant of plasma sex steroids is sex hormone–binding globulin (SHBG). SHBG increases during pregnancy, and because SHBG binds testosterone most avidly, plasma testosterone levels increase to the normal male range by the end of the first trimester. Free testosterone levels, however, are actually lower than in the nonpregnant state. DHEA does not bind to SHBG, and DHEA levels actually decrease during pregnancy. This is probably due to increased placental metabolism.

SUMMARY

The maternal adrenal cortex is dramatically affected by pregnancy. This is characterized by a marked increase in cortisol and aldosterone and a less marked increase in DHEA synthesis. The augmentation of cortisol synthesis is probably due to placental production of CRH and POMC-related peptides. This would explain the lack of normal glucocorticoid suppression with intact stress and stress responses and diurnal cortisol rhythm. The increases in aldosterone production are even more marked than those of cortisol. The renin-angiotensin system is increased in pregnancy as well as potential placental production of POMC peptides, which may have aldosterone-stimulating properties. Although adrenal androgen synthesis is increased, DHEA levels are lower during pregnancy owing to an increased placental uptake and metabolism. The overall increase in adrenal corticosteroid biosynthesis in pregnancy may be important for metabolic and fluid and electrolyte changes that occur in pregnancy as well as an appropriate response to the antagonistic actions of increased progesterone levels.

Acknowledgment

This work was supported by Grants-in-Aid R37DK12027-20 and HL-40123-01A1 from the National Institutes of Health.

REFERENCES

1. Arduini D, Rizzo G, Parlati E, et al. Modifications of ultradian and circadian rhythms of fetal heart rate after fetal-maternal adrenal gland suppression: a double blind study. Prenat Diagn 1986;6:409.
2. Armanini D, Zennaro CM, Martella L, et al. Mineralocorticoid effector mechanism in preeclampsia. J Clin Endocrinol Metab 1992;74:946.
3. Bay WH, Ferris TF. Factors controlling plasma renin and aldosterone during pregnancy. Hypertension 1979;1:410.
4. Casey ML, Guerami A, Winkel CA, MacDonald PC. The origin of and metabolic fate of deoxycorticosterone and deoxycorticosterone sulfate in pregnant women and their fetuses. J Steroid Biochem 1984; 20:237.
5. Challis J, Patrick J, Richardson B, Tevaarwerk G. Loss of diurnal rhythm in plasma estrone, estradiol, and estriol in women treated with synthetic glucocorticoids at 34 to 35 weeks' gestation. Am J Obstet Gynecol 1981;139:338.
6. Charnvises S, Fencl MD, Osathanondh R, et al. Adrenal steroids in maternal and cord blood after dexamethasone administration at midterm. J Clin Endocrinol Metab 1985;61:1220.
7. Cunningham FG, Lindheimer MD. Hypertension in pregnancy. N Engl J Med 1992;326:927.
8. Dalle M, Pradier P, Delost P. The conversion of cortisol into its principal metabolites, their tissular concentrations and transplacental transfer during 3H-cortisol infusion of mother and fetal guinea-pigs. Steroids 1983;42:511.
9. Demey Ponsart E, Foidart JM, Sulon J, Sodoyez JC. Serum CBG, free and total cortisol and circadian patterns of adrenal function in normal pregnancy. J Steroid Biochem 1982;16:165.
10. Dorr HG, Heller A, Versmold HT, et al. Longitudinal study of progestins, mineralocorticoids, and glucocorticoids throughout human pregnancy. J Clin Endocrinol Metab 1989;68:863.
11. Dunlap CE 3d, Sundberg DK, Rose JC. Characterization of opioid peptides from maternal and fetal sheep adrenal glands. Peptides 1985;6:483.
12. Gormley MJ, Hadden DR, Kennedy TL, et al. Cushing's syndrome in pregnancy—treatment with metyrapone. Clin Endocrinol (Oxf) 1982;16:283.
13. Griffing GT. The pregnant patient: how to distinguish diabetes and other disorders from normal endocrine changes. Consultant 1991;31:60.
14. Hercz P, Ungar L, Siklos P, Farquharson RG. Serum DHAS in the maternal-fetoplacental system during the 28th–40th weeks of pregnancy. Eur J Obstet Gynaecol Reprod Biol 1988;29:1.
15. Nolten WE, Lindheimer MD, Oparil S, Ehrlich EN. Desoxycorticosterone in normal pregnancy. I. Sequential studies of the secretory patterns of desoxycorticosterone, aldosterone, and cortisol. Am J Obstet Gynecol 1978;132:414.
16. Nolten WE, Holt LH, Rueckert PA. Desoxycorticosterone in normal pregnancy. III. Evidence of a fetal source of desoxycorticosterone. Am J Obstet Gynecol 1981;139:477.
17. Nolten WE, Rueckert PA. Elevated free cortisol index in pregnancy: possible regulatory mechanisms. Am J Obstet Gynecol 1981;139:492.
18. Novy MJ, Walsh SW. Dexamethasone and estradiol treatment in pregnant rhesus macaques: effects on gestational length, maternal plasma hormones, and fetal growth. Am J Obstet Gynecol 1983;145:920.
19. Smith R, Thomson M. Neuroendocrinology of the hypothalamo-pituitary-adrenal axis in pregnancy and the puerperium. Baillieres Clin Endocrinol Metab 1991;5:167.
20. Wacker J, Mistry NE, Bauer H, et al. Mineralocorticoids and mineralocorticoid receptors in mononuclear leukocytes in patients with pregnancy-induced hypertension. J Clin Endocrinol Metab 1992;74:946.
21. Weinberg J, Bezio S. Alcohol-induced changes in pituitary-adrenal activity during pregnancy. Alcohol Clin Exp Res 1987;11:274.
22. Wood CE. Are fetal adrenocorticotropic hormone and renin secretion suppressed by maternal cortisol secretion? Am J Physiol 1988;255:R412.

CHAPTER
10

The Maternal Ovaries

Gerson Weiss

A discussion of the maternal ovaries should start with a discussion of the corpus luteum because conception occurs coincident with corpus luteum formation. Under normal circumstances, the corpus luteum is maintained structurally intact and endocrinologically functional throughout pregnancy. The corpus luteum forms from the graafian follicle after ovulation. It functions for only 14 days unless a pregnancy results in its rescue and maintenance. The corpus luteum prepares the uterus for implantation and is necessary for the maintenance of early pregnancy. Classically its products are thought to be the steroids estradiol and progesterone. The surge of luteinizing hormone (LH) that induces ovulation also causes the formation of the corpus luteum. LH binds to cell membrane receptors and causes luteinization of granulosa cells. Working primarily through an adenyl cyclase mechanism, LH is responsible for the conversion of cholesterol to pregnenolone, then to progesterone, and finally to estrogen. Low-density lipoprotein (LDL) cholesterol is the precursor of progesterone production by the corpus luteum. LDL cholesterol binds to specific membrane receptors, which are internalized and processed by lysosomes, yielding the cholesterol necessary for steroidogenesis.[28]

The function of the corpus luteum is species specific. Products vary from species to species as do control mechanisms. For instance, it is clear that prolactin is a luteotropic hormone in the rat.[46] This is apparently not the case with the human corpus luteum. The function of the corpus luteum also depends on its age. A young corpus luteum may be hormonally responsive, whereas an older one may respond to different hormones or none at all.[39] For some hormones, an older, more mature corpus luteum responds better than a younger, less developed corpus luteum.

CELL TYPES IN THE CORPUS LUTEUM

The corpus luteum contains large cells that secrete most of the progesterone. The corpus luteum also contains small cells that are responsive to LH. This has best been worked out in the bovine species but seems true for all species. The large cells are greater than 20 μm in diameter. There are fewer large cells, but they have greater aromatase activity stimulated by follicle-stimulating hormone (FSH) and are unresponsive to LH/human chorionic gonadotropin (hCG). They have higher basal progesterone secretion. In contrast, the small cells, less than 20 μm in diameter, have low basal progesterone secretion, are very LH/hCG responsive, are more plentiful, and have lower aromatase activity, unstimulated by FSH.[37]

PRODUCTS OF THE CORPUS LUTEUM

Although the corpus luteum has traditionally been thought to be a steroidogenic organ, it also produces a wide variety of peptides. The classic hormones produced are progesterone, estradiol, and 17-hydroxyprogesterone. The corpus luteum secretes relaxin, a peptide hormone structurally analogous to insulin, in small quantities throughout the luteal phase. Oxytocin, an octapeptide, is also produced by the corpus luteum. During the menstrual cycle, oxytocin and relaxin are both detectable in the blood draining the corpus luteum.[29] The corpus luteum has also been shown to secrete inhibin.[1] The human corpus luteum has been thought to secrete growth hormone–releasing hormone-like substances as well.[8] The corpus luteum contains insulin-like growth factor-1 (IGF-1) and IGF-2. Insulin-like growth factor binding protein-1 (placental protein-12) is produced by human granulosa-luteal cells. This substance is regulated by both protein kinase C and adenylate cyclase–dependent pathways.[26] Other growth factors, such as transforming growth factor-β and epidermal growth factor, are mediators of rodent luteal function and may be present in the human corpus luteum as well.[32] Pregnancy-associated plasma protein A, a high-molecular-weight glycoprotein product of the syncytiotrophoblast, is also a luteal product. Its concentration in luteal cells depends on the reproductive state of the woman. It is present only in large luteal cells.[11]

The granulosa cells do not have a blood supply, but there is a rich blood supply to the corpus luteum. The development of this blood supply is due to the secretion of angiogenic factors. There are likely many angiogenic factors, some of which may be peptide in nature. The structure of most of these agents has not been determined.

Prostaglandins are produced by the corpus luteum.[6] Components of the renin-angiotensin system are also produced by the corpus luteum.[51] These substances are stimulated by hCG and may be related to early pregnancy recognition and maintenance.

MAINTENANCE OF THE CORPUS LUTEUM

LH/hCG is necessary for progesterone secretion. Withdrawal of LH support results in a loss of secretion of progesterone. Owing to the elegant studies of Hutchinson and Zeleznik,[25] we now understand that structure and function of the corpus luteum are dissociable. Luteal structural integrity appears to be preprogrammed and is designed to be maintained for roughly 2 weeks unless a pregnancy extends the duration of luteal maintenance. To demonstrate the dissociation of luteal structure and function, Hutchinson and Zeleznik used the rhesus monkey model. The animals had lesions placed in the arcuate nucleus of their hypothalamus to abolish production of GnRH. In turn, lack of LH production occurs with subsequent inhibition of corpus luteum maintenance. For normal reproductive function, it was necessary to connect these animals to an *artificial hypothalamus*. This consists of a pump providing 1 mg per minute GnRH for 6 minutes every hour. Connected to this pump, the animal would function normally. When the pump was disconnected in the middle of the luteal phase, there was a prompt decrease in LH secretion followed by a prompt drop in progesterone secretion. After several days when the pump was turned on again, LH secretion resumed. This resulted in a resumption of progesterone secretion to a level at which progesterone would have been secreted had the corpus luteum been allowed to continue functioning by leaving on the pump. This finding was true whether the pump was turned off in the early, middle, or late luteal

phase. In other words, the corpus luteum was structurally maintained, but its progesterone secretion was decreased in the absence of LH. Evidence suggests that luteal function can be restimulated by high doses of hCG in the follicular phase of the next cycle.[30] The role of prolactin in the maintenance of the human corpus luteum is not clear. There is some evidence in the rhesus monkey that prolactin can contribute to the maintenance of an already existing corpus luteum.[44] It is clear, however, that, in contrast to other species, prolactin is not a major luteotropic hormone in women. Prostaglandins I_2 and D_2 have been shown to stimulate cyclic adenosine monophosphate (cAMP) and progesterone production by human luteal cells in vitro.[6] These local hormones may play a role in luteal development and maintenance.

Although estradiol has been shown to contribute to the maintenance of luteal cells in vitro, it is not clear whether it subserves this function in vivo. The corpus luteum contains catecholamine receptors, and they may contribute to its maintenance. Some prostaglandins may have also been implicated in luteal maintenance. Epidermal growth factor and IGF-1 have both been shown to contribute to hormone production by the corpus luteum. It is likely that other growth factors may also synergize with gonadotropins in the maintenance of luteal function and hormone secretion.[17]

The factors responsible for the demise of the corpus luteum are also not well understood. There is significant evidence that the life span of the corpus luteum is specifically preprogrammed and it will self-destruct unless it is rescued in early pregnancy. There has been some evidence that estradiol in high concentration can cause luteolysis. Hoffmann[24] demonstrated that intraovarian crystals of estradiol cause luteal demise, but cholesterol crystals, as a control substance, did not. The mechanism of action of estradiol, however, may not be a direct action on the corpus luteum. Estradiol is not luteolytic in vitro, and there is no accumulation of estradiol in the corpus luteum. There is evidence in sheep and cows that oxytocin is luteolytic.[10] In women, it is possible that the oxytocin secreted by the corpus luteum has a regulatory role as well.

Locally produced oxytocin may regulate luteal demise.[5] Prostaglandin $F_2\alpha$ is luteolytic in many species, and there are some data to suggest that it may have this role in women as well.[2] Other peptides, including the LHRH-like peptides, may also contribute to luteal regression.

CORPUS LUTEUM OF PREGNANCY

If pregnancy occurs, a stimulus from the blastocyst, hCG, rescues the corpus luteum and allows it to be maintained to support the early pregnancy hormonally. This early stimulus for luteal maintenance occurs on approximately day 9 to 10 of the luteal phase. The levels of hCG necessary to rescue the corpus luteum are so small that they are difficult to detect in the maternal circulation. As can be seen from monkey data, the corpus luteum can be rescued by as little as 25 IU of hCG per day.[35]

In women, the corpus luteum is necessary to maintain pregnancy for approximately 4 weeks. After that time, pregnancies can be maintained without hormonal support even after luteectomy.[15] The corpus luteum, however, is maintained throughout pregnancy. At the time of cesarean section, the corpus luteum can be observed in the ovary.[57] The ovary may have to be transilluminated, however, because in late pregnancy the corpus luteum occupies a more internal portion of the ovary. The pituitary is not necessary for luteal maintenance in pregnancy because pregnancy can be maintained after the first trimester following hypophysectomy.[27] Women without pituitary glands can become pregnant if ovulation is induced with human menopausal gonadotropins.

hCG alone cannot maintain the corpus luteum of nonpregnant women for more than 2 to 3 weeks, suggesting that other luteotropic substances function during pregnancy. From 3 to 4 weeks after ovulation, the corpus luteum becomes refractory to hCG stimulation.[55] The maintenance of the corpus luteum of pregnancy is poorly understood. It is possible that there may be serial luteotropins during pregnancy. It is clearly known that the response to a stimulus by the corpus luteum is determined by the age of that structure. For instance, a 3-day-old corpus luteum responds poorly to CG, and its progesterone secretion is not increased. The same stimulus given on the ninth day of the luteal phase results in a prompt increase in progesterone secretion, maintenance of the corpus luteum for a longer period of time, and induction of the secretion of relaxin.[39]

The ultrastructure of the corpus luteum of pregnancy differs from that of the corpus luteum of the menstrual cycle in that the pregnancy corpus luteum, among other changes, has extensive granular endoplasmic reticulum, suggesting a greater capacity for peptide or protein production.[13]

STEROID SECRETION BY THE CORPUS LUTEUM OF PREGNANCY

For 3 to 4 weeks after luteal rescue, the corpus luteum continues to secrete progesterone, estrogen, and 17-hydroxyprogesterone. This is followed by a decrease in function.[34] The corpus luteum, however, continues to secrete progesterone at low levels for the duration of pregnancy. The corpus luteum of term pregnancy is qualitatively different from the corpus luteum of the menstrual cycle in that the corpus luteum of term pregnancy secretes little estradiol compared with the cycle corpus luteum.[58]

LUTEAL PLACENTAL SHIFT

After the fourth week of gestation, 17-hydroxyprogesterone declines. Because this hormone is produced by the corpus luteum but not the placenta, this indicates a decrease in luteal function. Progesterone, however, declines only slightly at this time. This is due to lowered luteal production but an increasing placental contribution to the production of progesterone.[34] At this point, the placenta takes over steroidogenesis, and progesterone continues to rise through the duration of pregnancy. This switch from luteal to placental steroid secretion is called the *luteal placental shift*. After the luteal placental shift, the corpus luteum is no longer necessary for pregnancy maintenance. Csapo et al.[15] demonstrated that removal of the corpus luteum before, but not after, the seventh week of gestation resulted in a decline in progesterone secretion and spontaneous abortion. This could be prevented by progesterone administration but only at supraphysiologic levels.[15]

RELAXIN

Relaxin is a peptide of approximately 6000 dalton molecular weight. It consists of dissimilar A and B chains linked by two disulfide linkages. There is an additional intrachain disulfide link in the A chain. There is remarkable structural similarity to insulin but less than a 25% amino acid homology.[3] Relaxin has no insulin activity. There are two nonallelic genes for human relaxin, both located on the ninth chromosome.[12] Only one of these genes, H2, is expressed in the corpus luteum. The corpus luteum is the source of circulating relaxin in pregnancy. Relaxin is present in the maternal circulation throughout pregnancy, but its concentrations are highest in the first trimester[4] (Fig. 10–1). At the time of term ce-

sarean section, simultaneous peripheral blood samples and ovarian vein blood samples were obtained for relaxin assay. Relaxin concentrations were similar in peripheral blood and in the blood draining the ovary not containing the corpus luteum of pregnancy. Relaxin concentrations were substantively higher in the ovarian vein draining the ovary containing the corpus luteum of pregnancy.[57] Mathieu et al.[31] immunohistochemically localized relaxin to the corpus luteum during pregnancy. These investigators were not able to demonstrate relaxin in adjacent ovarian tissue. Luteectomy at term pregnancy results in a prompt fall in levels of circulating relaxin. In contrast, in the absence of luteectomy after delivery, there is a gradual fall of relaxin secretion over 72 hours.[56]

In conception cycles, relaxin rises in maternal blood by the time of the missed menses.[42] There appears to be no diurnal variation in serum relaxin concentrations in pregnancy. There are no significant changes noted between antepartum and intrapartum relaxin concentrations. There appears to be no significant prelabor surge of circulating relaxin such as occurs in some other species.[41]

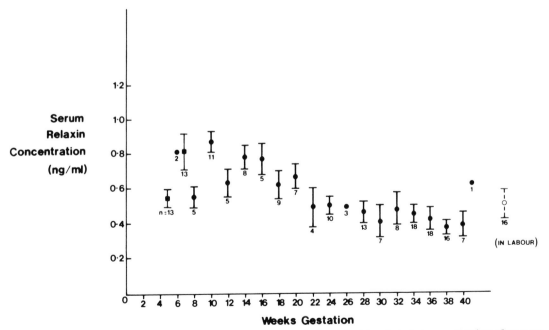

FIGURE 10–1. Relaxin levels in 19 normal pregnant women studied serially (closed circles). n = Number of measurements. Closed squares are 13 women measured twice. Open circle represents term pregnancy levels in labor. (From Bell RJ, Eddie LW, Lester AR, et al. Relaxin in human pregnancy serum measured with an homologous radioimmunoassay. Obstet Gynecol 1987;69:585–589. With permission.)

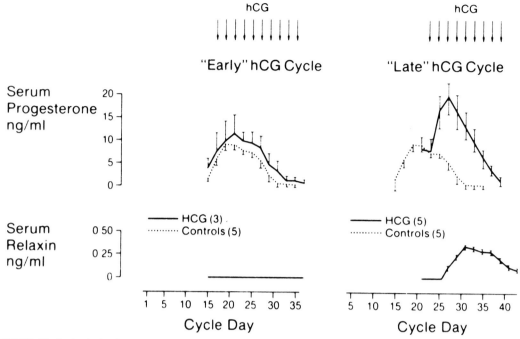

FIGURE 10–2. Ovulation has been standardized to day 14. hCG injections (2500 IU intramuscularly, every 2 days) are shown as arrows. (From Quagliarello J, Goldsmith L, Steinetz B, et al. Induction of relaxin secretion in nonpregnant women by human chorionic gonadotropin. J Clin Endocrinol Metab 1980;51:74–77. With permission.)

Relaxin concentrations in toxemic pregnancies are similar to those of normal pregnancies in the third trimester. In contrast, relaxin concentrations in pregnancies beyond 43 weeks' gestation and in women with premature labor were significantly lower than levels in normal women during the third trimester of pregnancy.[52] Serum relaxin concentrations were similar in normal patients and patients treated with human menopausal gonadotropin who had singleton pregnancies. Women given human menopausal gonadotropins with multiple fetuses, however, have significantly higher concentrations of relaxin, probably as a result of the presence of multiple corpora lutea. Because this latter group demonstrates a high incidence of premature birth, this may represent a human syndrome of hyperrelaxinemia, which may result in cervical incompetence early in pregnancy.[22] Using relaxin as an indicator of luteal activity and hCG as an indicator of placental function, women were prospectively studied in early pregnancies. Some of these women had spontaneous abortions. In women destined to abort, hCG levels fell before relaxin levels did. In fact, in some of these

women, relaxin levels were normal, but hCG levels were subnormal. This indicates that, at least in the pregnancies studied, the loss of the pregnancy was preceded by an initial loss of placental rather than luteal function.[43]

To test the hypothesis that an early blastocyst signal induced luteal relaxin secretion, Quagliarello et al.[39] gave hCG injections to normal women every other day starting on day 8 of the luteal phase. This resulted in a prompt rescue of the corpus luteum and then an abrupt rise in progesterone secretion (Fig. 10–2). Relaxin became detectable only 2 to 6 days later, but it continued to rise, while progesterone concentrations in the serum were falling for several days. Thus hCG can induce relaxin secretion in nonpregnant women, but as shown in the previous experiment, there may be different control mechanisms for relaxin and progesterone secretion by the corpus luteum even though the same exogenous hormone hCG is the stimulus for both.

The timing of the hCG stimulus is critical to relaxin secretion. When an identical experimental paradigm was used, starting hCG injections on day 2 or 3 of the luteal phase, no relaxin was detectable. This suggested that the corpus luteum is a dynamic structure and must be in the appropriate condition to respond to hCG with relaxin secretion. Although relaxin is present throughout pregnancy, administration of hCG is incapable of maintaining relaxin secretion from the nonpregnancy corpus luteum for more than 2 weeks. Thus other factors must also contribute to the relaxin secretion of pregnant women. These other factors are not known. Some investigators demonstrated that GnRH was capable of inducing relaxin secretion in nonpregnant women.[54] The patterns of decline of circulating relaxin in lactating and nonlactating women patients are similar, suggesting that the higher prolactin concentrations seen in nursing mothers are not luteotropic.[40] Radiolabeled placental lactogen does not bind in vitro to corpora lutea of pregnancy. This suggests that the lactogenic hormones may not have a role in the maintenance of the human corpus luteum of pregnancy. Prostaglandins $F_2\alpha$ and E_2 as well as oxytocin in concentrations high enough to induce labor did not cause alteration in circulating relaxin concentration.[23, 38]

ACTIONS OF RELAXIN IN PREGNANCY

Szlachter et al.[53] demonstrated that human relaxin can decrease the amplitude of spontaneous contractions in human myometrial strips obtained from nonpregnant premenopausal women. In a rat uterine segment model, oxytocin and endothelin have been shown to stimulate uterine contractions. This stimulation can be antagonized for both of these agents by relaxin. The effect of these agents can be modulated by progesterone. It has been postulated that both relaxin and progesterone work in synergy to control uterine activity and promote uterine quiescence in early pregnancy.[20, 50] The mechanism of action of relaxin is not fully known. In vitro relaxin stimulates prostacyclin secretion by human myometrial cells. Prostacyclins decrease myometrial contractility.[45] In a rat model, uterine cAMP is increased by relaxin. Nishikori et al.[36] have suggested a mechanism of action of relaxin on myometrial activity, demonstrating

that myosin light chain kinase activity, myosin light chain phosphorylation, and calcium-activated adenosine triphosphatase activity are decreased by relaxin. Relaxin stimulates calcium efflux and inhibits calcium influx.[19] The synergistic effect of relaxin and progesterone is modulated via an adenyl cyclase mechanism.[21]

The in vivo activity of relaxin on the human cervix is not known. It is clear, however, that exogenous relaxin is capable of softening and ripening the pregnant cervix as well as advancing Bishop score.[18] Relaxin significantly influences tritiated hydroxyproline incorporation by cervical tissues in vitro.[59] In vivo relaxin stimulates water inhibition of the primate cervix. There is radiographic evidence that there are changes in the pubic symphysis during early pregnancy. These changes (laxity of many joints) are likely due to relaxin. In several systems, relaxin has been shown to alter collagenase and proteoglycanase.

PREGNANCY IN ALUTEAL WOMEN

The advent of assisted reproductive technology has allowed the occurrence of pregnancy via egg donation. Thus human pregnancy can be initiated and maintained without the presence of maternal ovaries. The process is as follows: Recipients, women with premature ovarian failure, are treated with exogenous estrogen and progesterone in a manner that simulates circulating levels in the natural cycle. To prove a normal uterine response to the exogenous steroids, late luteal phase endometrial biopsies are performed. After egg donors are identified, they are hyperstimulated to produce multiple oocytes as one would do for in vitro fertilization. Oocytes are harvested and fertilized in vitro. Fertilized oocytes at the four to eight cell stage are transferred to the uteri of recipient women. These women are on day 18 of their induced cycles, a time that has been shown to produce a receptive endometrium. Resultant pregnancies are maintained with exogenous estrogen and progesterone until the ninth week of pregnancy, when exogenous hormones are decreased and eliminated as endogenous placental hormones rise. Most protocols of exogenous hormone secretion produce significantly higher levels of estrogen and progesterone than would be seen in natural pregnancies. Given this caveat, it is clear that pregnancies do well in the total absence of maternal ovaries.[16] Studying patients who are pregnant by egg donation allows a greater understanding of the role of the ovary in normal human pregnancy. Women who are pregnant without ovaries have no circulating relaxin. Relaxin, however, is also a product of human decidua during pregnancy.[48] In a baboon model, there is evidence that there is feedback between circulating and decidual relaxin such that aluteal baboons have higher levels of decidual relaxin than intact controls.[9]

Women pregnant without corpora lutea have no circulating inhibin until the eighth week of pregnancy. This is in contrast to normal women. This suggests that the corpus luteum is the source of circulating inhibin in early pregnancy in normal women.[49]

Estrogen stimulates growth hormone secretion.[33] Women pregnant by egg donation have higher levels of estrogen in early pregnancy than normal women because they are replaced with higher concentrations of exogenous estrogen. These women, however, have lower levels of circulating growth hormone than intact, normally pregnant women.[16] This suggests that an ovarian factor is present that normally stimulates growth hormone secretion in pregnancy. It has been shown in vitro that relaxin stimulates cAMP production in rat pituitary cells.[14] Exogenous relaxin has stimulated prolactin and growth hormone secretion in rhesus monkeys.[7] Thus it is likely that relaxin is a stimulus for growth hormone secretion in pregnant women. It has been shown that growth hormone is a major lactogenic hormone in women.[47] Thus relaxin may have effects on the initiation of lactation.

POSTPARTUM OVARIAN FUNCTION

After delivery, there is a decrease in luteal function that lasts 2 to 3 days until luteal function ceases. If there is no lactation, normal ovarian function resumes in roughly 6 weeks. Active nursing significantly delays the resumption of ovarian function, likely because of a suppression of gonadotropin secretion. In societies in which most of the nutrition of the infant is from nursing, the postpartum lactational amenorrhea results in effective contraceptive activity that may last for well over a year. Gradually there is a resumption of ovarian function as nursing decreases. Lactation and nursing can occur in the absence of ovaries.

REFERENCES

1. Abe Y, Hasegawa Y, Mujamoto K, et al. High concentration of plasma immunoreactive inhibin during normal pregnancy in women. J Clin Endocrinol Metabol 1990;71:133.
2. Auletta FJ, Flint APF. Mechanisms controlling corpus luteum function in sheep, cow, nonhuman primate, and women especially in relation to the time of luteolysis. Endocr Rev 1988;9:88.
3. Bedarkar S, Blundell T, Gowan LW, et al. On the three-dimensional structure of relaxin. Ann NY Acad Sci 1982;380:22.
4. Bell RJ, Eddie LW, Lester AR, et al. Relaxin in human pregnancy serum measured with a homologous radioimmunoassay. Obstet Gynecol 1987;69:585.
5. Bennegard B, Hahlin M, Dennefors B. Antigonadotropic effect of oxytocin on the isolated human corpus luteum. Fertil Steril 1987;47:431.
6. Bennegard B, Hahlin M, Hamberger L. Luteotropic effects of prostaglandins I$_2$ and D$_2$ on isolated human corpora luteum. Fertil Steril 1990;54:459.
7. Bethea CL, Cronin MJ, Galuska GJ, Novy MJ. The effect of relaxin infusion on prolactin and growth hormone secretion in monkeys. J Clin Endocrinol Metab 1989;69:956.
8. Bramley TA. GnRH peptides and regulation of the corpus luteum. J Reprod Fertil 1989;37(suppl):205.
9. Castracane VD, Lessing J, Brenner S, Weiss G. Relaxin in the pregnant baboon: evidence for local production in reproductive tissues. J Clin Endocrinol Metab 1985;60:133.
10. Chandrasekher YA, Fortune JE. Effects of oxytocin on steroidogenesis by bovine theca and granulosa cells. Endocrinol 1990;127:926.
11. Chegini N, Lei ZM, Rao Ch V, Bischof P. The presence of pregnancy-associated plasma protein-A in human corpora luteum: cellular and subcellular distribution and dependence on reproductive state. Biol Reprod 1991;44:201.
12. Crawford RJ, Hudson P, Shine J, et al. Two human relaxin genes on chromosome 9. EMBO J 1984;3:2343.
13. Crisp TM, Dessouky DA, Denys FR. The fine structure of the human corpus luteum of term pregnancy. Am J Obstet Gynecol 1973;115:901.
14. Cronin MJ, Malaska T, Bakhit C. Human relaxin increases cyclic AMP levels in cultured anterior pituitary cells. Biochem Biophys Res Commun 1987;148:1246.
15. Csapo AI, Pulkkinen MO, Wiest WG. Effects of luteectomy and progesterone replacement therapy in early pregnant patients. Am J Obstet Gynecol 1973;115:759.
16. Emmi AM, Skurnick J, Goldsmith LT, et al. Ovarian control of pituitary hormone secretion in early human pregnancy. J Clin Endocrinol Metabol 1991;72:1359.

17. Erickson GF, Garzo VG, Magoffin DA. Insulin-like growth factor-1 regulates aromatase activity in human granulosa and granulosa luteal cells. J Clin Endocrinol Metab 1989;69:716.

18. Evans MI, Dougan MB, Moawad AH, et al. Ripening of the human cervix with porcine ovarian relaxin. Am J Obstet Gynecol 1983;147:410.

19. Ginsburg F, Rosenberg C, Schwartz M, et al. The effect of relaxin on calcium fluxes in the rat uterus. Am J Obstet Gynecol 1988;159:1395.

20. Goldsmith LT, Skurnick JH, Wojtczuk AS, et al. The antagonistic effect of oxytocin and relaxin on rat uterine segment contractibility. Am J Obstet Gynecol 1989;161:1644.

21. Grazi RV, Goldsmith LT, Schmidt CL, et al. Synergistic effect of relaxin and progesterone on cyclic adenosine 3′,3′-monophosphate levels in rat uterus. Am J Obstet Gynecol 1988;159:1402.

22. Haning RV, Steinetz BG, Weiss G. Elevated serum relaxin levels in multiple pregnancy after menotropins treatment. Obstet Gynecol 1985;66:42.

23. Hochman J, Weiss G, Steinetz BG, O'Byrne EM. Serum relaxin concentrations in prostaglandin and oxytocin-induced labor in women. Am J Obstet Gynecol 1978;130:473.

24. Hoffmann F. Untersuchungen uber die hormonale Beeinflussung des Lebensdauer des Corpus Luteum in Zyklus der Frau. Geburtsh Frauenheilk 1960; 20:1153.

25. Hutchinson JS, Zeleznik AJ. The corpus luteum of the primate menstrual cycle is capable of recovering from a transient withdrawal of pituitary gonadotropin support. Endocrinol 1985;117:1043.

26. Jalkanen J, Suikkari A-M, Koistinen R, et al. Regulation of insulin-like growth factor-binding protein-1 production in human granulosa-luteal cells. J Clin Endocrinol Metab 1989;69:1174.

27. Kaplan NM. Successful pregnancy following hypophysectomy during the twelfth week of gestation. J Clin Endocrinol Metab 1961;21:1139.

28. Keyes PL, Wiltbank MC. Endocrine regulation of the corpus luteum. Ann Rev Physiol 1988;50:465.

29. Khan-Dawood Y, Goldsmith LT, Weiss G, Dawood M. Human corpus luteum secretion of relaxin, oxytocin and progesterone. J Clin Endocrinol Metab 1989;68:627.

30. Koulianos GT, Castillo RA, Goldsmith LT, et al. Ability to rescue the corpus luteum with hCG persists into the subsequent follicular phase (abstr 426). Presented at the Society for Gynecologic Investigation, St Louis, Mo, 1990.

31. Mathieu PH, Rahier J, Thomas K. Localization of relaxin in human gestational corpus luteum. Cell Tissue Res 1981;219:213.

32. Matsuyawa S, Shiota K, Takahashi M. Possible role of transforming growth factor-beta as a mediator of luteotropic action of prolactin in rat luteal cell cultures. Endocrinol 1990;127:1561.

33. Merimee TJ, Feinberg SE. Studies of the sex based variation of human growth hormone secretion. J Clin Endocrin Metabol 1971;33:851.

34. Mishell DR, Thorneycroft IH, Nagata Y, et al. Serum gonadotropin and steroid patterns in early human gestation. Am J Obstet Gynecol 1973;117:631.

35. Neill JD, Knobil E. On the nature of the initial luteotropic stimulus of pregnancy in the rhesus monkey. Endocrinol 1972;90:34.

36. Nishikori K, Weisbrodt NW, Sherwood OD, Sanborn BM. Relaxin alters rat uterine myosin light chain phos-

37. Niswender GD, Schwall RH, Fitz TA, et al. Regulation of luteal function in domestic ruminants: New concepts. Rec Prog Horm Res 1985;41:101.

38. Quagliarello J, Cederqvist L, Steinetz BG, Weiss G. Serum relaxin levels in prostaglandin E_2 induced abortions. Prostaglandins 1978;16:1003.

39. Quagliarello J, Goldsmith LT, Steinetz BG, et al. Induction of relaxin secretion in non-pregnant women by human chorionic gonadotropin. J Clin Endocrinol Metab 1980;51:74.

40. Quagliarello J, Goldsmith LT, Szlachter N, et al. Absence of luteotropic effect of prolactin and human placental lactogen on the human corpus luteum of pregnancy. In: Goldstein M, ed. Ergot compounds and brain function: neuroendocrine and neuropsychiatric aspects. New York: Raven Press, 1980:229.

41. Quagliarello J, Lustig DS, Steinetz BG, Weiss G. Absence of a prelabor relaxin surge in women. Biol Reprod 1980;22:202.

42. Quagliarello J, Steinetz BG, Weiss G. Relaxin secretion in early pregnancy. Obstet Gynecol 1979;53:62.

43. Quagliarello J, Szlachter BN, Nisselbaum JS, et al. Serum relaxin and human chorionic gonadotropin concentration in spontaneous abortions. Fertil Steril 1981;36:399.

44. Richardson DW, Goldsmith LT, Pohl CR, et al. The role of prolactin in the regulation of the primate corpus luteum. J Clin Endocrinol Metab 1985;60:501.

45. Richardson M, Mitchell MD, MacDonald PC, Casey ML. Effect of relaxin on prostacyclin production by human myometrial cells in monolayer culture. In: Society for Gynecologic Investigation Annual Program, Washington, DC, 1983.

46. Rothchild I. The regulation of the mammalian corpus luteum. Rec Prog Horm Res 1981;37:183.

47. Ruan WF, Feldman M, Newman CV, Kleinberg DL. Growth hormone is superior to prolactin in stimulating mammary development (abstr 908). Presented at Endocrinol Society Annual Meeting, Atlanta, Ga, 1990.

48. Sakbrun V, Ali SM, Greenwood FC, Bryant-Greenwood DG. Human relaxin in the amnion, chorion decidua parietalis, basal plate and placental trophoblast by immunocytochemistry and northern analysis. J Clin Endocrinol Metab 1990;70:508.

49. Santoro N, Ibrahim J, Schmidt CL, Schneyer A. Pituitary placental and luteal gonadotropin and inhibin secretion in early pregnancy in women without corpora lutea (abstr 665). Presented at Endocrinol Society Annual Meeting, Washington, DC, 1991.

50. Sarosi P, Schmidt CL, Essig M, et al. The effect of relaxin and progesterone on rat uterine contractions. Am J Obstet Gynecol 1983;145:402.

51. Sealy JE, Glorioso, N, Itskovitz J, Laragh JH. Prorenin as a reproductive hormone: a new form of the renin system. Am J Med 1986;81:1041.

52. Szlachter BN, Quagliarello J, Jewelewicz R, et al. Relaxin in normal and pathogenic pregnancies. Obstet Gynecol 1982;59:167.

53. Szlachter N, O'Bryne EM, Goldsmith LT, et al. Myometrial-inhibiting activity of relaxin containing extracts of human corpora lutea of pregnancy. Am J Obstet Gynecol 1980;136:584.

54. Thomas K, Loumaye E, Ferin J. Relaxin in non-pregnant women during ovarian stimulation. Gynecol Obstet Invest 1980;11:75.

55. Tu BK. Effect of hCG on human corpus luteum of

menstruation and early gestation. Endocrinol Jap 1978;25:569.

56. Weiss G, O'Byrne EM, Hochman JA, et al. Secretion of progesterone and relaxin by the human corpus luteum of midpregnancy and at term. Obstet Gynecol 1977;50:679.

57. Weiss G, O'Byrne EM, Steinetz BG. Relaxin: a product of the human corpus luteum of pregnancy. Science 1976;194:948.

58. Weiss G, Rifkin I. Progesterone and estrogen secretion by puerperal human ovaries. Obstet Gynecol 1975;46:556.

59. Wiqvist I, Norstrom S, O'Byrne EM, Wiqvist N. Regulating influence of relaxin on human cervical and uterine connective tissue. Acta Endocrinol (Copenh) 1984;106:127.

Postpartum Lactation and Resumption of Reproductive Functions

Dan Tulchinsky

PHYSIOLOGIC CHANGES

The postpartum period is marked by major physiologic, anatomic, and endocrinologic changes. There are changes in blood volume, blood flow, and intercompartmental fluid distribution. Involutional changes of the uterus occur simultaneously with proliferative changes of the breast. The pituitary gland, which enlarged in pregnancy, recedes to its normal size after lactation has been discontinued.

The endocrine changes that take place in the puerperium are due to two main events. First, the delivery of the fetus and placenta brings about a sudden withdrawal of hormones of fetoplacental origin, resulting in changes in the function of various physiologic and endocrinologic systems. Second, the continuous production of prolactin (PRL) in the presence of this placental withdrawal brings about the onset of lactation as well as exerting an inhibitory influence on other endocrine systems. As these changes subside, the normal physiologic and endocrine relationships characteristic of the nonpregnant state are restored.

HORMONAL CHANGES

Disappearance of Circulating Hormones

Following delivery, hormones that originate from the fetoplacental unit rapidly disappear (Table 11–1). The rate of disappearance depends on their half-life in blood. The disappearance rate of each hormone from blood can be expressed as two components: one rapid (first half-life), representing the phase of removal from an inner or vascular compartment, and a more prolonged one (second half-life), representing removal from the outer compartment, including extravascular and intracellular space. Hormones such as human chorionic gonadotropin (hCG) with a prolonged second half-life of 7 to 37 hours can be detected in plasma up to 3 to 4 weeks' postpartum[69, 154] (see Chapter 2). In contrast, human placental lactogen, with a short second half-life of 13 to 30 minutes, disappears from plasma within a day or two.[36, 69] Pregnancy-associated proteins (PAPS), which are believed to be of placental origin, disappear from blood within a few days after delivery.[113] Pregnancy zone proteins, such as α-fetoproteins and oxytocinase, can be detected in plasma many weeks' postpartum, suggesting that they are not derived solely from placenta.[36, 167] The plasma concentrations of steroid-binding proteins, such as corticosteroid-binding globulin, return to the nonpregnancy range within 2 weeks, whereas the mean plasma concentration of sex hormone–binding globulin at the same time is still 1.7-fold higher than that of nonpregnant patients.[182] Other substances are cleared at different rates.[85] By and large, the nonpregnant endocrine state is reached at 6 weeks' postpartum, but there are a few exceptions. Cholesterol in low-density lipoprotein may remain elevated longer than 6 weeks' postpartum,[150] and thyroglobulin levels may remain abnormally high beyond 6 weeks in up to 40% of patients.

The expulsion of the placenta, which is the main source of circulating estrogens and pro-

TABLE 11–1. Mean Serum Concentration of Various Hormones at Term Pregnancy Compared with Those Observed at 24 Hours' Postpartum and in the Nonpregnant State

	Serum Concentration (ng/mL)						DHEAS (μg/ml)	17-P (ng/mL)	P (ng/mL)	hPL (μg/mL)	hCG (mIU/mL)	PRL (ng/mL)
	E_1	E_2	E_3	A	T	DHEA						
Term pregnancy	7	17	13	5.3	1.4	4.1	0.8	6	170	6.5	7000	200
24 hours postpartum	0.3	0.2	0.2	3.2	1.4	2.3	0.9	0.4	7.0	0.1	2000	200
Early follicular phase levels	0.08	0.07	<25	2.0	0.3	5.0	1.6	0.4	<10	—	—	<25

E_1 = Estrone; E_2 = estradiol; E_3 = estriol; A = androstenedione; T = testosterone; DHEA = dehydroepiandrosterone; DHEAS = dehydroepiandrosterone sulfate; 17-P = 17-α-hydroxyprogesterone; P = progesterone; hPL = human placental lactogen; hCG = human chorionic gonadotropin; PRL = prolactin.

gesterone at term pregnancy, is associated with a rapid fall of the plasma concentrations of reproductive steroid hormones. Plasma estradiol, which has an initial half-life of approximately 20 minutes, with a second half-life of 6 to 7 hours,[183] disappears from plasma rapidly, and at 24 hours following delivery, its concentration reaches levels less than 2% of prepartum values[183] (Fig. 11–1). Estradiol reaches follicular phase levels (less than 100 pg/mL) within 1 to 3 days after delivery,[183] and at that time unconjugated estriol becomes undetectable (less than 50 pg/mL). The clearance rate of conjugated estrogens varies, depending on the type of conjugate. Thus the disappearance rate of sulfated estrogens such as estrone sulfate from serum is much slower than that of estrogen glucuronidates or unconjugated estrogens because of their much slower metabolic clearance rate.[36, 160]

The half-life of progesterone in plasma is rather rapid (second half-life of 20 minutes),[112] yet progesterone plasma concentration does not reach follicular phase levels as rapidly as plasma estradiol. This is because the corpus luteum of pregnancy continues to secrete progesterone in the first few days' postpartum.

The removal of the corpus luteum immediately after delivery results in a prompt fall of plasma progesterone to the nonpregnancy range.[194] Under normal conditions, luteal phase levels of progesterone (5 to 25 ng/mL) are reached within 1 day of delivery,[148, 195] and follicular phase levels (<1 ng/mL) may be reached as early as 72 hours or as late as 1 week after delivery (see Chapter 10).

Pituitary-Hypothalamic Controlled Functions

Prolactin Secretion

The increase in the number of PRL-secreting cells (galactotropes) during pregnancy brings about an increase in PRL plasma concentration as pregnancy progresses[10, 65] (see Chapter 7). The onset of labor leads to a significant decline in PRL levels,[76, 155] but delivery may be associated with a short-lived rise in PRL concentration.[155] In the absence of suckling, this would be followed within 7 to 14 days by a rapid fall of serum PRL levels to the nongravid range.[19, 44, 184] Wide fluctuations, however, in individual levels exist. The mean basal serum

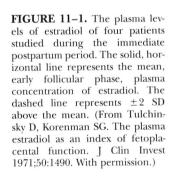

FIGURE 11–1. The plasma levels of estradiol of four patients studied during the immediate postpartum period. The solid, horizontal line represents the mean, early follicular phase, plasma concentration of estradiol. The dashed line represents ±2 SD above the mean. (From Tulchinsky D, Korenman SG. The plasma estradiol as an index of fetoplacental function. J Clin Invest 1971;50:1490. With permission.)

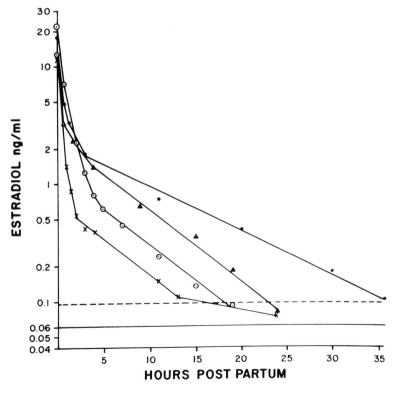

PRL concentration of breast-feeding women gradually returns toward the nonpregnancy range. It remains significantly higher, however, than that of nonnursing mothers after 90 days' postpartum and often after 6 months.[24, 156, 158, 177, 184]

In addition, a secondary pattern of PRL release (Fig. 11–2) is developed, which can be triggered in breast-feeding mothers by suckling.[89, 140, 184] Distinct bursts of PRL separated by an interval of secretory quiescence can be observed.[102] During the first 10 to 40 days of the puerperium, the maximal PRL levels that are reached after suckling approximate those seen in the first week postpartum. After the first 6 weeks of the puerperium, however, a trend of gradual reduction of the surges of serum PRL occurs despite continued successful breast-feeding. The rapidity with which baseline PRL returns to normal and the spikes of PRL following suckling disappear seems to be directly related to the frequency and intensity of nursing. In mothers who breast-feed fewer than 4 times a day, serum PRL returns to normal within 6 months, whereas in mothers who breast-feed 6 times a day, serum PRL may remain higher than normal for more than a year.[46, 156] Moreover, the most pronounced rise of PRL in response to suckling occurs after the last breast-feeding of the day. This physiologic hyperprolactinemia is achieved by increase in endogenous secretory rate of each release episode, not by change in frequency.[142] The increase in concentration is accompanied by a shift in release of lower molecular weight nonglycosylated species of PRL.[115] The nocturnal rise of PRL is maintained during the puerperium, with peak concentrations occurring between midnight and 6:00 PM.[50, 116, 174]

Gonadotropin Secretion

Suppression of pituitary gonadotropin secretion, which is characteristic of pregnancy, continues into the early puerperium. Serum follicle-stimulating hormone (FSH) as well as luteinizing hormone (LH) concentrations remain subnormal or undetectable during the first and second postpartum weeks, and pulsatility remains suppressed in both lactating and nonlactating patients.[29, 89, 92, 93, 110, 121, 131, 138, 158] A single infusion of gonadotropin-releasing hormone (GnRH) (Fig. 11–3) results in a negligi-ble or subnormal rise of LH and FSH during the first 2 weeks of the puerperium, indicating pituitary refractoriness to GnRH infusion.[29, 30, 64, 138]

Studies by Ishizuka et al.[87] showed that during the puerperium women exhibit a neuroendocrine feature similar to puberty before the start of menstrual cyclicity in that the FSH to LH ratio is close to 1, and FSH levels rise to surpass LH in response to GnRH administration. Mean LH pulse frequency, determined at 20-minute intervals, was 7.2 per 24 hours at both 10 and 24 to 26 days' postpartum. This frequency is much lower than that of patients in the early follicular phase (16 to 20 per 24 hours) which suggests reduced GnRH pulsatility postpartum. Nunley et al.,[141] however, reported normal mean frequency of LH release with attenuated peaks. During sleep, LH pulse frequency is decreased further in the presence of an increased amplitude so the overall LH secretion does not change.

After the first 2 weeks of the puerperium, gonadotropin pituitary function of nonlactating patients resumes gradually.[72] In lactating women, however, the reduction in the frequency and amplitude of LH pulses lasts longer.[73] At the end of the second postpartum week, an LH rise can be elicited by estradiol administration: After the third postpartum week, an increasing number of patients have normal FSH and LH levels, normal pulsatile LH release,[73, 102] and a normal pituitary response to GnRH infusion.[71]

The exact time for the resumption of normal pituitary function varies from one individual to another and depends on whether or not the patient is lactating.[73] By and large there is an agreement that by the fourth to sixth weeks of the puerperium, most nonlactating women have normal pituitary functions.[93, 110, 128, 138]

Possible Causes for Sluggish Puerperal Pituitary Response to Gonadotropin-Releasing Hormone

Although the precise cause for sluggish pituitary gonadotropin release during the early puerperium is not known, a considerable body of evidence suggests that several mechanisms may be involved. First, it has been noted that pituitary responsiveness to GnRH infusion is resumed earlier after termination of pregnancy in the first than in the second or third trimester of pregnancy.[52, 90] This suggests that

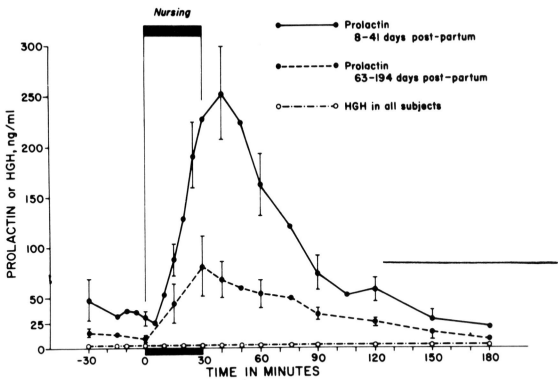

FIGURE 11–2. Plasma prolactin and growth hormone concentrations (hGH) (mean ± SE) during nursing in the 8th to 41st and in the 63rd to 194th day's postpartum. (From Noel GL, Suh HK, Frantz AG. Prolactin release during nursing and breast stimulation in postpartum and nonpostpartum patients. J Clin Endocrinol Metab 1974;38:413. With permission.)

either the duration of pregnancy or the larger amounts of hormones produced by a term pregnancy have an inhibitory influence on the pituitary-hypothalamic axis. More specifically, the large concentrations of the circulating estrogens have been implicated as causing pituitary hypothalamic suppression during pregnancy. Yet a rapid return of plasma estradiol to normal within a day or 2 after term delivery is not associated with an immediate resumption of pituitary function.

Second, it may well be that replenishing pituitary LH and FSH stores that have been depleted during pregnancy requires a period of time and delays the resumption of normal pituitary function. Here a delay in the resumption of the secretion of endogenous luteinizing hormone–releasing hormone (LHRH), which is required for building up such stores, may be responsible for the slow pituitary recovery. Indeed, priming the pituitary with multiple doses of GnRH during the first postpartum week has been shown to enhance FSH re-

sponse to GnRH administration, which supports the latter contention.[108, 178] Because the increase in LH and FSH following multiple doses of GnRH is still smaller than that of normally menstruating women, however, other inhibitory mechanisms must be considered.

It is possible that the high levels of circulating hCG would inhibit pituitary release of LH.[130] Alternatively, PRL, which is circulating in high concentrations, could exert an inhibitory influence on the gonadotropes, perhaps via activating dopaminergic neurons. This latter contention is a bit confusing, speculative, and perhaps unlikely.

Whether a reciprocal relationship between PRL and gonadotropins actually exists is not presently clear. Several observations, however, suggest that the relationship between the two is not casual. For instance, the resumption of normal pituitary function is usually observed at a time when baseline plasma PRL levels have returned to normal.[121] Moreover, weaning is associated with a rapid fall of basal circulating

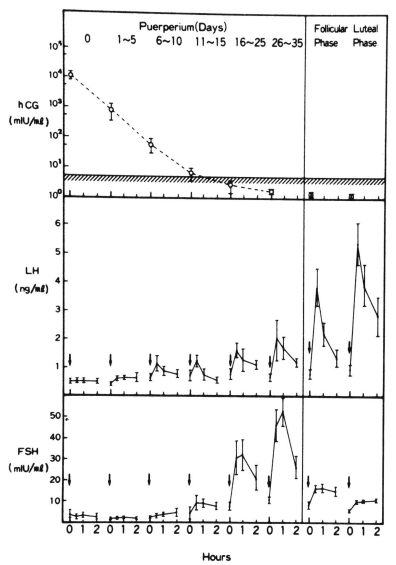

FIGURE 11–3. The serum concentration (mean ± SE) of hCG, FSH, and LH after a 100-μg bolus intravenous injection of GnRH in puerperal women as compared with normal menstruating women. (From Miyake A, Tanizawa D, Aono T, Kurachi K. Pituitary LH response to LHRH during the puerperium. Obstet Gynecol 1978; 51:37. With permission.)

PRL concentration and a simultaneous increase in LH. Further, the suppression of plasma PRL by the administration of bromocriptine is usually associated with a rapid recovery of basal FSH.[98, 136, 168, 191] Most investigators agree that the return of serum LH and estradiol to normal as well as the resumption of ovulation in lactating bromocriptine-treated patients is more prompt than that of nontreated lactating patients.[44, 136, 158] Because pituitary response to stimuli may be augmented even in the immediate postpartum period when serum PRL levels are high, one can argue that if PRL inhibits gonadotropin release, its action would have to be exerted at the hypothalamic rather than the pituitary level.

The suppression of GnRH secretion in the immediate postpartum period is not significantly due to opioid inhibition, which is known to be increased during pregnancy. Although elevated endorphin levels may decrease gonadotropin stores and secretion in the presence of elevated PRL levels, the administration of opioid inhibitors has no effect on gonadotropin levels on days' 7 to 10 postpartum.[87, 102, 129] Between day 13 and 25, however, it causes a significant rise in both gonadotropins.[87]

There appears to be a relationship between suckling and the resumption of pituitary function. In women, suckling has been reported to cause no change in baseline plasma LH and

FSH,[37] but studies in monkeys have suggested an inverse relationship between the two. Moreover, several investigators have reported that during the first 2 postpartum weeks FSH levels of lactating women are significantly lower than those of nonlactating women[27, 29, 37, 163, 177] and that the reduced frequency and amplitude of LH pulses last longer,[73] whereas some investigators have found no difference between nursing and nonnursing women in LH and FSH response to GnRH infusion.[5, 89] Others have reported a smaller rise of LH and FSH in nursing women during the first 3 weeks' postpartum.[151, 178] Moreover, hypothalamic refractoriness to stimuli has been suggested[71] because administration of pulsatile GnRH to lactating women 6 weeks' postpartum resulted in follicular development but failed to bring about normal ovulation.

Ovarian Function

Resumption of Ovulation in Nonbreast-Feeding Women

After delivery, the ovaries remain dormant for several weeks, in part because of delayed pituitary recovery and in part because of direct ovarian refractoriness to gonadotropin stimulation.[1, 209, 210] After the first 2 postpartum weeks, a decrease in ovarian refractoriness to gonadotropin stimulation occurs. Plasma estradiol concentrations, which are rather low (less than 50 pg/mL) during the first 2 weeks of the puerperium,[136, 158, 162] start to rise.[91, 177] Ovarian response to exogenous gonadotropins is also gradually restored. The administration of GnRH to anovulatory nursing women is likely to be associated with ovarian stimulation, as evidenced by the presence of follicular development at laparotomy.[171]

Resumption of ovulation seldom occurs before the 25th or 26th postpartum day.[75] The return of ovulation and menstruation is much more prompt after abortion than after term pregnancy. As many as half of all nonnursing women, however, resume ovulation by 45 days' postpartum, and more than 90% resume their menstrual periods by 12 weeks' postpartum. It should be pointed out that in the majority of women receiving bromocriptine for suppression of lactation the resumption of ovulation occurs earlier, usually by days' 23 to 28 postpartum.[103] The first menstruation is often anovulatory, and in the first ovulatory cycles many patients would be found to have luteal phase deficiency as evidenced by low urinary pregnanediol and serum progesterone concentration or abnormal endometrial biopsy.[17, 70, 75, 86, 111] Nevertheless, it is usually recommended that contraceptives be used after the third week postpartum. It is of interest that in one study the use of GnRH-agonist and in another one the use of progestogens were contemplated as contraceptive.[63, 169]

Effect of Breast-Feeding on Return of Ovulation

Women who breast-feed their infants show delayed resumption of menses, a high incidence of anovulatory cycles, and a decreased fertility rate compared with nonnursing mothers.[14, 100] Further, the duration of lactational amenorrhea and infertility is more prolonged in women who rely exclusively on breast-feeding for the nutrition of their infants, compared with those who alternatively use breast-feeding and bottle feeding. This is most likely due to increased PRL release resulting from more breast-feeding. In women in Zambia, where lactation is prolonged and no contraceptives are used, pregnancy is usually delayed for at least 12 months, and the peak in new conceptions occurs between 25 and 27 months after the last pregnancy.[197] Australian women had a mean of 322 days of anovulation and less than 20% ovulation by 6 months' postpartum.[17, 111] Eskimo women who continue breast-feeding while starting supplemental feeding when the infant is 6 months of age had 50% chance of resuming menstruation after 10 months' postpartum.[14] Although most nursing women are unlikely to ovulate before the 10th postpartum week, occasional ovulation may occur as early as the 35th day postpartum.[170] This would explain the 5 to 7% occurrence of pregnancy in breast-feeding women during the first 12 months following delivery.[171]

THE BREAST

The surge of breast milk in the postpartum period marks the culmination of a preparatory period that requires the collaboration of many endocrine systems. It has traditionally been differentiated into three phases: the phase of mammary growth (mammogenesis), the initiation of milk secretion (lactogenesis), and maintenance of established milk secretion (galactopoiesis). Information concerning the hormonal milieu necessary for human breast development is scant; our knowledge is based mainly on studies using animal models or in vitro studies of the mammary glands.

Mammary Growth in Preparation for Lactation (Mammogenesis)

The mammary glands are quiescent during childhood. Their growth begins during puberty, and further enlargement occurs during pregnancy. Pregnancy is marked by the continued proliferation of the epithelial cells of the alveoli and the formation of lobular alveolar architecture, which is the functional secretory unit of the mammary glands. At the end of the gestational period, the stroma tissue of the mammary gland has been largely replaced by growth of the lobules of newly formed alveoli and ducts. Dilatation of the lumina with accumulation of secretory materials is evident in many but not all animal species.[164] The proliferation of the mammary parenchyma continues into the period of early lactation. There is ample evidence of the importance of hormones in controlling the growth of the mammary glands during pregnancy (Fig. 11–4). Early investigations focused on the importance of estrogen and progesterone for growth and differentiation of the mammary gland during pregnancy. Relaxin may also aid growth and differentiation of mammary tissue.[8, 80] Studies in hypophysectomized animals have revealed, however, that estrogen alone or in combination with progesterone would not stimulate mammary growth and have suggested the intimate involvement of other hormones. Primary mammogenic activity, however, is reinstated when pituitary hormones, PRL, and growth hormone[120] are supplemented with synergistic activities coming from adrenal corticoids. The placenta is also important in supplying not only estrogen and progesterone, but also perhaps other mammogenic hormones, including growth factors; in the human, however, there is little evidence that placental lactogen is of major importance.[96] Women undergoing incomplete hypophysectomy or treatment with usual dose bromocriptine to suppress PRL during pregnancy, however, reportedly develop functional mammary glands during pregnancy.

Initiation of Milk Secretion (Lactogenesis)

In the early puerperium, the human mammary glands show a marked enlargement of the lobular architecture. This is due not only to vascular engorgement, but also to the continued increase in the size of alveoli and ductules.[164] A dramatic increase in the amounts of certain enzymes within the alveolar cells is associated with the initiation of the synthesis of milk con-

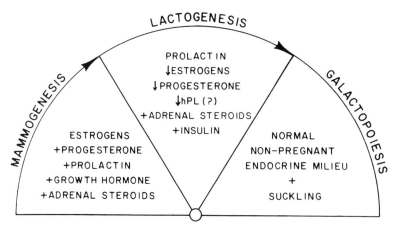

FIGURE 11–4. Multihormonal interaction on the growth of the mammary gland and in the initiation of lactogenesis and lactation delineated in animal models or in vitro experiments.

stituents, such as lactose, casein, and a-lactal-bumin, by the alveolar epithelium. The milk constituents, once formed, are moved to the Golgi body, where they appear in vesicles that then migrate to the luminal surface. By a process of reverse pinocytosis, the contents escape into the lumina of the alveoli.

Abundant milk secretion does not normally occur until 4 to 6 days' postpartum. Colostrum, which has a protein composition that differs from milk, however, is being secreted during the first 48 to 72 hours' postpartum. The sudden surge of milk is initiated by an interaction of several hormones and requires an environment in which circulating estrogen is low and PRL is high. Specific hormonal requirements for the induction of lactogenesis vary among species, but, in general, include PRL, insulin, and adrenal glucocorticoids (see Fig. 11–4).

PRL is considered an obligatory hormone for breast milk formation; in its absence, breast milk secretion does not occur. In vitro studies have shown that PRL induces synthesis of protein kinase, which, in turn, stimulates transcription and synthesis of RNAs that are essential for new protein synthesis. In organ culture of the mammary gland, PRL synergizes with insulin and corticosteroids to act on newly differentiated alveolar cells to induce the production of specific milk proteins and fats.[179] The importance of PRL is also underlined by the striking increase in the absolute number of PRL receptors observed immediately postpartum. This may well be initiated by the high levels of circulatory PRL because PRL is capable of increasing the levels of its own receptors;[16, 51] and the administration of a PRL antagonist, such as bromocriptine, has been shown to cause a decrease in the number of specific mammary receptors of PRL.

Although PRL and other hormones are considered obligatory for lactogenesis, lactation is not induced until a rapid fall of plasma estrogens and progesterone has occurred. The rapid fall in the plasma levels of the estrogens after delivery is thought to be associated with the removal of their blocking effect on breast tissue, thus enabling PRL to initiate breast milk production.[179] The role that the diminution in plasma progesterone plays in the initiation of lactation is less clear. The inhibitory effect of progesterone on the biosynthesis of lactose and a-lactalbumin in vitro has previously been documented, and in cows the fall of its peripheral concentration toward the end of pregnancy is associated with milk let-down just before parturition.

Because normal lactation does not occur until after delivery, however, it must be concluded that positive as well as negative factors are necessary for the initiation of normal lactogenesis. Moreover, exogenous progesterone administration to the pig in amounts sufficient to prolong pregnancy does not influence the onset of prepartum lactation, thus suggesting that progesterone plays no important role in the initiation of lactation.

The rapid fall of plasma human placental lactogen (hPL) that occurs following delivery may also be important for enhancing the effect of PRL on lactation. hPL competes with PRL on the same breast receptor sites; the rapid disappearance of hPL from blood in the early puerperium may open up more receptor sites for the binding action of PRL. Because PRL is a potent lactogenic hormone, whereas hPL is not, this may enhance lactogenesis.[182]

Maintenance of Established Milk Secretion (Galactopoiesis)

Hormonal Requirements

The continued maintenance of established milk secretion requires the establishment of periodic suckling as well as the actual removal of breast milk.[202] It also requires a hormonal milieu that includes PRL,[185] growth hormone,[68] corticoids, thyroxin, and insulin.[202] The importance of growth hormone in the human is questionable because ateliotic dwarfs with congenital absence of human growth hormone have lactated successfully. The importance of thyroxin in the human is also questionable[66] because hypothyroid patients have successfully breast-fed their infants. Also unclear is the importance of PRL for the long-term maintenance of lactation. The gradual fall of serum PRL during the puerperium indicates that high levels of this hormone are not mandatory for the successful continuation of breast milk production.[45, 47, 49, 50, 83, 86] Never-

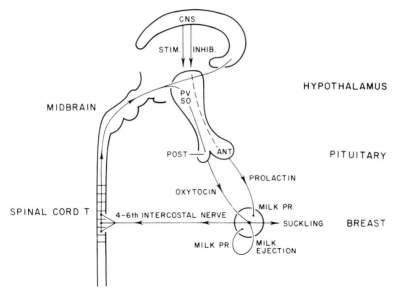

FIGURE 11–5. The neuroendocrine reflexes that are initiated by suckling. Stimulatory (Stim.) as well as inhibitory (Inhib.) influences leading to milk production (PR.) are shown. PV = Paraventricular nucleus; SO = supraoptic nucleus; T = thoracic region.

theless, some PRL must be present for lactation to take place. This is supported by the observation that bromocriptine administration in the late puerperium inhibits milk excretion.[19, 189] Further, in vitro studies have demonstrated the importance of PRL for continued milk production. In rats, it influences enzymes involved in fat metabolism in the mammary gland, leading to enhanced uptake of fat by the mammary gland. In the human, the rise of PRL that follows suckling is thought to be responsible for the increase in the milk volume and in the protein and fat content of milk secreted in the subsequent nursing period occurring 8 to 12 hours later. The amount of PRL required to maintain established lactation, however, appears to be small.

Nursing

During pregnancy, PRL response to breast stimulation is inhibited. The changes in responsiveness after delivery may reflect changes in central neuroendocrine response possibly mediated by withdrawal of peripheral hormones.[114, 202] In addition, breast nipple sensitivity is maximal at 3 days' postpartum. The suckling-induced rise of PRL, which is more pronounced in the immediate than in the late postpartum period, is responsible for generating milk for subsequent breast feedings[12] (see Fig. 11–3). In addition, suckling induces insulin secretion[203] as well as release of other sub-

stances, such as vasoactive intestinal polypeptide, gastrin, and somatostatin.[144, 157, 204] The frequency of suckling is an important determinant of successful lactation. When the nonsuckling interval exceeds 12 hours, breast milk production decreases, with subsequent refractoriness. Suckling evokes a neurohormonal reflex that is important for the maintenance of galactopoiesis[202] (Fig. 11–5). The nipples contain mechanical receptors that are responsive to suction and pressure. Stimulation of these sensory nerves in the nipples evokes a reflex release not only of PRL from the adenohypophysis, but also of oxytocin from the neurohypophysis[40, 53, 107, 118, 126, 187, 196] (see Chapter 13). Oxytocin release in response to suckling continues unabated during the first 6 months' postpartum, and basal and maximal levels do not decrease with time.[94]

The release of oxytocin by the neurohypophysis in response to suckling is thought to be transmitted by afferent nerve fibers that connect the mammary gland to the roots of the spinal cord and the midbrain. Destruction of this root at the level of the spinal cord or the brain stem suppresses lactation and milk ejection in the goat. The paraventricular and supraoptic neurons of the hypothalamus constitute the final afferent pathway of the milk ejection reflex. Other afferent pathways for milk ejection, however, have also been found distributed throughout the brain stem.

In addition, the central nervous system can

influence milk ejection, as shown by the observation that stress or fear may inhibit milk ejection, whereas the cry of an infant may provoke it. This is thought to be modulated via altering oxytocin release. Inhibition of oxytocin release by a very high dose of alcohol results in abolition of the milk ejection activity that is invoked by suckling. In contrast to the milk ejection caused by suckling, however, that which is caused by the cry of an infant is not followed by a rise in serum PRL.[140] Oxytocin release may not be absolutely necessary for successful lactation, however, because continued lactation has been achieved in patients with diabetes insipidus; in several animal species, suckling is not important for initiating and maintaining lactation.

The mechanism by which suckling affects PRL release from the pituitary during lactation is not well known. It is not mediated, however, by endogenous opioids.[32, 67, 77, 117] It may well be that suckling elicits PRL release by inhibiting the synthesis of hypothalamic PRL-inhibiting factor, most likely dopamine. Alternatively, because simulated changes in dopamine secretion usually fail to manipulate breast-induced PRL release, it is possible that PRL-releasing factor also exists, perhaps thyrotropin-releasing hormone and hypothalamic serotonin, and that suckling will stimulate its release. It should also be noted that both insulin and vasoactive intestinal polypeptide are released in breast-feeding women.[144, 203, 204] The process of the release of PRL from the pituitary during suckling is rather complicated, consisting of two phases. The first is depletion without release. This is followed by transformation into a releasable form. The second phase of release is not thought to be PRL-inhibiting factor regulated.

The secretory activity of the mammary gland is destined to decline and eventually to cease with time. The functional capacity of the breast to produce milk depends on the hormone release and responsiveness of the target organ. When this relationship is disrupted by changes in either the timing or the nature of the stimuli, the functional capacity of the system breaks down.

Effect of Prostaglandins

There are conflicting reports on the effect that prostaglandins may have on milk ejection.

Prostaglandin $F_{2\alpha}$ ($PGF_{2\alpha}$) administered to rats before suckling inhibits milk ejection, and this effect is considered to be central because it can be overcome by the simultaneous administration of oxytocin, which has peripheral effects. In lactating women, however, the intravenous infusion of PGE_2 and $PGF_{2\alpha}$ releases oxytocin intermittently and results in milk ejection activity, suggesting a central effect,[33, 70] whereas oral PGE_2 decreases prolactin levels.[26, 57, 180] The observation of a prolonged latency period between the intravenous administration of $PGF_{2\alpha}$ to breast-feeding mothers and milk ejection also suggests a central effect.[27] One must not rule out, however, a possible direct effect of prostaglandin on the mammary gland because in vitro studies have demonstrated the direct contractile effect of prostaglandins on the smooth muscle of the myoepithelium.

Hormonal Inhibition of Lactation

Estrogens

Attempts to block lactation (Table 11–2) and breast engorgement are related to the desire of many parturients to rid themselves of the discomfort associated with engorgement and breast-feeding, which usually begins on the third postpartum day and in the absence of breast-feeding persists for at least 1 week. Beginning in 1933, when Smith and Smith[172] demonstrated that estrogens would inhibit postpartum lactation in the rabbit, there have been numerous attempts to use estrogens for breast milk suppression. Several double-blind, controlled studies have shown that stilbestrol is more effective than placebo in reducing breast engorgement and lactation in hospitalized patients,[19, 39, 40, 189, 192] but that rebound engorgement and lactation may occur after discontinuance of estrogens. Other estrogens, such as chlorotrianisene (TACE) and quinestrol, have also been used successfully.[74, 135] The best clinical results and the diminution of late postpartum engorgement have been achieved when long-acting steroid esters in the form of estradiol valerate and testosterone enanthate were used.[135, 167a] Similarly good results were achieved with the use of long-acting estrogens

TABLE 11-2. Effects of Drugs on Serum Prolactin and Lactation

	Serum Prolactin	Lactation	Comments	References
Estrogen	↑	↓		39, 74, 135, 168, 193
Progesterone	—	→	May change milk composition	79, 97, 176, 208
Estrogen and progestin	—	→	Dose dependent	78, 79
		↓		
Testosterone and estrogen	—	→	Controversial	135, 167a
Clomiphene citrate	→	→		27, 39, 122, 193a, 212
	↓			
Tamoxifen	↓	↓		123
Pyridoxine	→	→	Controversial	28, 60, 61, 119
Bromocriptine	↓	↓		19, 30, 173, 189, 193, 193a, 205, 207
Ergometrine	→	→	Controversial	44
Metergoline	↓	↓		35, 43

alone.[74] Because of an increase in the incidence of thromboembolism in postpartum patients receiving estrogens, however, this treatment modality has fallen into disfavor and is rarely used.

The mechanism by which estrogens inhibit breast engorgement and lactation is not fully understood. Several studies have shown that estrogen administration does not change or may even increase serum PRL concentration[38, 192] (see Table 11–2). Thus the effectiveness of estrogens in suppressing breast engorgement and lactation in hospitalized patients has been attributed to their inhibitory influence on the breast tissue itself.[18] Support for this peripheral effect of estrogen is derived from the observation that mammary implants of estradiol in rats inhibit lactation, whereas pituitary implants stimulate lactation.[18] In addition, the administration of estradiol to postpartum rats decreases the number of PRL-binding sites in mammary tissue, thus rendering PRL a less potent stimulator of lactation.[16] Similarly, estradiol and progesterone, when administered to rats, prevent the hormonally induced rise of mammary DNA and RNA content.[59]

Progestins

The potential effectiveness of other drugs on breast engorgement and lactation has also been studied. Medroxyprogesterone acetate may cause an alteration in milk composition with some reduction in milk yield.[97, 176, 208] Breast-feeding can successfully be continued, however, despite the continuous administration of medroxyprogesterone acetate in contraceptive doses. No changes in the quantity of milk can be observed in women receiving norgestrol.[79]

Contraceptives

Contraceptive pills containing an estrogen-progesterone combination inhibit lactation if given in a large enough dose.[79] The duration of lactation and the quantities of milk produced, however, are not significantly affected by the administration of a combination of norethindrone, 1.0 mg, and ethinyl estradiol, 0.05 mg.[78, 79] Moreover, in the combination of norethynodrel and mestranol, a reduction in the progesterone dose reduces the degree of lactational inhibition.

Antiestrogens

Evidence suggests that antiestrogens may interfere with the secretion of PRL (see Table 11–2). Tamoxifen inhibits the estrogen-induced release of PRL in rats.[95] It blunts the response of PRL to thyrotropin-releasing hormone in nonpregnant women and moderately reduces PRL levels in postpartum patients.[122] Its administration at a dose of 10 mg 4 times daily effectively suppresses breast engorgement and milk production in more than 90% of patients and is not associated with rebound engorgement after the medication has been discontinued. Tamoxifen was also shown to suppress PRL release induced by mechanical breast stimulation.

The effectiveness of another antiestrogen, clomiphene citrate, in suppressing lactation is less clear.[27] Its administration does not ordinarily suppress serum PRL levels or alter PRL response to thyrotropin-releasing hormone. When a 5 day course of Clomid, 100 mg per day, is administered, however, the PRL rise that would ordinarily occur 30 minutes after mechanical breast emptying is completely abolished.[122] Although some investigators claim that clomiphene administration may relieve breast engorgement,[212] others have shown no beneficial effect on breast engorgement and milk secretion.[193a] Moreover, the safety of the use of these antiestrogens in the puerperium has not been established.

Bromocriptine

Bromocriptine (2-bromoergocryptine; 2-bromo-a-ergokryptin; CB-154) is effective in reducing the serum PRL level and in preventing lactation, breast engorgement, and pain.[11, 19, 30, 42, 54, 57, 149, 189, 193, 193a] It is a specific inhibitor of PRL secretion and inhibits its release from human pituitary tissue cultures. Administration of bromocriptine, 5 mg daily, results in a dramatic fall in serum PRL by the second or third day of treatment, with an excellent clinical response.[205] In animals, bromocriptine has been shown to reduce the number of PRL receptors in the mammary gland and to inhibit lactation and other PRL-dependent functions.[189] In humans, bromocriptine causes a reduction in the production of breast milk constituents.[105] When the effectiveness of 5 mg of bromocriptine given daily for 14 days was compared in a double-blind study with that of estrogens, the former was found to be equally[189] or more effective than estrogens[109, 173, 193, 193a, 207] in preventing breast engorgement and lactation in hospitalized patients. Its discontinuation on the 14th day of the puerperium, however, was associated with rebound lactation, albeit of a much less degree than that caused by the withdrawal of estrogens.[173] Bromocriptine, in contrast to estrogens, has also been reported to be capable of inhibiting lactation when lactation has already begun and serum PRL levels have returned to the normal range.[19, 189] Side effects to bromocriptine include significant hypotension as well as headache and nausea. Therefore if it is at all to be used, the first dose should not be given until vital signs have stabilized after delivery.

Other Drugs

Although the effect of bromocriptine on lactation is quite convincing, other ergot alkaloids are also effective. Either these compounds have dopamine-agonist activity (lisuride),[41, 188, 190] or they are serotonin antagonist (metergoline). Dopaminergic drugs, such as piribedil, have also been reported to suppress puerperal lactation. Metergoline,[149] a serotonin antagonist, and cabergoline[127] have also been reported to cause a decrease in plasma PRL and to suppress lactation and breast engorgement.[25] Pyridoxine effect is controversial.[28, 60, 61, 119]

Hormone Excretion in Milk

Various drugs given to the mothers and several endogenous hormones have been detected in human milk. Some of these drugs may exert undesirable effects on the infant. Diffusion due to a gradient between plasma and milk may be the primary mechanism to promote transport of such substances. The greater acidity of whole milk (pH 6.8) than plasma (pH 7.4), however, would facilitate the transport of basic compounds and hinder the passage of acid ones. Fat solubility may also be important because fat-soluble drugs can be transferred into milk more easily. Active transport mechanisms may also exist to explain why the concentrations of some drugs are higher in milk than in blood. It is also conceivable that unbound steroids enter into milk much more freely than those that are bound to plasma protein carriers.

Progestins

Sex steroids contained in contraceptive pills reach the human milk.[165] When radiolabeled steroids of the types contained in oral contraceptives are given orally to lactating but non-nursing women, the radioactivity appears in milk.[106] The measurement of D-norgestrel and megesterol acetate concentrations in plasma and milk of lactating women revealed that those in milk were 15 and 80% of those in plasma.[139] In another study, after injection of 150 mg of medroxyprogesterone acetate, the levels of this hormone in breast milk were similar to those in plasma, whereas levels of D-norgestrel and norethisterone in milk of women taking oral contraceptives were approximately 16% less than those found in plasma. The highest concentrations were achieved within 3 hours of the drug administration. The amounts of D-norgestrel and megesterol acetate that were transferred with 600 mL of milk were calculated to be 0.3 μg and 1.9 μg with the daily intake of 250 μg of D-norgestrel or 4 mg of megestrol acetate, respectively. No D-norgestrel could be detected in the milk of women receiving 30 μg per day.[139] Other investigators have estimated the amounts of gestagens appearing in 500 mL of milk to be as low as 0.004% or as high as 1.5% of the administered oral dose.[106]

Estrogens

Estrogens can also be excreted in milk.[84, 124] Stilbestrol ingested by cows can be detected in their milk. Estrogens such as mestranol contained in low-dose contraceptive pills are also excreted in milk, but the amounts ingested by the fetus are considered small. If larger amounts of the sex steroid are absorbed from ingested milk into the infant's circulation, however, they may compete with bilirubin for hepatic glucuronyl transferase activity, thereby causing hyperbilirubinemia. There are also anecdotal reports of proliferation of vaginal epithelium in female nurslings or gynecomastia in male nurslings following maternal ingestion of comparatively high-dose contraceptive preparations. Normal human milk, however, contains only small amounts of estradiol.

Thyroid Hormones

Iodine is actively concentrated by mammary tissue, and considerable quantities are secreted in human milk. The concentration of triiodothyronine (T_3) and thyroxine (T_4) in the breast milk of primates, both women and monkeys, is reported to be sufficient to prevent the development of hypothyroidism in infants.[132, 133, 143, 165, 175] The low concentrations of T_4 observed in the milk expressed in the first postpartum day has been shown to rise subsequently and reach mean levels of 4.3 μg/dL, suggesting that the lactating mother can secrete up to 40 to 50 μg of T_4 per day in her milk. The ingestion of these amounts of T_4 may be a significant source of T_4 for the infant because they approximate the therapeutic dose recommended for hypothyroid infants. This may therefore mask the clinical symptoms of congenital hypothyroidism and delay its diagnosis.

Corticosteroids

Milk contains a corticosteroid-binding globulin (CBG) that is quite similar to that isolated from plasma.[145, 159] A decrease in milk CBG in the first 2 weeks' postpartum occurs simultaneously with that observed in maternal plasma CBG. Cortisol in milk, however, in contrast to CBG, does not vary systematically with time after delivery and invariably exceeds the binding capacity of CBG. Thus the cortisol environment of the breast is maintained at a relatively constant level[3] with some changes.[104] This might be important for the continued formation of milk because cortisol is essential for the synthesis of the two major milk proteins, casein and a-lactalbumin. The concentration of cortisol in breast milk varies from 0.8 to 3.5 μg/dL, amounting to approximately 1 to 4% of the reported concentrations in maternal plasma at term pregnancy.[159] Thus it can be estimated that 500 mL of breast milk would contain approximately 10 μg of cortisol.

Synthetic corticosteroids can also be detected in milk.[125] In a mother taking 10 μg of prednisone daily, the concentrations of milk prednisone and prednisolone were found to be 0.16 and 2.67 μg/dL 2 hours after its ingestion. An infant taking 0.5 L of milk could receive approximately 15 μg of the two steroids per day, which is probably an insignificant dose.[99]

Other Hormones and Substances

Hypothalamic gonadotropin-releasing hormone (GnRH) has been found in the milk of women, cows, and rats.[49, 137] The concentration ranges from 0.2 to 3 ng/mL and is much higher than that in serum, implying either an active concentration mechanism in the mammary gland or the existence of an additional extrahypothalamic production of the peptide. Because the serum LH of female pups is significantly lower when suckling is prevented, it has been suggested that this milk GnRH is absorbed from the gut of the immature rat in a biologically active form and that this milk GnRH may influence the secretion of gonadotropin hormones in neonates. The GnRH-agonist buserelin, however, when given to a mother, would have no biologic activity in breast milk.[48] Other hypothalamic hormones, including thyrotropin-releasing hormone and growth hormone releasing factor, are present in milk at much lower concentrations.[4, 198, 199]

The presence of PRL in the milk of women throughout lactation has also been reported.[2, 65a, 82, 206] In contrast to serum, however, more than 90% of milk PRL is "little" PRL, and the concentration of PRL found in milk is 30% of that in serum on the fourth postpartum day. Whether this "little" PRL is biologically active and whether it can be absorbed by the human infant and induce any physiologic changes in the neonate are presently unknown. Other hormones and neurotransmitters are present in milk.[81, 101, 146, 166] Epidermal growth factors, insulin, and somatomedin-C/insulin-like growth factors are present in human milk;[31, 34, 88, 105, 134, 146, 147, 152, 153] however, whether they can be absorbed and act as neonatal growth factor is doubtful.[13] Other substances found in human milk include relaxin,[55] calcitonin,[7, 20, 21, 22, 201] bombesin, neurotensin and melanotropin,[56] high levels of vasoactive intestinal peptide,[15, 200] β-endorphin-like and α-MSH-like hormones,[58, 211] and parathyroid hormone.[23]

Absence of Milk Production

Deficient secretion of PRL has been associated with the failure of lactation in two clinical syndromes. In the syndrome described by Sheehan, pituitary infarction is often secondary to profound hypotension owing to massive postpartum hemorrhage. For further review, see Chapter 7.

Patients with the rare syndrome of isolated deficiency of PRL secretion also fail to lactate. In this case, the pituitary reserve for the secretion of adrenocorticotropic hormone and growth hormone is intact, whereas the serum PRL level is undetectable, and no rise of PRL can be elicited by any provocative test.

More common is the finding of poor or partial failure to lactate (lactational insufficiency). This may be caused by several abnormalities. Aono et al.[6] found that although the basal PRL levels of such patients did not differ from those of normally lactating patients, their postnursing increase in PRL was absent but could be initiated by a breast pump, suggesting that this disorder is caused by abnormalities in the nipples, which prevent initiation of the normal suckling reflex. Others have reported that in two such patients the oral administration of thyrotropin-releasing hormone increases PRL concentrations as well as breast engorgement and milk let-down.[186] Further, the administration of dopaminergic antagonists raises serum PRL and enhances milk production in patients who exhibit partial failure to lactate. Administration of thyrotropin-releasing hormone to another group of patients, however, could not elicit a rise of PRL, suggesting that in some patients there is an impairment in PRL release. In some animal species, a decreased parathormone secretion has also led to diminished milk output.

Persistent Galactorrhea

In the absence of suckling, the continued secretion of milk is pathologic and should arouse suspicion of an endocrinologic abnormality. In many cases, continued galactorrhea may be caused by continued breast manipulation. The ingestion of phenothiazides, methyldopa, reserpine, haloperidol, and other drugs could inhibit dopaminergic transmission and result in elevated PRL levels.

Pathologic galactorrhea is usually classified into several syndromes. These classifications should be discouraged because they are often misleading. For example, many patients with the Chiari-Frommel syndrome, which describes postpartum patients having amenorrhea and persistent galactorrhea in the absence of suckling, might eventually be proved to have pituitary tumors. These patients may have either elevated or normal serum PRL levels. Although in the past this disorder has been attributed to functional pituitary or hypothalamic abnormality, modern radiologic techniques should be employed to rule out the existence of a pituitary tumor (see Chapter 7).

Elevated PRL levels have also been reported in patients with chromophobe adenoma and, rarely, with hypothalamic tumors, in which depression of the normal hypothalamic inhibitory influence has been implicated in causing pathologic lactation.

REFERENCES

1. Acar B, Fleming R, Macnaughton MC, Coutts JR. Ovarian function in women immediately postpartum. Obstet Gynecol 1981;57:468.
2. Adamopoulus DA, Kapolla N. Prolactin concentration in milk and plasma of puerperal women and patients with galactorrhea. J Endocrinol Invest 1984;7:273.
3. Alexandrova M, Macho L. Glucocorticoids in human, cow and rat milk. Endocrinol Exp 1983;17:183.
4. Amarant T, Fridkin M, Koch Y. Luteinizing hormone-releasing hormone and thyrotropin-releasing hormone in human and bovine milk. Eur J Biochem 1982;127:647.
5. Andreassen B, Tyson JE. Role of the hypothalamic-pituitary-ovarian axis in puerperal infertility. J Clin Endocrinol Metab 1976;42:1114.
6. Aono T, Shioji T, Shoda T, Kurachi K. The initiation of human lactation and prolactin response to suckling. J Clin Endocrinol Metab 1977;44:1101.
7. Arver S, Bucht E, Sjoberg HE. Calcitonin-like immunoreactivity in human milk, longitudinal alterations and divalent cations. Acta Physiol Scand 1984;122:461.
8. Bani G, La Malfa A, Petrucci F, Bigazzi M. Effects of relaxin on mammary gland growth in female mice. In: Bigazzi M, Greenwood FC, Gasparri F, eds. Biology of relaxin and its role in the human. Amsterdam: Excerpta Medica, 1983:106.
9. Baram T, Koch Y, Hazum E, Fridkin M. Gonadotropin-releasing hormone in milk. Science 1977;18:300.
10. Barberia JM, Abu-Fadil S, Kletsky OA, et al. Serum prolactin patterns in early human gestation. Am J Obstet Gynecol 1975;121:1107.
11. Barbieri RL, Ryan KJ. Bromocriptine: endocrine pharmacology and therapeutic applications. Fertil Steril 1983;39:727.
12. Battin DA, Marrs RP, Fleiss PM, Mishell DR. Effect of suckling on serum prolactin, luteinizing hormone, follicle-stimulating hormone, and estradiol during prolonged lactation. Obstet Gynecol 1985;65:785.
13. Baxter RC, Zaltsman Z, Turtle JR. Immunoreactive somatomedin-C/insulin-like growth factor I and its binding protein in human milk. J Clin Endocrinol Metab 1984;58:955.
14. Berman ML, Hanson K, Hellman IL. Effect of breast-feeding on postpartum menstruation, ovulation, and pregnancy in Alaskan Eskimos. Am J Obstet Gynecol 1972;114:524.
15. Berseth CL, Michener SR, Nordyke CK, Go VL. Postpartum changes in pattern of gastrointestinal regulatory peptides in human milk. Am J Clin Nutr 1990;51:985.
16. Bohnet HG, Gomez F, Friesen HG. Prolactin and estrogen binding sites in the mammary gland of the lactating and non-lactating rat. Endocrinology 1977;101:1111.
17. Brown JB, Harrison P, Smith MA. A study of returning fertility after childbirth and during lactation by measurement of urinary oestrogen and pregnanediol excretion and cervical mucus production. J Biosoc Sci 1985;9(suppl):5.
18. Bruce JO, Ramirez VD. Site of action of the inhibitory effect of estrogen upon lactation. Neuroendocrinology 1970;6:19.
19. Brun del Re R, del Pozo E, de Grandi P, et al. Prolactin inhibition and suppression of puerperal lactation by a Br-ergocryptine (CB 154). Obstet Gynecol 1973;41:884.
20. Bucht E, Arver S, Sjoberg HE, Low H. Heterogeneity of immunoreactive calcitonin in human milk. Acta Endocrinol 1983;103:572.
21. Bucht E, Sjoberg HE. Evidence for precursors of calcitonin/PDN 21 in human milk. Regul Pept 1987;19:65.
22. Bucht E, Telenius-Berg M, Lundell G, Sjoberg HE. Immunoextracted calcitonin in milk and plasma from totally thyroidectomized women. Evidence of monomeric calcitonin in plasma during pregnancy and lactation. Acta Endocrinol 1986;113:529.
23. Budayr AA, Halloran BP, King JC, et al. High levels of a parathyroid hormone-like protein in milk. Proc Natl Acad Sci USA 1989;86:7183.
24. Bunner DL, Vanderlaan EF, Vanderlaan WP. Prolactin levels in nursing mothers. Am J Obstet Gynecol 1978;131:250.
25. Caballero-Gordo A, Lopez-Nazareno N, Calderay M, et al. Oral cabergoline. Single-dose inhibition of puerperal lactation. J Reprod Med 1991;36:717.
26. Caminiti F, DeMurtas M, Parodo G, et al. Decrease in human plasma prolactin levels by oral prostaglandin E2 in early puerperium. J Endocrinol 1980;87:333.
27. Canales ES, Lasso P, Soria J, Zarate A. Effect of clomiphene on prolactin secretion and lactation in puerperal women. Br J Obstet Gynaecol 1977;84:758.
28. Canales ES, Soria J, Zarate A, et al. The influence of pyridoxine on prolactin secretion and milk production in women. Br J Obstet Gynaecol 1976;83:387.
29. Canales ES, Zarate A, Garrido J, et al. Study on the recovery of the pituitary FSH function during puerperium using synthetic LRH. J Clin Endocrinol Metab 1974;38:1140.
30. Canales ES, Zarate A, Soria J, et al. Further observations on postpartum ovarian refractoriness: effect of gonadal stimulation in women receiving bromocriptine. Clin Endocrinol 1976;5:127.
31. Carpenter G. Epidermal growth factor is a major growth-promoting agent in human milk. Science 1980;210:198.
32. Cholst IN, Wardlaw SL, Newman CB, Frantz AG. Prolactin response to breast stimulation in lactating women is not mediated by endogenous opioids. Am J Obstet Gynecol 1984;150:558.
33. Cobo E, Rodriguez A, De Villamizar M. Milk-ejecting

activity induced by prostaglandin $F_{2\alpha}$. Am J Obstet Gynecol 1974;118:831.

34. Connolly JM, Rose DP. Epidermal growth factor-like proteins in breast fluid and human milk. Life Sci 1988;42:1751.

35. Crosignani PG, Lombroso GC, Caccamo A, et al. Suppression of puerperal lactation by metergoline. Obstet Gynecol 1978;51:113.

36. Crystle CD, Breuning F, Dubin NH, et al. Blood disappearance rates of certain hormones and enzymes advocated as fetoplacental function tests. Obstet Gynecol 1974;43:41.

37. Crystle CD, Powell J, Stevens VC. Plasma gonadotropins during the postpartum period. Obstet Gynecol 1970;36:887.

38. Crystle CD, Sawaya GA, Stevens VC. Effects of ethinyl estradiol on the secretion of gonadotropins and estrogens in postpartum women. Am J Obstet Gynecol 1973;116:616.

39. David A, Romem I, Lunenfeld B, et al. Stilbestrol administration in the puerperium and its effect on the prolactin excretion of non-lactating patients. Acta Obstet Gynecol Scand 1977;56:211.

40. Dawood MY, Khan-Dawood FS, Wahl RS, Fuchs F. Oxytocin release and plasma anterior pituitary and gonadal hormones in women during lactation. J Clin Endocrinol Metab 1981;52:678.

41. DeCecco L, Venturini PL, Ragni N, et al. Effect of lisuride on inhibition of lactation and serum prolactin. Br J Obstet Gynaecol 1979;86:905.

42. Defoort P, Thiery M, Baele G, et al. Bromocriptine in an injectable retard form for puerperal lactation suppression: comparison with estandron prolongatum. Obstet Gynecol 1987;70:866.

43. Delitala G, Masala A, Alagna S, et al. Metergoline in the inhibition of puerperal lactation. BMJ 1977;1:744.

44. del Pozo E, Brun del Re R, Hinselmann M. Lack of effect of methyl-ergonovine on postpartum lactation. Am J Obstet Gynecol 1975;123:845.

45. Delvoye P, Delogne-Desnoeck J, Robyn C. Hyperprolactinaemia during prolonged lactation: evidence for anovulatory cycles and inadequate corpus luteum. Clin Endocrinol 1980;13:243.

46. Delvoye P, Demaegd M, Delogne-Desnoeck J, Robyn C. The influence of the frequency of nursing and of previous lactation experience on serum prolactin in lactating mothers. J Biosoc Sci 1977;9:447.

47. Delvoye P, Demaegd M, Uwayitu-Nyampeta, Robyn C. Serum prolactin, gonadotropins, and estradiol in menstruating and amenorrheic mothers during two years' lactation. Am J Obstet Gynecol 1978;130:635.

48. Dewart PJ, McNeilly AS, Smith SK, et al. LRH agonist buserelin as a post-partum contraceptive: lack of biological activity of buserelin in breast milk. Acta Endocrinol 1987;114:185.

49. Diaz S, Cardenas A, Brandeis A, et al. Early difference in the endocrine profile of long and short lactational amenorrhea. J Clin Endocrinol Metab 1991;72:196.

50. Diaz S, Seron-Ferre M, Cardenas H, et al. Circadian variation of basal plasma prolactin, prolactin response to suckling and the length of amenorrhea in nursing women. J Clin Endocrinol Metab 1989;68:946.

51. Djiane J, Durand P, Kelly PA. Evolution of prolactin receptors in rabbit mammary gland during pregnancy and lactation. Endocrinology 1977;100:1348.

52. Domenzain ME, Shapiro AG, Bezjian AA, et al. Pituitary response to luteinizing hormone-releasing hormone after induced abortion in the first and second trimesters. Fertil Steril 1977;28:531.

53. Drewett RF, Bowen-Jones A, Dogterom J. Oxytocin levels during breast-feeding in established lactation. Horm Behav 1982;16:245.

54. Duchesne C, Leke R. Bromocriptine mesylate for prevention of postpartum lactation. Obstet Gynecol 1981;57:464.

55. Eddie LW, Sutton B, Fitzgerald S, et al. Relaxin in paired samples of serum and milk from women after term and preterm delivery. Am J Obstet Gynecol 1989;161:970.

56. Ekman R, Ivarsson S, Jansson L. Bombesin, neurotensin, and pro-gamma-melanotropin immunoreactants in human milk. Reg Pept 1985;10:99.

57. England MJ, Tjalinks A, Hofmeyr J, Harber J. Suppression of lactation: a comparison of bromocriptine and prostaglandin E2. J Reprod Med 1988;33:630.

58. Ferrando T, Rainero I, De Gennaro T, et al. β-endorphin-like and alpha-msh-like immunoreactivities in human milk. Life Sci 1990;47:633.

59. Ferreri LF, Griffith DR. Inhibition of experimental lactational mammary gland growth in the rat with exogenous estrogen and progesterone. Proc Soc Exp Biol Med 1977;155:429.

60. Fleming JS. Inhibition of puerperal lactation: pyridoxine of no benefit. Aust N Z J Obstet Gynaecol 1977;17:131.

61. Foukas MD. An antilactogenic effect of pyridoxine. J Obstet Gynaecol Br Comm 1973;80:718.

62. Fox SR, Smith MS. The suppression of pulsatile luteinizing hormone secretion during lactation in the rat. Endocrinology 1984;115:2045.

63. Fraser HM, Dewart PJ, Smith SK, et al. Luteinizing hormone releasing hormone agonist for contraception in breast feeding women. J Clin Endocrinol Metab 1989;69:996.

64. Friedman C, Gaeke ME, Fang V, Kim MH. Pituitary responses to LRH in the postpartum periods. Am J Obstet Gynecol 1976;124:75.

65. Friesen HG, Fournier P, Desjardins P. Pituitary prolactin in pregnancy and normal and abnormal lactation. Clin Obstet Gynecol 1973;16:25.

65a. Gala RR, Van De Walle C. Prolactin heterogeneity in the serum and milk during lactation. Life Sci 1977;21:99.

66. Gautvik KM, Tashjian AH Jr, Kourides IA, et al. Thyrotropin-releasing hormone is not the sole physiologic mediator of prolactin release during suckling. N Engl J Med 1974;290:1162.

67. Genazzani AR, Facchinetti F, Parrini D, et al. Puerperal breast feeding does not stimulate circulating opioids in humans. J Endocrinol Invest 1982;5:367.

68. Gertler A, Cohen N, Maoz A. Human growth hormone but not ovine or bovine growth hormones exhibits galactopoietic prolactin-like activity in organ culture from bovine lactating mammary gland. Mol Cell Endocrinol 1983;33:169.

69. Gieger W. Radioimmunological determination of human chorionic gonadotropin, human placental lactogen growth hormone and thyrotropin in the serum of mother and child during the early puerperium. Horm Metab Res 1973;5:342.

70. Gillespie A, Brummer HC, Chard T. Oxytocin release by infused prostaglandin. BMJ 1972;1:543.

71. Glasier A, McNeilly AS, Baird DT. Induction of ovarian activity by pulsatile infusion of LHRH in women

with lactational amenorrhoea. Clin Endocrinol 1986;24:243.

72. Glasier A, McNeilly AS, Howie PW. Fertility after childbirth: changes in serum gonadotrophin levels in bottle and breast feeding women. Clin Endocrinol 1983;19:493.

73. Glasier A, McNeilly AS, Howie PW. Pulsatile secretion of LH in relation to the resumption of ovarian activity postpartum. Clin Endocrinol 1984;20:415.

74. Grant K, Rabello Y, Freeman AG, et al. Comparison of quinestrol and TACE for relief of postpartum breast discomfort. Obstet Gynecol 1978;51:636.

75. Gray RR, Campbell OM, Zacur HA, et al. Postpartum return of ovarian activity in nonbreastfeeding women monitored by urinary assays. J Clin Endocrinol Metab 1987;64:645.

76. Gregoriou O, Pitoulis S, Coutifaris B, et al. Prolactin levels during labor. Obstet Gynecol 1979;53:630.

77. Grossman A, West S, Williams J, et al. The role of opiate peptides in the control of prolactin in the puerperium, and TSH in primary hypothyroidism. Clin Endocrinol 1982;16:317.

78. Guiloff E, Ibarra-Polo A, Zanartu J, et al. Effect of contraception on lactation. Am J Obstet Gynecol 1974;118:42.

79. Gupta AN, Mathur VS, Garg SK. Effect of oral contraceptives on quantity and quality of milk secretion in human beings. Ind J Med Res 1974;62:964.

80. Harness JR, Anderson RR. Effect of relaxin and somatotropin in combination with ovarian steroids on mammary glands in rats. Biol Reprod 1977;17:599.

81. Hazum E. Hormones and neurotransmitters in milk. Trends Pharmacol Sci 1983;4:454.

82. Healy DL, Rattigan S, Hartmann PE, et al. Prolactin in human milk: correlation with lactose, total protein, and alpha-lactalbumin levels. Am J Physiol 1980;238:83.

83. Hennart P, Delogne-Desnoeck J, Vis H, Robyn C. Serum levels of prolactin and milk production in women during a lactation period of thirty months. Clin Endocrinol 1981;14:349.

84. Holdsworth RJ, Chamings RJ. Measurement of progestogen and oestrogen levels in human breast milk. Br Vet J 1983;139:59.

85. Holst N, Jenssen TG, Burhol PG, et al. Plasma vasoactive intestinal polypeptide, insulin, gastric inhibitory polypeptide, and blood glucose in late pregnancy and during and after pregnancy. Am J Obstet Gynecol 1986;155:126.

86. Howie PW, McNeilly AS, Houston MJ, et al. Fertility after childbirth: infant feeding patterns, basal PRL levels and post-partum ovulation. Clin Endocrinol 1982;17:315.

87. Ishizuka B, Quigley ME, Yen SSC. Postpartum hypogonadotrophinism: evidence for increased opioid inhibition. Clin Endocrinol 1984;20:573.

88. Jansson L, Karlson FA, Westermark B. Mitogenic activity and epidermal growth factor content in human milk. Acta Paediatr Scand 1985;74:250.

89. Jeppsson S, Nilsson KO, Rannevik G, Wide L. Influence of suckling and of suckling followed by TRH or LH-RH on plasma prolactin, TSH, GH and FSH. Acta Endocrinol 1976;82:246.

90. Jeppsson S, Rannevik G. Studies on the gonadotropin response after administration of LH/FSH releasing hormone (LRH) during pregnancy and after therapeutic abortion in the second trimester. Am J Obstet Gynecol 1976;125:484.

91. Jeppsson S, Rannevik G, Kullander S. Studies on the

decreased gonadotropin response after administration of LH/FSH-releasing hormone during pregnancy and the puerperium. Am J Obstet Gynecol 1974;120:1029.

92. Jeppsson S, Rannevik G, Thorell JI, Wide L. Influence of LH/FSH releasing hormone (LRH) on the basal secretion of gonadotrophins in relation to plasma levels of oestradiol, progesterone and prolactin during the postpartum period in lactating and in nonlactating women. Acta Endocrinol 1977;84:713.

93. Jequier AM, Vanthuyne C, Jacobs HS. Gonadotrophin secretion in lactating women: response to luteinizing hormone releasing hormone/follicle-stimulating hormone releasing hormone in the puerperium. J Endocrinol 1973;59:14.

94. Johnston JM, Amico JA. A prospective longitudinal study of the release of oxytocin and prolactin in response to infant suckling in long term lactation. J Clin Endocrinol Metab 1986;62:653.

95. Jordan VC, Koerner S, Robinson C. Inhibition of oestrogen-stimulated prolactin release by anti-oestrogens. J Endocrinol 1975;65:151.

96. Josimovich JB, Archer DF. The role of lactogenic hormones in the pregnant woman and the fetus. Am J Obstet Gynecol 1977;129:777.

97. Kader-Abdel AM, Aziz MTA, Bahgat MR, et al. Effect of two long acting injectable progestogens on lactation in the human. Acta Biol Med Ger 1975;34:1199.

98. Katsutoshi S, Mitsunori S, Toshiko I. Serum FSH rise induced by CB-154 (2Br-alpha-ergocryptine) in postpartum women. J Clin Endocrinol Metab 1974;39:184.

99. Katz FH, Duncan BR. Entry of prednisone into human milk (letter). N Engl J Med 1975;2:1154.

100. Kennedy KI, Wisness CM. Contraceptive efficacy of gestational amenorrhea. Lancet 1992;227:339.

101. Koldovsky O. Hormones in milk. Life Sci 1980; 26:1833.

102. Kremer JA, Borm G, Schellekens LA, et al. Pulsatile secretion of luteinizing hormone and prolactin in lactating and nonlactating women and the response to naltrexone. J Clin Endocrinol Metab 1991;72:294.

103. Kremer JA, Rolland R, VanderHeijden PF, et al. Return of gonadotropic function in postpartum women during bromocriptine treatment. Fertil Steril 1989;51:622.

104. Kulski JK, Hartmann PE. Changes in the concentration of cortisol in milk during different stages of human lactation. Aust J Exp Biol Med Sci 1981;59:769.

105. Kulski JK, Hartmann PE. Milk insulin, GH and TSH: relationship to changes in milk lactose, glucose, and protein during lactogenesis in women. Endocrinol Exp 1983;17:317.

106. Laumas KR, Malkani PK, Bhatnagar S, Laumas V. Radioactivity in the breast milk of lactating women after oral administration of ³H-norethynodrel. Am J Obstet Gynecol 1967;98:411.

107. Leake RD, Waters CB, Rubin RT, et al. Oxytocin and prolactin responses in long-term breast-feeding. Obstet Gynecol 1983;62:565.

108. Lee LR, Paul SJ, Smith MS. Dose response effects of pulsatile GnRH administration on restoration of pituitary GnRH receptors and pulsatile LH secretion during lactation. Neuroendocrinology 1989;49:664.

109. Leleux D, Merveille JJ, Capel P, et al. Bromocriptine compared to long-acting estrogens in lactation prevention: clinical efficacy, prolactin secretion and co-

agulation parameters. Eur J Obstet Gynecol Reprod Biol 1981;12:235.

110. LeMarie WJ, Shapiro AG, Riggall F, Yang ST. Temporary pituitary insensitivity to stimulation by synthetic LRF during the postpartum period. J Clin Endocrinol Metab 1974;38:916.

111. Lewis PR, Brown JB, Renfree MB, Short RV. The resumption of ovulation and menstruation in a well-nourished population of women breastfeeding for an extended period of time. Fertil Steril 1991;55:529.

112. Lin TJ, Lin SC, Erlenmeyer F, et al. Progesterone production rates during the third trimester of pregnancy in normal women, diabetic women, and women with abnormal glucose tolerance. J Clin Endocrinol Metab 1972;34:287.

113. Lin TM, Halbert SP, Spellacy WN, Gall S. Human pregnancy-associated plasma proteins during the postpartum period. Am J Obstet Gynecol 1976;124:382.

114. Lincoln DW, Paisley AC. Neuroendocrine control of milk ejection. J Reprod Fertil 1982;65:571.

115. Liu JH, Lee DW, Markoff E. Differential release of prolactin variants in postpartum and early follicular phase women. J Clin Endocrinol Metab 1990;71:605.

116. Liu JH, Park KH. Gonadotropin and prolactin secretion increases during sleep during the puerperium in nonlactating women. J Clin Endocrinol Metab 1988;66:839.

117. Lodico G, Stoppelli I, Delitala G, Maioli M. Effects of naloxone infusion on basal and breast-stimulation-induced prolactin secretion in puerperal women. Fertil Steril 1983;40:600.

118. Lucas A, Drewett RB, Mitchell MD. Breast feeding and plasma oxytocin concentrations. BMJ 1980;281:834.

119. MacDonald HN, Collins YD, Tobin MJW, Wijayaratne DN. Use of pyridoxine in suppression of puerperal lactation. Br J Obstet Gynaecol 1976;83:54.

120. Macleod JN, Worsley I, Ray J, et al. Human growth hormone-variant is a biologically active somatogen and lactogen. Endocrinology 1991;128:1298.

121. Marrs RP, Kletzky OA, Mishell DR. Functional capacity of the gonadotrophs during pregnancy and the puerperium. Am J Obstet Gynecol 1981;141:658.

122. Masala A, Delitala G, LoDico G, et al. Effect of clomiphene on release of prolactin induced by mechanical breast emptying in women postpartum. J Endocrinol 1977;74:501.

123. Masala A, Delitala G, LoDico G, et al. Inhibition of lactation and inhibition of prolactin release after mechanical breast stimulation in puerperal women given tamoxifen or placebo. Br J Obstet Gynaecol 1978;85:134.

124. McGarrigle HH, Lachelin GC. Oestrone, oestradiol and oestriol glucosiduronates and sulphates in human puerperal plasma and milk. J Steroid Biochem 1983;18:607.

125. McKenzie SA, Selley JA, Agnew JE. Secretion of prednisolone into breast milk. Arch Dis Child 1975;50:894.

126. McNeilly AS, Robinson ICAF, Houston MJ, Howie PW. Release of oxytocin and prolactin in response to suckling. BMJ 1983;286:257.

127. Melis GB, Mais V, Paoletti AM, et al. Prevention of puerperal lactation by a single oral administration of the new prolactin-inhibiting drug, cabergoline. Obstet Gynecol 1988;71:311.

128. Messinis I, Souvatzoglou A, Stefos T, et al. Relationships between serum prolactin levels and follicle stimulating hormone response to luteinizing hormone-releasing hormone during early puerperium. Acta Endocrinol 1983;104:143.

129. Messinis I, Souvatzoglou A, Stefos T, et al. Naloxone effect on FSH response to LRH in early puerperium. Acta Endocrinol 1984;265(suppl):36.

130. Miyake A, Tanizawa O, Aono T, et al. Suppression of luteinizing hormone in castrated women by the administration of human chorionic gonadotropin. J Clin Endocrinol Metab 1976;43:928.

131. Miyake A, Tanizawa O, Aono T, Kurachi K. Pituitary LH response to LHRH during the puerperium. Obstet Gynecol 1978;51:37.

132. Mizuta H, Amino N, Ichihara K, et al. Thyroid hormones in human milk and their influence on thyroid function of breast-fed babies. Pediatr Res 1983;17:468.

133. Moller B, Bjorkhem I, Falk O, et al. Identification of thyroxine in human breast milk by gas chromatography-mass spectrometry. J Clin Endocrinol Metab 1983;56:30.

134. Moran JR, Courtney ME, Orth DN, et al. Epidermal growth factor in human milk: daily production and diurnal variation during early lactation in mothers delivering at term and at premature gestation. J Pediatr 1983;103:402.

135. Morris JA, Creasy RK, Hohe PT. Inhibition of puerperal lactation: double blind comparison of chlorotrianisene and testosterone enanthate with estradiol valerate and placebo. Obstet Gynecol 1970;36:107.

136. Nader S, Kjeld JM, Blair CM, et al. A study of the effect of bromocriptine on serum oestradiol, prolactin and follicle stimulating hormone levels in puerperal women. Br J Obstet Gynaecol 1975;82:750.

137. Nair RM, Sarda AK, Barnes MA, Phansey S. Elevated LHRH levels in human milk. Endocrinol Exp 1983;17:335.

138. Nakano R. Pituitary responsiveness to luteinizing hormone-releasing hormone (LH-RH) during pregnancy and the postpartum period. Am J Obstet Gynecol 1976;126:518.

139. Nilsson S, Nygren KG, Johansson EDB. Megestrol acetate concentrations in plasma and milk during administration of an oral contraceptive containing 4 mg megestrol acetate to nursing women. Contraception 1977;16:615.

140. Noel GL, Suh HK, Frantz AG. Prolactin release during nursing and breast stimulation in postpartum and nonpostpartum patients. J Clin Endocrinol Metab 1974;38:413.

141. Nunley WC, Urban RJ, Evans WS, Veldhuis JD. Preservation of pulsatile luteinizing hormone release during postpartum lactation amenorrhea. J Clin Endocrinol Metab 1991;73:629.

142. Nunley WC, Urban RJ, Kitchin JD, et al. Dynamics of pulsatile prolactin release during the postpartum lactational period. J Clin Endocrinol Metab 1991;72:287.

143. Oberkotter LV. Analysis of term human milk concentrations of 3.5.3′-triiodo-L-thyronine by high-performance liquid chromatography and radioimmunoassay: correlation with circulating serum levels in lactating women. J Chromatogr 1989;487:445.

144. Ottesen B, Schierup L, Bardrum B, Fahrenkrug J. Release of vasoactive intestinal polypeptide (VIP) in breast-feeding women. Eur J Obstet Gynecol Reprod Biol 1986;22:333.

145. Pearlman WH. Glucocorticoids in milk: a review. Endocrinol Exp 1983;17:165.

146. Pearlman WH. Hormones and tissue growth factors

in milk: evolutionary implications. Endocr Regul 1991;25:4.

147. Petrides PE, Hosang M, Shooter E, et al. Isolation and characterization of epidermal growth factor from human milk. FEBS Lett 1985;187:89.

148. Poindexter AN, Ritter MB, Besch PK. The recovery of normal plasma progesterone levels in the postpartum female. Fertil Steril 1983;39:494.

149. Pontiroli AE, DiMicco R, Sartani A, et al. Puerperal lactation, gonadotropin release and estradiol release: effects of metergoline and bromocriptine. Gynecol Obstet Invest 1987;24:179.

150. Potter JM, Nestel PJ. The hyperlipidemia of pregnancy in normal and complicated pregnancies. Am J Obstet Gynecol 1979;133:165.

151. Rastogi GK, Sialy R, Thomas Z, Vasista K. Hormonal response to LHRH and combined LHRH-TRH in postpartum lactating and nonlactating women. Ind J Med Res 1977;65:105.

152. Read LC, Francis GL, Wallace JC, Ballard FJ. Growth factor concentrations and growth-promoting activity in human milk following premature birth. J Dev Physiol 1985;7:135.

153. Read LC, Upton FM, Francis GL, et al. Changes in the growth-promoting activity of human milk during lactation. Pediatr Res 1984;18:133.

154. Reyes FI, Winter JSD, Faiman C. Postpartum disappearance of chorionic gonadotropin from the maternal and neonatal circulations. Am J Obstet Gynecol 1985;153:486.

155. Rigg LA, Yen SSC. Multiphasic prolactin secretion during parturition in human subjects. Am J Obstet Gynecol 1977;128:215.

156. Robyn O, Delvoye P, Badawi M, et al. Introduction to the physiology of human prolactin. Acta Endocrinol 1977;85(suppl 212):16.

157. Rolandi E, Ragni N, Fanceschini R, et al. Possible role of vasoactive intestinal polypeptide on prolactin release during suckling in lactating women. Horm Res 1987;27:211.

158. Rolland R, DeJong FH, Schellekens LA, Lequin R. The role of prolactin in the restoration of ovarian function during the early postpartum period in the human female. Clin Endocrinol 1975;4:27.

159. Rosner W, Beers PC, Awan TT, Khan MS. Identification of corticosteroid binding globulin in human milk: measurement with a filter disk assay. J Clin Endocrinol Metab 1976;42:1064.

160. Ruder HJ, Loriaux L, Lipsett MB. Estrone sulfate: production rate and metabolism in man. J Clin Invest 1972;51:1020.

161. Sack J, Amado O, Lunenfeld B. Thyroxine concentration in human milk. J Clin Endocrinol Metab 1977;45:171.

162. Said S, Johansson EDB, Gemzell C. Serum oestrogens and progesterone after normal delivery. J Obstet Gynaecol Br Comm 1973;80:542.

163. Said S, Johansson EDB, Gemzell C. Return of ovulation during the postpartum period. Acta Obstet Gynecol Scand 1974;53:63.

164. Salazar H, Tobon H, Josimovich JB. Developmental, gestational and postgestational modifications of the human breast. Clin Obstet Gynecol 1975;18:113.

165. Saxena BN, Shrimanker K, Grudzinskas JG. Levels of contraceptive steroids in breast milk and plasma of lactating women. Contraception 1977;16:605.

166. Schams D, Karg H. Hormones in milk. Ann N Y Acad Sci 1986;464:75.

167. Schoultz B. A quantitative study of the pregnancy zone protein in the sera of pregnant and puerperal women. Am J Obstet Gynecol 1974;119:792.

167a. Schwartz DJ, Evans PC, Garcia CR, et al. A clinical study of lactation suppression. Obstet Gynecol 1973;42:599.

168. Seki K, Seki M, Okumura T. Serum FSH rise induced by CB-154 (2-Br-alpha-ergocryptine) in postpartum women. J Clin Endocrinol Metab 1974;39:184.

169. Shaaban MM. Contraception with progestogens and progesterone during lactation. J Steroid Biochem Mol Biol 1991;40:705.

170. Sharman A. Postpartum regeneration of the human endometrium. J Anat 1953;87:1.

171. Sheehan KL, Yen SSC. Activation of pituitary gonadotropic function by an agonist of luteinizing hormone-releasing factor in the puerperium. Am J Obstet Gynecol 1979;135:755.

171a. Short RV, Lewis PR, Renfree MD, Shaw G. Contraceptive effects of extended lactational amenorrhea: beyond the Bellagio consensus. Lancet 1991;337:715.

172. Smith GVS, Smith OW. The inhibition of lactation in rabbits with large amounts of estrin. Am J Physiol 1933;103:356.

173. Steenstrup EK, Steenstrup OR. Prevention of puerperal lactation with bromocriptine (CB 154). A double blind comparison with diethylstilbestrol. Obstet Gynecol Surv 1977;32:642.

174. Stern JM, Reichlin S. Prolactin circadian rhythm persists throughout lactation in women. Neuroendocrinology 1990;51:31.

175. Strbak V, Giraud P, Resetkova E, et al. Thyroliberin (TRH) and TRH free acid (TRH-OH) present in milk do not originate from local synthesis in mammary gland. Endocr Regul 1991;25:134.

176. Toddywalla VS, Joshi L, Virkar K. Effect of contraceptive steroids on human lactation. Am J Obstet Gynecol 1977;127:245.

177. Tolis G, Guyda H, Pillorger R, Friesen HG. Breast feeding: effects on the hypothalamic pituitary gonadal axis. Endocr Res Commun 1974;1:293.

178. Tolis G, Guyda H, Rochefort JG. Pituitary responsiveness to gonadotrophin releasing factor (GnRH) in puerperium. Endocr Res Commun 1975;2:521.

179. Topper YJ. Multiple hormone interactions in the development of mammary gland in vitro. Rec Prog Horm Res 1970;26:287.

180. Tulandi T, Gelfand MM, Maiolo L. Effect of prostaglandin E2 on puerperal breast discomfort and prolactin secretion. J Reprod Med 1985;30:176.

181. Tulchinsky D, Abraham GE. Radioimmunoassay of plasma estriol. J Clin Endocrinol Metab 1971;33:775.

182. Tulchinsky D, Chopra IJ. Competitive ligand-binding assay for measurement of sex hormone binding globulin (SHBG). J Clin Endocrinol Metab 1973;37:873.

183. Tulchinsky D, Korenman SG. The plasma estradiol as an index of fetoplacental function. J Clin Invest 1971;50:1490.

183a. Turkington RW, Majumder GC, Kadohama N, et al. Hormonal regulation of gene expression in mammary cells. Rec Prog Horm Res 1973;29:417.

184. Tyson JE, Hwang P, Guyda H, Friesen HG. Studies of prolactin secretion in human pregnancy. Am J Obstet Gynecol 1972;113:14.

185. Tyson JE, Khojandi M, Huth J, Andreassen B. The influence of prolactin secretion on human lactation. J Clin Endocrinol Metab 1975;40:764.

186. Tyson JE, Perez A, Zanartu J. Human lactational response to oral thyrotropin releasing hormone. J Clin Endocrinol Metab 1976;43:760.

187. Uvnas-Moberg K, Widstrom AM, Werner S, et al. Oxytocin and prolactin levels in breast-feeding women: correlation with milk yield and duration of breast-feeding. Acta Obstet Gynecol Scand 1990;69:301.

188. Van Dam LJ, Rolland R. Lactation-inhibiting and prolactin-lowering effect of lisuride and bromocriptine: a comparative study. Eur J Obstet Gynecol Reprod Biol 1981;12:323.

189. Varga L, Lutterbeck PM, Pryor JS, et al. Suppression of puerperal lactation with an ergot alkaloid: a double-blind study. BMJ 1972;2:743.

190. Venturini PL, Horowski R, Maganza C, et al. Effects of lisuride and bromocriptine on inhibition of lactation and on serum prolactin levels: comparative double blind study. Eur J Obstet Gynecol Reprod Biol 1981;11:395.

191. Villalobos H, Canales ES, Zarate A, et al. Effect of prolactin suppression on gonadotrophic secretion in the puerperium. Acta Endocrinol 1976;83:236.

192. Walker S. A comparison of 2-bromo-a-ergocryptine, quinoestrol and placebo in suppression of puerperal lactation. Br J Clin Pharmacol 1975;2:368.

193. Walker S, Groom G, Hibbard BM, et al. Controlled trial of bromocriptine, quinestrol and placebo in suppression of puerperal lactation. Lancet 1975;2:842.

193a. Weinstein D, Ben David M, Polishuk WZ. Serum prolactin and suppression of lactation. Br J Obstet Gynaecol 1976;83:679.

194. Weiss G, O'Byrne EM, Hochman JA, et al. Secretion of progesterone and relaxin by the human corpus luteum at mid pregnancy and at term. Obstet Gynecol 1977;50:697.

195. Weiss G, Rifkin I. Progesterone and estrogen secretion by puerperal human ovaries. Obstet Gynecol 1975;46:557.

196. Weitzman RE, Leake RD, Rubin RT, Fisher DA. The effect of nursing on neurohypophyseal hormone and prolactin secretion in human subjects. J Clin Endocrinol Metab 1980;51:836.

197. Wenlock RW. Birth spacing and prolonged lactation in rural Zambia. J Biosoc Sci 1977;9:481.

198. Werner H, Amarant T, Fridkin M, Koch Y. Growth hormone releasing factor-like immunoreactivity in human milk. Biochem Biophys Res Commun 1986;135:1084.

199. Werner H, Katz P, Fridkin M, et al. Growth hormone releasing factor and somatostatin concentrations in the milk of lactating women. Eur J Pediatr 1988;147:252.

200. Werner H, Koch Y, Fridkin M, et al. High levels of vasoactive intestinal peptide in human milk. Biochem Biophys Res Commun 1985;133:228.

201. Werner S, Widstrom AM, Wahlberg V, et al. Immunoreactive calcitonin in maternal milk and serum in relation to prolactin and neurotensin. Early Hum Dev 1982;6:77.

202. Whitworth NS. Lactation in humans. Psychoneuroendocrinology 1988;13:171.

203. Widstrom AM, Winberg J, Werner S, et al. Suckling in lactating women stimulates the secretion of insulin and prolactin without concomitant effects on gastrin, growth hormone, calcitonin, vasopressin or catecholamines. Early Hum Dev 1984;10:115.

204. Widstrom AM, Winberg J, Werner S, et al. Breast feeding-induced effects on plasma gastrin and somatostatin levels and their correlation with milk yield in lactating females. Early Hum Dev 1988;16:293.

205. Willmott MP, Colhoun EM, Bolton AE. The suppression of puerperal lactation with bromocriptine. Acta Obstet Gynecol Scand 1977;56:145.

206. Yuen BH. Prolactin in human milk: the influence of nursing and the duration of postpartum lactation. Am J Obstet Gynecol 1988;158:583.

207. Yuen BH, Pendleton HJ, Blair S. Efficacy of bromocriptine and chlorotriansene in preventing postpartum lactation. Can Med Assoc J 1977;117:919.

208. Zanartu J, Aguilera E, Munoz G, Peliowsky H. Effect of long-acting contraceptive progestogen on lactation. Obstet Gynecol 1976;47:174.

209. Zarate A, Canales ES, Soria J, et al. Ovarian refractoriness during lactation in women: effect of gonadotropin stimulation. Am J Obstet Gynecol 1972;112:1130.

210. Zarate A, Canales ES, Soria J, et al. Refractory postpartum ovarian response to gonadal stimulation in nonlactating women. Obstet Gynecol 1974;44:819.

211. Zivny J, Kobilkova J, Vorlicek F, et al. Plasma beta-endorphin-like immunoreactivity during pregnancy, parturition, puerperium and in newborn. Acta Obstet Gynecol Scand 1986;65:129.

212. Zuckerman H, Carmel S. The inhibition of lactation by clomiphene. J Obstet Gynaecol Br Comm 1973;80:822.

The Human Fetal Hypothalamus and Pituitary Gland:
The Maturation of Neuroendocrine Mechanisms Controlling the Secretion of Fetal Pituitary Growth Hormone, Prolactin, Gonadotropins, Adrenocorticotropin-Related Peptides, and Thyrotropin

———

Melvin M. Grumbach

Peter D. Gluckman

———

The extraordinary advances in our understanding of the mammalian fetal endocrine system over the past two decades collectively constitute an especially notable achievement of modern biomedical science. A remarkable increase transpired in our knowledge of the ontogenesis of the human fetal endocrine system and the role of fetal hormones in morphogenesis, in the regulation of metabolic processes and homeostatic mechanisms in the fetus, and during parturition. Historically the modern era of fetal endocrine research began more than four decades ago. Its origin was in the pioneering experiments by Jost,[281–284] Moore,[375] Wells,[555] and Raynaud and Frilley,[450] which involved ablation of fetal endocrine glands in experimental animals as well as the administration of hormones to the mother and the fetus. The development of methods for the measurement of minute quantities of hormones, including growth factors and hormone-binding proteins, gave a major impetus to studies on the development and regulation of hormone secretion in the human fetus. These advances, coupled with techniques for implanting long-term, indwelling vascular catheters into the intact fetus and pregnant animal made possible new experimental approaches in determining the role of the fetal endocrine system and its regulation, through the use of large domestic animals and nonhuman primates as experimental models. More recently, the exploitation of advances in cell biology and the application of the power of molecular genetics, including the development of transgenic animals, have led to new insights into the differentiation, maturation, integration, and function of the human maternal-placental-fetal network and to the action of hormones at the molecular level.

The endocrine system is characterized by a hierarchy of function. For pituitary hormones, this includes the central nervous system (CNS) regulation of the adenohypophysis mediated through the hypothalamic hypophysiotropic hormones (and their plasma membrane receptors), transmitted to the pituitary gland by a private conduit—the hypothalamic hypophyseal portal vascular system (Fig. 12–1); the secretion of pituitary hormones into the systemic circulation and their transport to peripheral tissues and endocrine glands; and finally bind-

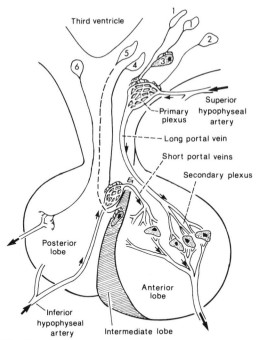

FIGURE 12–1. The mature hypothalamohypophyseal unit. Secretion of hormones by the adenohypophysis is regulated by hypothalamic peptides, which are released into the portal circulation. Neuron 3 represents a hypothalamic peptidergic neuron, which secretes into the primary plexus of the portal circulation within the median eminence. The secreted peptide reaches the adenohypophysis via the long portal vessels and is distributed through the gland in the secondary plexus. Neuron 4 is a similar peptidergic neuron, which terminates lower in the infundibular stalk and secretes into the portal circulation fed by the inferior hypophyseal artery and drains into the adenohypophysis by the short portal vessels. The hypothalamic peptidergic neurons are in turn regulated by monoaminergic neurons (neuron 1). Dopamine, a prolactin inhibitory factor (PIF), is secreted directly into the portal circulation (neuron 2). The intermediate lobe hormones are regulated mainly by a monoaminergic neuronal system directly regulating the cells within the intermediate lobe (neuron 5). The neurohypophysis secretes peptidergic hormones from nerve ends of neurons with their cell bodies in the supraoptic and paraventricular nuclei (neuron 6); the axons of these neurons form the tuberohypophyseal tract. (Modified from Gay VL. The hypothalamus: Physiology and clinical use of releasing factors. Fertil Steril 1972; 23:50.)

ing to receptors on the cell surface of target tissues to initiate the peripheral action of these hormones.

The fetus is exposed to hormones secreted by the mother, the placenta, and the fetus itself. In addition to differences in concentration of many hormones between fetal and postnatal life, some important qualitative differences have been described apart from the presence of placental hormones in the fetus.

For example, arginine vasotocin, a neurohypophyseal hormone of lower vertebrates, is a major posterior pituitary peptide in the human fetus early in gestation that gradually diminishes as the fetus matures and is replaced by arginine vasopressin; the α-glycoprotein hormone subunit appears earlier than the β subunits of the pituitary glycoprotein hormones and is the major glycoprotein hormone component in the fetal pituitary gland through midgestation; α-melanocyte-stimulating hormone (α-MSH) and peptides with a portion of the sequence of amino acids in adrenocorticotropic hormone (ACTH) (e.g., corticotropin-like intermediate lobe peptide [CLIP]) present in the human fetal pituitary gland are for all purposes absent in the adult gland.

Parathyroid hormone-related protein (PTHrP), synthesized and secreted mainly by the placenta and also by the fetal parathyroid glands, is expressed in a wide variety of tissues. It has a critical but poorly understood role in fetal growth and development ("knockout of the PTHrP gene is lethal in the newborn mouse"), it is the putative "fetal parathyroid hormone," and it affects placental calcium and phosphorus transport. This is in contrast to its role in the normal adult, in whom plasma PTHrP levels are exceedingly low. Similarly, calcitonin circulates at high levels in the fetus but in low concentrations in the normal child and adult. Proinsulin and prorenin are increased relative to insulin and renin in the fetal pancreas and kidney. Finally, reverse triiodothyronine, an apparently inactive thyroxine metabolite, is the predominant circulating fetal triiodothyronine.

Autocrine and paracrine mechanisms play an important role in the action of fetal hormones. Differences exist in the cellular origin of certain hormones and their action in the fetus and adult, e.g., the inhibin/activin system; a pituitary cell with the capacity to secrete both growth hormone and prolactin, the somatomammotrope, is more prevalent in the fetal pituitary than that of the adult. The generation of insulin-like growth factor 1 (IGF-1) is growth hormone dependent postnatally but only to a minor degree in the fetus. The fetal Leydig cell differs morphologically and functionally from the adult Leydig cell; e.g., it does not exhibit down-regulation of testosterone synthesis after chronic stimulation by human chorionic gonadotropin/luteinizing hormone (hCG/LH). Somatostatin is a much less effective inhibitor of pituitary growth hormone release in the fetus than postnatally, in contrast to the brisk growth hormone response to growth hormone–releasing factor (GRF).

New insight has been gained of the morphogenesis of hormone-specific cell differentiation of the adenohypophysis by the ascertainment of the role of the pituitary transcription factor, Pit-1. The discovery of the extra-CNS origin of luteinizing hormone–releasing factor (LRF) neurons from the ectodermally derived olfactory placode and the action of the KAL gene, which encodes a protein with structural homology to neural cell adhesion molecules, fibronectin, and other proteins involved in neuronal migration and axon pathfinding and targeting of LRF neurons from the nose to the forebrain provides a new model for studying fundamental mechanisms of neural cell migration and histogenesis.

This chapter mainly addresses the differentiation and function of the fetal hypothalamic unit and the ontogenesis of the regulation of pituitary function by the CNS. By the 12th week of gestation, organogenesis of the hypothalamus and the pituitary gland is well advanced, hypothalamic hypophysiotropic hormones are detectable in the medial basal hypothalamus, the hypophyseal portal system is intact, and the pituitary gland can synthesize most of the major pituitary hormones. The secretion of pituitary hormones by the fetus is regulated principally by fetal and not maternal influences, with little exchange of peptide hormones across the placenta. Moreover, the developmental pattern of the secretion of fetal pituitary hormones exhibits independent secretory patterns.

Neurosecretion is a primitive regulatory system, and neuroendocrine mechanisms differentiate and function from early in fetal life. The complex developmental changes in the essence and extent of hypothalamic regulation (the *final common pathway* for the influence of the CNS) on the function of the fetal adenohypophysis are incompletely understood. The hypothalamus is an interface between the environment and the "interval milieu," and a site at which the neuroendrocrine system, the autonomic nervous system, and the CNS, especially its limbic system, interact. Previously we advanced the concept that in early fetal life, there is relatively autonomous and unrestrained secretion of certain hypothalamic hypophysiotropic factors and pituitary hormones.[229, 230, 290] With advancing gestation, the maturation of inhibitory influences, mediated, at least in part, via the CNS and acting on the hypothalamus and its neurosecretory neurons, modulates pituitary secretion.

Increased understanding of the ontogeny of the endocrine system; of the developmental processes influenced by hormones; and of maternal, placental, and fetal factors that adversely affect their normal and harmonious maturation offers the promise of new insights into the adaptation to postnatal life of preterm and full-term infants and into the prenatal antecedents of morbidity in later life. Further, the potential now exists to recognize and modify impaired growth in the fetus as well as abnormalities of the fetal endocrine system.

In this chapter, we discuss the embryology and development of the fetal hypothalamus and adenohypophysis, the development of neurotransmitters and neurosecretory factors within the hypothalamus, the appearance of hormones in the anterior and intermediate lobe of the pituitary, and the regulation of pituitary secretion in the fetus. Thyroid-stimulating hormone (TSH) is discussed separately in Chapter 16. The placenta is a miniature of the endocrine system. In addition to the pituitary-like hormones, it synthesizes a variety of hypothalamic neuropeptides, the inhibin/activin class of gonadal hypophysiotropic peptides, and a large number of growth factors and their receptors. It is now recognized that the placental secretion of protein and steroid hormones is not simply autonomous but is influenced by many factors, including placental hypothalamic-like neuropeptides and a complex intraplacental paracrine-autocrine autoregulatory communication system. We consider selected interrelationships and interactions of the placental, the decidua, and the fetal endocrine systems. Chapter 2 considers in detail the peptide hormones of the placenta. Finally, clinically important congenital disorders that involve the hypothalamic-pituitary unit are discussed.

EMBRYOGENESIS OF THE FETAL HYPOTHALAMIC-PITUITARY UNIT

Hypothalamus

The hypothalamus develops from the prosencephalon (forebrain), the most caudal part of the neural tube. Early in embryogenesis (approximately 22 days postconception), the primitive forebrain develops as the anterior neuropore closes. By 34 days, the forebrain can be morphologically separated into the cerebral hemispheres and the diencephalon.[312] The most ventral part of the diencephalon develops into the hypothalamus, and at this stage, primitive fiber tracts and neuroblasts are already being differentiated in the primordial hypothalamus.[44, 302, 400, 554] Between 35 and 100 days after conception, the hypothalamic nuclei differentiate within the hypothalamus[268, 302, 407] (Table 12–1). The infundibular bulb, the primitive neurohypophysis, first appears at 37 days,[407, 555, 572] and by 60 days, the supraoptic hypophyseal tract, which is formed by the axons of the neurosecretory neurons that secrete neurohypophyseal hormones, is developed.[555] At this time (60 days), the median eminence is distinguishable.[268] The primary plexus of the portal circulation penetrates the median eminence, and the hypothalamic-hypophyseal portal vascular system is intact by at least 11.5 weeks.[532] By 100 days' gestation, the hypothalamic nuclei are fully differentiated. (The appearance and development of neurotransmitter and neurohormone systems is discussed in the section on Neurosecretions and Neurotransmitters of the Fetal Hypothalamus.) Further, the human hypothalamus, as well as other parts of the brain, exhibits a sex dimorphism (reviewed in Swaab et al.[518]).

More than 30 releasing factors that influence pituitary secretion have been isolated from the hypothalamus and their chemical structures established. All are peptides except one, dopamine, the main prolactin-release inhibiting factor. Of the classic hypothalamic neuropeptides, GRF or growth hormone–releasing hormone (GRH), somatostatin, thyrotropin-releasing factor (TRF) or thyrotropin-releasing hormone (TRH), and corticotropin-releasing factor (CRF) or corticotropin-releasing hormone (CRH) are synthesized and se-

TABLE 12–1. Early Development of the Human Fetal Pituitary and Hypothalamus

Gestational Age (weeks)	Hypothalamus	Pituitary	Portal Circulation
3	Forebrain appears		
4		Rathke pouch in contact with stomodeum	
5	Diencephalon differentiated	Rathke pouch separated from stomodeum and in contact with infundibulum; pituitary in culture can secrete ACTH, prolactin, GH, FSH	
6	Premamillary preoptic nucleus; LHRH detected	Intermediate-lobe primordia: cell cords penetrate mesenchyme around Rathke pouch	
7	Arcuate, supraoptic nucleus	Sphenoidal plate forms	
8	Median eminence differentiated: TRH detected*	Basophils appear	Capillaries in mesenchyme
9	Paraventricular nucleus; dorsal medial nucleus	Pars tuberalis formed: β-endorphin detected*	
10	Serotonin and norepinephrine detected*	Acidophils appear	
11	Mamillary nucleus; primary (hypothalamic) portal plexus present; β-endorphin and opioidergic neurons detected*	Secondary (pituitary) portal plexus present catecholamines (IF)†	Functional hypothalamic-hypophyseal portal system
12	Dopamine present		
13	Corticotropin-releasing hormone detected*	α-Melanocyte-stimulating hormone detected	
14	Fully differentiated hypothalamus	Adult form of hypophysis developed	

Hormone detected at this gestational age but may be present earlier.
†*IF, detected by immunofluorescence.*

creted by neurosecretory neurons that originate from ventricular zones within the embryonic forebrain with the single exception of the luteinizing hormone–releasing factor (luteinizing hormone–releasing hormone [LH-RH], LRF, or gonadotropin-releasing hormone [Gn-RH]) neurons and their distinctive peregrination.

In contrast to the other major hypothalamic hypophysiotropic neurosecretory neurons, LH-RH neurons arise in the embryo from the epithelium of the medial olfactory pit and migrate from the olfactory placode in the nose, along the pathway of the olfactory nerve–nervus terminalis–vomeronasal complex to the forebrain to seed the hypothalamus (Fig. 12–2). As discovered in mice by Schwanzel-Fukuda and Pfaff[486] and by Wray et al.,[568, 569] the LRF neurosecretory neurons migrate in a rostrocaudal direction across the nasal cavity and cribriform plate to the forebrain. The nasal origin of LRF neurons is established in species from amphibians to the human.[484, 485] The migrating LRF neurons are associated with a *scaffolding* of immunoreactive neural cell adhesion molecule (NCAM)[158] fibers that may serve as a

guide to the migration of LRF neurosecretory neurons and the olfactory neuron complex.[483] Another class of cell surface glycoconjugate recognized by antiserum to CC_2 may play a role in this process.[536]

In Kallmann's syndrome, a genetically heterogeneous disorder characterized by hypothalamic hypogonadism and anosmia (see the section on Kallman's Syndrome and Hypogonadotropic Hypogonadism), the loss of the X-linked KAL gene (in the Xp22.3 region) or its mutation (see review in Petit[425] and Prager and Braunstein[439] leads to arrest of LRF neuron migration in the nose and outside the dura and aplasia or hypoplasia of the olfactory bulbs and tracts.[484] The KAL gene encodes a 680 amino acid glycoprotein with characteristics of an extracellular neural adhesion molecule that could serve as a pathfinder in the guidance of LRF neurons and the olfactory nerve.[176, 310, 425, 470] In the developing and mature chicken, the KAL gene is expressed in the mitral cells of the olfactory bulb and in the Purkinje cells of the cerebellar cortex, regions that are affected in Kallmann's syndrome.[470]

LRF is present in human embryonic brain

extracts by 4.5 weeks of gestation[561] and thereafter in hypothalamic extracts.[33, 290, 561] LRF neurons that also contain LRF prohormone are detectable in the medial basal fetal hypothalamus by 9 weeks, and by 11 weeks, axon fibers that contain LRF have reached the median eminence[75] and terminate in contact with the capillaries of the primary plexus of the hypophyseal-portal system.[90–92, 414] In the ovine fetus, LRF neurosecretory neurons, present in the hypothalamus by at least 58 days of gestation,[231] secrete LRF in a pulsatile manner, indicating a functional LRF pulse generator by at least midgestation.[105]

Adenohypophysis

The pituitary gland arises from two primordia: the ectoderm of the primitive oral cavity (stomadeum) and the neuroectoderm of the infundibulum, a vertical diverticulum of the floor of the diencephalon (Fig. 12–3). The classic description of the development of the adenohypophysis suggests that Rathke's pouch, the precursor of the adenohypophysis, develops as a diverticulum of the primitive stomadeum and is, therefore, ectodermal in origin.[30, 117, 125, 126, 192, 535] Studies, however, initially in avian and amphibian embryos, have challenged this concept and suggested that Rathke's pouch is not derived from stomodeal ectoderm but rather from neuroectoderm of the caudal region of the ventral neural ridge. In the chick embryo, the earliest precursor of the adenohypophysis appears as a sulcus in the ventral neural ridge. Then, as the developing brain begins to fold, it later extends as far as the oral plate to form the classic Rathke pouch. Because of the process of head-enfolding, the pouch secondarily appears to be a cranial extension of the stomadeum.[524] This issue remains unresolved. In vertebrates, most cells that produce hormonal peptides belong to a family of cells known as the amine content or precursor uptake and decarboxylation (APUD) series; the acronym is derived from some of the cells' most important and constant cytochemical properties.[420] These cells, widely distributed in the body, were at first considered to be solely of neuroectodermal, primarily neural crest, origin.[418, 419] This concept, how-

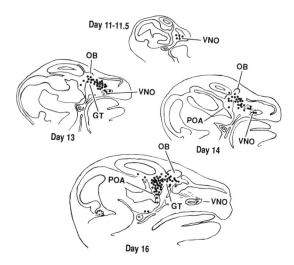

FIGURE 12–2. Ontogeny of LRF neurons in the mouse. The migratory route of LRF neurosecretory neurons (black dots) in the mouse embryo is shown from their origin in the medial olfactory placode in the primitive nose through the forebrain into the hypothalamus and its preoptic areas. At embryonic day (ED) 11 to 11.5, LRF cells are in the anlage of the vomeronasal organ and medial wall of the olfactory placode. By ED 13, the number of LRF neurons has increased, and most are in the nasal septum with the nervus terminalis and the vomeronasal nerves; only a few neurons have reached the brain. By ED 14, the majority of LRF cells are in the ganglion terminale and the central root of the nervus terminalis and arch through the forebrain to the hypothalamus. By ED 16, most of the LRF neurons are in the hypothalamus and its preoptic areas, and the migration is almost complete. GT = Ganglion terminale; OB = olfactory bulb; POA = preoptic area; VNO = vomeronasal organ. (Adapted from Schwanzel-Fukuda M, Pfaff DW. Nature 1989; 338:161. From Grumbach MM, Styne DM. Puberty: Ontogeny, neuroendocrinology, physiology, and disorders. In: Wilson JD, Foster DW, eds. Williams textbook of endocrinology, ed 8. Philadelphia: WB Saunders, 1992:1139.

ever, is no longer tenable.[50, 183] The hypothesis that Rathke's pouch is of neuroectodermal rather than ectodermal origin has its advocates.[399, 418–420, 537] The caudal region of the ventral neural ridge contributes to the embryonic diencephalon,[420, 524] and it remains possible that both the hypothalamus and the adenohypophysis are embryologic derivatives of a common neuroectodermal anlage. In any event, both the mesoderm beneath the ectoderm and the brain influence the early development of the pituitary primordium.[270, 303]

In the human fetus, the craniopharyngeal invagination that forms Rathke's pouch is apparent by 22 days.[30, 125, 126, 166, 399] One report provocatively suggests that Rathke's pouch arises as a solitary vesicle unconnected with the

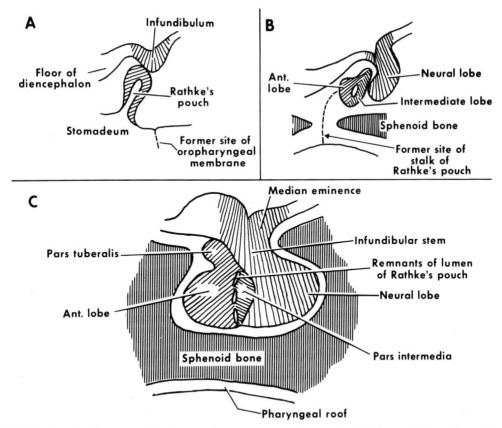

FIGURE 12–3. *A,* Development of Rathke pouch by 5 weeks' postconception. Rathke pouch is no longer in open connection with the stomadeum, but remnants of the regressing stalk are present and may persist into adult life. By 5 weeks, Rathke pouch is in contact with the primitive infundibular process, which forms as a diverticulum from the floor of the diencephalon. The oropharyngeal membrane ruptures in the fourth week to bring the stomadeum or primitive oral cavity and the foregut into contact. The posterior limb of Rathke pouch in contact with the infundibulum develops into the pars intermedia and the anterior limb into the adenohypophysis. By 5 weeks, the hypothalamus is a histologically distinct portion of the diencephalon. *B,* The sphenoid bone begins to develop as a cartilaginous plate by about 7 weeks. By 14 weeks, the pituitary has attained its adult form, with the lumen of Rathke pouch largely obliterated and only a few clefts remaining to separate the intermediate lobe from the anterior lobe. *C,* The pituitary fossa is formed, and the hypothalamus is fully differentiated. (Modified from Moore KL. The developing human: Clinically oriented embryology. Philadelphia: WB Saunders, 1973.)

stomadeum (oral cavity).[537] In any event, by 35 days it is elongated and separated from the stomadeum (oral cavity) (Figs. 12–4 and 12–5), and the posterior wall of the pouch is in contact with the primitive infundibular process of the embryonic diencephalon, the future neurohypophysis.[166, 270] The cells forming the wall of Rathke's pouch appear similar to neural tube cells.[270] The two limbs of the thin-walled Rathke's pouch develop differently. The posterior limb between the lumen of the pouch and the neurohypophysis forms the intermediate lobe and the pars tuberalis.[26, 482, 565] The anterior limb gives rise to the adenohypophysis. By 40 days, Rathke's pouch is lined

with small cuboidal epithelial cells, but soon thereafter, the cells proliferate and penetrate the surrounding mesechyme to form the cell cords that make up the bulk of the anterior lobe.[18, 117] The pituitary gland is readily identifiable by 7 weeks (Fig. 12–5); cartilage of the primordial sphenoid bone separates the primordium of the pituitary gland and Rathke's pouch from the stomadeum.[270]

As early as 35 days, the primitive adenohypophysis in vitro can secrete growth hormone (GH), prolactin, follicle-stimulating hormone (FSH), LH, and ACTH,[435, 498] although histologically the cells appear undifferentiated until 8 to 9 weeks, when ACTH containing basophils

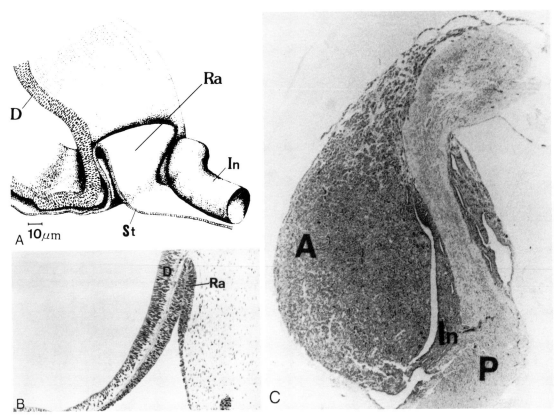

FIGURE 12–4. *A,* Three-dimensional reconstruction of the differentiation of the human embryonic pituitary gland of a 5-week-old embryo (ovulation age); midsagittal section as seen from the left side. The expression of the α-glycoprotein subunit occurs before the formation of Rathke pouch and is a marker for the onset of organogenesis of the pituitary gland. D = Diencephalon; In = internal carotid artery; Ra = Rathke diverticulum; St = stomadeum. *B,* Sagittal section of hypophyseal region of a human embryo at 5 weeks' gestation. H&E × 400. *C,* Sagittal section of the pituitary gland of a 21-week-old human fetus. Note the remnant of Rathke pouch between the anterior and intermediate lobes. H&E, × 66. A = Anterior lobe; In = intermediate lobe; P = posterior lobe. (From Ikeda H, Suzuki J, Sasano N, Niizuma H. The development and morphogenesis of the human pituitary gland. Anat Embryol 1988; 178:327.)

are apparent.[270] Acidophils appear at 9 to 12 weeks,[126, 166] and by 14 weeks, the classic shape and arrangement of the pituitary are present (see Fig. 13–3). During the remainder of gestation, the pituitary gland increases 30-fold in weight.[125, 126, 293]

The pharyngeal hypophysis, located on the pharyngeal roof,[354, 362] arises from vestiges of the stomodeal stalk (see Fig. 12–5) that before linked Rathke's pouch to the stomadeum.[79, 353] Compared with the adenohypophysis, it is small but vascular and densely innervated. It grows only during fetal development and is enlarged in anencephaly.[355] Both GH and prolactin have been detected in the pharyngeal pituitary[355, 362] as well as other pituitary cell types.[104] The role, if any, of the pharyngeal hypophysis in the function of the fetal endocrine system is unknown.

GENE REGULATION OF PITUITARY CELL-SPECIFIC DIFFERENTIATION. A remarkable development is the new insight gained into molecular mechanisms that regulate cell-specific differentiation and development of the final hormone-producing cell types of the anterior pituitary gland arising from ectodermal cells in Rathke's pouch. A transcriptional regulator, Pit-1 (GHF-1),[77, 99, 271, 273, 530, 545] a protein containing 291 amino acids, is encoded by a gene that is part of the large POU-homeodomain family of genes, originally described in certain *Drosophila* homeotic* and

---

*Homeotic genes: "master control genes" that regulate the development of various body parts of the fly and contain homeoboxes, DNA boxes with a fixed number of nucleotides. These tightly clustered genes are arranged sequentially in the order they are expressed along the body axis.

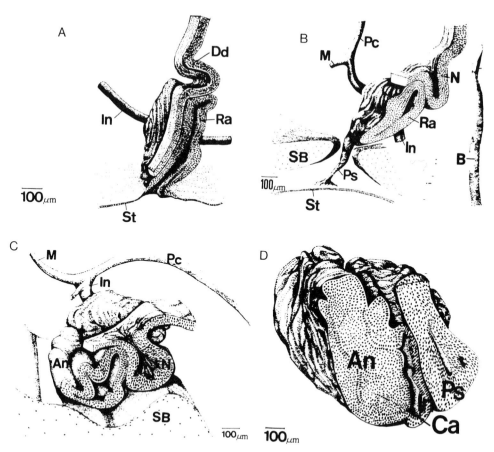

FIGURE 12–5. *A,* Three-dimensional microstructure of the pituitary region of a 6-week-old human embryo; left side of a midsagittal section. Dd = Diencephalon diverticulum; In = internal carotid artery; Ra = Rathke diverticulum; St = stomadeum. *B,* A 6- to 7-week-old human embryo; left side of a midsagittal section, nasal side at left. During the seventh fetal week with further development of the primordial sphenoid bone, Rathke pouch is separated from the stomadeum. B = Basilar artery; In = internal carotid artery; M = middle cerebral artery; N = neurohypophysis primordium; Pc = posterior communicating artery; Ps = pharyngohypophyseal stalk; Ra = Rathke pouch; St = stomadeum; SB = primordium of sphenoid bone. *C,* A 9-week-old human fetus; midsagittal section, left side. Both the tip of Rathke pouch and the upper half of its posterior wall are in close opposition to the infundibulum. An = Anterior lobe. *D,* Three-dimensional microstructure of the pituitary region of a 13-week-old human fetus; midsagittal section, left side. Contact between Rathke pouch and the diencephalon is limited to the superior central portion of the posterior wall and the lateral portions of the pouch. An = Anterior lobe; Ca = cavity of Rathke pouch; It = intermediate lobe; Ps = posterior lobe. (From Ikeda H, Suzuki J, Sasano N, Niizuma H. The development and morphogenesis of the human pituitary gland. Anat Embryol 1988; 178:327.)

segmentation genes, which are important regulators of mammalian development.[250] Pit-1 has a critical role in the activation and expression of the genes encoding GH and prolactin[150, 174, 271–273, 338] and the transcriptional activation of the β subunit of thyrotropin.[509] The POU proteins share two homologous DNA binding domains: the POU homeodomain, a conserved 60 amino acid region related to the DNA-binding domain of homeobox proteins, and the POU-specific domain, a 70 to 78 amino acid sequence that is common to Pit-1 and two other mammalian transcription factors, Oct_1 and Oct_2; the two domains are separated by a nonconserved region (Fig. 12–6).

In studies of the ontogeny of phenotypic-specific differentiation of anterior pituitary hormone-secreting cells, the application of molecular biologic and immunochemical techniques in the rat and mouse, the use of transgenic mouse models, and the identification of mutations in the Pit-1 gene in dwarf mice,[97, 317] and more recently in the human,[395, 409, 431, 445, 529] have clarified the spatial and temporal differentiation of the somatotrope, lactotrope, and thyrotrope.[502]

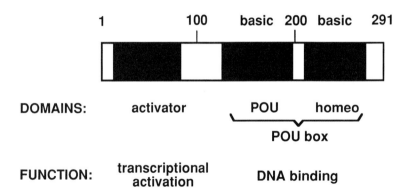

FIGURE 12–6. The Pit-1 (GHF-1) protein illustrating its functional domains (see text). Missense and nonsense mutations in the POU-specific domain, the POU-homeo domain, or the transcriptional activator domain are described in patients with combined GH, PRL, and TSH deficiency. Similarly, Snell (dw) and Jackson (dw′) dwarf mice, which lack somatotropes, lactotropes, and thyrotropes, have mutations in the Pit-1 gene.

A surprising observation is the expression of the α-glycoprotein subunit on embryonic day (ED) 11 of the rat in the columnar epithelium ectoderm, part of the anterolateral ridge ectoderm lying directly beneath the neural tube between the hypothalamus and the primitive gut.[502] The α-glycoprotein subunit is the first marker for cells of the nascent anterior pituitary placode. By ED 12, the transcripts are limited to the definitive Rathke's pouch (see Fig. 12–4); later in development, the α subunit transcript is restricted to gonadotropes and thyrotropes.

Pit-1 gene transcripts are first detected on ED 15 in many pituitary cells—all five pituitary cell types express Pit-1 mRNA. Pit-1 protein, in contrast, is limited to the nuclei of somatotropes, lactotropes, and thyrotropes. It seems that the absence of Pit-1 protein in corticotropes and gonadotropes is due to a cell–type specific inhibitory mechanism. Using additional in situ techniques, the order of differentiation of the cells of the rat anterior pituitary was defined[502] (Fig. 12–7). The first differentiated cells were the corticotrope and thyrotrope on ED 13 to 14, followed by the LH-containing gonadotrope on ED 16.5. After the appearance of Pit-1 protein (ED 15 to 16), somatotrope and lactotrope cells were detected on ED 17 to 18, as were cells containing beta FSH mRNA. GH and prolactin gene ablation experiments in transgenic mice support the derivation of the lactotrope from a GH-expressing stem cell that gives rise to both somatotropes and lactotropes[78] and in the fetus a transient somatomammotrope. The sequence of appearance of immunoreactive hormones in the human fetal pituitary cells is similar.[28]

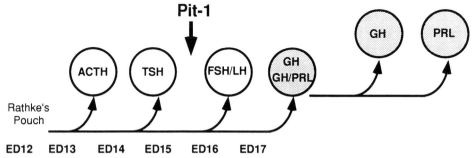

FIGURE 12–7. The sequence of differentiation of the five distinct cell types of the rat anterior pituitary gland. The α-glycoprotein subunit appears before differentiation of Rathke pouch. Expression of POMC mRNA (ACTH prohormone) is detectable by embryonic day (ED) 13.5. Pit-1 protein is expressed initially on ED 15. On ED 17, GH and PRL transcripts are present. Pit-1 activates, directly or indirectly, expression of the GRF receptor gene, a critical regulator of somatotrope proliferation (see text). An estrogen response element is located in the distal PRL enhancer. Estrogen receptors on the lactotrope increase strikingly after birth in the rat and correlate with the increased expression of PRL postnatally. The temporal pattern of differentiation of cell types in the human fetal pituitary gland is comparable to that in the rat and mouse when related to the length of gestation. (Diagrammatic scheme courtesy of Holly A. Ingraham, University of California, San Francisco, California. Data from Simmons DM, Voss JW, Ingraham HA, et al. Pituitary cell phenotype involve cell-specific Pit-1 mRNA translation and synergistic interaction with other class of transcription factors. Genes Dev 1990; 4:695.)

A large body of evidence supports the critical role during development of the protein product of the Pit-1 transcription activator in the cell-specific activation of the GH and prolactin genes by binding to components of their promoters and in the differentiation and proliferation of somatotropes and lactotropes as well as the survival of thyrotropes. Hence the pleiotropic action of the Pit-1 gene may prevent programmed cell death (apoptosis) of these three pituitary cell types.

The expression of the GRF receptor gene, an important regulator of somatotrope proliferation when stimulated by GRF, is activated directly or indirectly by Pit-1;[320] it is not expressed in dw/dw or df/df dwarf mice. This action may explain in part the lack of proliferation of somatotropes in Pit-1 mutations in the human and mouse.

The discovery of the pleiotropic Pit-1 gene is a first step in defining the complex molecular mechanisms that govern the development of final differentiated specific cell types in the anterior pituitary gland. It is likely that a network of trans-acting factors interact to determine the pattern of activation of the hormone-secreting anterior pituitary cell types.[502] The expression of another homeobox-containing gene, Hox-7, was detected in Rathke's pouch of the 10.5-day mouse embryo.[332]

Studies of the ontogeny of the somatotrope and lactotrope by a variety of techniques, including novel gene ablation experiments in transgenic mice,[60, 78] support the hypothesis of the derivation of the fetal lactotrope from a presomatotrope stem cell. The presomatotrope cell that expresses GH is the precursor of the differentiated somatotrope and lactotrope and a population of transient fetal somatomammotropes.[28, 180, 382]

From experimental evidence[57, 210, 435, 498, 553] and consideration of the anencephalic human fetus, the differentiation of the fetal adenohypophysis does not seem to depend on hypothalamic influences, although the fetal hypothalamus is essential for many fetal pituitary secretions.

Intermediate Lobe

Advances in our knowledge of ACTH-related peptides have led to an increasing awareness of the possible physiologic role of the intermediate lobe. The relative prominence of this lobe in the human fetus may reflect the potential significance of its secretions in utero. The posterior limb of Rathke's pouch, the primordium of the intermediate lobe, comes into contact with the developing neurohypophysis early in gestation[166, 270] (see Figs. 12–3 and 12–4). By 50 days, this region of Rathke's pouch can be differentiated morphologically.[30, 125, 126, 270] The intermediate lobe is relatively much larger in the human fetus than in the adult, although in other species a distinct intermediate lobe may persist.[558] In the fetus, the intermediate lobe is separated from the pars distalis by a cleft, which is a remnant of Rathke's pouch[30, 166, 270] (see Fig. 12–5). After birth, this cleft is usually reduced to a zone of discontinuous lumina, and the lobe itself regresses so that only a discontinuous layer represents the intermediate lobe in the adult.[558] A pars intermedia is not present in the pharyngeal pituitary.[270]

Hypothalamohypophyseal Portal System

The functional link between the hypothalamus and the adenohypophysis is the hypothalamohypophyseal portal system. Blood entering the median eminence region of the hypothalamus via the superior hypophyseal arteries passes through a capillary network (the primary plexus) into which hypothalamic factors are secreted. Blood then leaves the median eminence via the portal vessels to enter the anterior hypophysis and to be distributed within the gland in a secondary plexus of capillaries (see Fig. 12–1). The demonstration of retrograde blood flow from the pituitary to the brain[65, 395] suggests a further potential mechanism of pituitary hypothalamic interaction, the significance of which is as yet uncertain.

It is likely that in all stages of human development, the adenohypophyseal blood supply arises solely from the developing portal circulation; the adenohypophysis lacks an arterial blood supply. Vascularization of Rathke's pouch is evident by 8 weeks.[30, 166] The median eminence is distinguishable by 9 weeks.[268] An intact hypothalamohypophyseal portal system is demonstrable using perfusion techniques by 11.5 weeks of gestational age, the youngest fetus studied,[532] and may well be present earlier. This observation indicates that in the human fetus, vascular connections between the median eminence of the hypothalamus (the site of the primary capillary plexus) and the anterior lobe of the pituitary gland (the site of the secondary capillary plexus) are linked by the portal venous channels by at least 11.5 weeks of gestation. Thus, by 0.3 gestation, the three components of the portal system are present, and the CNS and the fetal adenohypophysis are linked by a private vascular conduit. The capillary tufts of the primary and secondary plexus increase in number and by 28 weeks are numerous; portal trunks are well delineated by 13 weeks. Further, the hypothalamo-hypophyseal portal system may be functional before morphologic differentiation has occurred. Indeed, in the ovine fetus, an intact portal system is demonstrable by at least 48 days of gestation[348] (term is at 147 days), a fetal age that appears to coincide with or even precede release of hypothalamic neuropeptides at the median eminence.[210, 231, 290]

Immunocytochemical studies demonstrate that by 16 weeks or earlier, LRF, CRF, and somatostatin neurons within the human fetal hypothalamus terminate in the external layer of the median eminence in contact with capillary tufts of the primary plexus.

NEUROSECRETIONS AND NEUROTRANSMITTERS OF THE FETAL HYPOTHALAMUS

Biogenic Amines and Neuromodulators

The tuberohypophyseal neurons are the *final common pathway* of neural control of the anterior pituitary gland. These neurons are acted on by neurotransmitters (mainly biogenic amines but including excitatory amino acids such as glutamate and aspartate and the inhibitory amino acid gamma-aminobutyric acid [GABA]); neuromodulators, including a wide variety of brain peptides; circulating hormones of peripheral endocrine glands through feedback mechanisms; and even certain pituitary

peptide hormones acting through paracrine mechanisms.

Central biogenic amine pathways form a complex system. Of concern here are those pathways acting on the tuberohypophyseal neurons. The noradrenergic, adrenergic, and serotoninergic neurons originate in the midbrain as well as other CNS sites and are the origin of fibers containing these neurotransmitters in the hypothalamus and median eminence. In contrast, the dopaminergic neurons that affect anterior pituitary hormone secretions mainly arise in the arcuate nucleus of the hypothalamus and project fibers to the median eminence. The tuberohypophyseal dopamine pathway, for example, is the major inhibitory regulator of prolactin secretion.[304, 340] The majority of other dopaminergic neuronal tracts have their origin in the midbrain. The hypothalamic tuberohypophyseal dopaminergic neurons differ from other central dopaminergic systems in that they contain prolactin receptors but lack dopamine receptors.

Limited information is available on the ontogeny of neurotransmitter mechanisms in the human hypothalamus. In the rhesus monkey, brain stem monoamine neurons differentiate and send out fiber projections during the early fetal period (0.25 gestation).[315] A remarkable development of the human fetal catecholamine and serotonin neurotransmitter systems occurs between the seventh and 23rd weeks of gestation.[278, 389, 396, 434, 523] Dopamine, norepinephrine, serotonin, and 5-hydroxyindole acetic acid are present in the human fetal hypothalamus by 10 to 13 weeks.[195, 268]

In addition, evidence for the presence of other neurotransmitters and neuromodulators in the human fetal hypothalamus has been reported, including immunoreactive substance P;[413] endogenous opioids;[314, 448] the cholecystokinin/gastrin family;[151] and the main inhibitory neurotransmitter in the mammalian CNS, as reflected by its metabolite gamma-hydroxybutyric acid.[278, 506]

That these neurotransmitter and neuromodulator pathways may influence the function of the fetal hypothalamic hypophysiotropic neurosecretory neurons during the second half of gestation is well illustrated, for example, by studies in the chronic instrumented ovine fetus and the effect of stress on pituitary hormone secretion in the human fetus.[124, 210, 231]

TABLE 12–2. Studies on the Ontogeny of Hypothalamic Luteinizing Hormone–Releasing Factor

Investigator	Method	No. of Fetuses Studied	Gestational Age Range (weeks)	LRF Content ng/Hypo-thalamus	LRF Concentration pg/mg	Age First Detected (weeks)	Comment
Levina, 1970	Bioassay	28	19–40			19(F) 24(M)	
Minkina & Blushtein, 1973	Bioassay of acetone-HCl extract	39	13–32			13*	
Gilmore et al, 1978	Bioassay of HCl extract	16	11–21			11*	No relationship to gestational age
Bugnon et al, 1976, 1977	Immunocytochemistry	14	10–40			13	
Winters et al, 1974	RIA of methanolic whole brain extract	5	4.5–11		0.4–1.9	4.5*	Whole brain extract assayed
	RIA of methanolic hypothalamic extract	10	8–22		3.8–65.8	8*	No relationship to gestational age
{Kaplan & Grumbach, 1976 {Aubert et al, 1977	RIA of acetone/acetic acid extract	44	11–22	0–20(M) 0–3.2(F)	0.13(M) 0–6.5(F)	11*	No relationship to sex or gestational age
Aksel & Tyrey, 1977	RIA of methanolic extract	20	15–20		0.2–29.7(M) 0.12–22.8(F) 0.6–11.8	6 11* 14*	No sex difference, tend to rise with gestational age
Gilmore et al, 1978	RIA of HCl extract	8	11–19	11–23.3	20–97	14*	Maximum content in females at 22–25 weeks, in males at 34–38 weeks. In both sexes, concentration decreases with age
Siler-Khodr & Khodr, 1978	RIA of acetone/NaHCO₃ extract	45	14–38				

Present in youngest sample examined.
M = male; F = female; RIA = radioimmunoassay.

Hypothalamic Hypophysiotropic Factors

As discussed earlier, adenohypophyseal secretion is regulated by specific hypothalamic releasing or inhibitory factors. The chemical structure, biosynthesis, and action of the classic hypothalamic hypophysiotropic factors has been established and their pituitary receptors characterized. More recently, the genomic DNA structure for each of the factors and their receptors is known, and the regulation of gene expression, hormone biosynthesis, and secretion has become an exciting area of research.[462] The peptide factors arise from the posttranslational processing of prohormones.

Dopamine, secreted by the hypothalamic dopaminergic tuberohypophyseal neurons, is the major prolactin-inhibiting factor and is released at the median eminence into the hypophyseal-portal circulation.[304, 340]

Luteinizing Hormone–Releasing Factor

LRF neurosecretory neurons arise in the olfactory placode and migrate to the embryonic hypothalamus (see Fig. 12–2)[484] (see the section on Hypothalamus). Biologically active and immunoreactive LRF has been detected in the fetal hypothalamus by a number of techniques (Table 12–2). LRF has been detected by radioimmunoassay in a whole fetal brain homogenate at 4.5 weeks.[561] In most studies, no correlation with fetal sex or gestation age before 22 weeks has been noted.[10, 33, 110, 194, 290, 561] Fetal sex differences, however, were detected late in gestation; the highest hypothalamic LRF content was found in the female between 22 and 25 weeks and in the male between 34 and 38 weeks.[496]

Immunohistochemical studies of the fetal hypothalamus have shown that the distribution of LRF-containing neurons is similar to that in the adult primate—mainly localized to the medial basal hypothalamus and the preoptic region. By 11 weeks' gestation, fibers that stain for LRF are present in the median eminence and terminate in contact with capillaries of the median eminence.[75] Most of the LRF in the fetal hypothalamus can be recovered by differential centrifugation in the synaptosomal fraction (the fraction representing the nerve terminals), thereby suggesting that LRF is available for neurosecretion.[408] Thus, regulation of the fetal gonadotrope by LRF is present by the end of the first trimester.

Growth Hormone–Releasing Factor

Immunoreactive fetal hypothalamic GRF neurosecretory neurons and fibers are present in the fetal hypothalamus by 18 weeks of gestational age; the intensity of staining increases with advancing fetal age but decreases at the time of birth.[82] Studies of fetal GH secretion in the human and ovine fetus, however, suggest that hypothalamic GRF is present and secreted into the hypophyseal portal circulation much earlier in gestation (see the section on Pituitary Growth Hormone). We emphasize the importance of the limitations of immunocytochemical techniques. A negative result does not indicate the absence of a hormone antigen, only that it is not detected by the antiserum or technique used. The rat and mouse placenta contain immunoreactive GRF that exhibits biologic activity by 13 days of gestation in the rat.[35, 363] Different untranslated 5' sequences in rodent placental and hypothalamic GRF cDNA suggest organ-specific regulation of GRF gene expression. A placental form of human GRF mRNA, however, has not been detected. Further, the concentration of plasma GRF in the mother during pregnancy, which arises mainly from extrahypothalamic sites, is similar to nonpregnant levels and does not differ from that in umbilical cord blood despite the high concentration of GH in cord blood.[351]

Somatostatin

Somatostatin, the tetradecapeptide found widely in the brain and gastrointestinal system, is released by the hypothalamus into the portal circulation to inhibit GH secretion. Somatotropin-release inhibiting factor (SRIF) is detectable by immunofluorescence in the fetal hypothalamus at 16 weeks[415] and by radioimmunoassay in both the human fetal cerebral cortex and the hypothalamus from the earliest gestation studied (11 weeks).[33] Between 11 and 22 weeks, the SRIF content and concentration in the hypothalamus are correlated with gestational age.[33, 290] The relative amount of the biologically active forms of somatostatin in the

fetal hypothalamus—SRIF 1–14 and 1–28—increases between 12 and 28 weeks of gestation in relation to larger somatostatin precursors.[5] Circulating somatostatin, arising mainly from fetal sources outside the CNS,[356, 446] is present in umbilical cord blood and in early infancy.[301, 472] Somatostatin can cross the human placenta, at least when the maternal-fetal gradient is high.[467]

Thyrotropin-Releasing Factor

This tripeptide, which stimulates both pituitary TSH and prolactin release, has been detected in the whole brain homogenate of a 4.5-week fetus.[561] TRF is present in the fetal hypothalamus in substantial amounts between 8 and 22 weeks of gestation but shows no relationship to gestational age over this period.[33, 290] It can also be detected in other parts of the brain[33, 290, 361, 561] and the pancreas.[307, 446] Fetal pancreatic TRF colocalizes with insulin in B cells; it is present in high concentration in the fetal pancreas at 6 to 8 weeks of gestation and falls to relatively low levels after the 12th week.[307] The placenta contains TRF and TRF-like peptides. The fetal hypothalamus before 16 weeks may contain prolactin-releasing activity other than TRF.[361]

The high immunoreactive TRF concentrations in umbilical cord blood are mainly derived from extrahypothalamic sources,[324] and the levels decrease a few days after birth. TRF degrading activity, low in cord blood, increases within the first week.[23] TRF is transferred across the placenta.[377]

Corticotropin-Releasing Factor

Immunoreactive and bioactive CRF is detectable in the fetal hypothalamus as early as the 12th week of gestation.[6] In addition, a high-molecular-weight form of CRF (approximately 9000) is present until about 20 weeks. Immunoreactive fibers are at the median eminence by 16 weeks, and perikaryons are readily detectable by 19 weeks of gestation.[83, 93, 94] CRF neurons sending fibers to the median eminence arise mainly from parvocellular neurons in the paraventricular nucleus. Arginine vasopressin also is found in the fetal hypothalamus and colocalizes with CRF in some neurons. It has a synergistic action with CRF on the release of ACTH from human fetal pituitary glands in culture by at least 14 weeks of gestation.[76]

The placenta as well as the hypothalamus is a major source of CRF in pregnancy, and placental CRF mRNA is expressed by 7 weeks of gestation, mainly in the cytotrophoblast and intermediate trophoblast. In addition to a form identical to hypothalamic CRF, two higher molecular weight placental CRFs have been identified, neither of which stimulate ACTH release from the rat pituitary.[102, 458, 459, 476] The concentration of circulating CRF increases in the mother and fetus with advancing gestation, and the increase correlates with the concentration of placental CRF mRNA, amniotic fluid CRF, and the placental content of CRF but not with maternal or fetal concentrations of plasma ACTH or β-endorphin. Maternal plasma concentrations of CRF fall to nonpregnant values within the first day postpartum. CRF levels in fetal plasma are less (approximately 50%) than in maternal plasma. Placental CRF is not the principal regulator of maternal or fetal ACTH secretion.[157, 220] CRF circulates bound (approximately 90%) to a 37-kd CRF-binding protein[402] during pregnancy, which is synthesized by the placenta, mainly the syncytial layer of placental villi, fetal membranes, natural decidua, and the liver and brain. This binding protein increases in the mother during late pregnancy as well as in the fetus, where it may serve to protect the mother and fetus from the biologic effects of the placental CRF.[321, 475] Most of the placental CRF is secreted as a CRF-CRF-BP complex; evidence suggests that placental CRF-BP may regulate CRF through a paracrine mechanism.

ONTOGENY OF ADENOHYPOPHYSEAL HORMONES

It is necessary to be aware of the limitations of interpretation of observations made on the human fetus, in which most samples have been obtained after delivery or abortion.[199, 201, 210, 229, 290] More recently, a few data have become available from healthy fetuses by fetal blood sampling. Nevertheless, good agreement with studies in experimental animals has generally been noted. The pattern of differentiation of hormone-producing cells in the human fetal anterior pituitary by electron microscopy and ultrastructural immunochemistry has been reviewed.[28]

Growth Hormone

Pituitary Growth Hormone

Acidophils are first detectable histologically between 9 and 12 weeks,[166, 416, 417] and characteristic somatotropes with secretory granules are obvious by 12 weeks.[153, 316] There follows a rapid increase in the number of somatotropes within the gland through the remainder of gestation.[25, 36, 403] A proportion of GH-secreting cells in the fetal pituitary secrete both GH and prolactin (somatomammotropes), and these cells appear to be the precursor cell for lactotrope formation.[28, 180, 382, 545]

Immunoreactive GH is detectable in the fetal anterior pituitary between 7 and 9 weeks of gestation.[29, 55, 344, 416] The concentration of GH and of its mRNA[290, 293, 515] in the pituitary rises rapidly from 10 to 14 weeks and is maximal between 25 and 29 weeks; thereafter, it is constant to term[290, 293] (Fig. 12–8).

Although the human fetal pituitary at 5 weeks is primitive, fetal pituitary glands in culture at this stage secrete GH;[435, 498] the secretory capacity of the gland in culture increases with advancing age.[196] Thus, the capacity of the pituitary to secrete GH is present well before differentiation of the hypothalamic-adenohypophyseal portal system. Evidence indicates that the ability of the pituitary to initiate secretion of GH depends on the transcription factor Pit-1 discussed earlier[545] and that the development of the somatotrope, at least in vitro, is influenced by cortisol, thyroid hormone, and IGF-1.[252]

Plasma Growth Hormone

GH can be detected in fetal plasma by 70 days of gestation;[293] its concentration rises from 50 ng/mL at 10 to 14 weeks' gestation to a peak of 150 at 20 to 24 weeks then falls rapidly (Fig. 12–9). These values, which were originally obtained from abortuses, have been confirmed by fetal blood sampling.[257, 473]

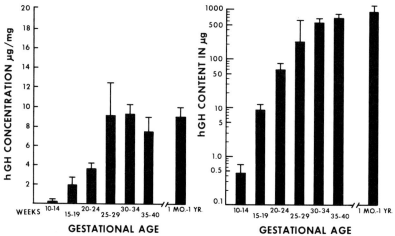

FIGURE 12–8. The mean (±SEM) concentration (*left panel*) and content (*right panel*) of hGH in pituitary glands of fetuses 68 days to term (plotted at 5-week intervals) and in infants aged 1 month to 1 year. The graph on the left indicates hGH in micrograms per milligram of pituitary gland on a linear scale; on the right, as hGH content in micrograms per pituitary gland on a semilogarithmic scale. The marked rise in glandular content and concentration of hGH between 20 and 30 weeks coincides with the fall in plasma GH concentrations (see Fig. 12–9), suggesting the development of inhibitory influences over GH release in the fetal hypothalamic-pituitary unit in this period of gestation. (From Kaplan SL, Grumbach MM, Shepard TH. The ontogenesis of human fetal hormones. I. Growth hormone and insulin. J Clin Invest 1972; 51:3080.)

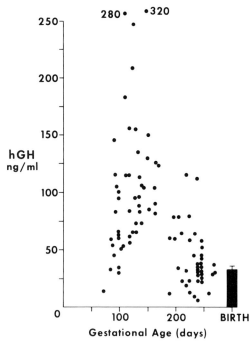

FIGURE 12–9. The concentration of hGH (ng/mL) in fetal serum is shown for the gestational period of 68 days to 260 days and in umbilical venous serum at delivery. (From Kaplan SL, Grumbach MM, Aubert M. The ontogenesis of pituitary hormones and hypothalamic factors in the human fetus: maturation of central nervous system regulation of anterior pituitary function. Recent Prog Horm Res 1976; 32:161; and Kaplan SL, Grumbach MM, Shepard TH. The ontogenesis of human fetal hormones. I. Growth hormone and insulin. J Clin Invest 1972; 51:3080.)

In experimental animals, in which multiple sampling is possible, fetal GH levels show marked pulsatility with exaggerated amplitude pulses and high interpulse nadirs,[12, 46] and the pulsatile secretion of GH and prolactin and of GH, LH, and FSH are temporarily coupled as shown by a significant number of coincident pulses.[12] The metabolic clearance rate of GH in preterm infants or in experimental animals is not different from that in the adult,[120, 438] and it seems unlikely that altered clearance is a major factor in the high fetal GH concentrations.

In cord blood at term, GH concentrations are 30 to 50 ng/mL[293, 386] (see Fig. 12–9). The premature and full-term neonate also has a high secretory rate for GH and exhibits striking pulsatile GH secretion with an increased pulse frequency and an elevated pulse amplitude—not due to decreased clearance of GH.[144, 570] The pattern of pulsatile secretion was unrelated to sleep.[570] At all times in gestation, fetal concentrations of plasma GH are much higher than maternal concentrations.[290] Maternal plasma pituitary GH levels are suppressed, especially in late gestation,[295] presumably by placental variant GH (hGH-V)[147, 177] and chorionic somatomammotropin.[295] There is no evidence of significant placental transfer of hGH,[197, 306] and hGH-V has not been detected in the fetal circulation.[177, 178] GRF does not stimulate hGH-V secretion, nor is it transferred across the placenta.[147]

The concentration of circulating GH-binding protein[48] is low in fetal blood, reflecting the lower levels of expression of GH receptor in fetal tissues.[129, 342] Consequently, less circulating GH is found in high-molecular-weight forms.

Regulation of Growth Hormone Secretion

In the adult, GH is under dual control by two hypothalamic factors: a hypothalamic-releasing hormone (GRF), a 44 amino acid peptide, which stimulates growth of the somatotrope as well as the synthesis and secretion of GH, and an inhibitory factor, somatostatin (SRIF), which is a tetradecapeptide. Hypothalamic GRF and somatostatin neurons have bidirectional synaptic connections that may serve to integrate their GH regulatory actions. These factors are modulated in turn by various biogenic amine systems, including adrenergic, serotoninergic, cholinergic, and dopaminergic pathways within the hypothalamus.[210] Although other brain peptides, including vasopressin, TRF, β-endorphin, enkephalin, substance P, and neurotensin, stimulate GH release, their physiologic significance is unclear.

Important questions concerning GH secretion in the fetus are: Why are the plasma concentrations so high? Why does pituitary secretion diminish in the second half of gestation despite rising pituitary content?

The onset of GH synthesis and secretion may be independent of hypothalamic influences, and the high concentration of plasma GH seen early in gestation may represent autonomous secretion by the pituitary gland. Alternatively, the pituitary may be regulated by hypothalamic GRF—this is certainly the case by midgestation. GRF could stimulate pituitary GH secretion via the portal system, which is established at least by 11.5 weeks' gestation, or earlier in gestation by this route, by simple diffusion from the hypothalamus to the adenohypophysis, or via the mantle plexus.[210, 290] As midgestation approaches, this unrestrained secretion of GRF and the relative resistance of

the somatotrope to SRIF lead to intensive stimulation of GH secretion and an increase in somatotropes. Further, the neonate exhibits a striking increase in GH release elicited by GRF[132, 492] but a blunted response to somatostatin.[133, 467]

There is now considerable evidence to suggest that the primary reason fetal GH levels are high in midgestation and late gestation is an immaturity within the somatotrope that leaves it relatively defective in its response to inhibitory control and partially resistant to somatostatin in particular.[142, 202, 206, 210, 217] Experimental and clinical studies clearly show that fetal GH secretion depends on fetal hypothalamic GRF secretion.[200, 210, 290] Infusion of somatostatin or agents that stimulate somatostatin release, however, only partially inhibit fetal GH release.[202, 206, 217] Initially somatostatin does not inhibit the fetal GH response to GRF. As gestation advances, however, the inhibitory action of somatostatin on the effect of GRF increases, and soon after birth, somatostatin effectively blocks the GH-releasing action of GRF.[142] Somatostatin acts via an inhibitory G (Gi) protein-linked receptor. Presumably it is the gradual maturation of one or more components of this inhibitory control system that is associated with the progressive reduction in GH secretion late in gestation. A similar mechanism involving the Gi protein system has been proposed for the lack of desensitization of the fetal Leydig cell to unrestrained hCG stimulation (see the section on Role of Fetal Gonadotropins). The rise in plasma glucocorticoids in late gestation may contribute to this change in sensitivity to somatostatin.[326]

Studies using dispersed ovine pituitary cells[501] and explant cultures of human fetal pituitary glands (9 to 19 weeks of gestation)[223, 224] support the in vivo observations in the ovine fetus on the predominant effect of GRF on the secretion of GH over that of somatostatin. Beginning as early as the ninth week, GRF stimulated GH release in a dose-related manner, indicating the presence of functional GRF receptors on the human somatotrope, and the GH response increased with advancing fetal age. The inhibitory effect of somatostatin on basal GH secretion, slight initially, increased from early to midgestation,[223] consistent with the in vivo studies in the ovine fetus. Further, evidence was obtained of an age-related increase in the stimulatory G protein–dependent signal transduction system induced by GRF in the fetal somatotrope; although Ca^{++} influx (another signal transduction pathway) was essential for GH release, no age-related change was detected. The inhibitory effect of somatostatin appeared to be mediated through an inhibitory G protein pathway.[224] Hence there is evidence of early maturation of at least one system of the GRF-induced signaling machine, whereas developmental changes in the maturation of the somatostatin-evoked signal transduction system are poorly understood.

Other factors are involved in the regulation of GH secretion. Circulating IGF-1 levels in the fetus are low, rising in late gestation.[208, 473] The ability of the fetal pituitary to respond to IGF-1 as reflected by suppression of GH secretion appears to mature relatively late,[71, 141] and it may be that this contributes to defective negative feedback on GH secretion. In addition, the GH receptor in most tissues is in lower concentration than postnatally and matures late in fetal life.[209, 299] Although the development of the GH receptor in the hypothalamic-pituitary unit has not been studied, immaturity of the receptor at this level might lead to defective shortloop feedback.

One factor that plays some role in the perinatal changes in GH secretion is the onset of nonshivering thermogenesis after umbilical cord separation. Free fatty acids inhibit the actions of GRF. The rise in free fatty acids after birth when thermogenesis is initiated clearly explains the initial fall in GH seen at birth in some experimental animals.[39]

Although there is ample evidence of neurotransmitter-mediated regulation of GH secretion in utero,[200, 206, 210] there is also evidence of immaturity of integrated hypothalamic regulation.[199, 206, 207, 210, 230, 286, 290] For example, GH is poorly suppressible by glucose in the neonate[120, 452, 510] but is suppressible by 1 month of age.[120] A paradoxic GH response to L-dopa, a blunted response to somatostatin, and increased GH release by TRF have also been reported in the neonate.[133] Further evidence for immaturity of hypothalamic integration is the lack of a sleep-associated rise of GH in the neonate,[168, 570] which does not develop until the third postnatal month.

There is evidence of homeostatic regulation of GH in fetal life.[146] Under conditions of undernutrition, GH levels both in the fetus[146, 473] and at birth are elevated.[132, 145, 185] By midgestation, the human fetus is able to respond to the stress of delivery with an increase in plasma GH.[540] Exogenous glucocorticoids suppress GH release in the fetus by 28 weeks, but it is uncertain whether this suppression is at the level of the hypothalamus or pituitary gland or both.[41]

Thyroid hormone affects GH gene transcription. The neonate with congenital hypothyroidism exhibits decreased GH secretion.[148]

Role of Growth Hormone in the Fetus

A definitive function for GH in the fetus has not been established. Transgenic mice and rats expressing the GH gene are normal size at birth and do not exhibit excessive growth until after 14 days of age.[406, 551] The evidence regarding the role of GH in human fetal growth is based on naturally occurring developmental defects. Although it has generally been considered that it is not essential to normal fetal growth,[154, 319] evidence has shown that GH does play a modest role in regulating linear growth in utero.[211, 564] Infants with neonatal GH deficiency have a reduced birth length by about 0.5 to 1.5 SD and are relatively heavy for length, being of normal birth weight.[14, 211, 564] The birth length was 0.8 SD below the mean value and the birth weight -0.3 SD in 220 children in whom the diagnosis of idiopathic GH deficiency was made in infancy or childhood, compared with a well-matched group of normal newborn infants.[14] The growth of anencephalic fetuses is not greatly retarded, but interpretation is difficult because pituitary tissue is always present, and often there are other anomalies.[319]

GH receptors are present in fetal tissues, including the liver and musculoskeletal tissues.[256, 557] In the liver, however, the concentration of mRNA coding for the GH receptor[299] and the degree of GH binding[209] is much less than in the postnatal period, thus providing a physiologic explanation for the relatively small effect of fetal GH on the IGFs[512] and on skeletal growth in utero. In the human fetus, however, there is a relatively high concentration of mRNA coding for the GH receptor in extrahepatic sites, including growth plate chondrocytes and osteoblasts, fetal skin, gastrointestinal tract, brain, and lung.[256, 556, 557]

The role of GH receptors in fetal tissues and the biologic effects mediated by these receptors are somewhat speculative. Although GH receptor transcripts are low in the fetal liver, GH receptors seem more prevalent in many other human fetal tissues. In addition, the correlation of growth with GH receptor concentration is uncertain; the circulating high-affinity, GH-binding protein derived from the human GH receptor, which appears to correlate with the expression of tissue GH receptors, is low in umbilical cord blood and in infancy[129, 260, 342, 365] at a time in development of rapid growth. The concentration of plasma GH-binding protein does not correlate with growth in infancy.

There is evidence that GH has a role in the regulation of fetal metabolism.[146] It plays a part in the development and function of the pancreatic islet cells.[519] GH stimulates the expression of the insulin gene in human fetal pancreatic islets in vitro obtained between 10 and 20 weeks of gestation[172] and the growth of differentiated B cells.[388] Hypoglycemia is well recognized in neonatal GH deficiency,[222, 325] and hepatic glycogen deposition is reduced. In experimental hypopituitarism, fetal insulin to glucose ratios are abnormal.[410]

Understanding the function of the GH receptor in utero is made more complex by a consideration of the potential role of placental hGH-V and chorionic somatomammotropin (placental lactogen) (hPL). In contrast to hGH-V,[177] the latter is secreted also into the fetal circulation.[232, 293] If there is a deletion involving the hPL genes or the hGH-V gene or both genes, the placenta may have the capacity to secrete a modified chimeric hGH or hGH-V into the maternal circulation.[177, 179] It is not clear whether the same occurs in the fetal compartment. Because hGH-V and perhaps hPL can bind to the GH receptor, neither clinical observation nor current experimental approaches have resolved the relative role of each of these somatogens in utero.

Insulin-like Growth Factors

The IGFs are evolutionarily related to insulin. IGF-1 is the primary mediator of the actions of GH on skeletal growth and anabolism. IGF-1 acts via both the endocrine route, secondary to hepatic secretion, and the paracrine route in tissues such as placenta, muscle, and the growth plate. The role of IGF-2 postnatally is less certain because it has weaker anabolic and somatogenic actions than IGF-1. Both IGFs circulate in association with six specific binding proteins, each of which has different endocrine or metabolic regulation.[49] The binding proteins are also found throughout tissues and may modulate the action of IGFs in both positive and negative manners. They may also act to target IGFs to specific sites of action.[259] As well as GH, the IGFs are influenced by other hormones, including glucocorticoids, thyroid hormones, and insulin. There are two classes of IGF receptor. The type 1 receptor is structurally related to the insulin receptor and is the receptor through which IGF-1 and IGF-2 exert insulin-like and somatogenic actions. The type 2 receptor is also the mannose-6-phosphate (M6P) receptor. The significance of the type 2 receptor with respect to IGF-2 is not certain, but it may be a clearance receptor. Interestingly in fetal life, a significant amount of type 2 receptor is cleaved from the cell membrane and circulates as a binding protein—it may bind as much as 40% of circulating IGF-2 in fetal life.[189, 254]

There is ample evidence that the IGFs play an important role in fetal development—it is less certain to what extent they are regulated by fetal GH.[210, 218, 512] The mRNAs for IGF-1 and IGF-2 can be detected in preimplantation blastocysts. Essentially all fetal tissues express both IGF-1 and IGF-2. In the ovine and rat fetus, the expression of IGF-2 mRNA is high in fetal life compared with postnatal life, whereas the expression of IGF-1 is lower.[7, 52, 87, 241, 330] Postnatally in these species, there is a switch to increased IGF-1 and decreased IGF-2 in the neonatal period. The placenta is also rich in both IGF-1 and IGF-2 mRNAs. Transgenic mice with disrupted alleles for IGF-2 show embryonic growth retardation, suggesting the constitutive importance of IGF-2 to fetal growth in this mammal.[131] In the human fetus, however, the concentrations of both plasma IGF-1 and IGF-2 are low until late in the last trimester, when they increase until term. A major switch in the ratio of IGF-2 to IGF-1 between fetal and neonatal life does not appear to occur in the human.[307]

More is known of the role of IGF-1 in late gestation fetal growth. There is in a variety of species, including the human, a good correlation between fetal size, gestational age, skeletal age, placental weight, and fetal chorionic somatomammotropin and circulating IGF-1 levels in fetal or cord blood.[63, 201, 212, 213, 309] Fetal mice expressing high levels of IGF-1 grow larger than those expressing low levels of IGF-1.[216] Infusions of IGF-1 into the fetal circulation in sheep show IGF-1 to be anticatabolic and to alter placental metabolism to favor fetal growth.[203] Fetal IGF-1 is clearly regulated by glucose availability perhaps mediated by insulin release.[47] Because placental function is the major determinant of fetal growth in late gestation, it is not surprising that IGF-1 should be under nutritional regulation.[203, 405] There is also evidence that the fetal IGF binding proteins are regulated in an analogous manner postnatally[49] with undernutrition leading to an elevation in binding protein 1 and 2 (the dominant fetal binding protein) and a reduction in binding protein 3 (the primary GH-dependent binding protein.[186, 404] Experimental observations in sheep[210, 368] and clinical observations suggest that IGF-1 is somewhat GH dependent in utero. In the GH insensitivity syndrome (Laron type dwarfism), caused by a mutation in GH receptor,[17, 64] birth length[305] and IGF-1 levels are reduced from birth.

Prolactin

Pituitary Prolactin

Prolactin secretion by the fetal pituitary develops later than does GH secretion. Lactotropes also depend on pit-1 for differentiation and prolactin gene expression. Lactotropes appear to be derived from a stem cell somatotrope (see the section on Gene Regulation of Pituitary Cell-Specific Differentiation). The development of the lactotrope in vitro is influenced by the α-glycoprotein hormone subunit.[59, 545] Radioimmunoassayable prolactin is detected in the fetal pituitary between 9 and 12 weeks.[29, 32] Pituitary prolactin content is low before 15 weeks, but between 15 and 23 weeks, mRNA levels and the pituitary content and

concentration of prolactin increase rapidly[290, 514] (Fig. 12–10). By this age, lactotropes are clearly detectable.[28, 29, 58] After 23 weeks, prolactin content increases slowly, and the concentration of pituitary prolactin remains rather constant and similar to that of the infant.[32] There may be a greater proportion of glycosylated prolactin in fetal life.[503]

Fetal pituitaries in vitro release prolactin into the culture media;[411] prolactin can be detected in the media of cultures obtained from embryos as early as 5 weeks of gestation. There is an increase in releasable prolactin in vitro as gestational age advances.[498]

Plasma Prolactin

Prolactin is present in fetal plasma by at least 12 weeks.[32, 290] Between 11 and 20 weeks, prolactin concentrations show little change (mean 20 ng/mL), but there is a sharp rise after 30 weeks, which is maintained until term.[32, 109, 560] The mean prolactin concentration in umbili-

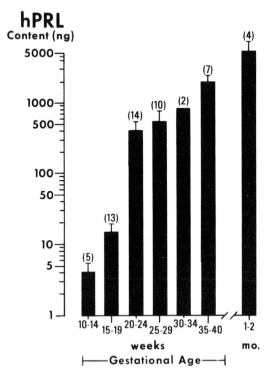

FIGURE 12–10. The content (mean ±SE) of hPRL in nanograms in the fetal pituitary plotted at 5-week intervals during gestation and for postnatal ages 1 to 2 months. (From Aubert ML, Grumbach MM, Kaplan SL. The ontogenesis of human fetal hormones. III. Prolactin. J Clin Invest 1975; 56:155.)

cal cord blood at term is 150 ng/mL.[32] Umbilical cord blood prolactin is usually greater than maternal concentrations, which also rise in late gestation[32, 244, 480] (Fig. 12–11). It has been suggested that there may be a diurnal rhythm in umbilical cord prolactin concentrations,[34] as is reported in the fetal sheep.[45, 359, 360, 543] Neonatal prolactin concentrations remain relatively high[31, 237, 517] for 2 to 3 months after birth. In contrast to the striking pulsatile pattern of GH secretion in the premature and full-term neonate, prolactin release in the neonate does not exhibit pulsatility.[144] The circu-

lating form of prolactin in the human fetus is predominantly monomeric, as in the adult.[290]

Regulation of Prolactin Secretion

Prolactin secretion in the adult is principally regulated by an inhibitory dopaminergic system.[304, 340] In addition, there are stimulatory mechanisms for prolactin secretion. The most important is TRF, which stimulates prolactin as well as TSH secretion. Estrogens, in addition to their mitogenic effect on lactotropes, also have a modulating action to increase prolactin secretion: They appear to act on several mechanisms affecting prolactin release at the level of both the pituitary gland and the hypothalamus,[32, 107, 210, 290, 304, 449] including stimulation of galanin synthesis and release by a population of lactotropes;[570a] galanin through a paracrine mechanism is critical in the regulation of basal and vasoactive intestinal polypeptide–stimulated prolactin release.

In the anencephalic fetus, concentrations of prolactin in cord blood are normal or near normal[32, 184, 230, 249, 560] (see Fig. 12–11). Thus, the hypothalamus is not essential in the fetus for the rise in prolactin secretion during gestation, and this is confirmed experimentally; it occurs independent of hypothalamic drive. In late gestation, levels of prolactin are higher than in normal postnatal life. It has been hypothesized that the principal influence on fetal concentrations of prolactin is circulating estrogen in the fetus.[32, 210, 379] Estrogens, particularly 17β-estradiol,[493] increase in parallel with rising fetal concentrations of prolactin in late gestation[32, 184, 210] (see Fig. 13–9) after an initial 3- to 4-week lag in the increase in prolactin.[32]

It is unlikely that immaturity of the inhibitory dopaminergic system is the cause of the high perinatal prolactin concentrations. In the fetal sheep, for example, tonic dopaminergic suppression of prolactin secretion is demonstrable even before the late gestation rise in plasma prolactin.[215] In the human, treatment of the pregnant mother with bromocriptine (a dopaminergic agonist) suppresses both maternal and fetal prolactin, suggesting that dopamine receptors are present in the human fetal pituitary gland.[135, 468] The human neonate responds to TRF with a rise in prolactin concentration,[134] and in the sheep fetus, a prolactin

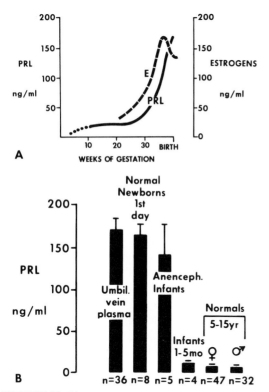

FIGURE 12–11. *A*, Comparison of the pattern of change of fetal plasma hPRL (solid line) and unconjugated estrogens (E) (broken line) during gestation. Estrogen data derived from Shutt DA, Smith ID, and Shearman RP. Oestrone, oestradiol-17β and oestriol levels in human foetal plasma during gestation and at term. J Endocrinol 1974; 60:333, and prolactin data from Aubert ML, Grumbach MM, and Kaplan SL. The ontogenesis of human fetal hormones. III. Prolactin. J Clin Invest 1975; 56:155. *B*, Plasma concentrations of PRL in normal and anencephalic newborns are compared with those of normal children and infants. The concentrations of PRL in anencephaly are similar to those in the normal infant, suggesting that the hypothalamus is not essential to maintain fetal PRL secretion. (From Aubert ML, Grumbach MM, Kaplan SL. The ontogenesis of human fetal hormones. III. Prolactin. J Clin Invest 1975; 56:155.)

response to TRF is present before the sharp rise in plasma prolactin in late gestation.[533] TRF crosses the human placenta and can stimulate fetal prolactin and thyroid hormone release.[377]

Prolactin in Amniotic Fluid

A variety of prolactin-like substances are produced by the uterus, fetal membranes, and placenta, but there are marked species differences.[507] In the human, prolactin is detectable in amniotic fluid in low concentrations at 8 weeks. Concentrations are highest at 15 to 17 weeks (1300 ng/mL) and gradually decline in the second half of gestation to 450 ng/mL[109, 480, 541] (Fig. 12–12). Amniotic fluid prolactin is indistinguishable from pituitary prolactin[61] and is primarily of decidual origin.[243, 251] In contrast to fetal and maternal serum prolactin, amniotic prolactin has been normal in instances in which the pregnant mother has been treated throughout pregnancy with dopaminergic agonists, such as bromocriptine.[135] Decidual prolactin release appears to be controlled by various local factors, including a peptidergic releasing factor, lipocortin-1, relaxin, and insulin.[242, 243] The function of amniotic prolactin is unclear. Because prolactin has an important osmoregulatory function in lower vertebrates, it has been suggested that it plays some part in regulating amniotic fluid volume.[279]

Role of Prolactin in the Fetus

As with GH, no definitive role for prolactin in the fetus has been established. There is in-

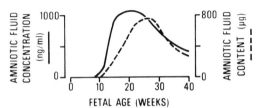

FIGURE 12–12. The pattern of amniotic fluid PRL content (broken line) and concentration (solid line) in human pregnancy. The rapid rise in PRL content and concentration in amniotic fluid at 10 to 20 weeks precedes the rise in fetal or maternal circulating PRL concentrations. (Modified from Studies on human sexual development. IV. Fetal pituitary and serum and amniotic fluid concentrations of prolactin. Clements JA, Reyes FI, Winter JSD, Faiman CJK. J Clin Endocrinol Metab 1977; 44:408.)

creasing evidence that prolactin has an effect on lung maturation. This hypothesis was based on, first, the temporal association between fetal prolactin concentrations and amniotic fluid surfactant content and, second, the association of low cord concentrations of prolactin with the occurrence of the respiratory distress syndrome.[205, 247] In hypophysectomized fetal lambs, replaced with various mixes of hormones, the combination of glucocorticoids, thyroxine, and prolactin was necessary to achieve maximal lung maturation.[479] Because maternally administered TRF crosses the placenta to release both thyroid hormone and PRL,[377] clinical trials have begun and suggest that prolactin does have a role in lung maturation. Osmotic influences can experimentally affect fetal prolactin release.[167] It has also been suggested that prolactin may play a role in perinatal sodium homeostasis.[160]

Luteinizing Hormone and Follicle-Stimulating Hormone

The glycoprotein hormones are composed of two noncovalently linked subunits: an α subunit, which has a similar amino acid sequence in FSH, LH, hCG, and TSH, and a β subunit, which confers immunologic and biologic specificity to each hormone. In the human, the α and β subunits for LH and FSH are synthesized in the same gonadotrope. LRF increases the expression of α-, LHβ-, and FSHβ-subunit transcripts. The formation of the β subunit limits the rate of biosynthesis of intact glycoprotein hormones. Descriptions of the ontogeny of pituitary FSH and LH are confounded by differences in assay specificity and sensitivity and by cross reaction in some immunoassay systems with the free α-glycoprotein subunit.

Pituitary Gonadotropins

GLYCOPROTEIN HORMONE SUBUNITS. It has been suggested that the initial secretion by the fetal pituitary may be limited to the α subunit alone[92, 152, 175, 238, 239, 290, 291, 412] rather than to the intact gonadotropin. Nevertheless, fetal pituitaries in culture can secrete intact LH as early as 5 to 7 weeks of gestation,[227, 435, 498] and intact LH has been detected in the fetal pituitary gland by 10 weeks.[286] Thus, although during early gestation the dominant glycoprotein fraction in the pituitary is α subunit, it is likely that at least small amounts of intact glycoprotein hormones are synthesized.[239, 291] Determination of the α subunit content of the pituitary, however, cannot determine the origin of the α subunit measured (α-LH, α-FSH, or α-TSH). The ratio of immunoreactive α subunit to intact LH is higher in pituitaries of less than 16 weeks' gestation and falls thereafter.[238, 239, 290, 291] In midgestation, α subunit is still the major glycoprotein component in the fetal pituitary.[286, 290, 291] The synthesis of intact LH and FSH is primarily determined by the rate of synthesis of β subunits.[290, 291] Only a small amount of free β subunit is detectable in either the fetal[412] or adult pituitary.

LUTEINIZING HORMONE AND FOLLI-CLE-STIMULATING HORMONE. With a variety of techniques, LH has been detected in the fetal pituitary by 10 weeks' gestation. The human fetal pituitary in culture secretes LH as early as 5 to 7 weeks.[226, 435, 498] Several studies have demonstrated sexual dimorphism, with higher pituitary LH content occurring in the female than in the male fetus (Table 12–3).

Using a radioimmunoassay that did not cross react with hCG, LH was detectable in fetal pituitaries of both sexes by 10 weeks' gestation. The content of LH in pituitary glands from both male and female fetuses rose sharply between 10 and 27 weeks with little change thereafter; however, LH content was higher in females between 10 and 29 weeks. The concentration of pituitary LH also rose to higher levels in the female, with the highest LH concentrations at 15 to 19 weeks, in contrast to 20 to 24 weeks in the male[229, 230, 286, 290] (Fig. 12–13). This sexual dimorphism is likely to be related, at least in part, to the higher concentrations of plasma testosterone in the male fetus (see the section on Role of the Fetal Gonadotropins).

FSH has also been detected in the fetal pituitary by a variety of techniques as early as 10 weeks' gestation (Table 12–4). Radioimmunoassayable FSH has been detected in the pituitaries of both sexes by 70 days. The presence of a sexual dimorphism is similar to that for LH. The FSH to LH ratio is higher in female fetuses, but in both sexes there is a striking rise in FSH content between 10 and 25 weeks; FSH remains constant thereafter. The concentration of FSH, however, decreases in both the female and the male in late gestation. Both the pituitary concentration and the content of FSH are higher in the female than in the male fetus[108, 230, 286, 290] (Fig. 12–14).

Plasma Gonadotropins

LUTEINIZING HORMONE AND FOLLI-CLE-STIMULATING HORMONE. Earlier studies of plasma LH are difficult to interpret because hCG cross reacts with LH in many radioimmunoassays. The development of radioimmunoassays using anti-βLH subunit sera makes specific measurement of LH possible. Specific, highly sensitive assays detected LH in fetal plasma by 100 days' gestation, about the same time as it appears in the fetal pituitary. Higher concentrations are found in midgestation with lower levels toward term; in cord blood, LH values are low.[286, 290] Higher plasma concentrations have been reported in female fetuses between 12 and 20 weeks,[108] and we found a similar trend.[230, 286]

FSH has been detected by radioimmunoassay in fetal plasma by 10 to 11 weeks,[108, 230, 286, 290] which is comparable to the gestational age that FSH appears in the fetal pituitary gland. Plasma concentrations of FSH in the female fetus rise to a peak concentration between 20 and 29 weeks and fall to low concentrations in cord blood. In midgestation, the FSH levels are comparable to those in castrated adults and higher than LH concentrations in male and female fetuses.

In the male fetus, FSH follows a pattern similar to that in the female fetus, with highest concentrations in midgestation, which are, however, significantly lower than in female fetuses[229, 230, 286, 454, 522] (Fig. 12–15). Thus, the pattern of plasma concentration of FSH in fetuses of both sexes is similar to the changing pituitary concentration of FSH with advancing gestation and the number of gonadotropes that are immunoreactive for FSH.[290]

CORDOCENTESIS. The use of fetal blood sampling and highly sensitive, specific gonadotropin immunoassays, although largely confirming earlier studies, has provided valuable

TALE 12–3. Ontogeny of Luteinizing Hormone in the Fetal Pituitary

Investigator	Method	No. of Pituitaries Studied	Gestational Age (weeks)	First Detected (weeks)	Comment
Levina, 1968	Bioassay	148	11–40	13	From 19 to 28 weeks, content and concentration in F>M
Pasteels et al, 1974	Immunocyto-chemistry	—	—	10	
Dubois & Dubois, 1974	Immunocyto-chemistry	—	7–40	16F, 20M	
Baker & Jaffe, 1975	Immunocyto-chemistry	21	6–23	10.5	
Bugnon et al, 1977	Immunocyto-chemistry	20	6–26	15	
Groom et al, 1971	Organ culture (1–6 days)	13	8–18	8†	
Pierson et al, 1973	Organ culture (1–14 days)	12F, 14M	7–42	7†	
Siler-Khodr et al, 1974	Organ culture (20–109 days)	16F, 17M	5–38	5†	From 17 to 28 weeks, females released more LH than males
Pasteels et al, 1977	Organ culture (1–84 days)	7M	13–27	13†	
Grumbach & Kaplan, 1973, 1974 Kaplan & Grumbach, 1976	RIA*	79	10–40	10†	Females, maximum content at 25–29 weeks; males, maximum content at 35–40 weeks. Females have higher content than males at 10–29 weeks
Hagen & McNeilly, 1975, 1977	RIA*	20	9.5–32	9.5†	
Clements et al, 1976	RIA*	30	9.5–20	9.5†	Females have higher content than males at 12–20 weeks
Pasteels et al, 1977	RIA*	9M	13–27	13†	
Skebelskaya & Kuznetsova, 1978	RIA	29	8–34	8†	Maximum LH content in females at 19–20 weeks; maximum LH content in males at 24–28 weeks. LH content in females greater than males at 21–24 weeks

*Using a β-LH–specific method.
†LH present in the earliest sample available.
M = Male; F = female; RIA = radioimmunoassay.

new information on the pattern of change in both immunoreactive and bioactive gonadotropins and sex steroids in fetuses between 17 weeks and term.[54] The serum concentration of FSH and LH and of bioactive FSH were significantly higher in female than male fetuses at 17 to 24 weeks' gestation, and in both sexes, FSH and LH decreased strikingly between 25 to 40 weeks' gestation. Bioactive FSH, which was higher than immunoreactive FSH, however, remained elevated toward term and 50-fold to 100-fold greater than immunoreactive FSH but did not exhibit a sex difference.

Serum free testosterone levels at midgestation were lower in female than male fetuses. Curiously and in contrast to earlier studies, the concentration of serum free testosterone was higher at 35 to 40 weeks in both sexes than at midgestation, and there was no sex difference.

Highly specific radioimmunoassays were used to study serum levels of FSH and LH in samples of umbilical cord blood obtained at birth from 112 fetuses between 26 and 40 weeks' gestation.[341] The mean concentration of serum FSH and LH was elevated at the beginning of the third trimester and fell with

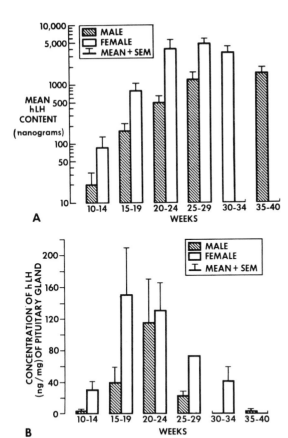

A

B

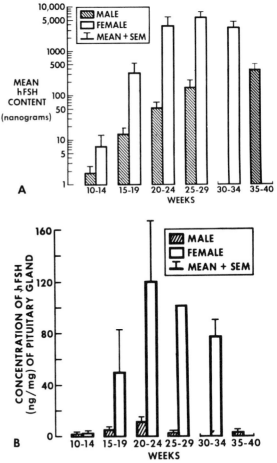

A

B

placental gonadotropin, is highest before 90 days then falls as gestation proceeds. The concentration of hCG in fetal plasma correlates with maternal levels, although fetal concentrations are much lower; at midgestation, the fetal level is about 1/1000 that of the mother.[54] hCG concentrations in the fetus also decrease before the fall in fetal plasma LH but are still detectable at birth.[128, 286]

As in the pituitary, the α-glycoprotein subunit is the dominant glycoprotein fraction present in fetal plasma and cord blood, with no sex difference noted.[291, 511] Measurement of the α-glycoprotein hormone subunit cannot deter-

FIGURE 12–13. The mean (±SE) content and concentration of hLH (LER-960) in fetal pituitary glands is plotted at 5-week intervals (68 days to term). *A*, The hLH content in ng/pituitary gland on a semilogarithmic scale. *B*, The hLH concentration in ng/mg pituitary gland on a linear scale. The values for males are indicated in shaded bars and for females in open bars. (From Kaplan SL, Grumbach MM. The ontogenesis of human foetal hormones. II. Luteinizing hormone (LH) and follicle stimulating hormone (FSH). Acta Endocrinol 1976; 81:808.)

advancing gestational age to undetectable levels in term births. The mean FSH concentration was higher in female fetuses between 26 and 32 weeks, whereas the mean LH level was higher in males (Fig. 12–16). These observations provide additional evidence for the continued secretion of fetal pituitary FSH and LH albeit in gradually decreasing amounts.

Most studies have found no sex difference at term in cord FSH levels, which are very low,[108, 229, 230, 286, 341, 372, 521] although a small sex difference was reported by Penny et al.[421] Several studies have shown that in the older neonate, FSH values in plasma are higher in the female than in the male.[164, 165, 521]

The maternal concentration of hCG, the

FIGURE 12–14. The mean (±SE) content and the concentration of hFSH (LER-869) in the pituitary glands of fetuses plotted at 5-week intervals (68 days to term). *A*, hFSH content in ng/pituitary gland on a semilogarithmic scale. *B*, hFSH concentration in ng/mg pituitary gland on a linear scale. The values for males are indicated in shaded bars and for females in open bars. (From Kaplan SL, Grumbach MM. The ontogenesis of human foetal hormones. II. Luteinizing hormone (LH) and follicle stimulating hormone. Acta Endocrinol 1976; 81:808.)

TABLE 12–4. Ontogeny of Follicle-Stimulating Hormone in the Fetal Pituitary

Investigator	Method	No. of Pituitaries Studied	Gestational Age (weeks)	First Detected (weeks)	Comment
Levina, 1968	Bioassay	98	11–40	13F, 20M	Between 20 and 28 weeks, FSH content greater in female
Bugnon et al, 1977	Immunocyto-chemistry	19	6–26	15	
Gitlin & Biasucci, 1969	Organ culture (2–4 days)	11	4.2–18	14	
Groom et al, 1971	Organ culture (1–6 days)	13	8–18	13	
Siler-Khodr et al, 1974	Organ culture (20–100 days)	17M, 16F	5–38	5F,* 7M*	Maximum secretion in culture occurred at 21–31 weeks (female) and 32 weeks (male). Between 17 and 30 weeks, secretion by female glands > by male glands
Grumbach & Kaplan, 1973, 1974 Kaplan & Grumbach, 1976	RIA	79	10–40	10*	In females, maximum content at 25–29 weeks; in males, maximum content at 35–40 weeks. Between 15 and 29 weeks, content of female glands > male
Hagen & McNeilly, 1975, 1977	RIA	20	9.5–32	13	
Clements et al, 1976	RIA	36	9.5–20	11	Between 12 and 20 weeks, content of female glands > male
Pasteels et al, 1977	RIA	9M	13–27	13*	

FSH present in the earliest sample available.
M = Male; F = female; RIA = radioimmunoassay.

mine the origin of the subunit. It may originate from cells that secrete LH, FSH, TSH, or hCG or any combination of these sources. The concentration of free α subunit in fetal serum is higher in midgestation and falls progressively to term.[238, 239, 291] The rapid postnatal fall in circulating concentrations of the free α subunit at a time when FSH and LH concentrations are rising suggests that at term α-hCG is the major contributor to circulating α subunit.[511]

Regulation of Gonadotropin Secretion

The primary regulator of pituitary gonadotropin secretion is the hypothalamic LRF pulse generator (Fig. 12–17). The pulsatile secretion of fetal LRF[12, 105, 231] and the response of the pituitary to it are modulated by gonadal steroids and possibly by inhibin. The anencephalic fetus has lower plasma concentrations of FSH and LH, suggesting that the fetal hypothalamus is important in regulating fetal pituitary gonadotropin secretion.[290] LRF is detectable in the fetal hypothalamic extracts by

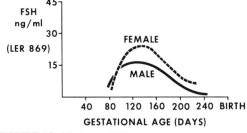

FIGURE 12–15. Serum hFSH (ng/ml, LER-869) concentration during gestation. The solid line represents the regression curve for male fetuses and the broken line for female fetuses. (Data recalculated from Kaplan SL, Grumbach MM. The ontogenesis of human foetal hormones. II. Luteinizing hormone (LH) and follicle stimulating hormone (FSH). Acta Endocrinol 1976; 81:808.)

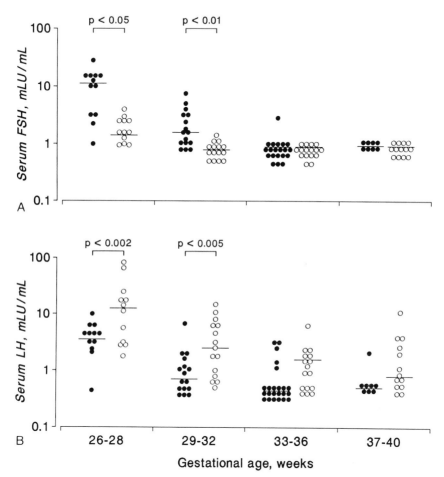

FIGURE 12–16. Serum concentrations of FSH (*A*) and LH (*B*) in 112 fetal cord blood samples collected at birth between 26 and 40 weeks of gestation determined by highly specific and sensitive solid-phase, enzyme-amplified immunoassays. The solid bar designates the median value; solid circles indicate levels in females and open circles levels in males. Note the log scale. (From Massa G, de Zegher F, Vanderschueren-Lodeweyckx M. Serum levels of immunoreactive inhibin, FSH and LH in human infants at preterm and term birth. Biol Neonate 1992; 61:150.)

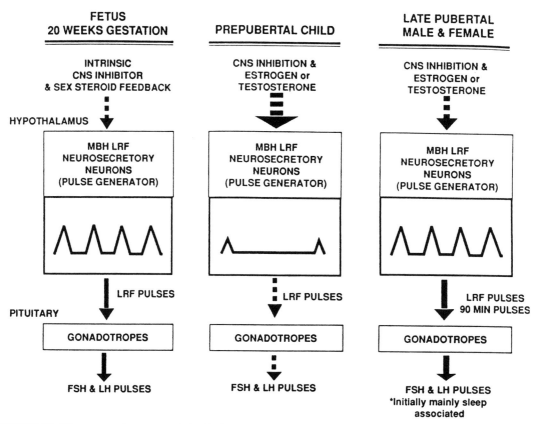

FIGURE 12–17. Postulated ontogeny of the dual mechanism for the inhibition of puberty. Note the highly active LRF pulse generator in the midgestation human fetus and the quiescent juvenile pause. MBH = medial basal hypothalamus. (Modified from Grumbach MM, Kaplan SL. The neuroendocrinology of human puberty: an ontogenetic perspective. In: Grumbach MM, Sizonenko PC, Aubert ML, eds. Control of the onset of puberty. Baltimore: Williams & Wilkins, 1990:1. From Grumbach MM, Styne DM. Puberty: ontogeny, neuroendocrinology, physiology, and disorders. In: Wilson JD, Foster DW, eds. Williams textbook of endocrinology, ed 8. Philadelphia: WB Saunders, 1992:1139.)

at least 10 weeks of gestation (see Table 12–2),[33, 110] and pulsatile release of LRF was demonstrated in midgestation human fetal mediobasal hypothalami.[448] The human fetal pituitary in vitro is responsive to LRF.[226, 412] The LRF-evoked release of LH is greater in second trimester cultured human fetal pituitary cells and greater in female than male pituitary glands;[98, 155] in pituitary glands from both sexes, the LH response is enhanced by estradiol.[155] Similar results were obtained in LRF-perfused fetal hemipituitaries.[465]

When synthetic LRF was administered in vivo to male and female fetuses in midgestation and late gestation in a dose of 2 μg/kg intramuscularly, there was both a FSH and a LH response in all by 16 weeks of gestation, with a much greater increase in plasma fetal FSH in the female. By late gestation, the mag-

nitude of the gonadotropin response to LRF was much less, and there was no sex difference.[522] In neonates less than 96 hours old, the response to LRF was similar to that in late gestation[478, 522] (Fig. 12–18). The anencephalic infant and infants with neonatal hypothalamic hypogonadotropic hypogonadism have an absent or diminished LH and FSH response to exogenous LRF.[231, 290] These results provide indirect evidence for the presence of LRF receptors in the human fetal pituitary by at least 15 weeks of gestation and for the critical role of hypothalamic LRF in regulating the secretion of fetal pituitary gonadotropins.

Fetal plasma concentrations of FSH and LH are high in midgestation and fall in late gestation; FSH and LH levels are higher in females than males. The high gonadotropin levels in midgestation apparently are a consequence of

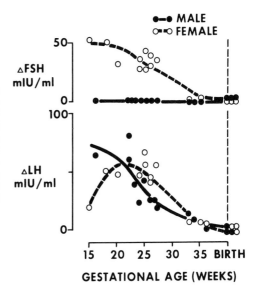

FIGURE 12–18. The effect of LRF 2 μg/kg administered to the human fetus intramuscularly, on plasma gonadotropins. The incremental response (Δ) between a baseline and a 15-minute post-LRF plasma sample is plotted as a function of gestational age. The FSH response is shown in the upper panel and the LH response in the lower panel. Males are represented by solid circles and females by open circles. The regression curve of the response versus gestational age is shown by a solid line for male fetuses and a broken line for female fetuses. (Data recalculated from Takagi S, Yoshida T, Tsubata K, et al. Sex differences in fetal gonadotropins and androgens. J Steroid Biochem 1977; 8:609.)

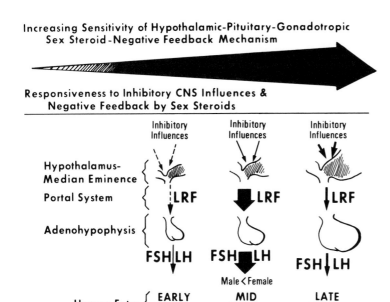

FIGURE 12–19. Schematic representation of the development of regulatory mechanisms for the control of FSH and LH secretion in the human fetus. (From Grumbach MM, Kaplan SL. In: Gluck L, ed. Modern perinatal medicine. Chicago: Year Book Medical Publishers, 1974:247.)

the unrestrained pulsatile release of LRF acting on the fetal gonadotropes and leading to pulsatile release of LH and FSH[12, 105, 229, 230, 231, 286, 290] (see Fig. 12–17). With the advance in fetal maturation, the negative feedback mechanism matures, and the hypothalamus secretes less LRF. This results in the decreased secretion of FSH and LH (Fig. 12–19). This inhibition of the fetal hypothalamic LRF pulse generator and pituitary gonadotropin secretion is postulated to result from the increased inhibitory effects on the fetal hypothalamic LRF-pituitary gonadotropin unit of the high concentrations of sex steroids, especially estrogens and progesterone, in both sexes, and the appearance of sex steroid receptors in the fetal hypothalamus and pituitary—the maturation of the negative feedback loop.[230, 231, 290]

The sex difference in the fetal pituitary content and circulating levels of FSH and LH, however, is not explained by the similar ambient concentration of estrogens and progesterone in both sexes. Two factors may explicate, at least in part, this sex difference. The higher concentration of plasma testosterone in the male fetus between 11 and 23 weeks of gestation and its postulated negative feedback effect and fundamental organizational actions influence the subsequent pattern of gonadotropin secretion and its regulation.[230, 231, 290, 366]

The second factor is the sex difference in the male and female fetus in the maturation of gonadal inhibins (a heterodimer glycoprotein consisting of an α subunit and one of two β subunits, β_A or β_B) and activins (a homodimer glycoprotein consisting of two inhibin β subunits, $\beta_A\beta_A$ or $\beta_B\beta_B$), members of the TGF-β superfamily, which includes the antimüllerian hormone (AMH).[571] At midgestation, immunoreactive inhibin activity is much greater in the human fetal testes than in the fetal ovary;[442, 443, 490] both FSH and hCG stimulate inhibin secretion by the midgestation human fetal testis in vitro. All three subunits of inhibin (α, β_A, and β_B) are present in the midgestation human fetal testis (18 to 23 weeks). Only α-inhibin subunit and its mRNA were detected in fetal Sertoli cells; all three subunits and their mRNAs were found in some interstitial cells, which indicates the capacity to synthesize both inhibin and activin by the latter cells.[442, 546] In contrast, in the late gestation fe-

tal monkey testis, both α and β_B subunits were localized in Sertoli cells, consistent with the putative principal site of inhibin synthesis in adult testes; only the β_B subunit, however, was found in both Sertoli and Leydig cells. Apparently a maturational shift occurs in the site of synthesis of these subunits during the development of the primate fetal testis from mainly interstitial cell production in the midgestation fetal testis to primarily seminiferous tubule synthesis in late gestation.[442]

Bioactive inhibin is present in the ovine fetal testis and ovary from 111 days of gestation to term (147 days), and the pulsatile administration of FSH to the fetus increases the content and concentration of gonadal inhibin bioactivity and decreases the content and secretion of gonadal testosterone.[11] Further, a crude inhibin preparation infused into the ovine fetus causes a gradual fall in circulating fetal FSH in both sexes.[13] In addition, in the male ovine fetus, the concentration of plasma immunoreactive inhibin increases from 55 days of gestation to term and is several times higher than in the female fetus at all stages of gestation; in the latter, plasma inhibin values fall between 55 days and term (147 days).[432] Taken together, along with the higher concentration of immunoreactive inhibin in the midgestation human fetal testis than the low amount in the fetal ovary,[490] these studies suggest that the fetal pituitary FSH-inhibin mechanism is active in the male ovine fetus and possibly in the human and may be a factor in the sex difference in fetal pituitary content and concentration of FSH and the circulating concentration of FSH in the fetus.

The human placenta synthesizes and secretes inhibin[350, 357, 358, 369, 426, 429] and synthesizes activin.[428] Further, inhibin and activin subunits (α, β_A, and β_B) and their mRNAs are expressed in midgestation and neonatal human fetal adrenal cells.[508] In addition to the postulated paracrine/autocrine action[69, 542] of inhibin and activin in the fetus and placenta,[428, 508] the human placenta (not the ovary) is the principal source of the high concentration of immunoreactive and bioactive inhibin in the maternal circulation from 10 weeks of pregnancy to term.[1, 297, 357, 440, 441, 520] The mean immunoreactive inhibin concentration in umbilical cord blood at term is about 2½ times the

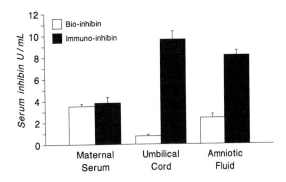

FIGURE 12–20. The mean concentration of bioactive inhibin and immunoreactive "inhibin" in maternal sera (n = 16), umbilical cord sera (n = 21), and amniotic fluid. Note the striking discordance in bioactive inhibin and immunoreactive inhibin in umbilical cord sera and amniotic fluid but not in maternal sera. The concentration of immunoreactive inhibin is greater in cord sera and amniotic fluid than in maternal sera, whereas the bioactive inhibin levels are higher in maternal sera than either umbilical cord sera or amniotic fluid. See text for discussion of this discrepancy. (Modified from Qu J, Thomas K. Changes in bioactive and immunoactive inhibin levels around human labor. J Clin Endocrinol Metab 1992; 74:1290.)

level in the maternal circulation, whereas the bioactive inhibin concentration was low in cord blood and about one-third the level in the maternal circulation; the striking discrepancy in immunoreactivity to bioactivity in cord blood is in contrast to the lack of discordance in maternal sera[440, 441] (Fig. 12–20). The occurrence of free α-inhibin subunit and other inhibin-like components (e.g., pro-α C subunit) in plasma quite likely explains the discordance in bioactive and immunoreactive activity as well as the variation reported in the plasma concentration of immunoreactive inhibin in maternal and umbilical cord blood.[1, 297, 520] Further, neither an umbilical arterial-venous gradient nor a sex difference is reported, which suggests that the major portion of the inhibin in the fetal circulation at term is of placental origin.

In the midgestation baboon fetus, plasma immunoreactive inhibin concentrations are exceedingly high and 16 times the elevated levels in maternal blood.[70] Serum levels of immunoreactive inhibin are elevated throughout the third trimester human fetus, falling modestly as gestation progresses (Fig. 12–21), and were highest in the 26- to 28-week male fetuses.[341] The higher immunoreactive inhibin values in the late gestation male fetus support a fetal testicular contribution to the extragonadal source(s) of inhibin, principally the placenta. Until more is known about the pattern of change in bioactive fetal plasma inhibin and the contribution of a variety of placental and fetal sources of inhibins and activins, the relative importance of inhibin in contrast to fetal plasma testosterone as an explication of the sex difference in circulating FSH at midgesta-

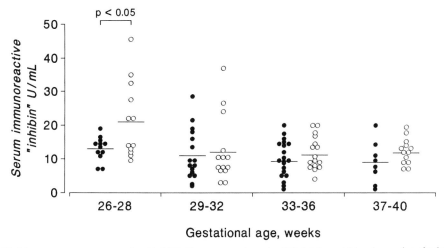

FIGURE 12–21. Serum immunoreactive "inhibin" concentrations in 112 fetal cord blood samples obtained at birth between 26 and 40 weeks of gestation. The solid bar indicates the mean value; closed circles designate female levels and open circles male levels. (From Massa G, de Zegher F, Vanderschueren-Lodeweyckx M. Serum levels of immunoreactive inhibin, FSH and LH in human infants at preterm and term birth. Biol Neonate 1992; 61:150.)

tion in the human fetus is uncertain and speculative.

Less fetal pituitary gonadotropin is secreted as negative feedback develops. This maturation may be the result of increasing sensitivity of the hypothalamic-pituitary unit to sex steroids of gonadal and extragonadal origin and the development of functional sex steroid receptors as well as the maturation of intrinsic inhibitory CNS mechanisms[229, 230, 233, 290] (see Fig. 12–19). The increasing concentrations of circulating fetal estrogens and progesterone in both sexes[454, 493] may be an important factor in the decreasing concentrations of gonadotropins in late gestation. Further, maturation of the negative feedback mechanism depends on the activation of and increase in sex steroid receptors in the hypothalamus and the pituitary gland. Gonadotropin concentrations remain high in the neonatal rat until estrogen receptors increase in the brain at puberty.[396] In the human fetus, estrogen receptors are demonstrable in hypothalamic and pituitary cytosol extracts at midgestation.[130] The role of testosterone and inhibin in negative feedback and the sex difference in pituitary and circulating gonadotropins is discussed later.

The midgestation hypothalamus has the ability to form the potent catechol-estrogens that bind to the hypothalamic estrogen receptor.[169] The ovine fetal pituitary can form 17β-estradiol from estrone sulfate.[275] The human fetal hypothalamus can also metabolize androgens; 5α-reductase is present from 12 weeks[276, 481] and is also found in the fetal pituitary gland. The fetal hypothalamus can aromatize testosterone to 17β-estradiol from at least 15 weeks.[385, 463] These data suggest that by midgestation, the fetal hypothalamus and pituitary have the capacity to metabolize gonadal sex steroids as they do in the adult, and they further support an important role of the fetal CNS in the regulation of gonadotropin secretion.

The higher concentration of pituitary FSH and LH and of plasma FSH in the female fetus is quite likely a consequence of the difference in concentrations of circulating sex steroids (and possibly inhibin)[341] in male and female fetuses.[229–231] Although there is no sex difference in circulating estrogens and progesterone,[493] the concentration of testosterone in the male fetus before 20 weeks' gestation is in the pubertal range.[4, 149, 454] Testosterone is secreted by the fetal testes early in gestation at the time of sexual differentiation. hCG is the main extragonadal regulator of testosterone production in early gestation, and plasma concentrations of testosterone fall in midgestation in parallel with fetal hCG[229, 230, 286, 290, 454] (Fig. 12–22).

The secretion of testosterone in the male fetus may advance maturation of the negative feedback mechanism by its action on the hypothalamic-pituitary apparatus and, as a consequence, lead to a sex difference in the pituitary content of gonadotropins and their secretion at midgestation.

Role of Fetal Gonadotropins

The human fetal gonad is under the influence of hCG and fetal pituitary LH and FSH. Early in gestation, hCG seems to have an important role in the secretion of testosterone by the fetal testes during the time of differentiation of the wolffian ducts and the masculinization of the urogenital sinus and external genitalia; fetal plasma hCG peaks at about 12 weeks and decreases to its nadir at 20 weeks.[54, 287, 290, 454] Leydig cells begin to differentiate from undifferentiated mesenchymal cells of the gonadal blastema during the eighth fetal week (30 to 35 mm stage of development) and by the 13th week compose about 50% of the fetal testicular mass and attain their maximum number, 48×10^6 Leydig cells per pair of fetal testes[112] (see Fig. 12–22). The absolute number remains fairly constant until about the 24th week, when the number of Leydig cells progressively decreases to 18×10^6 cells per pair of testes at the end of gestation.[112] The concentration of plasma testosterone in the male fetus correlates with the testosterone content and biosynthetic activity of the fetal testis;[495, 525] the peak concentration of fetal plasma testosterone occurs during the 12th to 16th week of gestation, when levels (230 to 1100 ng/dL) comparable to the adult male are attained (see Fig. 12–22). Between 16 and 20 weeks, the plasma testosterone concentration falls to about 100 ng/dL (about three times higher than in the female fetus), which is apparently due to decreased expression of mRNAs for

FIGURE 12–22. Comparison of the pattern of change of serum testosterone, hCG, and serum and pituitary LH (LER 960) and FSH (LER 869) concentrations in the human male fetus during gestation in relation to morphologic changes in the fetal testis. By the 13th week of gestation, Leydig cells make up about 50% of the fetal testicular mass and attain their maximum number, 48×10^6 Leydig cells per pair of fetal testes. After the 24th week, the number of Leydig cells progressively decreases to 18×10^6 cells per pair of testes at term. The top graph illustrates the hormonal response to LRF.[522] (Modified from Kaplan SL, Grumbach MM. Pituitary and placental gonadotropins and sex steroids in the human and sub-human primate fetus. Clin Endocrinol Metab 1978; 7:487.)

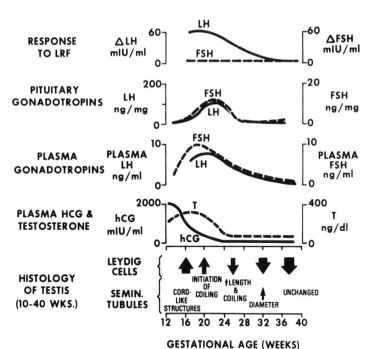

P450c17 (17 hydroxylase/17,20-lyase) and P450scc (cholesterol side-chain cleavage) by the fetal testes.[547] All of these changes correlate with the pattern of fetal plasma hCG.

Fetal Leydig cells exhibit remarkable morphologic and functional differences from that of adult-type cells:[265] (1) Human fetal Leydig cells form tightly opposed clusters joined by gap junctions and by the 15th week are the main testicular component; crystalloids of Reinke are absent. (2) They lack a number of the negative modulatory mechanisms of the adult Leydig cell and as a consequence have a greater steroidogenic capacity and compared with adult Leydig cells do not exhibit desensitization to high doses of LH or hCG[311] owing to loss of LH receptors, inhibition of LH receptor transcripts, and impaired testosterone biosynthesis. Fetal Leydig cells have little aromatase activity[528] and, in contrast to adult cells, do not exhibit estrogen-evoked suppression of testosterone synthesis; estrogen receptors in fetal Leydig cells are low or undetectable. The inhibitory guanine nucleotide binding protein (G_i) is coupled to the LH receptor in the adult Leydig cell and negatively regulates adenyl cyclase, inhibiting cyclic adenosine monophosphate (cAMP) production, and, as a result, LH-induced synthesis of testosterone is suppressed. The G_i protein is apparently not pres-

ent or functional in fetal Leydig cells.[265, 552] These studies suggest that LH/hCG stimulation is maximized in the fetal Leydig cell and serves to ensure optimal synthesis and secretion of testosterone for its critical action on male sex differentiation. The inhibitory mechanisms in the adult-type Leydig cell restrain overstimulation by LH and excessive testosterone synthesis.

Activin and inhibin have an autocrine/paracrine action on gonadal steroidogenesis: Inhibin stimulates and activin inhibits LH-induced testosterone synthesis,[343] and both affect other aspects of gonadal function and development. FSH stimulation of the ovine fetal ovary and testis was associated with a decrease in fetal gonadal and circulating testosterone,[11] possibly mediated by activin. The ontogeny and role of follistatin,[139, 343] an inhibin-binding and activin-binding protein present in a wide variety of tissues, including the pituitary gland and gonads, in fetal development are not yet known. In contrast, the critical role of the AMH (müllerian inhibitory factor) in sex differentiation is well established. AMH and its transcripts are present in the pre–Sertoli cell of the embryonic testis but not in the fetal ovary. High concentrations of serum AMF have been detected at 19 to 22 weeks of gestation (the earliest fetuses studied) in the male fetus, and the lev-

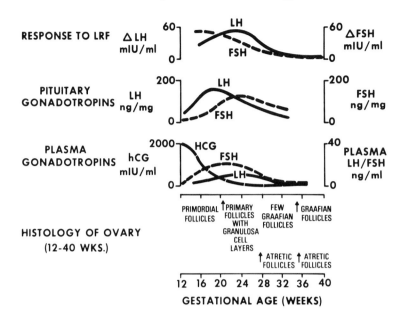

RESPONSE TO LRF ΔLH mIU/ml

PITUITARY GONADOTROPINS LH ng/mg

PLASMA GONADOTROPINS hCG mIU/ml

ΔFSH mIU/ml

FSH ng/mg

PLASMA LH/FSH ng/ml

HISTOLOGY OF OVARY (12–40 WKS.)

PRIMORDIAL FOLLICLES | PRIMARY FOLLICLES WITH GRANULOSA CELL LAYERS | FEW GRAAFIAN FOLLICLES | GRAAFIAN FOLLICLES

ATRETIC FOLLICLES | ATRETIC FOLLICLES

12 16 20 24 28 32 36 40
GESTATIONAL AGE (WEEKS)

FIGURE 12–23. A graphic comparison of the hormonal response to LRF[522] pituitary and plasma FSH and LH,[286] and plasma hCG,[286] with histologic changes in the ovary of the human female fetus during gestation. (Modified from Kaplan SL, Grumbach MM. Pituitary and placental gonadotropins and sex steroids in the human and sub-human primate fetus. Clin Endocrinol Metab 1978; 7:487.)

els remain high through term and in the perinatal period in the male. AMF was not detected in sera from female fetuses.[280]

The fetal testis contains hCG/LH receptors. hCG produced by the syncytiotrophoblast stimulates testosterone synthesis and secretion from the fetal Leydig cells; the concentration of fetal plasma hCG correlates with the circulating level and testicular content of testosterone as well as the pattern of Leydig cell maturation and regression. LH/hCG receptors have been detected in the human fetal testis during the second trimester (12 to 24 weeks).[262, 373] A controversial report suggests that testosterone secretion and adenyl cyclase activity in the early fetal testis are autonomous and independent of hCG.[567] Nevertheless, it is unresolved whether functional hCG/LH receptors are present before the 12th week of gestation and whether the early fetal testis responds to hCG. An additional factor is the detection of apparently local synthesis of hCG by the human fetal testis.

In the second trimester, high-affinity FSH receptors are present in the human fetal testis (in contrast to the fetal ovary), and during this period, the number of FSH receptors increases. When in gestation the human testicular FSH receptor becomes functional has not yet been determined.[267]

About the 11th to 12th week of gestation (80 mm stage), well after the indifferent gonad

differentiates as a testis in the male fetus, the progenitor oogonia enter meiotic prophase and undergo the transition to oocytes[37, 193, 228] (see Chapter 15). The peak number of germ cells is reached at 16 to 20 weeks.[37] Beginning about 20 weeks, primordial follicles and shortly thereafter primary follicles appear (Fig. 12–23); by 24 weeks, preantral follicles are seen followed by a few antral and graafian follicles near term[300, 424] (see review by Grumbach and Conte[228] and Rabinovici and Jaffe[443]). In contrast to fetal testes, FSH receptors have not been detected in midtrimester human fetal ovaries,[267] which may be a factor in the low amount of immunoreactive inhibin in the midtrimester fetal ovary.[490] Fetal pituitary FSH apparently is not required for the proliferation of oogonia, oocyte differentiation, or formation of human primordial follicles,[38] but it is involved in the formation and maintenance of preantral and antral follicles. It is not until the definitive thecal layer forms that the follicle has the capacity to synthesize estradiol. Although the primordial ovary has aromatase activity,[191] quite likely it is present in extra-follicular cell components. The fetal ovary does not contribute significantly to the large amount of circulating estrogens and immunoreactive inhibin in the human fetus.

Sexual differentiation does not depend on fetal pituitary gonadotropins. For about the first 14 weeks of gestation, during the critical period of male sex differentiation, hCG is the dominant stimulus to testosterone secretion by the fetal Leydig cells. In midgestation, as fetal hCG and testosterone concentrations fall, there is regression of the Leydig cells.[112, 193] In late gestation, a sex difference in the concentration of serum testosterone has not been found; however, a small difference has been described in cord blood and a larger sex difference in the peripheral blood of the neonate,[170, 171] suggesting that Leydig cell secretion, while still present, is largely suppressed in late gestation.

However, the male fetus with anencephaly or congenital hypopituitarism associated with gonadotropin deficiency often has hypoplastic male external genitalia, including micropenis and undescended testes.[51, 228, 325, 573, 574] The testes show a decreased number of Leydig cells, and the epididymis is underdeveloped despite the presence of low concentrations of hCG.[38, 103, 573, 574] The number of spermatogonia within the seminiferous tubules is usually little affected.[38] Similar findings are present in the decapitated monkey fetus.[539] The cynomolgus male monkey fetus given a long-acting LRF-agonist during midgestation has a smaller phallus and testes at birth than untreated male fetuses.[323] The weight of evidence suggests that, after midgestation, fetal pituitary gonadotropins influence the growth of the fetal testis and the male external genitalia.

The fetal ovary does not have a critical function in female sexual differentiation. In the late gestation anencephalic human female fetus, the ovaries after about 32 to 34 weeks' gestation are small and contain a decreased number and hypoplasia of primary follicles; antral follicles are absent, but ovarian hilar cells are abundant.[38, 103, 575] Similar findings have been described in the hypophysectomized female fetal monkey.[236] These observations suggest that the growth, development, and maintenance of the human fetal ovary are influenced significantly by fetal pituitary gonadotropins after 32 weeks of gestation.

ONTOGENY AND REGULATION OF GONADOTROPINS IN THE OVINE FETUS.

Even though studies in the human fetus contributed to our understanding of the ontogeny of the hypothalamic–pituitary gonadotropin-gonadal apparatus, they have provided little information on the mechanisms of the maturation of its regulation.[231] The pregnant sheep, in which chronic indwelling vascular catheters are placed in the fetus and pregnant ewe, has provided a useful model for carrying out mechanistic studies.[231] Term in the sheep fetus is at 147 days. The pattern of ontogeny of fetal gonadotropins, hypothalamic LRF, and gonadal maturation, including sex steroid secretion, is similar to that in the human fetus.[105, 106, 231, 380, 504] The hypothalamohypophyseal portal system is intact by at least 45 days of gestation.[348] The ovine fetal hypothalamus contains immunoreactive LRF by 58 days, the youngest fetus studied.[231]

The ovine fetal hypothalamic LRF pulse generator is operative early in gestation and by at least 80 days regulates the pulsatile secretion of LH and FSH—the secretion of FSH and LH is not autonomous.[12, 105, 106] By 0.6 gestation, the ovine fetal hypothalamic-pituitary gonadotropin unit has the capacity to respond to sex steroid negative feedback.[214] Evidence for an operative negative feedback system has been obtained as well in the fetal monkey.[159, 453]

There is a striking sex difference in the effect of fetal castration on pulsatile LH secretion and the mean concentration of plasma FSH.[366] Castration of the male ovine fetus from as early as 110 days increased LH pulse frequency and amplitude and the mean concentration of fetal plasma FSH. In contrast, castration of female fetuses had no effect on LH pulsatility or plasma FSH. These studies support an organizational effect of fetal testicular hormones, especially testosterone, on the development of the fetal hypothalamic-pituitary gonadotropin system.

Evidence was obtained for a tonic suppressive effect of opioidergic neurons on the pulsatile release of LRF by the fetus, especially during midgestation;[124] N-methyl-D-aspartate (NMDA), a potent excitatory amino acid analog, stimulated a LH pulse mediated by LRF in the fetus, which provides additional evidence for the functional integrity of the fetal LRF neurosecretory neurons and the capacity of the excitatory amino acids, glutamate and aspartate, to interact with the LRF pulse generator.[66] That this effect is a direct one is supported by the stimulatory effect of NMDA on LRF release by an immortalized LRF neuronal cell line and the identification of NMDA receptor transcripts in these LRF neurons.[337]

In addition, FSH induces bioactive inhibin synthesis in the ovine fetal testis and ovary,[11] and the infusion of an inhibin-rich extract into the ovine fetus inhibits fetal FSH but not LH release.[13] These studies, in light of the demonstration of immunoreactive inhibin in the fetal circulation,[432] support, at least in the ovine fetus, the potential function of the FSH-fetal gonadal inhibin feedback system.

These observations in the human and ovine fetus, along with those in the nonhuman primate,[437] are consistent with the hypothesis that the hypothalamic-pituitary gonadotropin unit is operative by at least 0.3 gestation in the human fetus and 0.4 gestation in the ovine fetus (quite likely earlier) and for the central role of the CNS in this process[231] (Table 12–5). The secretion of fetal gonadotropins is not autonomous; the pulsatile release of fetal pituitary LH and FSH is mediated by a functional hypothalamic LRF pulse generator.

HUMAN NEONATES. During the first few days after birth, the plasma concentration of hCG, α-glycoprotein subunit, and placental steroids, including estradiol, decrease remarkably in both sexes.[108, 128, 230, 239, 286, 291, 456, 511, 521, 522] In cord blood, the concentration of LH and FSH is low without a sex difference.[290] In both premature and full-term newborn males, the testosterone level in umbilical cord blood, although low, is higher than in females;[33a, 170, 526] the testosterone concentration is greater in the umbilical artery than in the vein, which suggests a contribution by the male fetus presumably from the testis. In contrast to the concentration of testosterone in cord blood, the peripheral level shortly after birth is about seven times higher than in the female and in the midpubertal range;[170] the concentration of free testosterone has a similar pattern[170] (Table 12–6). The low concentration of sex steroid–binding protein at birth[33a] increases to reach a plateau by about 1 month of age.[170] Within minutes after birth in the male but not female neonate, the concentration of serum LH increases rapidly and is followed within the first 3 hours by a sharp increase in plasma testosterone.[119] By 9 hours after birth, male neonates exhibit high-frequency pulsatile secretion of LH and testosterone concentrations

TABLE 12–5. Postulated Ontogeny of the Hypothalamic-Pituitary-Gonadal Circuit

Fetus
Medial basal hypothalamic LH-RH neurosecretory neurons (pulse generator) operative by 80 days
Pulsatile secretion of FSH and LH by 80 days of gestation
Initially unrestrained secretion of LH-RH (100–150 days)
Maturation of negative gonadal steroid feedback mechanisms by 150 days of gestation—sex difference
Low level of LH-RH secretion at term

Early Infancy
Hypothalamic LH-RH pulse generator functional in newborn
Prominent FSH and LH episodic discharges until approximately 6 months of age in males and 12 months of age in females with transient increase in plasma levels of testosterone and estradiol in males and females

Late Infancy and Childhood
Intrinsic CNS inhibition of hypothalamic LH-RH pulse generator operative; predominant mechanism in childhood; maximal sensitivity by approximately 4 years of age
Negative feedback control of FSH and LH secretion highly sensitive to gonadal steroids (low set point)
LH-RH pulse generator inhibited; low amplitude and frequency of LH-RH discharge
Low secretion of FSH, LH, and gonadal steroids

Late Prepubertal Period
Decreasing effectiveness of intrinsic CNS inhibitory influence and decreasing sensitivity of hypothalamic-pituitary unit to gonadal steroids (increased set point)
Increased amplitude and frequency of LH-RH pulses, initially most prominent with sleep (nocturnal)
Increased sensitivity of gonadotropes to LH-RH
Increased secretion of FSH and LH
Increased responsiveness of gonad to FSH and LH
Increased secretion of gonadal hormones

Puberty
Further decrease in CNS restraint of hypothalamic LH-RH pulse generator and of the sensitivity of negative feedback mechanism to gonadal steroids
Prominent sleep-associated increase in episodic secretion of LH-RH gradually changes to adult pattern of pulses about every 90 minutes
Pulsatile secretion of LH follows pattern of LH-RH pulses
Progressive development of secondary sexual characteristics
Spermatogenesis in males
Middle to late puberty—operative positive feedback mechanism and capacity to exhibit an estrogen-induced LH surge
Ovulation in females

Modified from Grumbach MM, Roth JC, Kaplan SL, et al: Hypothalamic-pituitary regulation of puberty in man: evidence and concepts derived from clinical research. In: Grumbach MM, Grave GD, Mayer FE, eds. Control of the onset of puberty. New York: John Wiley & Sons, 1974:115–166.

in the adult male range; in contrast, the female neonate has LH values less than the sensitivity of immunoradiometric assays. During the first neonatal day, FSH levels were low in both sexes.[143]

Plasma testosterone concentrations fall during the latter part of the first week in males, then increase again during the second to third week to reach peak values comparable to pubertal levels,[170, 559] and then gradually fall to prepubertal concentrations by 6 months of age (see Table 12–5). Testosterone concentrations

TABLE 12–6. Plasma Concentrations (nmol/L) of Sex Steroids (Mean ± 1 SD) at Birth and During Infancy

		Progestagens		Androgens				Estrogens	
		P	OHP	Total T	Unbound T	Δ⁴	DHT	E₂	E₁
At birth: Mother		500–610	23.7±6.9	3.6±1.5	0.008±0.002	8.3±2.9	0.62±0.12	64.5±33.7	47.3±21.9
Fetus: Cord vein*	M	1540±985†	56.4±31†	1.4±0.38†	0.038±0.009†	2.99±0.98	0.22±0.06†	29.6±14.7†	92.8±24†
	F		70.8±41	1.0±0.26	0.030±0.001	3.3±1.3	0.12±0.05		
Peripheral vein	M	12–32		9.5±3.1†	0.27±0.13†	6.7±3.2	0.17–1.7	1.4±0.07†	4±7.4†
(0–2 hours)	F	10–30	12.7±5.8†	1.6±0.48	0.04±0.001	6.1±2.6	<0.34		
Infancy									
4–8 days	M	0.75–3.5	3.2±1.8	1.15±0.15†	0.0114±0.006	1.22±0.6	0.39±0.2	0.007–0.018	0.007–0.045
	F	0.2–6.5	2.9±1.2	0.45±0.3	0.011±0.002	1.16±0.6	0.32±0.1	0.001–0.03	0.003–0.02
1–2 months	M	0.09–1.1	6.1±2.4	8.8±2.7†	0.06±0.01†	1.5 ±0.45†	2.25±1.2†	0.001–0.041†	0.003–0.015
	F	0.05–0.9	3.2±1.5	0.28±0.13	0.002±0.0007	0.66±0.24	0.29±0.18	0.001–0.02	0.004–0.015
7–9 months	M	0.09–0.5	0.88±0.63†	0.24±0.14	0.005±0.003	0.38±0.09	0.15±0.11	0.001–0.09	0.002–0.012
	F	0.12–0.8	1.82±1.27	0.21±0.11	0.002±0.0007	0.38±0.05	0.19±0.14	0.0015–0.01	0.0015–0.010
9–12 months	M	0.16–0.7	0.85±0.66	0.24±0.13	0.002±0.0003	0.38±0.2	0.13±0.11	0.001–0.009	ND–0.009
	F	0.11–0.8	1.30±0.75	0.24±0.13	0.002±0.0003	0.38±0.1	0.11±0.05	0.002–0.008	ND–0.01
Children: 1–2 years	M+F	0.1–0.5	0.77±0.3	0.22±0.1	0.0014±0.003	0.38±0.2	0.08±0.04	ND–0.03	ND–0.02
Adults: Male		0.3–0.6†	3.5–1.2†	19.8±4.7†	0.29±0.08†	3.7±0.9†	1.95±0.7†	0.09±0.03†	0.15±0.05
Female	FP	1.8±0.34	1.3±0.25	0.75±0.2	0.01±0.002	2.7±1.0	0.52±0.2	0.35±0.18	0.16±0.08
	LP	43±13	7.4±2	1.28±0.3		5.2±1.5	0.65±0.3	0.64±0.38	0.33±0.09†

*In most instances, mixed cord blood constituted mostly of venous blood.

†Pooled M and F values, no sex difference.

‡Sex difference.

P_4 = Progesterone; OHP = 17α-hydroxyprogesterone; T = testosterone; Δ⁴ = androstenedione; DHT = 5α-dihydrotestosterone; E_2 = estradiol-17β; E_1 = estrone; M = males; F = females; ND = not detectable; FP = follicular phase; LP = luteal phase.

From Forest MG. Pituitary gonadotropin and sex steroid secretion during the fist two years of life. In: Grumbach MM, Sizonenko PC, Aubert ML, eds. Control of the onset of puberty. Baltimore: Williams & Wilkins, 1990:451–477.

in the testis during infancy show a similar pattern of change to circulating testosterone.[67] During this period of high testosterone levels in early infancy, LH pulsatility is greater in the male than the female, and FSH values in the male are relatively low.[550] The LH response evoked by the administration of LRF increases to a pubertal LH response after the first week; it gradually decreases after 3 months of age to the prepubertal-type LH response.[187, 231, 526] Hence the neonatal hypothalamic LRF pulse generator–pituitary gonadotropin unit in the male is functional on the first day of life, becomes quiescent by the end of the first week, and then reaches a second peak of activity that persists for 3 to 6 months, when it is inhibited until its reactivation in the prepubertal period a decade later[231, 234] (see Table 12–5 and Fig. 12–7).

The pattern of gonadotropin secretion in the female neonate is different. After a period of low circulating gonadotropins for about the first week; FSH concentrations rise in the female earlier than in the male and remain elevated, reaching a peak in the menopausal range by 3 to 4 months of age, and then gradually fall to prepubertal levels at about 2 to 3 years of age. FSH pulse amplitude is much greater in the female than the male infant[550] and is associated with a larger FSH response to LRF throughout childhood.[187, 231, 233, 526] For example, in infants 1 to 2 months of age, the increase in FSH elicited by LRF was 8 to 10 times greater in the female than in the male. Further, the mean content and concentration of pituitary FSH is greater in female than in male infants 2 to 4 months of age.[290] In female infants, estradiol values are intermittently elevated but widely scattered during the first year of life and for part of the second year.[68, 559]

This striking sex difference in gonadotropin secretion is present as well in the infant rhesus monkey[437] and in agonadal male and female infants.[231, 331] The mechanism is uncertain but appears to be an effect of testosterone secretion on the fetal hypothalamic-pituitary gonadotropin unit by the surge in testosterone secretion in the male fetus.[231]

The importance of the neonatal hypothalamic LRF pulse generator–pituitary gonadotropin unit to gonadal sex steroid secretion in the infant is illustrated by the hypogonado-tropic-hypogonadism of the anencephalic infant and the congenital hypothalamic-hypopituitary deficient infant, including male infants with Kallmann's syndrome.[231, 234, 290, 325]

Adrenocorticotropic Hormone and Related Peptides

ACTH is derived from a larger pituitary peptide, proopiomelanocortin (POMC), of 31,000 daltons, which is the common precursor for a number of other anterior and intermediate lobe hormones, including ACTH and β-lipotropin (β-LPH)[505] (Fig. 12–24). ACTH and β-LPH themselves contain within their sequences biologically active fragments. β-LPH consists of a 91 amino acid peptide chain, which includes within its structure the sequence for β-endorphin ($\beta\text{-LPH}_{61-91}$), and metenkephalin ($\beta\text{-LPH}_{61-65}$). A variety of forms of endorphin can be found in the human fetal pituitary.[162, 163, 549] ACTH is a 39 amino acid peptide; at least the first 19 residues are required for corticotropic activity. ACTH_{1-39} is the major corticotropin peptide of the human fetal pituitary gland.[5] ACTH contains within its primary structure the sequences of α-melanotropic–stimulating hormone (α-MSH) or ACTH_{1-13} and corticotropin-like intermediate lobe peptide (CLIP) or ACTH_{18-39}, both of which are derived from ACTH by enzymatic cleavage. The processing of POMC differs in the anterior and intermediate lobes with the larger peptides ACTH, β-endorphin, and β-LPH being the primary products of the anterior lobe and the smaller peptides being products of the intermediate lobe (Fig. 12–24). Thus, although desacetyl-α-MSH and CLIP are present in the fetal pituitary gland, which has an intermediate lobe, they are not detected in the adult pituitary gland except during pregnancy.[161, 327]

Pituitary Adrenocorticotropic Hormone and Related Peptides

The corticotrope is the first pituitary cell type to differentiate.[25, 28, 270, 502, 545] By 9 weeks' gestation, the human fetal pituitary gland contains bioassayable corticotropic activity,[294, 416] and the content and concentration of ACTH in-

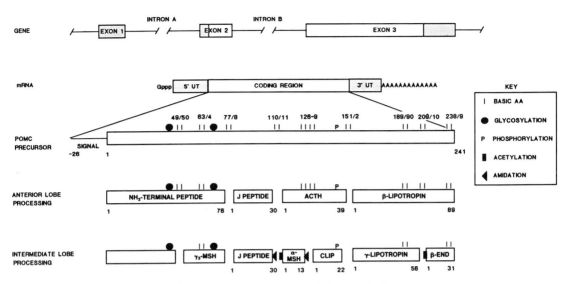

FIGURE 12–24. The structures of the human POMC gene and its mRNA, the POMC precursor, and the mature peptides derived from the POMC molecule by cleavage at basic dipeptides in the anterior lobe. The bottom scheme illustrates the POMC products derived by processing in the intermediate lobe of the human fetus (and the pregnant woman). UT = Flanking untranslated region; J PEPTIDE = joining peptide; CLIP = corticotropin-like intermediate-lobe peptide (see text). (From Orth DN, Kovacs WJ, Debold CR. The adrenal cortex. In: Wilson JD, Foster DW, eds. Williams textbook of endocrinology, ed 8. Philadelphia: WB Saunders, 1992:489.)

crease with gestational age. In culture, the fetal pituitary can secrete ACTH from as early as 5 weeks' gestation.[498]

α-MSH, a fetal intermediate lobe POMC derivative, is present in fetal pituitary glands at 12 weeks' gestation, at midgestation, and at term and in late-trimester fetal sera[349] but not in adult pituitaries:[499, 500] It is found mainly in the desacetyl form.[89, 111, 161] Even though α-MSH may have a unique role in the fetus,[349] perhaps as one tropin for the fetal zone of the adrenal cortex,[499, 500] its function remains uncertain.

β-LPH, an α-endorphin (β-LPH$_{61-76}$), and β-endorphin have been detected immunochemically as early as 8 weeks' gestation within the same pituitary cell, as would be expected if they were derived from a common precursor.[56, 74] There appear to be ontogenic changes in the histologic characteristics of the corticotrope with a uniquely fetal form of corticotrope present in midgestation.[384, 423] It is suggested that glucocorticoids themselves may enhance the maturation of the corticotrope.[20]

Plasma Adrenocorticotropic Hormone

Because of the difficulty of sampling and measurement, there is a paucity of data on the reg-

ulation of ACTH secretion in the human fetus. Even indirect assessment of the hypothalamic-pituitary-adrenal axis by measurement of plasma glucocorticoids is difficult because the sensitivity of the fetal adrenal cortex to ACTH varies with gestational age.[563] Although cortisol crosses the human placenta, most of the maternal cortisol that is transferred in the last trimester is converted by the placenta to cortisone. In contrast to earlier in gestation, the increased production of estrogen in the second half of gestation increases the oxidative function of placental 11β-hydroxydehydrogenase and as a consequence augments the placental conversion of cortisol to cortisone.[422] Thus, most data on the developing hypothalamic-pituitary-adrenal axis have been derived in animals and have been extrapolated to humans. A study of the concentrations of ACTH in fetal scalp blood, obtained during labor, showed increasing levels of ACTH as labor progressed, suggesting that the fetus responds to the stress of labor with augmented secretion of ACTH.[22]

ACTH is detectable by radioimmunoassay in human fetal plasma at 12 weeks' gestation. Concentrations are higher before 34 weeks' gestation, with a significant fall in late gestation;[562] however, the values are higher at all gestational ages and at term than in the normal adult[15, 371, 562] (Fig. 12–25). The pattern of secretion in the last few weeks of gestation is uncertain—in the fetal sheep, ACTH levels rise in late gestation. ACTH does not cross the placenta;[15, 371] however, the placenta is also a source of corticotropins of unknown biologic significance in the human fetus.

Melanotropic-Stimulating Hormone

The mean concentration of α-MSH peptides and other fetal intermediate lobe peptides in umbilical cord plasma progressively decreases during the last trimester and falls to low levels by 12 hours after birth. Desacetyl α-MSH, the predominant α-MSH form, decreases from about 75% of plasma total α-MSH immunoactivity at 25 to 30 weeks' gestation to 45% at term, with a proportionate increase in α-MSH and diacetyl α-MSH. Intrauterine stress during parturition increases all three forms of α-MSH.[349]

Regulation of Adrenocorticotropic Hormone Secretion

The low concentrations of ACTH in anencephaly[15, 371] suggest that the fetal hypothalamus is important in stimulating ACTH secretion. The major neuroendocrine factors regulating anterior pituitary ACTH release are CRF and arginine vasopressin (AVP). Both are stimulatory and are present in the fetal hypo-

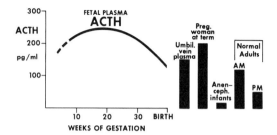

FIGURE 12–25. The pattern of ACTH (pg/mL) in the human fetus during gestation. Plasma ACTH levels (pg/mL) in maternal and cord serum at delivery and in anencephalic infants are shown as solid bars on the right. Data from Allen et al.[16] and Winters et al.[562] (From Grumbach MM, Kaplan SL. Fetal pituitary hormones and the maturation of central nervous system regulation of anterior pituitary function. In: Gluck L, ed. Modern perinatal medicine. Chicago: Year Book Medical Publishers, 1974:247.)

thalamus by 12 weeks,[6] with maturation of the neurohemal terminals by midgestation.[83, 93] CRF and AVP both independently and synergistically stimulate ACTH release from human fetal pituitary glands between 14 and 24 weeks of gestation in cell perfusion and cell culture systems,[76] whereas α-adrenergic and β-adrenergic agonists, prostaglandins E_1 and E_2, and indomethacin had no effect on ACTH release in contrast to their effects on adult pituitary cells. Indirect evidence suggests that glucocorticoids can inhibit ACTH secretion by the human fetus in late gestation. For example, maternal administration of betamethasone suppresses the concentration of ACTH, cortisol, and dehydroepiandiosterone sulfate in cord blood.[41, 190] Dexamethasone administered directly to the human fetus in midtrimester lowers maternal estrogens, a consequence of the suppression of the fetal pituitary-adrenal axis.[21]

A body of data is growing on the regulation of fetal ACTH secretion in the nonhuman primate[422] and especially in the chronically catheterized sheep fetus. ACTH levels rise in the last trimester and are associated in the partum period with a marked rise in glucocorticoid secretion. The initial rise in ACTH appears to be due to increased sensitivity to CRF,[329] but then, in the immediate prepartum period, there appears to be a reduction in responsivity to CRF,[391] perhaps as a result of the high circulating cortisol levels. AVP stimulates ACTH release by an independent pathway[8] and is synergistic with CRF.[390] Such synergism can also be demonstrated in the human fetal pituitary.[76] CRF originating in the paraventricular nucleus is essential to the release of ACTH in response to fetal hypotension and asphyxia.[352] Endogenous opioids may exert tonic stimulation in late gestation and play a role in the prepartum increase in ACTH.[86]

There is a marked increase in the ACTH response to hypoxemia and hypotension after 125 days of gestation in the fetal lamb.[9, 463] The persistence of high ACTH levels in late gestation in the presence of high cortisol levels might reflect relatively deficient negative feedback late in gestation. This may be related, in part, to the high levels of cortisol-binding globulin in the ovine fetal circulation,[100] which would decrease the amount of free cortisol. Earlier in gestation negative feedback appears quite efficient.[464, 566] The placenta is also a source of CRF as well as POMC-derived peptides.[100, 429] Whether these contribute to fetal adrenal activation is not resolved, but at present the evidence does not support a major effect.

Placental CRF, its localization and distribution in the human placenta[457] and fetal membranes, gene expression in the placenta[397] and decidua,[427] secretion, its regulation of placental ACTH by a dexamethasone-insensitive mechanism, and the CRF-binding protein in pregnancy are discussed in Chapter 2.

CRF-binding protein has been detected in human amniotic fluid by 15 weeks and in umbilical cord blood by 24 weeks of gestation.[513] About 90% of CRF in umbilical cord plasma is bound.[475] Circulating fetal as well as maternal CRF is almost exclusively of placental origin. The adrenal hypoplasia in anencephaly and in congenital hypothalamic hypopituitarism accompanied by ACTH deficiency suggests that CRF-binding protein prevents or impedes the action of placental CRF on the fetal pituitary gland.[321]

Role of Adrenocorticotropic Hormone and Related Peptides

ACTH stimulates cortisol production from the definitive zone of the fetal adrenal and dehydroepiandrosterone sulfate (DHEAS) secretion from the fetal zone.[422] ACTH is also important in adrenal growth; in the anencephalic fetus, the fetal zone of the adrenal develops normally up to about 17 weeks' gestation, suggesting that growth up to this fetal age is independent of fetal pituitary ACTH, and involutes by the 20th week.[62] The sensitivity of the adrenal to ACTH varies during fetal life.[156, 563] Cortisol itself induces adrenal maturation perhaps by an effect on the ACTH receptor.[101] ACTH stimulates IGF-2 transcripts in the human fetal adrenal gland,[548] and it affects other growth factors as well.[367] The IGFs and a variety of other growth factors appear to have a paracrine role possibly mediated by fetal ACTH in regulating fetal adrenal growth.[240, 328, 367, 422]

hCG has been reported to stimulate cortisol release in the perfused human fetal adrenal gland in vitro.[488] The anencephalic fetus, however, has adrenal hypoplasia despite a normal fetal concentration of hCG; therefore, it is unlikely that hCG is an important tropic agent to the fetal adrenal cortex in the second half of gestation. hCG administered intramuscularly to the anencephalic fetus in utero in late gestation had no effect on the fetal adrenal cortex.[261] Before 17 to 18 weeks' gestation, however, the fetal adrenal gland in the anencephalic fetus is normally developed,[19, 62] and to reconcile some of the aforementioned discrepancies, it has been suggested that hCG might be a tropic agent to the adrenal cortex during early but not late gestation.[62, 488]

PLACENTAL-DECIDUAL UNIT

The placental-decidual unit is a major site of peptide and steroid hormone production during pregnancy and contains counterpart hormones to the hypothalamus, pituitary, and gonads, including peptidergic-releasing factors and other neural peptides, peptide and glycoprotein hormones similar in structure to certain pituitary and gonadal hormones, biogenic amines, cytokines, and a variety of growth factors and their receptors.[72] This topic is discussed in Chapter 2 and was reviewed by Petraglia et al.[429] Although a variety of hypophysiotropic factors have been isolated from the placental-decidual unit, it is uncertain whether they directly influence pituitary function in the fetus. Despite the fact that the placenta synthesizes LRF and CRF, for example, placental LRF does not prevent hypothalamic hypogonadotropic hypogonadism in the fetus, nor does placental CRF or ACTH prevent regression of the adrenal cortex and its fetal zone in anencephaly. Our understanding, however, of the integrated function of the placenta, its diverse and newly recognized paracrine-autocrine mechanisms, and their impact on the fetus is at an early stage.

CONGENITAL HYPOPITUITARISM: ABNORMALITIES OF THE HYPOTHALAMIC-PITUITARY UNIT AND BRAIN MALFORMATIONS

The remarkable advances in neuroendocrinology; brain imaging technology; and the advent of immunoassays for peptide, steroid, and thyroid hormones and techniques of molecular biology have not only shed light on the ontogeny of the hypothalamus and pituitary gland, on the CNS regulation of pituitary function, and on the effect of hormones on the CNS and pituitary, but also they have had a striking effect on our understanding of the pathophysiology of hypothalamic and pituitary disorders arising in the fetus, their diagnosis, and management.

Five examples of CNS malformations and the function of the hypothalamic-pituitary unit are discussed: (1) anencephaly, (2) the holoprosencephaly-septo–optic dysplasia–optic nerve hypoplasia sequence or complex, (3) hypopituitarism and the abnormal (or dysgenetic, absent, or attenuated) infundibular stalk and ectopic neurohypophysis, (4) Kallmann's syndrome and hypogonadotropic-hypogonadism, and (5) hypothalamic hamartoma and true or central precocious puberty.

General Considerations

Neonatal hypopituitarism may be a consequence of either a hypothalamic or a primary pituitary defect or an absent or abnormal receptor for a pituitary hormone (e.g., the GH resistance syndrome). This discussion is limited to infants who manifest symptoms and signs of hypopituitarism in the neonatal period or early infancy.

Recurrent, severe, and persistent hypoglycemia and its manifestations—apneic spells, seizures, jitteriness, flaccidity, and temperature instability—especially in a neonate, most commonly on the first day after birth, or in older infants of normal birth weight may be due to GH or ACTH deficiency or both and occurred in all 27 of our patients with *idiopathic neonatal hypopituitarism*.[222, 288, 325] In addition, prolonged direct hyperbilirubinemia owing to cholestasis and giant cell hepatitis, micropenis, pendular nystagmus, a history of breech delivery (particularly in a male infant), perinatal anoxia, optic nerve hypoplasia, midline facial malformations such as cleft lip or palate, and evidence of excessive urination and dehydration consistent with central diabetes insipidus strongly support the diagnosis. In affected males, micro-

penis, a frequent clinical marker, facilitates the diagnosis. Although the mean birth length in neonatal hypopituitarism is modestly below the normal mean value (see the section on Role of Growth Hormone in the Fetus), clearly obvious growth retardation is usually not a major clinical feature for the first few months of life.

Congenital hypopituitarism when associated with ACTH deficiency is a cause of low maternal serum and urine estriol values; this diagnosis should be considered in pregnant women with low estriol values.

The diagnosis can be confirmed readily in the first days of life by finding a low concentration of plasma GH (in contrast to the strikingly elevated levels in the normal neonate), total or free thyroxine, and cortisol.[288, 325] The hypoglycemia is not accompanied by a disproportionate increase in plasma insulin, excluding disorders associated with hyperinsulin. In male infants who have gonadotropin deficiency, the postnatal increase in plasma testosterone does not occur. The concentration of plasma prolactin is low in infants with pituitary aplasia in contrast to those with hypothalamic hypopituitarism; after the first 8 weeks of life, an elevated plasma prolactin is consistent with a hypothalamic defect; in normal infants, there is a gradual fall in prolactin concentrations over the first month or so.

Neonatal hypopituitarism is life-threatening because of the risk of sudden death from hypoglycemia and cortisol deficiency.[325] It requires prompt initiation of diagnostic tests, correction of hypoglycemia, and replacement hormone therapy. The blood glucose level should be maintained at $\geq$70 mg/dL by the intravenous infusion of glucose (5 to 10 mg/kg per minute) to prevent CNS damage and neurodevelopmental delay from protracted hypoglycemia, while if possible continuing frequent feedings.

If the diagnosis is confirmed by the initial studies, more complex tests to assess hypothalamic-pituitary function can be carried out. Begin hormone replacement therapy without undue delay. If ACTH deficiency is present, oral cortisol (initially 25 mg/m^2 per day divided into three doses), should be given 24 hours before treatment of TSH deficiency with thyroxine (25 to 50 µg per day to maintain the plasma concentration of thyroxine between 10 and 15 µg/dL during the first 2 years) to prevent acute adrenal insufficiency. We initiate therapy with biosynthetic hGH (0.15 to 0.3 mg/kg per week subcutaneously divided into seven daily doses) at the time of diagnosis in all infants with documented neonatal hypopituitarism to correct or prevent recurrent hypoglycemia. Infants with associated central diabetes insipidus present an especially challenging problem in management. Fluid intake and the dose of DDAVP (0.025 µg/kg subcutaneously or 0.25 µg intranasally when necessary usually every 12 to 24 hours) need to be critically adjusted to avoid the morbidity of hypernatremia or hyponatremia and to ensure an adequate caloric intake for growth.

Pathogenesis

Neonatal hypopituitarism is most commonly of the so-called idiopathic type. It is now known that the interrupted or hypoplastic dysgenetic pituitary stalk syndrome is the usual cause, with hypothalamic hypopituitarism caused by the deficiency of hypothalamic hypophysiotropic factors or their impaired transmission to the often hypoplastic pituitary gland. Hypothalamic hypopituitarism can be caused by a variety of congenital malformations of diverse cause (Table 12–7). The cause may be genetic (autosomal recessive, X-linked recessive) or due to environmental factors or a combination of both. Perinatal trauma[122, 222, 288] and congenital infections, especially toxoplasmosis and cy-

TABLE 12–7. Midline Cleft Malformations of the Central Nervous System and Face Associated with Hypopituitarism

Dysgenesis of the pituitary stalk and ectopic neurohypophysis
Anencephaly
Holoprosencephaly ⎱ Prosencephalon
Septo-optic dysplasia ⎰ Dysgenesis
Optic nerve hypoplasia
Transsphenoidal encephalocele
Cleft lip and/or palate
Single central incisor
Congenital hypothalamic hamartoblastoma: Pallister-Hall syndrome
Rieger's syndrome
Anophthalmia, microphthalmia, cryptothalmia (Fraser's syndrome)

tomegalovirus infection, may be causes. Often, however, the etiology is unknown.

Less commonly, the defect resides at the level of the pituitary gland. Neonatal hypopituitarism may be due to a deleted or mutant gene that encodes a pituitary hormone—e.g., an autosomal recessive form of isolated GH deficiency[113, 433] as well as primary pituitary hypoplasia or aplasia with multiple hormone deficiencies, which can be familial and transmitted as an autosomal recessive trait.[471] A mutation in the GRF receptor is the cause of dwarfism in the "little" (lit/lit) dwarf mouse;[219] its counterpart in the human has not yet been detected.

Complete pituitary agenesis or aplasia, which may occur sporadically or in families,[471] is rare. The main distinguishing feature from congenital hypothalamic hypopituitarism is the low concentration of plasma prolactin. Body length is near normal, and in the male, penile size is reduced, and undescended testes are common. The adrenal glands are hypoplastic, and, in contrast to the anencephalic fetus, the thyroid glands of fetuses with pituitary aplasia are also hypoplastic.[73, 84, 376, 451] This suggests that, in the anencephalic fetus, fetal pituitary TSH is important in stimulating the fetal thyroid and that hCG alone cannot maintain normal thyroidal growth (see section on Anencephaly).

Pit 1 Gene Mutations and Familial Growth Hormone, Prolactin, and Thyroid-Stimulating Hormone Deficiency

A rare autosomal recessive form of multiple pituitary hormone deficiencies associated with GH, prolactin, and TSH deficiency owing to mutations in the Pit-1 gene, a member of the POU-homeodomain family of homeobox proteins, which act as transcription factors (see section on Gene Regulation of Pituitary Cell-Specific Differentiation). Patients with this disorder are the counterpart of the Snell and Jackson dwarf mice, which carry a mutation in the POU specific domain and POU homeodomain,[317] respectively (see Fig. 12–6). The mouse mutations are associated with pituitary hypoplasia and complete deficiencies of GH, prolactin, and TSH. The disorder in humans is more variable: Although all affected patients had striking short stature with severe GH and prolactin deficiencies, the degree of TSH deficiency varied from severe to mild, and pituitary hypoplasia was not an invariable finding.[392, 409, 431, 445, 529] One patient had a Pit-1 missense mutation in the transactivating domain,[392] whereas all of the others had a missense or nonsense mutation in the POU-specific domain or POU-homeodomain. Some mutations appeared to act as a dominant negative with autosomal dominant rather than autosomal recessive transmission.[392, 445] These reports of Pit-1 mutations are an example of the rapid exploitation of advances in molecular biology to increase our understanding of human disorders.

Anencephaly

Anencephaly is a disorder with an incidence of about 1 per 1000 births. It results from failure of closure of the rostral opening of the neural tube early in embryogenesis (23 to 26 days). The cause is heterogeneous; undernutrition, drug ingestion, and other teratogenic environmental factors have been implicated as well as a susceptible genotype.[96, 118] Screening during pregnancy by the measurement of maternal serum concentrations of α-fetoprotein and follow-up studies of high maternal levels with sonography and determination of amniotic fluid α-fetoprotein have made prenatal diagnosis a reality. An important development is the compelling evidence of the value of folate supplementation before and during pregnancy in preventing neural tube defects.[378]

The morphologic features of the syndrome are not constant;[313] e.g., the amount of diencephalic remnant is quite variable. The sella turcica is present but greatly deformed; the clinoid processes are hypoplastic, and there is no diaphragma sella.[19, 103, 313] The anterior lobe is always present, although reduced in size.[103] The neurohypophysis is present in about 25% of anencephalics;[313] when present, it is hypoplastic and deformed. An absence of neurosecretory material in the neural lobe has been noted.[436] The posterior limb of

Rathke's pouch (the primitive intermediate lobe) is found when the neurohypophysis is also present but is poorly developed.[403] The anencephalic fetus is a unique model, albeit one with important limitations, to study the neuroendocrine regulation of fetal pituitary function.[229, 230, 290, 531]

Although the size of the pituitary is reduced in anencephaly,[103] the cell cords are well developed.[477] Somatotropes, lactotropes, gonadotropes, and thyrotropes occur in the anencephalic pituitary in similar proportions to the distribution in normal fetal pituitaries.[246, 403, 474, 477] In contrast, corticotropes are considerably reduced in number.[55, 403, 477]

The GH content of the pituitary of one anencephalic fetus at term was 140 µg, equivalent to that observed at 14 to 24 weeks' gestation in human fetuses without a CNS abnormality.[229, 230, 290] In another single anencephalic fetus, the prolactin content of the pituitary was low and similar to that of a normal 20-week fetus.[230, 290] Similarly, the pituitary content of FSH and LH was low in three term anencephalic fetuses and comparable to that of fetuses between 10 and 20 weeks.[229, 230, 290] In a single anencephalic pituitary, α subunit was the dominant glycoprotein hormone fraction.[239] A constant feature of anencephaly is the regression of the adrenal cortex, particularly of the fetal zones, especially after 20 weeks' gestation;[3, 19, 62, 103, 277, 477] in contrast, the thyroid gland appears normal.[19, 103, 246, 274] The abnormalities of the fetal gonads and the hypoplastic male genitalia in anencephaly have already been discussed.

Thus, morphologic as well as hormonal studies of anencephalic fetuses indicate failure of the hypothalamic-pituitary-adrenal and gonadotropic axes. It is also apparent from these studies that the fetal hypothalamus is not essential for the development and differentiation of the anterior pituitary, with the possible exception of corticotropes.

In the fetal rat, evidence suggests that Rathke's pouch differentiates into corticotropes, somatotropes, lactotropes, thyrotropes, and gonadotropes when cultured in the absence of hypothalamic tissue;[553] however, hypothalamic mediation is required for full maturation of granular cells, as demonstrated both in vivo and in vitro.[127, 491]

Similarly, in the human anencephalic fetus, pituitary hormone secretion is abnormal even though cell differentiation occurs. There are low concentrations of plasma GH in anencephaly at birth.[16, 229, 230, 235, 249, 290] In nine anencephalic infants at term, the mean concentration of plasma GH was 7.0 ng/mL (1.0 to 17.0 ng/mL), significantly less than in normal infants (33.5 ± 4.3 ng/mL).[229, 230] Two anencephalic infants with very low basal GH concentrations showed no GH response to insulin or arginine infusion; however, one with a basal GH of 17 ng/mL responded to both stimuli with a rise in GH concentration. This suggests that the hypothalamic defect in anencephaly is variable and that, in some cases, there is sufficient functional hypothalamic tissue to affect pituitary hormone secretion.[229, 290]

In anencephalic infants at birth, the concentration of plasma prolactin is normal, indicating that hypothalamic stimulation is not required for differentiation and proliferation of lactotropes or prolactin secretion.[32, 173, 230, 249, 560] Exogenous TRF stimulates prolactin and TSH secretion in the anencephalic infant, suggesting the presence of TRF receptors in the pituitary.[32, 173, 230, 430, 465a]

Plasma ACTH has generally been reported to be low in anencephalic fetuses,[16, 371] and the pituitary content of ACTH is reduced;[16] however, lysine vasopressin stimulates ACTH release.[16] As discussed, the normal concentrations of plasma hCG, placental ACTH, and prolactin do not prevent adrenocortical hypoplasia.

The plasma concentration of TSH is normal on the day of birth in anencephaly,[16, 225] but it does not exhibit the characteristic increase shortly after delivery[225] and is low by the second to third postnatal day.[290] TRF induces a brisk, prolonged rise in TSH.[32, 230, 249, 430] Thus, the anencephalic infant is highly sensitive to TRF and has a pool of readily releasable TSH. The pituitary contains thyrotropes; the morphology of the thyroid is normal, as is the thyroxine concentration in umbilical cord blood.[16, 225] In contrast, infants with pituitary aplasia and some with Pit-1 mutations have a hypoplastic thyroid gland and severe hypothyroidism. These observations suggest that the thyroid gland of the anencephalic fetus is stimulated by TSH but that the secretion of fetal pituitary TSH is not regulated by hypothalamic TRF but by extrahypothalamic factors. Further, in blood samples obtained by cordocentesis from nine anencephalic fetuses between 17 and 26 weeks of gestation, the plasma concentrations of immunoreactive and bioactive TSH and free thyroxine did not differ from those of normal fetuses of comparable gestational age.[53]

The increased concentration of circulating TRF in the human fetus[324] is due to increased synthesis by extrahypothalamic tissues, especially the fetal pancreatoenteric system, and to the low TRF degrading enzyme activity of fetal blood.[23] Even though TRF can be transferred across the placenta,[465a, 466] maternal levels are exceedingly low and would not be a significant source of TRF in the anencephalic fetus. Hence it is possible that extrahypothalamic TRF stimulates sufficient pituitary TSH secretion to maintain the integrity of the anencephalic thyroid gland. It is unlikely that the thyroid is functioning autonomously because it is usually hypoplastic in infants with pituitary aplasia and in some infants with Pit-1 mutations.[27] hCG has less than 1/1000 the activity of TSH,[253] and the circulating concentration of hCG in the fetus, in contrast to in the mother during the first trimester, is insufficient to stimulate the thyroid. Moreover, fetal plasma hCG does not prevent the thyroid hypoplasia associated with pituitary aplasia. Extrahypothalamic TRF, for the present, seems a likely possibility as the mediator of TSH secretion in the anencephalic fetus. Further, TRF has been detected in the tissue that occupies the base of the cranial vault in an anencephalic fetus.[274]

In the normal fetus, the available evidence suggests that hypothalamic TRF by its action on the fetal thyrotrope has a role in the regulation of fetal thyroid function in midgestation and late gestation as evidenced by, for example, the capacity of goitrogens administered to the mother, including the thionamide class of antithyroid drugs, to induce fetal goiter[374, 465a, 534] and the fetal goiter associated with some mutations of thyroid hormone biosynthesis. Complete autonomous function of the fetal thyroid, independent of fetal TSH, does not explicate the hypoplastic thyroid gland of the fetus with primary pituitary aplasia or with a Pit-1 mutation.

Holoprosencephaly, Septo-optic Dysplasia, Optic Nerve Hypoplasia

Holoprosencephaly

Holoprosencephaly is a malformation complex whose basic characteristic is defective cleavage of the embryonic forebrain and usually craniofacial anomalies. The prosencephalon fails to cleave sagittally into cerebral hemispheres, transversely into telencephalon and diencephalon, and horizontally into optic and olfactory bulbs. Holoprosencephaly can be classified by severity as alobar, semilobar and lobar. Facial dysmorphism of varying degree is common, and there is a general but not invariable correlation between the severity of the brain malformation and the facial abnormalities.[121, 137, 138, 269, 383, 401, 460, 494]

Of interest is the absence of the septum pellucidum and, in some instances, the corpus collosum in the lobar or "incomplete" form; the often absent or minor facial abnormalities; and the occurrence of optic and olfactory hypoplasia. The pituitary gland and stalk may be absent or hypoplastic.[269, 461]

The etiology is exceedingly heterogeneous, varying from chromosome abnormalities, especially trisomy 13, deletion of the short arm of chromosome 18, and trisomy 18, to a variety of single gene defects and teratogenic factors, including substance abuse.[494, 544] There are a host of syndromic forms as well as nonchromosomal nonsyndromic holoprosencephaly.[115, 116] The vast majority of cases are sporadic.

Microforms of the disorder have been described in families of probands. These include a variety of CNS abnormalities, including microcephaly and mental retardation, short stature, hypopituitarism,[461] anosmia/hyposmia, single central maxillary incisor, cleft lip or palate, and hypotelorism.

Septo-optic Dysplasia; Optic Nerve Hypoplasia

The syndrome of septo-optic dysplasia was defined by de Morsier in 1956,[136] and in 1970, our group reported a high prevalence of hypopituitarism in this disorder.[292, 288] This midline malformation syndrome is heterogeneous

and the etiology diverse. Familial cases are rare; there is a strong association with young maternal age and a possible relationship to substance abuse.[544]

Hypothalamic-pituitary deficiencies are commonly associated with septo-optic dysplasia and with optic nerve dysplasia with an intact septum pellucidum.[24, 288, 339] In our group of more than 25 patients with the syndrome who had hypothalamic-pituitary deficiencies, about 50% of the patients with optic nerve hypoplasia had an absent septum pellucidum.[288] About 50% of children with severe, bilateral optic nerve hypoplasia have hypopituitarism, whereas only 10 to 20% with severe unilateral optic nerve dysplasia have an endocrine abnormality. Mental retardation, seizure disorders, and other neurologic abnormalities are common, but many patients have minimal or no neurologic deficits. About 25% of affected individuals are blind. Poor vision and pendular or seesaw nystagmus are frequent.

More than 90% of our patients had one or more anterior pituitary hormone deficiencies, most commonly pituitary GH deficiency.[288] About 30% had diabetes insipidus; the occurrence of anterior and posterior pituitary deficiencies is almost always indicative of a hypothalamic or pituitary neoplasm, but in this instance, it is due to a malformation involving the hypothalamus. Less commonly, diabetes insipidus may be the only endocrine manifestation.

In patients with septo-optic dysplasia and hypopituitarism, diffuse white matter hypoplasia is common.[42] The occurrence of porencephaly, encephalocele, and microcephaly, among other CNS abnormalities, is increased.[43, 85] Seizure disorders are more common when schizencephaly is present.[85]

Seizures may be due to hypoglycemia and CNS injury resulting from recurrent unrecognized hypoglycemia, or they may be due to a CNS anomaly. In some patients, both hypoglycemia and the brain malformations are the cause.

In the affected newborn and infant, pendular or rotary nystagmus, sluggish pupillary reaction to light, and the detection of a small optic disc, commonly with a "halo" or "double ring" sign, should suggest the diagnosis of optic nerve hypoplasia. The affected newborn and infant with associated hypopituitarism often presents with evidence of hypoglycemia, including apnea, hypotonia, and seizures, and with prolonged jaundice and, in some male infants, microphallus.[288] A varying degree of developmental delay may be present. If unrecognized in infancy, children with hypopituitarism present with short stature with or without neurologic deficits.

The occurrence of nystagmus in an infant should raise the possibility of optic nerve hypoplasia and the need for studies of hypothalamic-pituitary function, as should a short, blind child. A small proportion of affected individuals develop true or central precocious puberty as a consequence of the hypothalamic defect.

With the advent of magnetic resonance imaging (MRI), the CNS and optic nerve abnormalities have been defined more precisely and definitively[42, 85, 296] (Fig. 12–26). Three of our patients have had an attentuated or absent infundibular stalk and an ectopic neurohypophysis. Although in some patients septo-optic dysplasia is probably a variant of holoprosencephaly, in most patients, the pathogenesis is different.

CLEFT LIP AND PALATE. These malformations with or without other congenital anomalies can be associated with hypopituitarism either as isolated GH deficiency or with multiple pituitary hormone deficiencies. In short children with this isolated malformation (12.5% in one series), about 30% have GH deficiency with or without other pituitary hormone deficits owing to a hypothalamic abnormality.[469]

SINGLE CENTRAL INCISOR. This is another usually sporadic congenital anomaly that can be associated with impaired growth owing to hypopituitarism.[447]

Idiopathic Hypopituitarism with a Hypoplastic or Interrupted Stalk and Ectopic Neurohypophysis (Dysgenesis of the Pituitary Stalk)

The application of synthetic hypothalamic hormones (TRF, LRF, GRF, CRF) to test anterior pituitary function has provided a large body of evidence that pituitary hormone deficiencies in more than 80% of patients with idiopathic hypopituitarism are due to a failure of synthesis, secretion, or delivery of hypothalamic hypophysiotropic hormones to the pituitary gland.

The application of MRI to the study of the hypothalamic-pituitary region of patients with idiopathic hypopituitarism has brought to light a striking observation: A high proportion of affected individuals have on T1-weighted MRI an ectopic neurohypophysis located near or in apposition with the median eminence identified by the characteristic *bright spot* of the posterior pituitary gland and an absent, attenuated, or abnormal infundibular stalk, often associated with a small anterior pituitary gland (Fig. 12–27). This observation was first described by Fujisawa, Kikuchi, and their associates in 1987[181, 298] and confirmed in many subsequent studies.[2, 88, 95, 335]

Two large series of patients with idiopathic multiple pituitary hormone deficiencies (MPHD) or isolated GH deficiency (IGHD) have had MRI studies.[2, 95] In 38 patients with idiopathic MPHD, 79% had an ectopic neurohypophysis in contrast to 5% of 62 patients with IGHD. The infundibular stalk was absent in 68% and interrupted or attenuated in 26% of MPHD patients versus 3% of IGHD patients. The anterior pituitary gland was small (34%) or not visualized (42%) in MPHD in contrast to 15% and 2% in IGHD (Table 12–8). These observations strongly suggest that more than 90% of patients with so-called idiopathic neonatal hypopituitarism have a malformation involving the infundibular stalk of the pituitary gland that arises from the infundibular diverticulum of the diencephalon (see Figs. 12–3, 12–4, and 12–5), and as a consequence, 80% have an ectopic neurohypophysis, whereas only a small proportion of patients with IGHD have this abnormality. Similarly, the occurrence of a small or not visualized anterior pituitary gland was four times more frequent in patients with MPHD.

Even though the incidence of breech presentation and birth asphyxia is increased in idiopathic MPHD[122, 222] and a possible cause of the syndrome, for a number of reasons, it is more likely that the malformation more commonly arose earlier in gestation, and perinatal

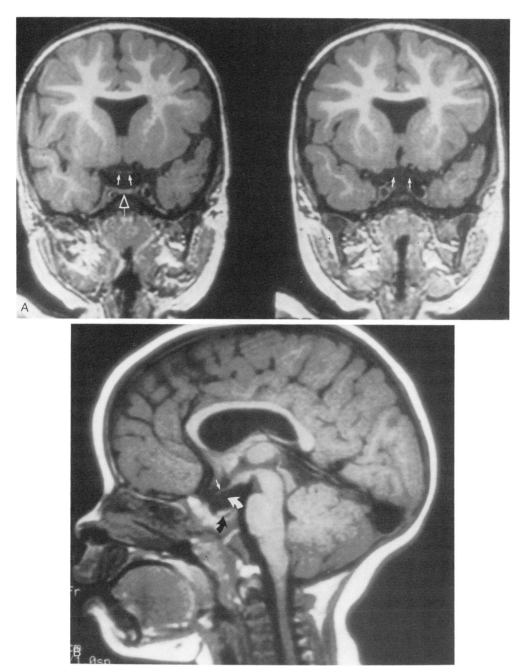

FIGURE 12–26. An infant with septo-optic dysplasia and multiple pituitary hormone deficiencies, an attenuated pituitary stalk, and a hypoplastic pituitary gland. *A,* Coronal T1-weighted MRI scan. Note absent septum pellucidum. Solid white arrows indicate intraorbital portions of hypoplastic optic nerves. The open white arrow designates the small pituitary gland. *B,* Sagittal T1-weighted image. Small white arrow indicates the hypoplastic optic chiasm; the curved, solid white arrow the attenuated pituitary stalk; and the solid black arrow the hypoplastic pituitary gland.

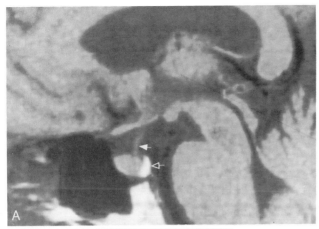
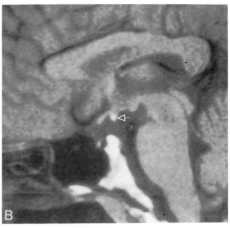
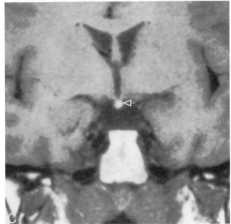

FIGURE 12–27. *A*, Midline sagittal T1-weighted MRI scan of a 4-year-old boy showing a normal pituitary stalk (solid white arrow) and a normal pituitary gland with the characteristic bright spot (open white arrow) of the posterior pituitary gland. *B*, Midline sagittal T1-weighted scan of a 2-year-old boy with multiple pituitary hormone deficiencies illustrating an ectopic posterior pituitary bright spot in opposition with the median eminence of the hypothalamus (open white arrow), absent pituitary stalk, and a hypoplastic pituitary gland. *C*, Coronal T1-weighted scan illustrating the ectopic posterior pituitary lobe (open white arrow) and the absent pituitary stalk.

difficulties were a consequence and not a cause of the abnormality. Infants with a variety of malformations, including brain anomalies, musculoskeletal disorders of diverse etiology, chromosomal abnormalities, and point mutations, have a strikingly increased prevalence of breech delivery.[81, 123] In our series of 27 patients with idiopathic neonatal hypopituitar-

ism, none appeared to be caused by birth trauma. Three infants presented in a breech or transverse position but were delivered by cesarean section before the onset of labor. Three other infants had major complications at birth, but all three were males with a micropenis, which we regard as evidence of prenatal and long-standing hypopituitarism. Our data

TABLE 12–8. Prevalence of Infundibular Stalk and Ectopic Neurohypophysis in So-called Idiopathic Hypopituitarism

Hypopituitarism	n	Ectopic Neurohypophysis	Absent Posterior Pituitary Bright Spot	Infundibular Stalk		Anterior Pituitary	
				Absent	*Transected*	*Small*	*Not Visualized*
Multiple pituitary hormone deficiencies	23*	17	6	13	10	3	16
	15†	13	0	13	0	10	0
	38	30 (79%)	6 (16%)	26 (68%)	10 (26%)	13 (34%)	16 (42%)
Isolated growth hormone deficiency	42*	1	0	0	1	4	1
	20†	2	0	2	1 (Hypoplastic)	5	0
	62	3 (5%)	0	2 (3%)	2 (3%)	9 (15%)	1 (2%)

*E. Cacciari et al.[95]
†Abrahams et al.[2]

are consistent with the hypothesis that fetal hypopituitarism per se may lead to birth complications, including malposition of the fetus, and that the deficiency of fetal pituitary hormones may prevent an adequate homeostatic response to the stress of delivery.

A similar view has been advanced by others.[333] Further, some of our patients with septo-optic dysplasia complex have exhibited the same type of defect,[296] which provides some support for the possibility of a developmental field defect[397, 398] in idiopathic MPHD with dysgenesis of the infundibular stalk as one feature of the field defect, as does the association with the type I Arnold-Chiari syndrome and syringomyelia.[182] Of interest, observations[383, 494] in holoprosencephaly had suggested earlier the possibility of impaired development of the anterior pituitary gland if it failed to fuse with the infundibular diverticulum of the diencephalon. An *ectopic* neurohypophysis can arise as a consequence of a low transection of the pituitary stalk in the adult human as well as the monkey and other experimental animals within a few weeks to months of the procedure.[20a, 127a] Our proposal is that in most infants with idiopathic MPHD, whatever untoward event in the fetus resulted in an ectopic posterior pituitary gland occurred remote from and unrelated to parturition. It is our view that the weight of evidence favors a malformation and not the birth injury theory[182, 255] as the cause of most cases of idiopathic neonatal hypopituitarism.

Kallmann's Syndrome and Hypogonadotropic Hypogonadism

In this inherited syndrome, the most common form of isolated hypogonadotropic hypogonadism with delayed puberty, anosmia or hyposmia resulting from agenesis or hypoplasia of the olfactory bulbs and tracts is associated with hypothalamic LRF deficiency as a consequence of a defect in neuronal migration.[234, 439] The extent of the defect in olfaction seems to correlate with the degree of LRF deficiency; in turn, the degree of LRF deficiency correlates with the size of the testes. Affected individuals often do not notice impaired olfaction; formal testing is necessary. The agenesis or hypoplasia of the olfactory nerve complex (olfactory sulci, bulbs, and tracts) can be detected by MRI even in the affected infant[234, 538] (Fig. 12–28). Undescended testes and micropenis are common features that are present at birth in affected males. Associated defects inconstantly present are cleft lip or palate, imperfect facial fusion, seizure disorders, unilateral renal agenesis, short metacarpals, pes cavus, and a variety of neurologic abnormalities, including mirror movements, sensorineural deafness, cerebellar ataxia, seizure disorders, and ocular motor abnormalities.[439]

This genetically heterogeneous syndrome is about four times as common in males as females and can be transmitted as an X-linked,[245] autosomal dominant or autosomal recessive trait. X-chromosome linked KAL gene has been mapped to Xp 22.3.[40] Contiguous gene deletions in this region of the X chromosome can lead to an association of Kallmann's syndrome with, for example, X-linked ichthyosis caused by steroid sulfatase deficiency, mental retardation, and chondroplasia punctata.

In *Kallmann's syndrome*, fetal LRF neurosecretory neurons fail to migrate from the olfactory placode, where they arise, to the medial basal hypothalamus,[484] where they constitute the LRF pulse generator. The defect may be absolute or relative. The fetal LRF-containing cells and neurites are arrested in their migration to the forebrain from the nose and end in a tangle around the cribriform plate and in the dural layers adjacent to the meninges beneath the forebrain (see Fig. 12–27). Defective migration of the olfactory nerve complex from the olfactory placode leads to agenesis or hypoplasia of the olfactory bulbs and anosmia or hyposmia; both the olfactory neurons and the LRF neurosecretory neurons migrate to the forebrain in embryonic life along a common pathway. The isolation of the KAL gene[176, 310] in X-linked Kallmann's syndrome indicates that its predicted product has properties of a neural cell adhesion molecule, which may act as a scaffold for the migration of LRF and olfactory neurons[176, 310, 470, 483] (see the section on Hypothalamus).

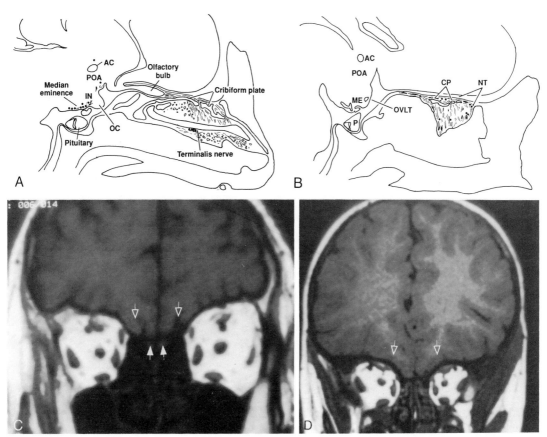

FIGURE 12–28. *A* and *B,* Comparison of brain and nasal cavities of a normal 19-week-old male fetus (*A*) and those of a male fetus of similar age with Kallmann's syndrome caused by an X chromosome deletion at Xp22.3 (*B*). In the normal fetal brain, the LRF neurosecretory neurons (black dots) are located in the hypothalamic area mainly in the medial basal hypothalamus as well as the anterior hypothalamic area and (of interest, in relation to an LRF-secreting hypothalamic hamartoma as a cause of true or central precocious puberty as an ectopic LRF pulse generator) in the premamillary and retromamillary areas. A small cluster of LRF neurons is present among the fibers of the nervus terminalis on the floor of the nasal septum. In the male fetus with Kallmann's syndrome (*B*), no LRF neurons are located in the hypothalamic region, including the basal hypothalamus, median eminence, and preoptic area. The LRF cells fail to migrate to and enter the brain from their origin in the medial olfactory placode in the nose; instead these cells end in a tangle beneath the forebrain on the dorsal surface of the cribriform plate and in the nasal cavity. The failure of olfactory nerve fibers to migrate from the lateral olfactory placode to reach the telencephalon leads to failure of induction of the olfactory bulbs and the development of the olfactory tract. The mitral cells of the olfactory bulb in the chick embryo express the KAL gene but not the olfactory placode (see text). *AC* = Anterior commissure; CG = cristal galli; IN = infundibular nucleus; NT = nervus terminalis; OC = optic chiasm; POA = preoptic area. *C* and *D,* MRI scans of brain (coronal, T1-weighted images). *C,* Normal olfactory sulci (open white arrows) and bulbs (solid white arrows) in a 15-year-old boy. *D,* Absent olfactory sulci (open white arrows) and bulbs (solid white arrows) in a 17-year-old anosmic, sexually infantile boy with Kallmann's syndrome. In a multiplex family with X-linked transmission of the syndrome, we have detected the same MRI findings in a 4-month-old affected boy. (*A* and *B,* adapted from Schwanzel-Fukuda M, Bick D, Pfaff DW. Luteinizing hormone–releasing hormone (LHRH)–expressing cells do not migrate normally in an inherited hypogonadal (Kallmann) Syndrome. Mol Brain Res 1989; 6:311. From Grumbach MM, Styne DM. Puberty: ontogeny, neuroendocrinology, physiology, and disorders. In: Wilson JD, Foster DW, eds. Williams textbook of endocrinology, ed 8. Philadelphia: WB Saunders, 1992:1139–1221. *C* and *D* from Grumbach MM, Styne DM. Puberty: ontogeny, neuroendocrinology, physiology, and disorders. In: Wilson JD, Foster DW, eds. Williams textbook of endocrinology, ed 8. Philadelphia: WB Saunders, 1992:1139–1221.)

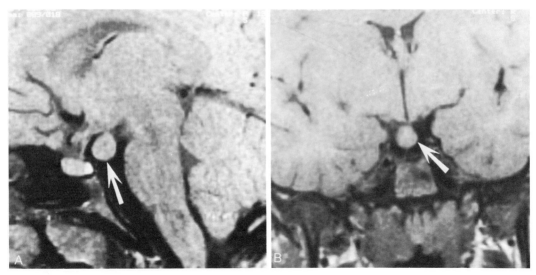

FIGURE 12–29. Cranial MRI of an LRF-secreting hypothalamic hamartoma in a 4-year-old girl with true precocious puberty who developed breasts at 0.7 year and menses at 0.8 year. *A,* Sagittal T1-weighted image. *B,* Coronal T1-weighted image. The white arrows indicate the pedunculated hamartoma, which measures 10 mm in its largest diameter. Note the normal pituitary stalk and gland and the posterior pituitary bright spot. The hypothalamic hamartoma has not increased in size during a 5-year follow-up by neuroimaging studies.

HYPOTHALAMIC HAMARTOMA AND TRUE OR CENTRAL PRECOCIOUS PUBERTY

Hamartomas of the tuber cinereum, congenital malformations composed of a heterotypic mass of neurosecretory neurons, fiber bundles, and glial cells, are frequently associated with true precocious puberty (when they contain LRF neurons),[258, 285] often before the patient is 3 years of age.[234, 289] Hypothalamic hamartomas that cause true or central precocious puberty can be associated with laughing (gelastic), petit mal, or generalized seizures; mental retardation; behavioral disturbances; and dysmorphic syndromes.[336] With computed tomography (CT) and MRI brain scans,[80] hamartomas of the tuber cinereum are now being detected in young boys and girls previously thought to have idiopathic central precocious puberty; before 1980, there were reports of about 37 patients in the literature with hamartomas of the tuber cinereum, and since 1980, more than 60 additional cases have been reported.[336]

Hamartomas of the tuber cinereum are not neoplasms but rather congenital, nonneoplastic heterotopic nests of cells arising from the third ventricle and composed of disordered but mature and differentiated neural elements.[336] Usually the hamartomas are pedunculated, connected with the posterior portion of the tuber cinereum by a distinct stalk; less commonly they are sessile. On CT scan they appear as an isodense, abnormal fullness of the interpeduncular, prepontine, and posterior suprasellar cisterns, occasionally with distortion of the anterior third ventricle. They characteristically have a collar button appearance and do not exhibit enhancement with contrast material. MRI gives the best visualization of the lesion (Fig. 12–29).

Analysis of hamartomas associated with true precocious puberty has revealed the presence of LRF neurosecretory neurons[258, 285] similar to the LRF-containing neurons (the LRF pulse generator) in their normal location in the medial basal hypothalamus. This heterotopia exerts its endocrine effects by the elaboration and pulsatile release of LRF. Indeed LRF-containing fibers have been identified passing from the hamartoma toward the median eminence. We have suggested that the LRF-neurosecretory neurons in the hamartoma are unrestrained by the intrinsic CNS mechanism that inhibits the normally situated LRF pulse generator and acts as an ectopic LRF pulse generator, either independently or in synchrony with the LRF neurosecretory neurons in the medial basal hypothalamus, to produce intermittent secretory bursts of LRF.[231, 234, 336] The LRF is transported to the pituitary by way of the hypophyseal portal circulation and elicits pulsatile release of LH and FSH. Hamartomas can be considered a counterpart of the transplantation of mouse LRF neurosecretory neurons into the third ventricle, which rescues and restores reproductive endocrine function in the hypogonadal/hypogonadal (hpg/hpg) mouse. The hpg/hpg mouse has a mutation in the gene encoding the LRF-prohormone, which leads to severe LRF deficiency and hypogonadotropic hypogonadism. Although sought, a comparable mutation in the human has not yet been identified.

The location of hypothalamic hamartomas makes surgical removal difficult and risky. Although there are cases in which removal of the mass led to a reversal of the pubertal process, the mortality and morbidity are high. Hamartomas grow slowly, if in fact they do enlarge, and any change (for example, the remote possibility of transformation into a hamartoblastoma) can be detected readily on periodic CT or MRI scans. Further, the precocious sexual development can be easily controlled by treatment with potent LRF-agonists.[234] Neurosurgical extirpation is contraindicated in the absence of evidence of rapid growth of the hamartoma.

PRENATAL AND NEONATAL OVARIAN CYSTS

As discussed earlier, the onset of meiosis in the oogonia of the fetal ovary begins during the 11th week of gestation[221] and gives rise to oocytes, a process that continues until birth. The first follicles marked by the appearance of granulosa cells appear about the 16th week of gestation, and by late gestation, numerous late preantral and antral follicles surrounded by a definitive theca layer are present, which now have the capacity to synthesize estradiol. Even though folliculogenesis is associated with the rise in fetal pituitary gonadotropins, the role of fetal FSH in the initiation and maintenance

of this process before late in gestation is uncertain because functional FSH receptors have not been detected in the midtrimester human fetal ovary.[267]

The advent of routine fetal sonography has led to the detection of large ovarian cysts as early as the 28th week of gestation. The prevalence is not known; in one report, more than 85% of the cysts were greater than 3 cm in diameter,[516] and torsion has been reported in 15 to 30% without an effect on fetal well-being. With rare exceptions, the presence of a large follicular cyst is not an indication for cesarean section. After delivery, the size of the cyst should be monitored by clinical observation, careful assessment, and serial sonograms. The natural history is one of spontaneous regression usually within 6 months, sometimes with disappearance of the cyst in a few weeks but in other instances not for months. An indeterminate number are functional and secrete estradiol. Fetal and neonatal ovarian follicular cysts are usually asymptomatic. Rupture of the cyst is rare; however, torsion with infarction of the ovary, more commonly involving the right ovary, is a risk, but it can be suspected by the sonographic appearance of the cyst. Torsion of the cyst requires immediate surgical intervention. Percutaneous aspiration guided by sonography is a useful first approach to reducing the size of a large untorsed follicular cyst (if it is sufficiently symptomatic to warrant intervention) and to preserving the ovary.[188] Treatment of large asymptomatic follicular cysts with medroxyprogesterone acetate should be considered; if the cyst secretes increased amounts of estradiol, a trial on a LRF-agonist may be useful. It is important to inform the parents of the symptoms of torsion and the necessity of seeking prompt medical attention.

A new syndrome has been defined characterized by estradiol-secreting ovarian cysts in preterm infants less than 30 weeks' gestation associated with edema of the labia majora and in some cases of the abdominal wall. In four preterm neonates, the syndrome first appeared weeks after birth and about 1 to 4 weeks before the expected full-term date. The follicular cysts may be unilateral or bilateral and are readily detected by sonography.[114] The LH and FSH rise induced by LRF suggested that the cysts were LRF and gonadotropin dependent. Medroxyprogesterone acetate treatment was associated with regression of the cysts.[487]

The size and appearance of the ovaries in normal neonates and infants has been defined by pelvic sonography. The mean ovarian volume is 1.06 cm^3 in infants age 1 day to 3 months. Twenty-eight percent of ovaries have follicular cysts, of which one-fourth are macrocysts (longer than 0.9 cm [range 0.1 to 1.4 cm in diameter]).[114] This prevalence approximates that found at autopsy in neonatal deaths.[140]

REFERENCES

1. Abe Y, Miyamoto HK, Yamaguchi M, et al. High concentrations of plasma immunoreactive inhibin during normal pregnancy. J Clin Endocrinol Metab 1990; 71:133.
2. Abrahams JJ, Trefelner E, Boulware SD. Idiopathic growth hormone deficiency: MR findings in 35 patients. Am J Neuroradiol 1991; 12:155.
3. Abramovitch DR. Physiologic and endocrinologic study of the anencephalic syndrome. Obstet Gynecol 1977; 38:869.
4. Abramovitch DR, Rowe P. Foetal plasma testosterone levels at mid pregnancy and at term. J Endocrinol 1973; 56:621.
5. Ackland J, Ratter S, Bourne GL, Rees LH. Characterization of immunoreactive somatostatin in human fetal hypothalamic tissue. Regul Pept 1983; 5:95.
6. Ackland JF, Ratter SJ, Bourne GL, Rees LH. Corticotropin-releasing factor-like immunoreactivity and bioactivity of human fetal and adult hypothalami. J Endocrinol 1986; 108:171.
7. Adamo M, Lowe WL Jr, LeRoith D, Roberts CT. Insulin-like growth factor I messenger ribonucleic acids with alternative 5'-untranslated regions are differentially expressed during development of the rat. Endocrinology 1989; 124:2737.
8. Akagi K, Berdusco ETM, Challis JRG. Cortisol inhibits ACTH but not the AVP response to hypoxemia in fetal lambs at d125-130 of gestation. J Dev Physiol 1991; 14:319.
9. Akagi K, Challis JRG. Hormonal and biophysical responses to acute hypoxemia in fetal sheep at 0.7–0.8 gestation. Can J Physiol Pharmacol 1990; 68:1527.
10. Aksel S, Tyrey L. Luteinizing hormone-releasing hormone in the human fetal brain. Fertil Steril 1977; 28:1067.
11. Albers N, Bettendorf M, Hart CS, et al. Hormone ontogeny in the ovine fetus. XXIII. Pulsatile administration of follicle-stimulating hormone stimulates inhibin production and decreases testosterone synthesis in the ovine fetal gonad. Endocrinology 1989; 124:3089.
12. Albers N, Bettendorf M, Herrmann H, et al. Hormone ontogeny in the ovine fetus. XXVII. Pulsatile and copulsatile secretion of luteinizing hormone, follicle stimulating hormone, growth hormone, and prolactin in late gestation: A new method for the analysis of copulsatility. Endocrinology 1993; 132:701.
13. Albers N, Hart CS, Kaplan SL, Grumbach MM. Hormone ontogeny in the ovine fetus. XXIV. Porcine follicular fluid "inhibins" selectively suppress plasma follicle-stimulating hormone in the ovine fetus. Endocrinology 1989; 125:675.
14. Albertsson-Wikland K, Nicklasson A, Karlberg P. Birth data for patients who later develop growth hormone deficiency: preliminary analysis of a national register. Acta Paediatr Scand 1990; 370(suppl):115.
15. Allen JP, Cook DM, Kendall JW, McGilvra R. Maternal-fetal ACTH relationship in man. J Clin Endocrinol Metab 1973; 37:230.
16. Allen JP, Greer MA, McGilvra R, et al. Endocrine function in an anencephalic infant. J Clin Endocrinol Metab 1974; 38:94.
17. Amselem S, Sobrier M-I, Duquesnoy P, et al. Recurrent nonsense mutations in the growth hormone receptor from patients with Laron dwarfism. J Clin Invest 1991; 87:1098.
18. Andersen H, von Bülow FA, Mollgard K. The early development of the pars distalis of human foetal pituitary gland. Z Anat Entw 1971; 135:117.
19. Angevine DM. Pathological anatomy of hypophysis and adrenals in anencephaly. Arch Pathol 1938; 26:507.
20. Antolovich GA, McMillen IC, Perry RA, et al. The development of corticotrophs in the fetal sheep pars distalis. The effect of cortisol infusion or adrenalectomy or hypothalamo-pituitary disconnection (HPD). In: Jones CT, ed. Research in perinatal medicine. Ithaca, NY: Perinatology Press, 1988:243.
20a. Antunes JL, Louis KM, Huang S, et al. Section of the pituitary stalk in the rhesus monkey: morphological and endocrine observations. Ann Neurol 1980; 8:308.
21. Arai K, Kuwabara Y, Okinaga S. The effect of adrenocorticotrophic hormone and dexamethasone, administered to the fetus in utero on maternal and fetal oestrogens. Am J Obstet Gynecol 1972; 113:316.
22. Arai K, Yanaihara T, Okinaga S. Adrenocorticotrophic hormone in human fetal blood at delivery. Am J Obstet Gynecol 1976; 125:1136.
23. Araten-Spire S, Czernichow P. Thyrotropin releasing hormone degrading activity of neonatal human plasma. J Clin Endocrinol Metab 1980; 50:88.
24. Arslanian SA, Rothfus WE, Foley TP Jr, Becker DJ. Hormonal, metabolic, and neuroradiologic abnormalities associated with septo-optic dysplasia. Acta Endocrinol (Copenh) 1984; 107:282.
25. Asa SL, Kovacs K. Functional morphology of the human fetal pituitary. Pathol Annu 1984; 19:275.
26. Asa SL, Kovacs K, Bilbao JM. The pars tuberalis of the human pituitary. Virchows Arch (A) 1983; 399:49.
27. Asa SL, Kovacs K, Halasz A, et al. Absence of somatotrophs, lactotrophs, and thyrotrophs in the pituitary of two dwarfs with hypothyroidism: deficiency of pituitary transcription factor-1? Endocr Pathol 1992; 3:93.
28. Asa SL, Kovacs K, Horvath E, et al. Human fetal adenohypophysis: electron microscopic and ultrastructural immunocytochemical analysis. Neuroendocrinology 1988; 48:423.
29. Asa SL, Kovacs K, Laszlo FA, et al. Human fetal adenohypophysis: histologic and immunocytochemical analysis. Neuroendocrinology 1986; 43:308.
30. Atwell WJ. The development of the hypophysis cerebri in man, with special reference to the pars tuberalis. Am J Anat 1926; 37:159.
31. Aubert ML, Grumbach MM, Kaplan SL. Heterolo-

gous radioimmunoassay for human prolactin (hPRL): values in normal subjects, puberty, pregnancy and in pituitary disorders. Acta Endocrinol 1974; 77:460.

32. Aubert ML, Grumbach MM, Kaplan SL. The ontogenesis of human fetal hormones. III. Prolactin. J Clin Invest 1975; 56:155.

33. Aubert ML, Grumbach MM, Kaplan SL. The ontogenesis of human fetal hormones. IV. Somatostatin, luteinizing hormone releasing factor, and thyrotropin releasing factor. J Clin Endocrinol Metab 1977; 44:1130.

33a. August GP, Tkachuk M, Grumbach MM. Plasma testosterone-binding affinity and testosterone in umbilical cord plasma, late pregnancy, prepubertal children and adults. J Clin Endocrinol Metab 1969; 29:891.

34. Badawi M, Van Exter C, Delogne-Desnoeck J, et al. Cord serum prolactin in relation to the time of the day, the sex of the neonate and the birth weight. Acta Endocrinol 1978; 87:241.

35. Baird A, Wehrenberg B, Bohlen P, Ling N. Immunoreactive and biologically active growth hormone-releasing factor in the rat placenta. Endocrinology 1985; 117:1598.

36. Baker RL, Jaffe RB. The genesis of cell types in the adenohypophysis of the human fetus as observed with immunocytochemistry. Am J Anat 1975; 143:137.

37. Baker TG. A quantitative and cytological study of germ cells in human ovaries. Proc Roy Soc Lond [Biol] 1963; 158:417.

38. Baker TG, Scrimegeour JB. Development of the gonad in normal and anencephalic human fetuses. J Reprod Fertil 1980; 60:193.

39. Ball KT, Power GG, Gunn TR, et al. Modulation of growth hormone (GH) secretion by thermogenically-derived free fatty acids (FFA) in the perinatal lamb. Endocrinology 1992; 131:337.

40. Ballabio A, Bardoni B, Carrozzo R, et al. Contiguous gene syndromes due to deletions in the distal short arm of the human X chromosome. Proc Natl Acad Sci USA 1989; 86:10001.

41. Ballard PL, Gluckman PD, Liggins GC, et al. Steroid and growth hormone levels in premature infants after prenatal betamethasone therapy to prevent respiratory distress syndrome. Pediatr Res 1980; 14:122.

42. Barkovich AJ, Fram EK, Norman D. Septo-optic dysplasia: MR imaging. Radiology 1989; 171:189.

43. Barkovich AJ, Norman D. Absence of the septum pellucidum: a useful sign in the diagnosis of congenital brain malformations. Am J Neuroradiol 1988; 9:1107.

44. Bartelmez GW, Dekaban AS. The early development of the human brain. Contrib Embryol Carnegie Inst 1962; 37:13.

45. Bassett NS, Bennet L, Ball KT, Gluckman PD. Circulating prolactin (PRL) in the ovine fetus demonstrates a diurnal rhythm and is influenced by maternal nutrition. Biol Neonate 1989; 55:164.

46. Bassett N, Gluckman PD. Pulsatile growth hormone release in the ovine fetus and neonatal lamb. J Endocrinol 1986; 109:307.

47. Bassett NS, Oliver MH, Breier BH, Gluckman PD. The effect of starvation on fetal IGF-1. Pediatr Res 1990; 27:401.

48. Baumann G. Growth hormone heterogeneity: genes, isohormones, variants, and binding proteins. Endocr Rev 1991; 12:424.

49. Baxter RC. Circulating binding proteins for the insu-

lin-like growth factors. Trends Endocrinol Metab 1993; 4:91.

50. Baylin SB. "APUD" cells: fact and fiction. Trends Endocrinol Metab 1990; 1:198.

51. Bearn JG. Anencephaly and the development of the male genital tract. Acta Paediatr Acad Sci Hung 1968; 9:159.

52. Beck F, Samani NJ, Byrne S, et al. Histochemical localization of IGF-I and IGF-II mRNA in the rat between birth and adulthood. Development 1988; 104:29.

53. Beck-Peccoz P, Cortelazzi D, Persani L, et al. Maturation of pituitary-thyroid function in the anencephalic fetus. Acta Med Austriaca 1992; 19(suppl. 1):72.

54. Beck-Peccoz P, Padmanabhan V, Baggiani AM, et al. Maturation of hypothalamic-pituitary-gonadal function in normal human fetuses: circulating levels of gonadotropins, their common α-subunit and free testosterone, and discrepancy between immunological and biological activities of circulating follicle-stimulating hormone. J Clin Endocrinol Metab 1991; 73:525.

55. Begeot M, Dubois MP, Dubois PM. Growth hormone and ACTH in the pituitary of normal and anencephalic human fetuses: immunocytochemical evidence for hypothalamic influences during development. Neuroendocrinology 1977; 24:208.

56. Begeot M, Dubois MP, Dubois PM. Localisation par immunofluorescence de l'hormone β-lipotrope (βLPH) et de la β-endorphine dans l'antehypophyse de foetus humains normaux et anencephales. C R Acad Sci Paris 1978; 286:213.

57. Begeot M, Dubois MP, Dubois PM. Influence de l'hypothalamus sur la differenciation des cellules presentant une immunoreactive de type ACTH, β-LPH (β-lipotropine), α- et β-endorphines dans les ebauches antehypophysaires de foetus de rat en culture organotypique. J Physiol (Paris) 1979; 75:27.

58. Begeot M, Dubois MP, Dubois PM. Evolution of lactotropes in normal and anencephalic human fetuses. J Clin Endocrinol Metab 1984; 58:726.

59. Begeot M, Hemming FJ, Combarnous Y, Dubois MP, Aubert ML. Induction of pituitary lactotrope differentiation by luteinizing hormone α-subunit. Science 1984; 226:566.

60. Behringer RR, Mathews LS, Palmiter RD, Brinster RL. Dwarf mice produced by genetic ablation of growth hormone expressing cells. Genes Dev. 1988; 2:453.

61. Ben-David M, Chrambach A. Preparation of bio- and immunoactive human prolactin in milligram amounts from amniotic fluid in 60% yield. Endocrinology 1977; 101:250.

62. Benirschke K. Adrenals in anencephaly and hydrocephaly. Obstet Gynecol 1956; 8:412.

63. Bennett A, Wilson DM, Liu F, et al. Levels of insulin-like growth factors I and II in human cord blood. J Clin Endocrinol Metab 1983; 57:609.

64. Berg MA, Argente J, Chernausek S, et al. Diverse growth hormone receptor gene mutations in Laron syndrome. Am J Hum Genet 1993; 52:998.

65. Bergland RM, Page RB. Can the pituitary secrete directly to the brain? (affirmative anatomical evidence). Endocrinology 1978; 102:1325.

66. Bettendorf M, Albers N, de Zegher F, et al. A neuroexcitatory amino acid analog, N-methyl D-aspartate (NMDA), elicits LH and FSH release in the ovine fetus by a central mechanism (abstr.). Program of the 70th Annual Meeting of The Endocrine Society, New Orleans, 1988.

67. Bidlingmaier F, Dorr HG, Eisenmenger W, et al. Testosterone and androstenedione concentrations in human testis and epididymis during the first two years of life. J Clin Endocrinol Metab 1983; 57:311.

68. Bidlingmaier F, Knorr D. Oestrogens. Physiological and clinical aspects. In: Laran Z, ed. Pediatric and Adolescent Endocrinology, Vol 4. Basel: S. Karger, 1978.

69. Bilezikjian LM, Vale WV. Local extragonadal roles of activins. Trends Endocrinol Metab 1992; 3:218.

70. Billiar RB, Rohan R, Henson MC, et al. Regulation of immunoreactive inhibin patterns in baboon pregnancy: maternal, placental, and fetal considerations. J Clin Endocrinol Metab 1992; 75:1345.

71. Blanchard MM, Goodyer CG, Charrier J, Barenton B. In vitro regulation of growth hormone (GH) release from ovine pituitary cells during fetal and neonatal development: effects of GH-releasing factor, somatostatin, and insulin-like growth factor I. Endocrinology 1988; 122:2114.

72. Blay J, Hollenberg MD. The nature and function of polypeptide growth factor receptors in the human placenta. J Dev Physiol 1989; 12:237.

73. Blizzard RM, Alberts M. Hypopituitarism, hypoadrenalism and hypogonadism in the newborn infant. J Pediatr 1956; 48:782.

74. Bloch B, Bugnon C, Lenys D, Fellman D. Description des neurones immunoreactifs à un immunosérum anti β-endorphine présents dans le noyau infundibulaire chez l'Homme. C R Acad Sci Paris 1978; 287:309.

75. Bloch B, Gaillard RC, Culler MD, Negro-Villar A. Immunohistochemical detection of proluteinizing hormone-releasing hormone peptides in neurons in the human hypothalamus. J Clin Endocrinol Metab 1992; 74:135.

76. Blumenfeld Z, Jaffe RB. Hypophysiotropic and neuromodulatory regulation of adrenocorticotropin secretion in the human fetal pituitary gland. J Clin Invest 1986; 78:288.

77. Bodner M, Castrillo J-L, Theill LE, et al. The pituitary-specific transcription factor GHF-1 is a homeobox-containing protein. Cell 1988; 55:505.

78. Borrelli E, Heymann RA, Arias C, et al. Transgenic mice with inducible dwarfism. Nature 1989; 339:538.

79. Boyd JD. Observations on human pharyngeal hypophysis. J Endocrinol 1956; 14:66.

80. Boyko OB, Curnes JT, Oakes WJ, Burger PC. Hamartomas of the tuber cinereum: CT, MR, and pathologic findings. Am J Neuroradiol 1991; 12:309.

81. Braun FHT, Jones KL, Smith DW. Breech presentation as an indicator of fetal abnormality. J Pediatr 1975; 86:419.

82. Bresson J-L, Clavequin M-C, Fellmann D, Bugnon C. Ontogeny of the neuroglandular system revealed with HPGRF-44 antibodies in human hypothalamus. Neuroendocrinology 1984; 39:68.

83. Bresson J-L, Clavequin M-C, Fellmann D, Bugnon C. Human corticolibrin hypothalamic neuroglandular system: comparative immunocytochemical study with anti-rat and anti-ovine corticotropin-releasing factor sera in the early stages of development. Dev Brain Res 1987; 32:241.

84. Brewer DB. Congenital absence of the pituitary gland and its consequences. J Pathol Bacteriol 1957; 73:59.

85. Brodsky MC, Glasier CM. Optic nerve hypoplasia: Clinical significance of associated central nervous system abnormalities on magnetic resonance imaging. Arch Ophthalmol 1993; 111:66.

86. Brooks AN, Challis JRG. Effects of naloxone on the preparturient increase in ACTH and cortisol in fetal sheep. J Neuroendocrinol 1991; 3:419.

87. Brown AL, Graham DE, Nissley SP, et al. Developmental regulation of insulin-like growth factor II mRNA in different rat tissues. J Biol Chem 1986; 261:13144.

88. Brown RS, Bhatia V, Hayes E. An apparent cluster of congenital hypopituitarism in central Massachusetts: magnetic resonance imaging and hormonal studies. J Clin Endocrinol Metab 1991; 72:12.

89. Brubaker PL, Baird AC, Bennett HPJ, et al. Corticotropic peptides in the human fetal pituitary. Endocrinology 1982; 111:1150.

90. Bugnon C, Bloch B, Fellmann D. Mise en evidence cytoimmunologique de neurones à LH-RF chez le foetus humain. C R Acad Sci Paris 1976; 282:1625-Series D.

91. Bugnon C, Bloch B, Fellmann D. Étude immunocytologique des neurones hypothalamiques à LH-RH chez le foetus humain. Brain Res 1977; 128:249.

92. Bugnon C, Bloch B, Fellmann D. Cyto-immunological study of the ontogenesis of the gonadotropic hypothalamo-pituitary axis in the human fetus. J Steroid Biochem 1977; 8:565.

93. Bugnon C, Fellmann D, Bresson J-L, Clavequin MC. Etude immunocytochimique de l'ontogenese du systeme neuroglandulaire a CRF chez l'Homme. C R Acad Sci Paris 1982; 294:491.

94. Bugnon C, Fellmann D, Gouget A, et al. Corticolibrin neurons: cytophysiology, phylogeny, and ontogeny. J Steroid Biochem 1984; 20:183.

95. Cacciari E, Zucchini S, Carla G, et al. Endocrine function and morphological findings in patients with disorders of the hypothalamopituitary area: a study with magnetic resonance. Arch Dis Child 1990; 65:1199.

96. Campbell LR, Dayton DH, Sohal GS. Neural tube defects: a review of human and animal studies on the etiology of neural tube defects. Teratology 1986; 34:171.

97. Camper SA, Saunders TL, Katz RW, Reeves RH. The pit-1 transcription factor gene is a candidate for the murine Snell dwarf mutation. Genomics 1990; 6:586.

98. Castillo RH, Matteri RL, Dumesic DA. Luteinizing hormone synthesis in cultured fetal human pituitary cells exposed to gonadotropin-releasing hormone. J Clin Endocrinol Metab 1992; 75:318.

99. Castrillo J-L, Theill LE, Karin M. Function of the homeodomain protein GHF1 in pituitary cell proliferation. Science 1991; 253:197.

100. Challis JRG, Brooks AN. Maturation and activation of hypothalamic-pituitary-adrenal function in fetal sheep. Endocr Rev 1989; 10:182.

101. Challis JRG, Huhtanen D, Sprague C, et al. Modulation by cortisol of ACTH-induced activation of adrenal function in fetal sheep. Endocrinology 1985; 116:2267.

102. Chan EC, Thompson M, Madsen G, et al. Differential processing of corticotropin-releasing hormone by human placenta and hypothalamus. Biochem Biophys Res Commun 1988; 153:1229.

103. Ch'in KY. The endocrine glands of anencephalic foetuses. Chinese Med J 1938; 2(suppl.):63.

104. Ciocca DR, Puy LA, Stati AO. Identification of seven hormone-producing cell types in the human pharyngeal hypophysis. J Clin Endocrinol Metab 1985; 60:212.

105. Clark SJ, Ellis N, Styne DM, et al. Hormone ontogeny in the ovine fetus. XVII. Demonstration of pulsatile

luteinizing hormone secretion by the fetal pituitary gland. Endocrinology 1984; 115:1774.

106. Clark SJ, Hauffa BP, Rodens KP, et al. Hormone ontogeny of the ovine fetus. XIX. The effect of a potent luteinizing hormone-releasing factor agonist on gonadotropin and testosterone release in the fetus and neonate. Pediatr Res 1989; 25:347.

107. Clements JA, Meites J. Control of prolactin secretion. In: Li CH, ed. Hormonal proteins and peptides. Vol 4. New York: Academic Press, 1977.

108. Clements JA, Reyes FI, Winter JSD, Faiman C. Studies on human sexual development. III. Fetal pituitary and serum and amniotic fluid concentrations of LH, CG and FSH. J Clin Endocrinol Metab 1976; 42:9.

109. Clements JA, Reyes FI, Winter JSD, Faiman C. Studies on human sexual development. IV. Fetal pituitary and serum and amniotic fluid concentrations of prolactin. J Clin Endocrinol Metab 1977; 44:408.

110. Clements JA, Reyes FI, Winter JSD, Faiman C. Ontogenesis of gonadotropin-releasing hormone in the human fetal hypothalamus. Proc Soc Exp Biol 1980; 163:437.

111. Coates PJ, Doniach I, Holly JMP, Rees LH. Demonstration of desacetyl α-melanocyte-stimulating hormone in fetal and adult human anterior pituitary corticotrophs. J Endocrinol 1989; 120:525.

112. Codesal J, Regadera J, Nistal M, et al. Involution of human fetal Leydig cells—an immunohistochemical, ultrastructural and quantitative study. J Anat 1990; 172:103.

113. Cogan JD, Phillips III JA, Sakati N, et al. Heterogeneous growth hormone (GH) gene mutations in familial GH deficiency. J Clin Endocrinol Metab 1993; 76:1224.

114. Cohen HL, Shapiro MA, Mandel FS, Shapiro ML. Normal ovaries in neonates and infants: a sonographic study of 77 patients 1 day to 24 months old. Am J Roentgenol 1993; 160:583.

115. Cohen MM Jr. Perspectives on holoprosencephaly. Part I. Epidemiology, genetics, syndromology. Teratology 1989; 40:211.

116. Cohen MM Jr. Perspectives on holoprosencephaly. Part III. Spectra, distinctions, continuities, and discontinuities. Am J Med Genet 1989; 34:271.

117. Conklin JL. The development of the human fetal adenohypophysis. Anat Rec 1968; 160:79.

118. Copp AJ, Brook FA, Estibeiro JP, et al. The embryonic development of mammalian neural tube defects. Prog Neurobiol 1990; 35:363.

119. Corbier P, Dehennin L, Castanier M, et al. Sex differences in serum luteinizing hormone and testosterone in the human neonate during the first few hours after birth. J Clin Endocrinol Metab 1990; 71:1344.

120. Cornblath M, Parker ML, Reisner SH, et al. Secretion and metabolism of growth hormone in premature and full-term infants. J Clin Endocrinol Metab 1965; 25:209.

121. Couly GF, LeDouarin NM. Mapping of the early neural primordium in quail-chick chimeras. II. The prosencephalic neural plate and neural folds: implications for the genesis of cephalic human congenital abnormalities. Dev Biol 1987; 120:198.

122. Craft WH, Underwood LE, Van Wyk JJ. High incidence of perinatal insult in children with idiopathic hypopituitarism. J Pediatr 1980; 96:397.

123. Cruikshank DP. Breech presentation. Clin Obstet Gynecol 1986; 29:255.

124. Cuttler L, Egli CA, Styne DM, et al. Hormone ontogeny in the ovine fetus. XXIII. The effect of an opioid antagonist on luteinizing hormone secretion. Endocrinology 1985; 116:1997.

125. Daikoku S. Studies on the human foetal pituitary. 1. Quantitative observations. Tokushima J Exp Med 1958; 5:200.

126. Daikoku S. Studies on the human foetal pituitary. 2. On the form and histological development, especially that of the anterior pituitary. Tokushima J Exp Med 1958; 5:214.

127. Daikoku S, Kinutani M, Watanabe YG. Role of hypothalamus on development of adenohypophysis: an electron microscopic study. Neuroendocrinology 1973; 11:284.

127a. Daniel PM, Pritchard MML. Studies of the hypothalamus and the pituitary gland, with special reference to the effects of transection of the pituitary stalk. Acta Endocrinol 1975; 80(suppl 201):1.

128. Danon M, Velez O, Ostrea T, et al. Dynamics of bioactive luteinizing hormone-human chorionic gonadotropin during the first 7 days of life. Pediatr Res 1988; 23:530.

129. Daughaday WH, Trivedi B, Andrews BA. The ontogeny of serum GH binding protein in man: a possible indicator of hepatic GH receptor development. J Clin Endocrinol Metab 1987; 65:1072.

130. Davies IJ, Naftolin F, Ryan KJ, Siu J. A specific, high-affinity, limited-capacity estrogen binding component in the cytosol of human fetal pituitary and brain tissues. J Clin Endocrinol Metab 1975; 40:909.

131. DeChiara TM, Robertson EJ, Efstratiadis A. Parental imprinting of the mouse insulin-like growth factor II gene. Cell 1991; 64:849.

132. Deiber M, Chatelain P, Naville D, et al. Functional hypersomatotropism in small for gestational age (SGA) newborn infants. J Clin Endocrinol Metab 1989; 68:232.

133. Delitata G, Meloni T, Masala A, et al. Action of somatostatin, levodopa and pyridoxine on growth hormone (GH) secretion in newborn infants. Biomedicine 1978; 29:13.

134. Delitata G, Meloni T, Masala A, et al. Dynamic evaluation of prolactin secretion during the early hours of life in human newborns. J Clin Endocrinol Metab 1978; 46:880.

135. Del Pozo E, Hiba J, Lancranjan I, Kunzig HJ. Prolactin measurements throughout the life cycle: endocrine correlations. In: Crosignani PG, Robyn C, eds. Prolactin and human reproduction. New York: Academic Press, 1977.

136. de Morsier G. Etudes sur les dysraphies cranio-encephaliques. III. Agenesie du septum lucidum avec malformation du tractus optique: La dysplasie septo-optique. Schweiz Arch Neurol Psychiatr 1956; 77:267.

137. DeMyer W. Holoprosencephaly (cyclopia-arhinencephaly). In: Vinken PJ, Bruyn GW, Klawans HL, eds. Handbook of clinical neurology. Revised Ser, Vol 6. Amsterdam: Elsevier, 1987:225.

138. DeMyer W, Zeman W, Palmer CG. The face predicts the brain: diagnostic significance of median facial anomalies for holoprosencephaly (arhinencephaly). Pediatrics 1964; 34:256.

139. De Paolo LV, Bicsak TA, Erickson GF, et al. Follistatin and activin: a potential intrinsic regulatory system within diverse tissues. Proc Soc Exp Biol Med 1991; 198:500.

140. de Sa DJ. Follicular ovarian cysts in still births and neonates. Arch Dis Child 1975; 50:45.

141. de Zegher F, Bettendorf M, Kaplan SL, Grumbach MM. Hormone ontogeny in the ovine fetus. XXI.

The effect of insulin-like growth factor-I on plasma fetal growth hormone, insulin and glucose concentrations. Endocrinology 1988; 123:658.

142. de Zegher F, Daaboul J, Grumbach MM, Kaplan SL. Hormone ontogeny in the ovine fetus and neonate. XXII. The effect of somatostatin on the growth hormone (GH) response to GH-releasing factor. Endocrinology 1989; 124:1114.

143. de Zegher F, Devlieger H, Veldhuis JD. Pulsatile and sexually dimorphic secretion of luteinizing hormone in the human infant on the day of birth. Pediatr Res 1992; 32:605.

144. de Zegher F, Devlieger H, Veldhuis JD. Properties of growth hormone and prolactin hypersecretion by the human infant on the day of birth. J Clin Endocrinol Metab 1993; 76:1177.

145. de Zegher F, Kimpen J, Raus J, Vanderschueren-Lodeweyckxz M. Hypersomatotropism in the dysmature infant at term and preterm birth. Biol Neonate 1990; 58:188.

146. de Zegher F, Styne DM, Daaboul J, et al. Hormone ontogeny in the ovine fetus and neonatal lamb. XX. Effect of age, breeding season, and twinning on the growth hormone (GH) response to GH-releasing factor: evidence for a homeostatic role of fetal GH. Endocrinology 1989; 124:124.

147. de Zegher F, Vanderschueren-Lodeweyckx M, Spitz B, et al. Perinatal growth hormone (GH) physiology: effect of GH-releasing factor on maternal and fetal secretion of pituitary and placental GH. J Clin Endocrinol Metab 1990; 71:520.

148. de Zegher F, Vanderschueren-Lodeweyckx M, Suarez P, et al. Congenital hypothyroidism and growth hormone deficiency (Letter). Lancet 1988; 2:1489.

149. Diez d'Aux KC, Murphy BEP. Androgens in the human fetus. J Steroid Biochem 1974; 5:207.

150. Dólle P, Castrillo JL, Theill LE, et al. Expression of GHF-1 protein in mouse pituitaries correlates both temporally and spatially with the onset of growth hormone gene activity. Cell 1990; 60:809.

151. Dorn A, Schmidt K, Schmidt W, et al. Localization of cholecystokinin immunoreactivity in the human brain with special reference to ontogeny. J Hirnforsch 1985; 26:167.

152. Dubois PM, Dubois MP. Mise en evidence par immunofluorescence de l'activité gonadotrope dans l'antehypophyse foetale humaine. International Symposium on Sexual Endocrinology of the Perinatal Period. INSERM 1974; 32:37.

153. Dubois PM, Dumont L. Observation en microscopie electronique du lobe anterieur de l'hypophyse embryonnaire humaine au troisieme mois de la vie intra-uterine. C R Soc Biol 1965; 159:1574.

154. Ducharme JR, Grumbach MM. Studies on the effects of human growth hormone in premature infants. J Clin Invest 1961; 40:243.

155. Dumesic DA, Goldsmith PC, Jaffe RB. Estradiol sensitization of cultured human fetal pituitary cells to gonadotropin-releasing hormone. J Clin Endocrinol Metab 1987; 65:1147.

156. Durand P. ACTH receptor levels in lamb adrenals at late gestation and early neonatal stages. Biol Reprod 1979; 20:837.

157. Economides D, Linton E, Nicolaides K, et al. Relationship between maternal and fetal corticotropin-releasing hormone-41 and ACTH levels in human midtrimester pregnancy. J Endocrinol 1987; 114:497.

158. Edelman GM, Crossin KL. Cell adhesion molecules: implications for a molecular histology. Annu Rev Biochem 1991; 60:155.

159. Ellinwood WE, Baughman WL, Resko JA. The effect of gonadectomy and testosterone treatment on luteinizing hormone secretion in fetal Rhesus monkeys. Endocrinology 1982; 110:183.

160. Ertl T, Sulyok E, Varga L, Csaba IF. Postnatal development of plasma prolactin level in premature infants with and without NaCl supplementation. Biol Neonate 1983; 44:219.

161. Facchinetti F, Storchi AR, Furani S, et al. Pituitary changes of des-acetyl alpha-melanocyte stimulating hormone throughout development. Biol Neonate 1988; 54:86.

162. Facchinetti F, Storchi AR, Petraglia F, et al. Ontogeny of pituitary β-endorphin and related peptides in the human embryo and fetus. Am J Obstet Gynecol 1987; 156:735.

163. Facchinetti F, Storchi AR, Petraglia F, Genazzani AR. Presence of acetylated and shortened endorphins in human fetal pituitary gland. Pediatr Res 1989; 25:652.

164. Faiman C, Reyes FI, Winter JSD. Serum gonadotropin patterns during the perinatal period in man and in the chimpanzee. International Symposium on Sexual Endocrinology of the Perinatal Period. INSERM 1974; 32:281.

165. Faiman C, Winter JSD. Sex differences in gonadotropin concentrations in infancy. Nature 1971; 232:130.

166. Falin LI. The development of human hypophysis and differentiation of cells of its anterior lobe during embryonic life. Acta Anat 1961; 44:188.

167. Figueroa JP, McDonald TJ, Gluckman PD, et al. Osmotic regulation of prolactin secretion in the fetal sheep. J Dev Physiol 1990; 13:339.

168. Finkelstein JW, Anders TR, Sachar EJ, et al. Behavioral state, sleep stage, and growth hormone levels in human infants. J Clin Endocrinol Metab 1971; 32:368.

169. Fishman J, Naftolin F, Davies IJ, et al. Catechol estrogen formation by the human fetal brain and pituitary. J Clin Endocrinol Metab 1976; 42:177.

170. Forest MG. Pituitary gonadotropin and sex steroid secretion during the first two years of life. In: Grumbach MM, Sizonenko PC, Aubert ML, eds. Control of the onset of puberty. Baltimore: Williams & Wilkins, 1990: 451.

171. Forest MG, Cathiard AM. Pattern of plasma testosterone and Δ⁴-androstenedione in normal newborn: evidence for testicular activity at birth. J Clin Endocrinol Metab 1975; 41:977.

172. Formby B, Ullrich A, Coussens L, et al. Growth hormone stimulates insulin gene expression in cultured human fetal pancreatic islets. J Clin Endocrinol Metab 1988; 66:1075.

173. Forsbach G, Ayala A, Soria J, et al. Secretion de prolactin en recien nacidos normales y anencefalos. Arch Invest Med 1976; 7:85.

174. Fox SR, Jong MTC, Casanova J, et al. The homeodomain protein, Pit-1/GHF-1, is capable of binding to and activating cell-specific elements of both the growth hormone and prolactin gene promoters. Mol Endocrinol 1990; 4:1069.

175. Franchimont P, Pasteels JL. Secretion independante des hormones gonadotropes et de leurs sous-unites. CR Acad Sci Paris 1972; 275:1799.

176. Franco B, Guioli S, Pragliola A, et al. A gene deleted in Kallmann syndrome shares homology with neural cell adhesion and axonal pathfinding molecules. Nature 1991; 353:529.

177. Frankenne F, Closset J, Gomez F, et al. The physiology of growth hormones (GHs) in pregnant women and partial characterization of the placental GH variant. J Clin Endocrinol Metab 1988; 66:1171.

178. Frankenne F, Rentier-Delrue F, Scippo M-L, et al. Expression of the growth hormone variant gene in human placenta. J Clin Endocrinol Metab 1987; 64:635.

179. Frankenne F, Scippo ML, Marcotty C, et al. Growth hormone and related peptides in human pregnancy (abstr.). Proceedings of the 9th International Congress of Endocrinology, Nice, France, 1992.

180. Frawley LS, Boockfor FR. Mammosomatotropes: presence and function in normal and neoplastic pituitary tissue. Endocr Rev 1991; 12:337.

181. Fujisawa I, Kikuchi K, Nishimura K, et al. Transection of the pituitary stalk: development of an ectopic posterior lobe assessed with MRI imaging. Radiology 1987; 165:487.

182. Fujita K, Matsuo N, Mori O, et al. The association of hypopituitarism with small pituitary, invisible pituitary stalk, type 1 Arnold-Chiari malformation and syringomyelia in seven patients born in breech position: a further proof of birth injury theory on the pathogenesis of "idiopathic hypopituitarism." Eur J Pediatr 1992; 151:266.

183. Fujita T. Present status of paraneuron concept. Arch Histol Cytol 1989; 52(suppl):1.

184. Fukaya T, Furuhashi N, Shinkawa O, et al. The human fetal prolactin and estradiol levels, and their co-relationship. Tohoku J Exp Med 1984; 143:87.

185. Furuhashi N, Fukaya T, Kono H, et al. Cord serum growth hormone in the human fetus. Sex difference and a negative correlation with birth weight. Gynecol Obstet Invest 1983; 16:119.

186. Gallaher BW, Breier BH, Oliver MH, et al. Ontogenic differences in the nutritional regulation of circulating IGF binding proteins in sheep plasma. Acta Endocrinol 1992; 126:49.

187. Garnier PE, Chaussain J-L, Binet E, et al. Effect of synthetic luteinizing hormone-releasing hormone (LH-RH) on the release of gonadotropins in children and adolescents. Acta Endocrinol 1974; 77:422.

188. Gaudin J, LeTreguilly C, Parent P, et al. Neonatal ovarian cysts: twelve cysts with antenatal diagnosis. Pediatr Surg Int 1988; 3:158.

189. Gelato MC, Rutherford C, Stark RI, Daniel SS. The insulin-like growth factor II/mannose-6-phosphate receptor is present in fetal and maternal sheep serum. Endocrinology 1989; 124:2935.

190. Gennser G, Ohrlander S, Eneroth P. Fetal cortisol and the initiation of labour in the human. In: Knight J, O'Connor M, eds. The fetus and birth. Ciba Foundation Series 47. Amsterdam: Elsevier-Excerpta Medica, 1977.

191. George FW, Wilson JD. Conversion of androgen to estrogen by the human fetal ovary. J Clin Endocrinol Metab 1978; 47:550.

192. Gilbert MS. Some factors influencing the early development of the mammalian hypophysis. Anat Rec 1935; 62:337.

193. Gillman J. The development of the gonads in man with a consideration of the fetal endocrines and the histogenesis of ovarian tumors. Contrib Embryol Carnegie Inst 1948; 32:81.

194. Gilmore DP, Dobbie HG, McNeilly AS, Mortimer CH. Presence and activity of LHRH in the mid-term human fetus. J Reprod Fertil 1978; 52:355.

195. Gilmore DP, Wilson CA. Indoleamine and catechol-amine concentrations in the mid-term human fetal brain. Brain Res Bull 1983; 10:395.

196. Gitlin D, Biasucci A. Ontogenesis of immunoreactive growth hormone, follicle stimulating hormone, thyroid stimulating hormone, luteinizing hormone, chorionic prolactin, and chorionic gonadotropin in the human conceptus. J Clin Endocrinol Metab 1969; 29:926.

197. Gitlin D, Kumate J, Morales C. Metabolism and maternofetal transfer of human growth hormone in the pregnant woman at term. J Clin Endocrinol Metab 1965; 25:1599.

198. Gluckman PD. The maturation of neuroendocrine systems in the fetus. In: Martini L, Besser GM, eds. Clinical neuroendocrinology II. New York: Academic Press, 1982: 1.

199. Gluckman PD. The fetal neuroendocrine axis. In: Martin L, James V, eds. Fetal endocrinology and metabolism. (Current Topics in Experimental Endocrinology No. 15.) New York: Academic Press, 1983: 1.

200. Gluckman PD. Neuroendocrine function in the ovine fetus: studies of the regulation of growth hormone and prolactin secretion. In: Ellendorff F, Gluckman PD, Parvizi N, eds. Fetal neuroendocrinology. Ithaca, NY: Perinatology Press, 1984: 193.

201. Gluckman PD. Fetal growth: an endocrine perspective. Acta Paediatr Scand 1989; 349(suppl):21.

202. Gluckman PD. Growth hormone and prolactin. In: Polin RA, Fox WW, eds. Fetal and neonatal physiology. Philadelphia: WB Saunders, 1992: 1785.

203. Gluckman PD. The regulation of fetal growth in late gestation. Journal of Japan Society of Premature and Newborn Medicine 1992; 4:13.

204. Gluckman PD. Intrauterine growth retardation: future research directions. Oxford Clinical Communications. Acta Paediatr 1993; 384(suppl.):96.

205. Gluckman PD, Ballard PL, Kaplan SL, et al: Prolactin in umbilical cord blood and the respiratory distress syndrome. J Pediatr 1978; 93:1011.

206. Gluckman PD, Bassett NS. The development of hypothalamic function in the perinatal period. In: Meisami E, Timeras P, eds. Handbook of human growth and developmental biology. Vol. II. Part A. Boca Raton: CRC Press, 1989: 3.

207. Gluckman PD, Bassett N, Ball K: The functional maturation of the somatotropic axis in the perinatal period. In: Kunzel W, Jensen A, eds. Endocrine control of the fetus. Physiologic and pathophysiologic aspects. Heidelberg: Springer Verlag, 1988:201.

208. Gluckman PD, Butler JH. Parturition related changes in insulin-like growth factors -I and -II in the perinatal lamb. J Endocrinol 1983; 99:223.

209. Gluckman PD, Butler JH, Elliott TB. The ontogeny of somatotropic binding sites in ovine hepatic membranes. Endocrinology 1983; 112:1607.

210. Gluckman PD, Grumbach MM, Kaplan SL. The neuroendocrine regulation and function of growth hormone and prolactin in the mammalian fetus. Endocr Rev 1981; 2:363.

211. Gluckman PD, Gunn AJ, Wray A, et al. Congenital idiopathic growth hormone deficiency is associated with prenatal and early postnatal growth failure. J Pediatr 1992; 121:920.

212. Gluckman PD, Harding JE. The regulation of fetal growth. In: Hernandez M, Argente J, eds. Human growth: basic and clinical aspects. International Congress Series 973. Amsterdam: Excerpta Medica, 1992: 253.

213. Gluckman PD, Johnson-Barrett JJ, Butler JH, et al.

Studies of insulin-like growth factor -I and -II by specific radioligand assays in umbilical cord blood. Clin Endocrinol 1983; 19:405.

214. Gluckman PD, Marti-Henneberg C, Kaplan SL, Grumbach MM. Hormone ontogeny in the ovine fetus. XIV. The effect of 17β-estradiol infusion on fetal plasma gonadotropins and prolactin and maturation of sex steroid-dependent negative feedback. Endocrinology 1983; 112:1618.

215. Gluckman PD, Marti-Henneberg C, Thomsett MJ, et al. Hormone ontogeny in the ovine fetus. VI. Dopaminergic regulation of prolactin secretion. Endocrinology 1979; 105:1173.

216. Gluckman PD, Morel PCH, Ambler GR, et al. Elevating maternal insulin-like growth factor-1 in mice and rats alters the pattern of fetal growth by removing maternal constraint. J Endocrinol 1992; 134:R1.

217. Gluckman PD, Mueller PL, Kaplan SL, et al. Hormone ontogeny in the ovine fetus. III. The effect of exogenous somatostatin. Endocrinology 1979; 104:974.

218. Gluckman PD, Uthne K, Styne DM, et al. Hormone ontogeny in the ovine fetus. IV. Serum somatomedin activity in the fetal and neonatal lamb and pregnant ewe: correlation with maternal and fetal growth hormone, prolactin and chorionic somatomammotropin. Pediatr Res 1979; 14:194.

219. Godfrey P, Rahal JO, Beamer WG, et al. GHRH receptor of *little* mice contains a missense mutation in the extracellular domain that disrupts receptor function. Nature Genet 1993; 4:227.

220. Goland RS, Wardlaw SL, Stark RI, et al. High levels of corticotropin-releasing hormone immunoactivity in maternal and fetal plasma during pregnancy. J Clin Endocrinol Metab 1986; 63:1199.

221. Gondos B, Westergaard L, Byskov A. Initiation of oogenesis in the human fetal ovary: ultrastructural and squash preparation study. Am J Obstet Gynecol 1986; 155:189.

222. Goodman HG, Grumbach MM, Kaplan SL. Growth and growth hormone. II. A comparison of isolated growth hormone deficiency and multiple pituitary hormone deficiencies in 35 patients with idiopathic hypopituitary dwarfism. N Engl J Med 1968; 278:57.

223. Goodyer CG, Branchaud CL, Lefebvre Y. Effects of growth hormone (GH)-releasing factor and somatostatin on GH secretion from early to midgestation human fetal pituitaries. J Clin Endocrinol Metab 1993; 76:1259.

224. Goodyer CG, Branchaud CL, Lefebvre Y. In vitro modulation of growth hormone (GH) secretion from early to midgestation human fetal pituitaries by GH-releasing factor and somatostatin: role of Gs-adenyl cyclase-Gi complex and Ca^{2+} channels. J Clin Endocrinol Metab 1993; 76:1265.

225. Grasso S, Filetti S, Mazzone D, et al. Thyroid-pituitary function in eight anencephalic infants. Acta Endocrinol 1980; 93:396.

226. Groom CV, Boyns AR. Effect of hypothalamic releasing factors and steroids on release of gonadotrophins by organ cultures of human foetal pituitaries. J Endocrinol 1973; 59:511.

227. Groom GV, Groom MA, Cooke ID, Boyns AR. The secretion of immunoreactive luteinizing hormone and follicle-stimulating hormone by the human foetal pituitary in organ culture. J Endocrinol 1971; 49:335.

228. Grumbach MM, Conte FA. Disorders of sex differentiation. In: Wilson JD, Foster DW, eds. Williams' text-book of endocrinology, ed 8. Philadelphia: WB Saunders, 1992:853.

229. Grumbach MM, Kaplan SL. Ontogenesis of growth hormone, insulin, prolactin and gonadotropin secretion in the human foetus. In: Cross KW, Nathanielsz P, eds. Foetal and neonatal physiology. Proceedings of Sir Joseph Barcroft Centenary Symposium. Cambridge: Cambridge University Press, 1973:462.

230. Grumbach MM, Kaplan SL. Fetal pituitary hormones and the maturation of central nervous system regulation of anterior pituitary function. In: Gluck L, ed. Modern perinatal medicine. Chicago: Year Book Medical Publishers, 1974:247.

231. Grumbach MM, Kaplan SL. The neuroendocrinology of human puberty: an ontogenetic perspective. In: Grumbach MM, Sizonenko PC, Aubert ML, eds. Control of the onset of puberty. Baltimore: Williams & Wilkins, 1990: 1.

232. Grumbach MM, Kaplan SL, Sciarra JJ, Burr IM. Chorionic growth hormone-prolactin (CGP): secretion, disposition, biologic activity in man, and postulated function as the "growth hormone" of the second half of pregnancy. Ann NY Acad Sci 1968; 148:501.

233. Grumbach MM, Roth JC, Kaplan SL, Kelch RP. Hypothalamic-pituitary regulation of puberty in man: evidence and concepts derived from clinical research. In: Grumbach MM, Grave GD, Mayer FI, eds. Control of onset of puberty. New York: John Wiley & Sons, 1974; 115.

234. Grumbach MM, Styne DM. Puberty: ontogeny, neuroendocrinology, physiology, and disorders. In: Wilson JD, Foster DW, eds. Williams' textbook of endocrinology, ed 8. Philadelphia: WB Saunders, 1992: 1139.

235. Grunt JA, Reynolds DW. Insulin, blood sugar, and growth hormone levels in an anencephalic infant before and after intravenous administration of glucose. J Pediatr 1970; 76:112.

236. Gulyas BJ, Hodgen GD, Tullner WW, Ross GF. Effects of fetal or maternal hypophysectomy on endocrine organs and body weight in infant rhesus monkeys (*Macaca mulatta*) with particular reference to oogenesis. Biol Reprod 1977; 16:216.

237. Guyda HJ, Friesen HG. Serum prolactin levels in humans from birth to adult life. Pediatr Res 1973; 7:534.

238. Hagen C, McNeilly AS. Identification of human luteinizing hormone, follicle stimulating hormone, luteinizing hormone β-subunit and gonadotropin α-subunit in foetal and adult pituitary glands. J Endocrinol 1975; 67:49.

239. Hagen C, McNeilly AS. The gonadotropins and their subunits in foetal pituitary glands and circulation. J Steroid Biochem 1977; 8:537.

240. Han VKM, Hill DJ, Strain AJ, et al. Identification of somatomedin/insulin-like growth factor immunoreactive cells in the human fetus. Pediatr Res 1987; 22:245.

241. Han VKM, Lund PK, Lee DC, D'Ercole AJ. Expression of somatomedin/insulin-like growth factor messenger ribonucleic acids in the human fetus: identification, characterization, and tissue distribution. J Clin Endocrinol Metab 1988; 66:422.

242. Handwerger S, Markoff E, Richards R. Regulation of the synthesis and release of decidual prolactin by placental and autocrine/paracrine factors. Placenta 1991; 12:121.

243. Handwerger S, Richards RG, Markoff E. The physiology of decidual prolactin and other decidual protein hormones. Trends Endocrinol Metab 1992; 3:91.

244. Haning RV, Barrett DA, Alberino SP, et al. Interrelationships between maternal and cord prolactin, progesterone, estradiol, 13,14-dihydro-15-keto-prostaglandin F2α, and cord cortisol at delivery with respect to initiation of parturition. Am J Obstet Gynecol 1978; 130:204.

245. Hardelin J-P, Levilliers J, Young J, et al. Xp22.3 deletions in isolated familial Kallmann's syndrome. J Clin Endocrinol Metab 1993; 76:827.

246. Hatakeyama S. Electron microscopic study of the anencephalic adenohypophysis with reference to the adenocorticotrophs and their correlation with the functional differentiation of the hypothalamus during the foetal life. Endocrinol Jpn 1969; 16:187.

247. Hauth JC, Parker CR, MacDonald PC, et al. A role of fetal prolactin in lung maturation. Obstet Gynecol 1978; 51:81.

248. Hay DL, Lopata A. Chorionic gonadotropin secretion by human embryos in vitro. J Clin Endocrinol Metab 1988; 67:1322.

249. Hayek A, Driscoll SG, Warshaw JB. Endocrine studies in anencephaly. J Clin Invest 1973; 52:1636.

250. He X, Treacy MN, Simmons DM, et al. Expression of a large family of POU-domain regulatory genes in mammalian brain development. Nature 1989; 340:35.

251. Healy DL, Kimpton WG, Muller HK, Burger HG. Human decidua-chorion synthesizes immunoreactive prolactin. Endocrinology 1978; 102:286A.

252. Hemming FJ, Begeot M, Dubois MP, Dubois PM. Fetal rat somatotropes in vitro: effects of insulin, cortisol and growth hormone-releasing factor on their differentiation: a light and electron microscopic study. Endocrinology 1984; 114:2107.

253. Hershman JM. Editorial: role of chorionic gonadotropin as a thyroid stimulator. J Clin Endocrinol Metab 1992; 74:258.

254. Hey AW, Browne CA, Thorburn GD. Fetal sheep serum contains a high molecular weight insulin-like growth factor (IGF) binding protein that is acid stable and specific for IGF-II. Endocrinology 1987; 121:1975.

255. Hibi I. The birth injury theory of "idiopathic" growth hormone deficiency. Clin Pediatr Endocrinol 1992; 1:1.

256. Hill DJ, Riley SC, Bassett NS, Waters MJ. Localization of the growth hormone receptor, identified by immunocytochemistry, in second trimester human fetal tissues and in placenta throughout gestation. J Clin Endocrinol Metab 1992; 75:646.

257. Hindmarch P. Hormonal levels in the human fetus between 14 and 22 weeks gestation. Early Hum Dev 1987; 15:253.

258. Hochmann HJ, Judge DM, Reichlin S. Precocious puberty and hypothalamic hamartoma. Pediatrics 1981; 67:236.

259. Hodgkinson SC, Spencer GSG, Bass JJ, et al. Distribution of circulating insulin-like growth factor-1 (IGF-1) into tissues. Endocrinology 1991; 129:2085.

260. Holl RW, Snehotta R, Siegler B, et al. Binding protein for human growth hormone: effects of age and weight. Horm Res 1991; 35:190.

261. Honnebier WJ, Jobsis AC, Swaab DF. The effect of hypophyseal hormones and human chorionic gonadotropin (hCG) on the anencephalic fetal adrenal cortex and on parturition in the human. J Obstet Gynaecol Br Comm 1974; 81:423.

262. Huhtaniemi IT, Korenbrot CC, Jaffe RB. hCG binding and stimulation of testosterone biosynthesis in the human fetal testis. J Clin Endocrinol Metab 1977; 44:963.

263. Huhtaniemi IT, Korenbrot CC, Jaffe RB. Content of chorionic gonadotropin in human fetal tissues. J Clin Endocrinol Metab 1978; 46:994.

264. Huhtaniemi I, Lautala P. Stimulation of steroidogenesis in human fetal testes by the placenta during perifusion. J Steroid Biochem 1979; 10:109.

265. Huhtaniemi I, Pelliniemi LJ. Fetal Leydig cells: cellular origin, morphology, life span, and special functional features. Proc Soc Exp Biol Med 1992; 201:125.

266. Huhtaniemi IT, Warren DW. Ontogeny of pituitary-gonadal interactions. Recent advances and controversies. Trends Endocrinol Metab 1990; 1:356.

267. Huhtaniemi IT, Yamamoto M, Ranta T, et al. Follicle-stimulating hormone receptors appear earlier in the primate fetal testis than in the ovary. J Clin Endocrinol Metab 1987; 65:1210.

268. Hyyppä M. Hypothalamic monoamines in human fetuses. Neuroendocrinology 1972; 9:257.

269. Ikeda H, Niizuma N, Suzuki J, et al. A case of cebocephaly-holoprosencephaly with an aberrant adenohypophysis. Childs Nerv Syst 1987; 3:251.

270. Ikeda H, Suzuki J, Sasano N, Niizuma H. The development and morphogenesis of the human pituitary gland. Anat Embryol 1988; 178:327.

271. Ingraham HA, Albert VR, Chen R, et al. A family of POU-domain and Pit-1 tissue-specific transcription factors in pituitary and neuroendocrine development. Ann Rev Physiol 1990; 52:773.

272. Ingraham HA, Chen R, Mangalam HJ, et al. A tissue-specific transcription factor containing a homeodomain specifies a pituitary phenotype. Cell 1988; 55:519.

273. Ingraham HA, Flynn SE, Voss JW, et al. The POU-specific domain of Pit-1 is essential for sequence-specific, high affinity DNA binding and DNA-dependent Pit-1—Pit1 interactions. Cell 1990; 61:1021.

274. Ishikawa H, Nagayama T, Kato C, Niizuma K. Establishment of a TSH-releasing-hormone secreting cell line from the area cerebrovasculosa of an anencephalic foetus. Am J Anat 1976; 145:143.

275. Jenkin G, Heap RB. Formation of oestradiol-17β from oestrone sulphate by sheep foetal pituitary in vitro. Nature 1976; 259:330.

276. Jenkins JS, Hall CJ. Metabolism of [14C] testosterone by human foetal and adult brain tissue. J Endocrinol 1977; 74:425.

277. Johannisson E. The foetal adrenal cortex in the human. Acta Endocrinol 1968; 58(suppl):7.

278. Johnston MV, Coyle JT. Development of central neurotransmitter systems. In: The fetus and independent life. Ciba Foundation Symposium 1981; 86:251.

279. Josimovich JB, Archer DF. The role of lactogenic hormones in the pregnant woman and the fetus. Am J Obstet Gynecol 1977; 129:777.

280. Josso N, Cate RL, Picard JV, et al. Anti-müllerian hormone: the Jost factor. Recent Prog Horm Res 1993; 48:1.

281. Jost A. Experiences de decapitation de l'embryon de lapin. CR Acad Sci Paris 1947; 225:322.

282. Jost A. Problems of fetal endocrinology: the gonadal and hypophyseal hormones. Recent Prog Horm Res 1953; 8:379.

283. Jost A. Anterior pituitary function in foetal life. In: Harris GW, Donovan BT, eds. The pituitary gland. Vol 2. London: Butterworth, 1966: 299.

284. Jost A, Picon L. Hormonal control of fetal develop-

ment and metabolism. Adv Metab Disorder 1970; 4:123.

285. Judge DM, Kulin HE, Santen R, Trapukdi S. Hypothalamic hamartoma: a source of luteinizing hormone releasing factor in precocious puberty. N Engl J Med 1977; 296:7.

286. Kaplan SL, Grumbach MM. The ontogenesis of human foetal hormones. II. Luteinizing hormone (LH) and follicle stimulating hormone (FSH). Acta Endocrinol 1976; 81:808.

287. Kaplan SL, Grumbach MM. Pituitary and placental gonadotropins and sex steroids in the human and sub-human primate fetus. Clin Endocrinol Metab 1978; 7:487.

288. Kaplan SL, Grumbach MM. Pathophysiology of GH deficiency and other disorders of GH metabolism. In: La Cauza C, Root AW, eds. Problems in pediatric endocrinology. Serono Symposia, Vol. 32. London: Academic Press, 1980: 45.

289. Kaplan SL, Grumbach MM. Pathogenesis of sexual precocity. In: Grumbach MM, Sizonenko PC, Aubert ML, eds. Control of the onset of puberty. Baltimore: Williams & Wilkins, 1990: 620.

290. Kaplan SL, Grumbach MM, Aubert ML. The ontogenesis of pituitary hormones and hypothalamic factors in the human fetus: maturation of central nervous system regulation of anterior pituitary function. Recent Prog Horm Res 1976; 32:161.

291. Kaplan SL, Grumbach MM, Aubert ML. α and β glycoprotein hormone subunits (hLH, hFSH, hCG) in the serum and pituitary of the human fetus. J Clin Endocrinol Metab 1976; 42:995.

292. Kaplan SL, Grumbach MM, Hoyt WF. A syndrome of hypopituitary dwarfism, hypoplasia of optic nerves, and malformation of the prosencephalon: report of six patients. Pediatr Res 1970; 4:480.

293. Kaplan SL, Grumbach MM, Shepard TH. The ontogenesis of human fetal hormones. I. Growth hormone and insulin. J Clin Invest 1972; 51:3080.

294. Kastin AT, Gennser G, Arimura A, et al. Melanocyte-stimulating and corticotrophic activities in human foetal pituitary glands. Acta Endocrinol 1968; 58:6.

295. Katz HP, Grumbach MM, Kaplan SL. Diminished growth hormone response to arginine in the puerperium. J Clin Endocrinol Metab 1969; 29:1414.

296. Kaufman LM, Miller MT, Mafee MF. Magnetic resonance imaging of pituitary stalk hypoplasia: a discrete midline anomaly associated with endocrine abnormalities in septo-optic dysplasia. Arch Ophthalmol 1989; 107:1485.

297. Kettel LM, Roseff SJ, Bangah ML, et al. Circulating levels of inhibin in pregnant women at term: simultaneous disappearance with estradiol and progesterone after delivery. Clin Endocrinol 1991; 34:19.

298. Kikuchi K, Fujisawa I, Momoi T, et al. Hypothalamic-pituitary function in growth hormone-deficient patients with pituitary stalk transection. J Clin Endocrinol Metab 1988; 167:817.

299. Klempt M, Bingham B, Breier BH, et al. Tissue distribution and ontogeny of growth hormone receptor mRNA and ligand binding to hepatic tissue in the midgestation sheep fetus. Endocrinology 1993; 132:1071.

300. Konishi I, Fujii S, Okamura H, et al. Development of interstitial cells and ovigerous cords in the human fetal ovary: an ultrastructural study. J Anat 1986; 148:121.

301. Koshimizu T, Ohyama Y, Yokota Y, Ohtsuka K. Peripheral plasma concentrations of somatostatin-like immunoreactivity in newborns and infants. J Clin Endocrinol Metab 1985; 61:78.

302. Kuhlenbeck H. The human diencephalon—a summary of development. Structure, function and pathology. New York: Karger, 1954.

303. Kusakabe M, Sakakura T, Sano M, Nishizuka Y. Epithelial-mesenchymal interaction in early development of the mouse pituitary gland. In: Yoshimura F, Gorbman A, ed. Pars distalis of the pituitary gland. Amsterdam: Elsevier, 1986: 15.

304. Lamberts SWJ, Macleod RM. Regulation of prolactin secretion at the level of the lactotroph. Physiol Rev 1990; 70:279.

305. Laron Z, Lilos P, Klinger B. Growth curves for Laron syndrome. Arch Dis Child 1993; 68:768.

306. Laron Z, Pertzelan A, Mannheimer S, et al. Lack of placental transfer of human growth hormone. Acta Endocrinol 1966; 53:687.

307. Lassare C, Hardouin S, Doffos F, et al. Serum insulin-like growth factors and insulin-like growth factor binding proteins in the human fetus: relationship with growth in normal subjects and in subjects with intrauterine growth retardation. Pediatr Res 1991; 29:219.

308. Leduque P, Aratan-Spire S, Czernichow P, Dubois PM. Ontogenesis of thyrotropin-releasing hormone in the human fetal pancreas. A combined radioimmunological and immunocytochemical study. J Clin Invest 1986; 78:1028.

309. Leech RW, Shuman RM. Holoprosencephaly and related cerebral midline anomalies: a review. J Child Neurol 1986; 1:3.

310. Legouis R, Hardelin J-P, Levilliers J, et al. The candidate gene for the X-linked Kallmann syndrome encodes a protein related to adhesion molecules. Cell 1991; 67:423.

311. Leinonen PJ, Jaffe RB. Leydig cell desensitization by human chorionic gonadotropin does not occur in the human fetal testis. J Clin Endocrinol Metab 1985; 61:234.

312. Lemire RJ. Embryology of the central nervous system. In: Davis JA, Dobbing J, eds. Scientific foundations of paediatrics. Philadelphia: WB Saunders, 1974: 547.

313. Lemire RJ, Beckwith JB, Warkany J. Anencephaly. New York: Raven Press, 1978.

314. Leonardelli J, Tramu G. Immunoreactivity for β-endorphin in LHRH neurons of the fetal human hypothalamus cell. Tissue Res 1979; 203:201.

315. Levitt P, Rakic P. The time of genesis, embryonic origin and differentiation of the brain stem monoamine neurons in the rhesus monkey. Dev Brain Res 1982; 4:35.

316. Li JY, Dubois MP, Dubois PM. Somatotrophs in the human fetal anterior pituitary. Cell Tissue Res 1977; 181:545.

317. Li S, Crenshaw EB III, Rawson EJ, et al. Dwarf locus mutants lacking three pituitary cell types result from mutations in the POU-domain gene pit-1. Nature 1990; 347:528.

318. Lieblich JM, Rosen SE, Guyda H, et al. The syndrome of basal encephalocele and hypothalamic-pituitary dysfunction. Ann Intern Med 1978; 89:910.

319. Liggins GC. The influence of the fetal hypothalamus and pituitary on growth. In: Elliott K, Knight J, eds. Size at birth. Ciba Foundation Symposium 27. Amsterdam: Elsevier-Excerpta Medica, 1974: 165.

320. Lin C, Lin S-C, Chang C-P, Rosenfeld MG. Pit-1-dependent expression of the receptor for growth hor-

mone releasing factor mediates pituitary cell growth. Nature 1992; 360:765.

321. Linton EA, Behan DP, Saphiec PW, Lowry PJ. Corticotropin-releasing hormone (CRH)-binding protein: reduction in the adrenocorticotropin-releasing activity of placental but not hypothalamic CRH. J Clin Endocrinol Metab 1990; 70:1574.

322. Lischka A. Investigation of peripheral androgen resistance in genital hypoplasia associated with congenital growth hormone deficiency. Andrologia 1987; 19:97.

323. Liu L, Cristiano AM, Southers JL, et al. Effects of pituitary-testicular axis suppression *in utero* and during the early neonatal period with a long-acting luteinizing hormone-releasing hormone analog on genital development, somatic growth, and bone density in male cynomolgus monkey in the first 6 months of life. J Clin Endocrinol Metab 1991; 73:1038.

324. Lombardi G, Lupoli G, Scopascasa F, et al. Plasma immunoreactive thyrotropin releasing hormone (TRH) values in normal newborns. J Clin Invest 1978; 1:69.

325. Lovinger RD, Kaplan SL, Grumbach MM. Congenital hypopituitarism associated with neonatal hypoglycemia and microphallus: four cases secondary to hypothalamic hormone deficiencies. J Pediatr 1975; 87:1171.

326. Lowe KC, Jansen CAM, Gluckman PD, Nathanielsz PW. Comparison of changes in ovine plasma chorionic somatomammotropin concentrations in the fetus and mother before spontaneous vaginal delivery at term and adrenocorticotropin induced premature delivery. Am J Obstet Gynecol 1984; 150:524.

327. Lowry PJ, Silman RE, Hope J, Scott AP. Structure and biosynthesis of peptides related to corticotropins and β-melanotropins. Ann NY Acad Sci 1977; 297:49.

328. Lü F, Bassett N, Yang KP, et al. Evidence for autocrine/paracrine mechanisms of action of insulin-like growth factors in the development of fetal sheep adrenal gland (abstr.). The Endocrine Society, San Antonio, TX, 1992.

329. Lü F, Yang K, Challis JRG. Characteristics and developmental changes of corticotrophin releasing hormone binding sites in the fetal sheep anterior pituitary. J Endocrinol 1991; 130:223.

330. Lund PK, Moats-Staats BM, Hynes MA, et al. Somatomedin-C/insulin-like growth factor-I and insulin-like growth factor-II mRNAs in rat fetal and adult tissues. J Biol Chem 1986; 261:14539.

331. Lustig RH, Conte FA, Kogan BA, Grumbach MM. Ontogeny of gonadotropin secretion in congenital anorchism: sexual dimorphism versus syndrome of gonadal dysgenesis and diagnostic considerations. J Urol 1987; 138:587.

332. MacKenzie A, Ferguson MW, Sharpe PT. Hox-7 expression during murine craniofacial development. Development 1991; 113:601.

333. Maghnie M, Larizza D, Triulzi F, et al. Hypopituitarism and stalk agenesis: a congenital syndrome worsened by breech delivery? Horm Res 1991; 35:104.

334. Maghnie M, Larizza D, Zuliani I, Severi F. Congenital central nervous system abnormalities, idiopathic hypopituitarism and breech delivery: What is the connection? Eur J Paediatr 1993; 152:175.

335. Maghnie M, Triulzi F, Larizza D, et al. Hypothalamic-pituitary dwarfism: comparison between MR imaging and CT findings. Pediatr Radiol 1990; 20:229.

336. Mahachoklertwattana P, Kaplan SL, Grumbach MM. The luteinizing hormone-releasing hormone-secreting hypothalamic hamartoma is a congenital malfor-

mation: natural history. J Clin Endocrinol Metab 1993; 77:118.

337. Mahachoklertwattana P, Sanchez J, Grumbach MM, et al. N-methyl-d-aspartate (NMDA) stimulates LHRH release via the NMDA receptor in an LHRH neuronal cell line (GT1-1) (abstr.). Fourth Joint Meeting of the Lawson Wilkins Pediatric Endocrine Society and the European Society for Paediatric Endocrinology, San Francisco. Pediatr Res 1993; 33(suppl):S34.

338. Mangalam HJ, Albert VR, Ingraham HA, et al. A pituitary POU domain protein, Pit-1, activates both growth hormone and prolactin promoters transcriptionally. Genes Dev 1989; 3:946.

339. Margalith D, Tze WJ, Jan JE. Congenital optic nerve hypoplasia with hypothalamic-pituitary dysplasia. Am J Dis Child 1985; 139:361.

340. Martinez de la Escalera G, Weiner RI. Dissociation of dopamine from its receptor as a signal in the pleiotropic hypothalamic regulation of prolactin secretion. Endocr Rev 1992; 13:241.

341. Massa G, de Zegher F, Vanderschueren-Lodeweyckx M. Serum levels of immunoreactive inhibin, FSH and LH in human infants at preterm and term birth. Biol Neonate 1992; 61:150.

342. Massa G, de Zegher F, Vanderschueren-Lodeweyckx M. Serum growth hormone-binding proteins in the human fetus and infant. Pediatr Res 1992; 32:69.

343. Mather JP, Woodruff TK, Krummen LA. Paracrine regulation of reproductive function by inhibin and activin. Proc Soc Exp Biol Med 1992; 201:1.

344. Matsuzaki F, Irie M, Shizume K. Growth hormone in human fetal pituitary glands and cord blood. J Clin Endocrinol Metab 1971; 33:908.

345. Matwijiw I, Faiman C. Control of gonadotropin secretion in the ovine fetus: the effects of specific gonadotropin-releasing hormone antagonist on pulsatile luteinizing hormone secretion. Endocrinology 1987; 121:347.

346. Matwijiw I, Faiman C. Control of gonadotropin secretion in the ovine fetus. II. A sex difference in pulsatile luteinizing hormone secretion after castration. Endocrinology 1989; 124:1352.

347. Matwijiw I, Faiman C. Control of gonadotropin secretion in the ovine fetus. III. Effect of castration on serum follicle-stimulating hormone levels during the last trimester of gestation. Endocrinology 1991; 129:1443.

348. Matwijiw I, Thliveris JA, Faiman C. Hypothalamo-pituitary portal development in the ovine fetus. Biol Reprod 1989; 40:1127.

349. Mauri A, Volpe A, Martellotta MC, et al. α-Melanocyte-stimulating hormone during human perinatal life. J Clin Endocrinol Metab 1993; 77:113.

350. Mayo KE, Cerelli GM, Spiess J, et al. Inhibin A-subunit cDNAs from porcine ovary and human placenta. Proc Natl Acad Sci USA 1986; 83:5849.

351. Mazlan M, Spence-Jones C, Chard T, et al. Circulating levels of GH-releasing hormone and GH during human pregnancy. J Endocrinol 1990; 125:161.

352. McDonald TJ, Rose JC, Figueroa JP, et al. The effect of hypothalamic paraventricular nuclear lesions on plasma ACTH concentrations in the fetal sheep at 108–110 days of gestational age. J Dev Physiol 1988; 10:191.

353. McGrath P. Volume and histology of the human pharyngeal hypophysis. Aust N Z J Surg 1967; 37:16.

354. McGrath P. Prolactin activity and human growth hormone in pharyngeal hypophysis from embalmed cadavers. J Endocrinol 1968; 42:205.

355. McGrath P. Aspects of the human pharyngeal hypophysis in normal and anencephalic fetuses and neonates and their possible significance in the mechanism of its control. J Anat 1978; 127:65.

356. McIntosh N, Pictet RL, Kaplan SL, Grumbach MM. The developmental pattern of somatostatin in the embryonic and fetal rat pancreas. Endocrinology 1977; 101:825.

357. McLachlan RI, Healy DL, Lutjen PJ, et al. The maternal ovary is not the source of circulating inhibin levels during human pregnancy. Clin Endocrinol 1987; 27:663.

358. McLachlan RI, Healy DL, Robertson DM, et al. The human placenta: a novel source of inhibin. Biochem Biophys Res Commun 1986; 140:485.

359. McMillen IC, Thorburn GD, Walker DW. Diurnal variations in plasma concentrations of cortisol, prolactin, growth hormone and glucose in the fetal sheep and pregnant ewe during late gestation. J Endocrinol 1987; 114:65.

360. McMillen IC, Walker DW, Young IR, Nowak R. A daily prolactin rhythm persists in the ewe, foetus and newborn lamb after maternal pinealectomy in late gestation. J Neuroendocrinol 1991; 3:369.

361. McNeilly AS, Gilmore D, Dobbie G, Chard T. Prolactin-releasing activity in the early human foetal hypothalamus. J Endocrinol 1977; 73:533.

362. McPhie JL, Beck JS. The histologic features and human growth hormone content of the pharyngeal pituitary gland in normal and endocrinologically-disturbed patients. Clin Endocrinol 1973; 2:157.

363. Meigan G, Sasaki A, Yoshinaga K. Immunoreactive growth hormone-releasing hormone in rat placenta. Endocrinology 1988; 123:1088.

364. Merker H-J. Morphology of development of the endocrine system in human embryos and fetuses. Adv Biosci 1974; 13:233.

365. Merrimee TJ, Russell B, Quinn S. Growth hormone-binding proteins of human serum: developmental patterns in normal man. J Clin Endocrinol Metab 1992; 75:852.

366. Mesiano S, Hart CS, Heyer BW, et al. Hormone ontogeny in the ovine fetus. XXVI. A sex difference in the effect of castration on the hypothalamic-pituitary gonadotropin unit in the ovine fetus. Endocrinology 1991; 129:3073.

367. Mesiano S, Mellon SH, Gospodarowicz D, et al. Basic fibroblast growth factor expression is regulated by ACTH in the human fetal adrenal: a model for adrenal growth regulation. Proc Natl Acad Sci USA 1991; 88:5428.

368. Mesiano S, Young IR, Baxter RC, et al. Effect of hypophysectomy with and without thyroxine replacement on growth and circulating concentrations of insulin-like growth factors I and II in the fetal lamb. Endocrinology 1987; 120:1821.

369. Meunier H, Rivier C, Evans RM, Vale W. Gonadal and extragonadal expression of inhibin α, βA and βB subunits in various tissues predicts diverse function. Proc Natl Acad Sci USA 1988; 85:247.

370. Miller JD, Wright NM, Esparza A, et al. Spontaneous pulsatile growth hormone release in male and female premature infants. J Clin Endocrinol Metab 1992; 75:1508.

371. Miyakawa I, Ikeda I, Maeyama M. Transport of ACTH across human placenta. J Clin Endocrinol Metab 1976; 39:440.

372. Miyake A, Tanizawa O, Aono T, Kurachi K. LH concentrations in human maternal and cord serum. Endocrinol Jpn 1977; 24:105.

373. Molsberry RL, Carr BR, Mendelson CR, Simpson ER. Human chorionic gonadotropin binding to human fetal testes as a function of gestational age. J Clin Endocrinol Metab 1982; 55:791.

374. Momotani N, Noh J, Oyanagi H. Anti-thyroid drug therapy for Graves' disease during pregnancy: optimal regimen for fetal thyroid status. N Engl J Med 1986; 315:24.

375. Moore CR. Embryonic sex hormones and sexual differentiation. In: Thompson WO, ed. A Monograph in American Lectures in Endocrinology. Springfield, IL: Charles C Thomas, 1947.

376. Mosier HD. Hypoplasia of the pituitary and adrenal cortex. J Pediatr 1956; 48:633.

377. Moya F, Mena P, Foradori A, et al. Effect of maternal administration of thyrotropin releasing hormone on the preterm fetal pituitary-thyroid axis. J Pediatr 1991; 119:966.

378. MRC Vitamin Study Research Group. Prevention of neural tube defects: results of the Medical Research Council vitamin study. Lancet 1991; 2:131.

379. Mueller PL, Gluckman PD, Kaplan SL, et al. Hormone ontogeny in the ovine fetus. V. Circulating prolactin in mid- and late gestation and in the newborn. Endocrinology 1979; 105:129.

380. Mueller PL, Sklar CA, Gluckman PD, et al. Hormone ontogeny of the ovine fetus. IX. Luteinizing hormone and follicle stimulating hormone response to luteinizing hormone-releasing factor in mid- and late gestation and in the neonate. Endocrinology 1981; 108:881.

381. Mulchahey JJ, DiBlasio AM, Martin MC, et al. Hormone production and peptide regulation of the human fetal pituitary gland. Endocr Rev 1987; 8:406.

382. Mulchahey JJ, Jaffe RB. Detection of a potential progenitor cell in the human fetal pituitary that secretes both growth hormone and prolactin. J Clin Endocrinol Metab 1988; 66:24.

383. Müller F, O'Rahilly R. Mediobasal prosencephalic defects, including holoprosencephaly and cyclopia, in relation to the development of the human forebrain. Am J Anat 1989; 185:391.

384. Mulvogue HM, McMillen IC, Robinson PM, Perry RA. Immunocytochemical localization of proγMSH, γMSH, ACTH and βendorphin/βlipotrophin in the fetal sheep pituitary: an ontogenetic study. J Dev Physiol 1986; 8:355.

385. Naftolin F, Ryan KJ, Davies IJ, et al. The formation of estrogens by central neuroendocrine tissues. Recent Prog Horm Res 1975; 31:295.

386. Nagashima K, Yagi H, Suzuki S, et al. Levels of growth hormone and growth-hormone-releasing factor in cord blood. Biol Neonate 1986; 49:307.

387. Nickel BE, Kardami E, Cattini PA. Differential expression of human placental growth hormone variant and chorionic somatomammotropin in culture. Biochem J 1990; 267:653.

388. Nielsen JH, Linde S, Wellinder BS, et al. Growth hormone is a growth factor for the differentiated pancreatic B-cell. Mol Endocrinol 1989; 13:165.

389. Nobin A, Björklund A. Topography of the monoamine neuron systems in the human brain as revealed in fetuses. Acta Physiol Scand 1973; 388(suppl):1.

390. Norman LJ, Challis JRG. Synergism between systemic CRF and AVP on ACTH release in vivo varies as a function of gestational age in the ovine fetus. Endocrinology 1987; 120:1052.

391. Norman LJ, Lye SJ, Wlodek ME, Challis JRG. Changes in pituitary responses to synthetic ovine corticotrophin releasing factor in fetal sheep. Can J Physiol Pharmacol 1985; 63:1398.

392. Ohta K, Nobukuni Y, Mitsubuchi H, et al. Mutations in the Pit-1 gene in children with combined pituitary hormone deficiency. Biochem Biophys Res Commun 1992; 189:851.

393. Ojeda SR, McCann SM. Development of dopaminergic and estrogenic control of prolactin release in the female rat. Endocrinology 1974; 95:1499.

394. Okamoto E, Takagi T, Azuma C, et al. Expression of the corticotropin-releasing hormone (CRH) gene in human placenta and amniotic membrane. Horm Metab Res 1990; 22:394.

395. Oliver D, Mical RS, Porter JC. Hypothalamic-pituitary vasculature. Evidence of retrograde blood flow in the pituitary stalk. Endocrinology 1977; 101:598.

396. Olson L, Boréus LO, Seiger A. Histochemical demonstration and mapping of 5-hydroxytryptamine and catecholamine-containing neuron systems in the human fetal brain. Z Anat Entwickl Gesch 1973; 139:259.

397. Opitz JM. The developmental field concept. A J Med Genet 1985; 21:1.

398. Opitz JM, Gilbert EF. Editorial comment: CNS anomalies and the midline as a "developmental field." A J Med Genet 1982; 12:433.

399. O'Rahilly R. The timing and sequence of events in the development of the human endocrine system during the embryonic period proper. Anat Embryol 1983; 166:439.

400. O'Rahilly R, Gardner E. The timing and sequence of events in the development of the human nervous system during the embryonic period proper. Z Anat Entwickl-Gesch 1971; 134:1.

401. O'Rahilly R, Müller F. Interpretation of some median anomalies as illustrated by cyclopia and symmelia. Teratology 1989; 40:409.

402. Orth DN, Mount CD. Specific high-affinity binding protein for human corticotropin-releasing hormone in normal human plasma. Biochem Biophys Res Commun 1987; 143:411.

403. Osamura RY. Functional prenatal development of anencephalic and normal anterior pituitary glands. Acta Pathol Jpn 1977; 27:495.

404. Osborn BH, Fowlkes J, Han VKM, Freemark M. Nutritional regulation of insulin-like growth factor-binding protein gene expression in the ovine fetus and pregnant ewe. Endocrinology 1992; 131:1743.

405. Owens JA. Endocrine and substrate control of fetal growth: fetal and maternal influences and insulin-like growth factors. Reprod Fertil Dev 1991; 3:501.

406. Palmiter RD, Norstedt G, Gelinas RE, et al. Metallothionein-human GH fusion genes stimulate growth of mice. Science 1983; 222:809.

407. Papez JW. The embryologic development of the hypothalamic area in mammals. Res Publ Assoc Nerv Ment Dis 1940; 20:31.

408. Parker CR, Porter JC, MacDonald PC. Subcellular localization of LHRH and TRH in the human fetal brain (abstr.). Society of Gynecologic Investigation, 25th Annual Meeting, Atlanta, 1978.

409. Parkes JS, Kinoshita E-I, Pfäffle RW. Pit-1 and hypopituitarism. Trends Endocrinol Metab 1993; 4:81.

410. Parkes MJ, Bassett JM. Antagonism by growth hormone of insulin action in fetal sheep. J Endocrinol 1985; 105:379.

411. Pasteels JL, Brauman H, Brauman J. Étude comparée de la secretion d'hormone somatotrope par l'hypophyse humain in vitro et de son activité lactogénique. C R Acad Sci Paris 1963; 256:2031.

412. Pasteels JL, Sheridan R, Gaspar S, Franchimont P. Synthesis and release of gonadotropins and their subunits by long-term organ cultures of human fetal hypophyses. Mol Cell Endocrinol 1977; 9:1.

413. Paulin C, Charnay Y, Chayvialle JA, et al. Ontogeny of substance P in the digestive tract, spinal cord and hypothalamus of the human fetus. Regul Pept 1986; 14:145.

414. Paulin C, Dubois MP, Barry J, Dubois PM. Immuno-fluorescence study of LH-RH producing cells in the human fetal hypothalamus. Cell Tissue Res 1977; 182:341.

415. Paulin C, Li J, Begeot M, Dubois PM. La somatostatine et la function somatotrope antehypophysaire chez le foetus humain. INSERM, Colloque de Synthese, Neuroendocrinologie, 1976: 129.

416. Pavlova EB, Pronina TS, Skebelskaya YB. Histostructure of adenohypophysis of human fetuses and contents of somatotrophic and adrenocorticotropic hormones. Gen Comp Endocrinol 1968; 10:269.

417. Pearse AGE. Cytological and cytochemical investigations on the foetal and adult hypophysis in various physiological and pathological states. J Pathol Bacteriol 1953; 65:355.

418. Pearse AGE. The diffuse neuroendocrine system: peptides, amines, placodes and the APUD theory. In: Hökfelt T, Fuxe K, Pernow B, eds. Progress in brain research. Vol 68. Amsterdam: Elsevier, 1986: 25.

419. Pearse AGE. The diffuse neuroendocrine system and the diencephalon. In: Scharrer B, Korf H-W, Hartwig H-G, eds. Functional morphology of neuroendocrine systems. Berlin: Springer, 1987: 133.

420. Pearse AGE, Takor Takor T. Neuroendocrinology, embryology and the APUD concept. Clin Endocrinol 1976; 5:229S.

421. Penny R, Olambiwonnu NO, Frasier SD. Follicle-stimulating hormone (FSH) and luteinizing hormone-human chorionic gonadotropin (LH-HCG) concentrations in paired maternal and cord serum. Pediatrics 1974; 53:41.

422. Pepe GJ, Albrecht ED. Regulation of the primate fetal adrenal cortex. Endocr Rev 1990; 11:151.

423. Perry RA, Mulvogue HM, McMillen IC, Robinson PM. Immunohistochemical localization of ACTH in the adult and fetal sheep pituitary. J Dev Physiol 1985; 7:397.

424. Peters H, Byskov AG, Grinsted J. Follicular growth in fetal and prepubertal ovaries of humans and other primates. Clin Endocrinol Metab 1978; 7:469.

425. Petit C. Molecular basis of the X-chromosome-linked Kallmann's syndrome. Trends Endocrinol Metab 1993; 4:8.

426. Petraglia F, Sawchenko PE, Lim ATW, et al. Localization, secretion, and action of inhibin in human placenta. Science 1987; 237:187.

427. Petraglia F, Tabanelli S, Galassi MC, et al. Human decidua and in vitro decidualized endometrial stromal cells at term contain immunoreactive corticotropin-releasing factor (CRF) and CRF messenger ribonucleic acid. J Clin Endocrinol 1992; 74:1427.

428. Petraglia F, Vaughn J, Vale W. Inhibin and activin modulate the release of gonadotropin-releasing hormone, human chorionic gonadotropin, and progesterone from cultured human placental cells. Proc Natl Acad Sci USA 1988; 86:5114.

429. Petraglia F, Volpe A, Genazzani AR, et al. Neuroen-

docrinology of the human placenta. Front Neuroendocrinol 1990; 11:6.

430. Pezzino V, Distefano G, Belfiore A, et al. Role of thyrotropin releasing hormone in the development of pituitary-thyroid function in eight anencephalic infants. Acta Endocrinol 1982; 101:538.

431. Pfäffle RW, DiMattia GE, Parks JS, et al. Mutation of the POU-specific domain of Pit-1 and hypopituitarism without pituitary hypoplasia. Science 1992; 257:1118.

432. Phillips DJ, Smith PR, Heath DA, et al. Bioactive and immunoreactive follicle-stimulating hormone and immunoreactive inhibin concentrations in the ovine fetus. J Endocrinol 1992; 134:287.

433. Phillips III JA. Inherited defects in growth hormone synthesis and action. In: Scriver CR, Beaudet AL, Sly WS, Valle D, eds. The metabolic basis of inherited disease. New York: McGraw Hill, 1989: 1965.

434. Pickel VM, Specht LA, Sumal KK, et al. Immunocytochemical localization of tyrosine hydroxylase in the human fetal nervous system. J Comp Neurol 1980; 194:465.

435. Pierson M, Malaprade D, Grignon G, et al. Étude de la secretion hypophysaire du foetus humain: correlations entre morphologie et activite secretoire. Ann Endocrinol 1973; 34:418.

436. Pinner-Poole B. Absence of neurosecretory material in the pituitary glands in anencephaly. J Neuropathol Exp Neurol 1967; 26:117.

437. Plant TM. Puberty in primates. In: Knobil E, Neill JD, eds. The physiology of reproduction. New York: Raven Press, 1988: 1763.

438. Power GC, Ball KT, Gluckman PD. Disappearance of growth hormone from plasma of fetal and newborn sheep. Am J Physiol 1988; 254:E318.

439. Prager D, Braunstein GD. Editorial: X-chromosome-linked Kallmann's syndrome: pathology at the molecular level. J Clin Endocrinol Metab 1993; 76:824.

440. Qu J, Thomas K. Changes in bioactive and immunoactive inhibin levels around human labor. J Clin Endocrinol Metab 1992; 74:1290.

441. Qu J, Vankrieken L, Brulet C, Thomas K. Bioactive levels during human pregnancy. Circulating inhibin. J Clin Endocrinol Metab 1991; 72:862.

442. Rabinovici J, Goldsmith PC, Robert VJ, et al. Localization and secretion of inhibin/activin subunits in the human and subhuman primate fetal gonads. J Clin Endocrinol Metab 1991; 73:1141.

443. Rabinovici J, Jaffe RB. Development and regulation of growth and differentiated function in human and subhuman primate fetal gonads. Endocr Rev 1990; 11:532.

444. Rabinovici J, Roberts VJ, Goldsmith PC, et al. Ontogeny of the site of production and regulation of inhibin/activin subunits in the primate fetal testis. Program of the 72nd Annual Meeting of The Endocrine Society, Atlanta, 1990: 392.

445. Radovick S, Nations M, Du Y, et al. A mutation in the POU-homeodomain of Pit-1 responsible for combined pituitary hormone deficiency. Science 1992; 257:1115.

446. Rahier J, Wullon J, Henquin JC. Abundance of somatostatin cells in the human neonatal pancreas. Diabetologia 1980; 18:251.

447. Rappaport EB, Ulstrom RA, Gorlin RJ, et al. Solitary central incisor and short stature. J Pediatr 1977; 91:924.

448. Rasmussen DD, Gambacciani M, Swartz WH, et al. Pulsatile GnRH release from the human mediobasal hypothalamus in vitro: opiate receptor mediated suppression. Neuroendocrinology 1989; 49:150.

449. Raymond V, Beaulieu M, Labrie F, Boissier J. Potent antidopaminergic activity of estradiol at the pituitary level on prolactin release. Science 1978; 200:1173.

450. Raynaud A, Frilley M. Developpement intrauterin des embryons de souris dont les ebauches de l'hypophyse ont ete detruites, au moyen des rayons X, au 13e jour de la gestation. I. Developpement de l'appareil genital. C R Acad Sci Paris 1947; 225:596.

451. Reid JD. Congenital absence of the pituitary gland. J Pediatr 1960; 56:658.

452. Reitano G, Grasso S, Distefano G, Messina A. The serum insulin and growth hormone response to arginine and to arginine with glucose in the premature infant. J Clin Endocrinol Metab 1971; 33:924.

453. Resko JA, Ellinwood WE. Negative feedback regulation of gonadotropin secretion by androgens in fetal rhesus macaques. Biol Reprod 1985; 33:346.

454. Reyes FI, Boroditsky RS, Winter JSD, Faiman C. Studies on human sexual development. II. Fetal and maternal serum gonadotropin and sex steroid concentrations. J Clin Endocrinol Metab 1974; 38:612.

455. Reyes FI, Winter JSD, Faiman C. Studies on human sexual development. I. Fetal gonadal and adrenal sex steroids. J Clin Endocrinol Metab 1973; 37:74.

456. Reyes FI, Winter JSD, Faiman C. Endocrinology of the fetal testis. In: Burger H, de Kretser D, eds. The testis, ed 2. New York: Raven Press, 1989: 119.

457. Riley SC, Walton JC, Herlick JM, Challis JR. The localization and distribution of corticotropin-releasing hormone in the human placenta and fetal membranes throughout gestation. J Clin Endocrinol Metab 1991; 72:1001.

458. Robinson BG, Arbiser JL, Emanuel RL, Majzoub JA. Species-specific placental corticotropin releasing hormone messenger RNA and peptide expression. Mol Cell Endocrinol 1989; 62:337.

459. Robinson BG, Emanuel RL, Frim DM, Majzoub JA. Glucocorticoid stimulates expression of corticotropin-releasing hormone gene in human placenta. Proc Natl Acad Sci USA 1988; 85:5244.

460. Roessmann U, Velasco ME, Small EJ, et al. Neuropathology of "septo-optic dysplasia" (DeMorsier syndrome) with immunohistochemical studies of the hypothalamus and pituitary gland. J Neuropathol Exp Neurol 1987; 46:597.

461. Romske C, Sotos JF. Hypothalamic-pituitary deformation in siblings with holoprosencephaly. J Pediatr 1973; 83:1088.

462. Rondeel JMM, Jackson IMD. Molecular biology of the regulation of hypothalamic hormones. J Endocrinol Invest 1993; 16:219.

463. Rose JC, MacDonald AA, Heymann MA, Rudolph AM. Developmental aspects of the pituitary adrenal axis response to hemorrhagic stress in lamb fetuses in utero. J Clin Invest 1978; 61:424.

464. Rose JC, Turner CS, de Wana R, Rawashdeh N. Evidence that cortisol inhibits basal adrenocorticotropin secretion in the sheep fetus by 0.70 gestation. Endocrinology 1988; 123:1307.

465. Rossmanith WG, Swartz WH, Tueros VS, et al. Pulsatile GnRH-stimulated LH release from the human fetal pituitary in vitro: sex-associated differences. Clin Endocrinol 1990; 33:719.

465a. Roti E. Regulation of thyroid-stimulating hormone (TSH) secretion in the fetus and neonate. J Endocrinol Invest 1988; 11:145.

466. Roti E, Gnudi A, Braverman LE, et al. Human cord

blood concentration of thyrotropin, thyroglobulin, and iodothyronines after maternal administration of thyrotropin-releasing hormone. J Clin Endocrinol Metab 1981; 53:813.

467. Roti E, Robuschi G, Alboni A, et al. Inhibition of foetal growth hormone and thyrotropin (TSH) secretion after maternal administration of somatostatin. Acta Endocrinol 1984; 106:393.

468. Roti E, Robuschi G, Alboni A, et al. Human foetal prolactin but not thyrotropin secretion is decreased by bromocriptine. Acta Endocrinol 1986; 112:35.

469. Rudman D, Davis GT, Preist JH, et al. Prevalence of growth hormone deficiency in children with cleft lip or palate. J Pediatr 1978; 93:378.

470. Rugarli EI, Lutz B, Kuratani SC, et al. Expression pattern of the Kallmann syndrome gene in the olfactory system suggests a role in neuronal targeting. Nature Genet 1993; 4:19.

471. Sadeghi-Nejad A, Senior B. A familial syndrome of isolated "aplasia" of the anterior pituitary. J Pediatr 1974; 84:79.

472. Saito H, Saito S, Sano T, et al. Fetal and maternal plasma levels of immunoreactive somatostatin at delivery: evidence for its increase in the umbilical artery and its arteriovenous gradient in the fetoplacental circulation. J Clin Endocrinol Metab 1983; 56:567.

473. Salardi S, Orsini LF, Cacciari E, et al. Growth hormone, insulin-like growth factor I, insulin and C-peptide during human fetal life: in-utero study. Clin Endocrinol 1991; 34:187.

474. Salazar H, MacAulay MA, Charles D, Pardo M. The human hypophysis in anencephaly. I. Ultrastructure of the pars distalis. Arch Pathol 1969; 87:201.

475. Salminen-Lappalainen K, Lautikuinen T. Binding of corticotropin-releasing hormone (CRH) in maternal and fetal plasma. Clin Chim Acta 1990; 195:57.

476. Sasaki A, Tempst P, Liotta AS, et al. Isolation and characterization of corticotropin-releasing hormone-like peptide from human placenta. J Clin Endocrinol Metab 1988; 67:768.

477. Satow Y, Okamoto N, Ikeda T, et al. Electron microscope studies of the anterior pituitaries and adrenal cortices of normal and anencephalic human fetuses. J Electron Microsc 1972; 21:29.

478. Sawada M. A study of functional development of hypothalamo-hypophyseogonadal system in human fetuses. Nichidai Igaku Zasshi 1976; 35:945.

479. Schellenberg J-C, Liggins GC, Manzai M, et al. Synergistic hormone effects on lung maturation in fetal sheep. J Appl Physiol 1988; 65:94.

480. Schenker JG, Ben-David M, Polishuk WZ. Prolactin in normal pregnancy: relationship of maternal, fetal and amniotic fluid levels. Am J Obstet Gynecol 1975; 123:834.

481. Schindler AE. Steroid metabolism in foetal tissues. IV. Conversion of testosterone to 5α-dihydrotestosterone in human foetal brain. J Steroid Biochem 1976; 7:97.

482. Schulze-Bonhage A, Wittkowski W. Cell types in the fetal pars tuberalis of the human adenohypophysis at mid-gestation. Cell Tissue Res 1991; 264:161.

483. Schwanzel-Fukuda M, Abraham S, Crossin KL, et al. Immunocytochemical demonstration of neural cell adhesion molecule (NCAM) along the migration route of luteinizing hormone-releasing hormone (LHRH) neurons in mice. J Comp Neurol 1992; 321:1.

484. Schwanzel-Fukuda M, Bick D, Pfaff DW. Luteinizing hormone-releasing hormone (LHRH)-expressing cells do not migrate normally in an inherited hypogonadal (Kallmann) syndrome. Mol Brain Res 1989; 6:311.

485. Schwanzel-Fukuda M, Jorgenson KL, Bergen HT, et al. Biology of normal luteinizing hormone-releasing hormone neurons during and after their migration from olfactory placode. Endocr Rev 1992; 13:623.

486. Schwanzel-Fukuda M, Pfaff DW. Origin of luteinizing hormone-releasing hormone neurons. Nature (Lond) 1989; 338:161.

487. Sedin G, Bergquist C, Lindgren PG. Ovarian hyperstimulation syndrome in preterm infants. Pediatr Res 1985; 19:548.

488. Seron-Ferre MC, Lawrence CC, Jaffe RB. Role of hCG in the regulation of the fetal zone of the human fetal adrenal zone. J Clin Endocrinol Metab 1978; 46:834.

489. Seron-Ferre M, Rose JC, Parer JT, et al. In vitro regulation of the fetal rhesus monkey adrenal gland. Endocrinology 1978; 103: 368.

490. Sheth JJ, Sheth AR, Vin FK. Bioimmunoreactive inhibin-like substance in human fetal gonads. Biol Res Pregnancy Perinatol 1983; 4:110.

491. Shiino M, Ishikawa H, Rennels EG. Accumulation of secretory granules in pituitary clonal cells derived from the epithelium of Rathke's pouch. Cell Tissue Res 1978; 186:53.

492. Shimano S, Suzuki S, Nagashima K, et al. Growth hormone responses to growth hormone releasing factor in neonates. Biol Neonate 1985; 47:367.

493. Shutt DA, Smith ID, Shearman RP. Oestrone, oestradiol-17β and oestriol levels in human foetal plasma during gestation and at term. J Endocrinol 1974; 60:333.

494. Siebert JR, Cohen Jr MM, Sulik KK, et al., eds. Holoprosencephaly: an overview and atlas of cases. New York: Wiley-Liss, 1990.

495. Siiteri PK, Wilson JD. Testosterone formation and metabolism during male sexual differentiation in the human embryo. J Clin Endocrinol Metab 1974; 38:113.

496. Siler-Khodr TM, Khodr GS. Studies in human fetal endocrinology. I. Luteinizing hormone-releasing factor content of the hypothalamus. Am J Obstet Gynecol 1978; 130:795.

497. Siler-Khodr TM, Khodr GS. Content of luteinizing hormone-releasing factor in the human placenta. Am J Obstet Gynecol 1978; 130:216.

498. Siler-Khodr TM, Morgenstern LL, Greenwood FC. Hormone synthesis and release from human fetal adenohypophyses in vitro. J Clin Endocrinol Metab 1974; 39:891.

499. Silman RE, Chard T, Landon J, et al. ACTH and MSH peptides in the human adult and fetal pituitary gland. Front Horm Res 1977; 4:179.

500. Silman RE, Chard T, Lowry PJ, et al. Human fetal pituitary peptides and parturition. Nature 1976; 260:716.

501. Silverman BL, Bettendorf M, Kaplan SL, et al. Regulation of growth hormone (GH) secretion by GH-releasing factor, somatostatin, and insulin-like growth factor I in ovine fetal and neonatal pituitary cells in vitro. Endocrinology 1989; 124:84.

502. Simmons DM, Voss JW, Ingraham HA, et al. Pituitary cell phenotype involve cell-specific Pit-1 mRNA translation and synergistic interaction with other class of transcription factors. Genes Dev 1990; 4:695.

503. Sinha YN, Klemcke HG, Maurer RR, Jacobsen BP. Ontogeny of glycosylated and nonglycosylated forms of prolactin and growth hormone in porcine pitui-

tary during fetal life. Proc Soc Exp Biol Med 1990; 194:293.

504. Sklar CA, Mueller PL, Gluckman PD, et al. Hormone ontogeny of the ovine fetus. VII. Circulating luteinizing hormone and follicle-stimulating hormone in mid and late gestation. Endocrinology 1981; 108:874.

505. Smith AI, Funder JW. Proopiomelanocortin processing in the pituitary, central nervous system and peripheral tissues. Endocrinol Rev 1988; 9:159.

506. Snead OC, Morley BJ. Ontogeny of gamma-hydroxybutyric acid I. Regional concentration in developing rat, monkey and human brain. Dev Brain Res 1981; 1:579.

507. Soares MJ, Faria TN, Roby KF, Deb S. Pregnancy and the prolactin family of hormones: coordination of anterior pituitary, uterine and placental expression. Endocr Rev 1991; 12:402.

508. Spencer SJ, Rabinovici J, Mesiano S, et al. Activin and inhibin in the human adrenal gland: regulation and differential effects in fetal and adult cells. J Clin Invest 1992; 90:142.

509. Steinfelder HJ, Radovick S, Mroczynski MA, et al. Role of a pituitary-specific transcription factor (pit-1/ GHF-1) or a closely related protein in cAMP regulation of human thyrotropin-beta subunit gene expression. J Clin Invest 1992; 89:409.

510. Stubbe P, Wolf H. Glucose loading and arginine infusions in newborn infants. Effect on growth hormone, blood sugar, fatty acids, and glycerin. Klin Wochenschr 1970; 48:918.

511. Styne DM, Kaplan SL, Grumbach MM. Plasma glycoprotein hormone α-subunit in the neonate and in prepubertal and pubertal children: effects of luteinizing hormone-releasing hormone. J Clin Endocrinol Metab 1980; 50:450.

512. Styne DM, Van Vliet G, Rudolph AM, et al. Somatomedin C in the ovine fetus and neonate. In: Raiti S, Tolman RA, eds. Human growth hormone. New York: Plenum Publishing Co, 1986: 635.

513. Suda T, Iwashita M, Sumitomo T, et al. Presence of CRH-binding protein in amniotic fluid and in umbilical cord plasma. Acta Endocrinol 1991; 125:165.

514. Suganuma N, Seo H, Yamamoto N, et al. Ontogenesis of pituitary prolactin in the human fetus. J Clin Endocrinol Metab 1986; 63:156.

515. Suganuma N, Seo H, Yamamoto N, et al. The ontogeny of growth hormone in the human fetal pituitary. Am J Obstet Gynecol 1989; 160:729.

516. Suita S, Handa N, Nakano H. Antenally detected ovarian cysts—a therapeutic dilemma. Early Human Dev 1992; 29:363.

517. Sultan C, Bonardet A, Bonnal B, et al. Evolution de la prolactine plasmatique chez l'enfant normal de la naissance á l'adolescence. C R Soc Biol 1977; 171:131.

518. Swaab DF, Gooren LJG, Hofman MA. The human hypothalamus in relation to gender and sexual orientation. Progr Brain Res 1992; 93:205.

519. Swenne I, Hill DJ, Strain AJ, Milner RDG. Growth hormone regulation of somatomedin C/insulin-like growth factor I production and DNA replication in fetal rat islets in tissue culture. Diabetes 1987; 36:288.

520. Tabei T, Ochiai K, Terashima Y, Takanashi N. Serum levels of inhibin in maternal and umbilical cord blood during pregnancy. Am J Obstet Gynecol 1991; 164:896.

521. Takagi S, Yoshida T, Tsubata K. An investigation of the materno-fetal hormonal milieu with special emphasis on the maternal influence. In: Notake Y, Su-

zuki S, eds. Biological and clinical aspects of the fetus. Baltimore: University Park Press, 1977: 134.

522. Takagi S, Yoshida T, Tsubata K, et al. Sex differences in fetal gonadotropins and androgens. J Steroid Biochem 1977; 8:609.

523. Takahashi H, Nakashima S, Ohama E, et al. Distribution of serotonin-containing bodies in the brainstem of the human fetus determined with immunohistochemistry using antiserotonin serum. Brain Dev 1986; 8:355.

524. Takor Takor T, Pearse AGE. Neuroectodermal origin of avian hypothalamo-hypophyseal complex: the role of the ventral neural ridge. J Embryol Exp Morphol 1975; 34:311.

525. Tapanainen J, Kellokumpu-Lehtinen P, Pelliniemi LJ, Huhtaniemi I. Age-related changes in endogenous steroids of human fetal testis during early and midpregnancy. J Clin Endocrinol Metab 1981; 52:98.

526. Tapanainen J, Koivisto M, Huhtaniemi I, Vihko R. Effect of gonadotropin-releasing hormone on pituitary-gonadal function of male infants during the first year of life. J Clin Endocrinol Metab 1982; 55:689.

527. Tapanainen J, Koivisto M, Vihko R, Huhtaniemi I. Enhanced activity of the pituitary-gonadal axis in premature human infants. J Clin Endocrinol Metab 1981; 52:235.

528. Tapanainen J, Voutilainen R, Jaffe RB. Low aromatase activity and gene expression in human fetal testes. J Steroid Biochem 1989; 33:7.

529. Tatsumi K-I, Miyai K, Notomi T, et al. Cretinism with combined hormone deficiency caused by a mutation in the PIT1 gene. Nature Genet 1992; 1:56.

530. Theill LE, Hattori K, Lazzaro D, et al. Differential splicing of the GHF1 primary transcript gives rise to two functionally distinct homeodomain proteins. Embo J 1992; 11:2261.

531. The Medical Task Force on Anencephaly. The infant with anencephaly. N Engl J Med 1990; 322:669.

532. Thliveris JA, Currie RW. Observations on the hypothalamohypophyseal portal vasculature in the developing human fetus. Am J Anat 1980; 157:441.

533. Thomsett MJ, Marti-Henneberg C, Gluckman PD, et al. Hormone ontogeny in the ovine fetus. VIII. The effect of thyrotropin-releasing factor on prolactin and growth hormone release in the fetus and neonate. Endocrinology 1980; 106:1074.

534. Thorpe-Beeston JG, Nicolaides KH, Felton CV, et al. Maturation of the secretion of thyroid hormone and thyroid-stimulating hormone in the fetus. N Engl J Med 1991; 324:532.

535. Tilney F. The development and constituents of the human hypophysis. Bull Neurol Inst N Y 1936; 5:387.

536. Tobet SA, Crandall JE, Schwarting GA. Relationship of migrating luteinizing hormone-releasing hormone neurons to unique olfactory system glycoconjugates in embryonic rats. Dev Biol 1992; 155:471.

537. Trandafir T, Sipot C, Froicu P. On a possible neural ridge origin of the adenohypophysis. Rev Roum Endocrinol 1990; 28:67.

538. Truwit CL, Barkovich AJ, Grumbach MM, Martini JJ. MR imaging of Kallmann syndrome, a genetic disorder of neuronal migration affecting the olfactory and genital systems. Am J Neuroradiol 1993; 14:827.

539. Tseng MT, Alexander NJ, Kittinger GW. Effects of fetal decapitation on the structure and function of Leydig cells in rhesus monkeys (*Macaca mulatta*). Am J Anat 1975; 349:214.

540. Turner RC, Schneeloch B, Paterson P. Changes in plasma growth hormone and insulin of the human

foetus following hysterotomy. Acta Endocrinol 1971; 66:577.

541. Tyson JE, Hwang P, Guyda H, Friesen HG. Studies of prolactin secretion in human pregnancy. Am J Obstet Gynecol 1972; 113:14.

542. Vale W, Hsueh A, Rivier C, Yu J. The inhibin/activin family of hormones and growth factors. Handb Exp Pharmacol 1990; 95(Part 2):211.

543. Vergara M, Parraguez VH, Riquelme R, et al. Ontogeny of the circadian variation of plasma prolactin in sheep. J Dev Physiol 1989; 11:89.

544. Volpe JJ. Effect of cocaine use on the fetus. N Engl J Med 1992; 327:399.

545. Voss JW, Rosenfeld MG. Anterior pituitary development: short tales from dwarf mice. Cell 1992; 70:527.

546. Voutilainen R, Erämaa M, Ritvos O. Hormonally regulated inhibin gene expression in human fetal and adult adrenals. J Clin Endocrinol Metab 1991; 73:1026.

547. Voutilainen R, Miller WL. Developmental expression of genes for the steroidogenic enzymes P450scc (20,22-desmolase), P450c17 (17-hydroxylase/17,20 lyase), and P450c21 (21-hydroxylase) in the human fetus. J Clin Endocrinol Metab 1986; 63:1145.

548. Voutilainen R, Miller WL. Coordinate tropic hormone regulation of mRNAs for insulin-like growth factor II and cholesterol side-chain cleavage enzyme, P450scc in human steroidogenic tissues. Proc Natl Acad Sci USA 1987; 84:1590.

549. Vuolteenaho O, Leppaluoto J, Hoyhtya M, Hirvonen J. β-endorphin-like peptides in autopsy pituitaries from adults, neonates and foetuses. Acta Endocrinol 1983; 102:27.

550. Waldhauser F, Weisenbacher G, Frisch H, Pollak A. Pulsatile secretion of gonadotropins in early infancy. Eur J Pediatr 1981; 137:71.

551. Wanke R, Wolf E, Hermanns W, et al. The GH-transgenic mouse as an experimental model for growth research: clinical and pathological studies. Horm Res 1992; 37(suppl):74.

552. Warren DW. Development of the inhibitory guanine nucleotide-binding regulatory protein in the rat testis. Biol Reprod 1989; 40:1208.

553. Watanabe YG, Daikoku S. Immunohistochemical study on adenohypophyseal primordia in organ culture. Cell Tissue Res 1976; 166:407.

554. Weill J, Bernfeld J. Le Syndrome Hypothalamique. Paris: Masson et Cie, Libraires de L'Acadame de Medicine, 1954.

555. Wells LJ. Progress studies designed to determine whether the foetal hypophysis produces hormones that influence development. Anat Rec 1947; 97:409.

556. Werther GA, Haynes KM, Barnard R, Waters MJ. Visual demonstration of growth hormone receptors on human growth plate chondrocytes. J Clin Endocrinol Metab 1990; 70:1725.

557. Werther GA, Haynes K, Waters MJ. Growth hormone (GH) receptors are expressed on human mesenchymal tissue—identification of messenger ribonucleic acid and GH-binding protein. J Clin Endocrinol Metab 1993; 76:1638.

558. Wingstrand KG. Microscopic anatomy, nerve supply and blood supply of the pars intermedia. In: Harris GW, Donovan BT, eds. The pituitary gland. Vol 3. London: Butterworths, 1966: 1.

559. Winter JSD, Faiman C, Hobson WC, et al. Pituitary-gonadal relations in infancy. I. Patterns of serum gonadotropin concentrations from birth to four years of age in man and chimpanzee. J Clin Endocrinol Metab 1975; 40:545.

560. Winters AJ, Colston C, MacDonald PC, Porter JC. Fetal plasma prolactin levels. J Clin Endocrinol Metab 1975; 41:626.

561. Winters AJ, Eskay RL, Porter JC. Concentration and distribution of TRH and LRH in the human fetal brain. J Clin Endocrinol Metab 1974; 39:960.

562. Winters AJ, Oliver C, Colston C, et al. Plasma ACTH levels in the human fetus and neonate as related to age and parturition. J Clin Endocrinol Metab 1974; 39:269.

563. Wintour EM, Brown EH, Denton DA, et al. The ontogeny and regulation of corticosteroid secretion by the ovine foetal adrenal. Acta Endocrinol 1975; 79:301.

564. Wit JM, Van Unen H. Growth of infants with neonatal growth hormone deficiency. Arch Dis Child 1992; 67:920.

565. Wittkowski WH, Schulze-Bonhage AH, Böckers TM. The pars tuberalis of the hypophysis: A modulator of the pars distalis? Acta Endocrinol 1992; 126:285.

566. Wood CE. Sensitivity of cortisol-induced inhibition of ACTH and renin in fetal sheep. Am J Physiol 1986; 250:R795.

567. Word RA, George FW, Wilson JD, Carr BR. Testosterone synthesis and adenylate cyclase activity in the early human fetal testis appear to be independent of human chorionic gonadotropin control. J Clin Endocrinol Metab 1989; 69:204.

568. Wray S, Grant P, Gainer H. Evidence that cells expressing luteinizing hormone-releasing hormone mRNA in the mouse are derived from progenitor cells in the olfactory placode. Proc Natl Acad Sci USA 1989; 86:8132.

569. Wray S, Nieburgs A, Elkabes S. Spatiotemporal cell expression of luteinizing hormone-releasing hormone in the prenatal mouse: evidence for an embryonic origin in the olfactory placode. Dev Brain Res 1989; 46:309.

570. Wright NM, Northington FJ, Miller JD, et al. Elevated growth hormone secretory rate in premature infants: deconvolution analysis of pulsatile growth hormone secretion in the neonate. Pediatr Res 1992; 32:286.

570a. Wynick D, Hammond PJ, Akinsanya KO, Bloom SR. Galanin regulates basal and oestrogen-stimulated lactotroph function. Nature 1993; 364:529.

571. Ying S-Y. Inhibins, activins, and follistatin: gonadal proteins modulating the secretion of follicle-stimulating hormone. Endocr Rev 1988; 9:267.

572. Yokoh Y. The early development of the nervous system in man. Acta Anat (Basel) 1968; 71:492.

573. Zondek LH, Zondek T. Observations on the testis in anencephaly with special reference to the Leydig cells. Biol Neonate 1965; 8:329.

574. Zondek LH, Zondek T. The influence of complications of pregnancy and of some congenital malformations on the reproductive organs of the male foetus and neonate. International Symposium on Sexual Endocrinology of the Perinatal Period. INSERM 1974; 32:79.

575. Zondek LH, Zondek T. Ovarian hilar cells and testicular Leydig cells in anencephaly. Biol Neonate 1983; 43:211.

The Fetal-Maternal Neurohypophyseal System

Rosemary D. Leake

Hormones synthesized in the hypothalamus and subsequently secreted by the neurohypophysis play a major role in maternal, fetal, and newborn salt and water homeostasis, adaptation to intrauterine stress, parturition, and transition to extrauterine life. Three neurohypophyseal hormones (NHP) have been identified in tissue or in plasma during the perinatal period in mammals: arginine vasotocin (AVT), arginine vasopressin (AVP), and oxytocin (OT).

CHEMISTRY OF MAMMALIAN NEUROHYPOPHYSEAL HORMONES

The amino acid sequences for AVT, AVP, and OT are shown in Figure 13–1. AVT, AVP, and OT have a similar amino acid sequence consisting of a six-member amino acid ring with a disulfide bridge from position 1 to position 6 and a three-member carboxyl terminal side chain; they differ only in the identity of the amino acids at positions 3 and 8. AVT has a "ring" identical to that of OT and a "tail" identical to AVP.

SYNTHESIS, SECRETION, AND CLEARANCE OF NEUROHYPOPHYSEAL HORMONES

The NHP are synthesized as large linear peptides in neural cell bodies in the supraoptic

and paraventricular nuclei. The preprohormone contains an N-terminal signal peptide, the nonapeptide (AVP or OT), and the specific AVP or OT neurophysin. In addition, the preprohormone for AVP terminates with a glycoprotein. Although both hormones are present in each nucleus, there are more AVP-secreting neurons in the supraoptic nucleus and more OT-secreting neurons in the paraventricular nucleus.[64] Each cell, however, appears to secrete only one hormone.[13, 111] Action potentials recorded in individual neuroendocrine cells may occur either irregularly (one to two spikes per second) or in intermittent bursts (phasic firing).[47] Data from simultaneous observations of single unit electrical activity and of target organ effects are consistent with the view that the random-firing neurons release OT and the phasic-firing neurons secrete AVP. Long axonal tracts extend from the neurons in the hypothalamus to nerve terminals in the posterior pituitary gland and median eminence. In the Golgi apparatus, the N-terminal signal peptide is removed; glycosylation of the AVP preprohormone occurs in the luminal space of the rough endoplasmic reticulum, resulting in prohormone formation. The prohormone is packaged into secretory granules and transported down the axon to the posterior pituitary. While in the granules, the prohormones are enzymatically converted to the nonapeptide hormones and their specific binding proteins or neurophysins. Intravesicular processing produces the nonapeptide hormone (AVP or OT), its neurophysin, and, in the case of vasopressin, a glycoprotein. The granules are then stored in terminal bulbs in the posterior pituitary gland, in release sites adjacent to the circulation. Depolarization of the neurosecretory neuron results in the fusion of the granules to the plasmalemma of the axon and their release into the circulation by exocytosis.[25]

The linkage between OT or AVP and their specific neurophysins is by means of a three-peptide bridge containing glycine, lysine, and arginine. Enzymatic cleavage by carboxypeptidase produces OT glycine (OT-gly) or AVP glycine (VP-gly) as intravesicular processing occurs. Both OT-gly and VP-gly have been identified in the ovine and human circula-

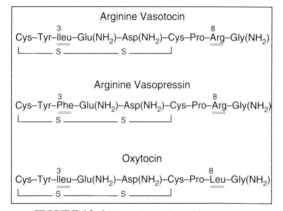

FIGURE 13–1. Neurohypophyseal hormones.

tion[4-6, 27] (see section on role of maternal NHP in parturition later).

Both the hormones and neurophysins circulate in the plasma, whereas the granule membrane is recaptured by pinocytosis. In addition to secretion into the circulation, neurosecretion of both hormones occurs directly into the third ventricle.[24] This pathway may be a part of the peptidergic neurosecretory system and may mediate some of the effects of AVP on behavior.[104]

Both OT and AVP circulate as free peptides in blood, with plasma half-lives varying from 3 to 6 minutes.[2, 29] In the adult, clearance occurs in both the kidney and the liver; neither the liver nor kidney appears to play a major role in fetal NHP clearance. In the pregnant guinea pig, the amniotic sac appears to be involved in AVP metabolism.[110] The primate (but not the nonprimate) placenta contains a system of enzymes, vasopressinases, or oxytocinases, produced by syncytiotrophoblastic cells.[88, 109] These degradative enzymes are present in human cord blood, maternal plasma, and amniotic fluid. The enzyme concentrations increase with advancing gestational age.[88] There is an increase in OT clearance rate during late gestation.[107] AVP clearance rate also increases between 8 weeks' postconception and midgestation, a time when there is also a marked increase in trophoblastic mass and plasma vasopressinase.[18] In the ovine model, AVP clearance is equivalent (on a per kilogram basis) in pregnant ewes, fetuses, and lambs.[103] Renal AVP clearance accounts for less than 8% of total body clearance in the fetus; thus the major site of AVP clearance in fetal life remains unclear.[17]

FUNCTION AND SECRETION OF NEUROHYPOPHYSEAL HORMONES (Table 13–1)

Arginine Vasotocin

AVT is found in fish, amphibians, and birds and to a lesser extent in mammals. In nonmammalian vertebrates, AVT is secreted following either osmotic or hypovolemic stimuli. In fish, amphibians, and birds, AVT regulates water reabsorption from the bladder, elevates blood pressure, and stimulates oviduct contraction.[95, 100] The human fetal hypothalamus contains AVT from 11 to 19 weeks' gestation and the human fetal pineal gland from 55 days' gestation.[65] AVT has also been identified (by radioimmunoassay or high-pressure liquid chromatography [HPLC]) in human amniotic fluid,[8] cord blood,[27] and newborn cerebrospinal fluid[8] as well as ovine fetal plasma. AVT does not appear to be secreted in the human adult; the timing of AVT disappearance following birth is unknown.

The regulation of secretion of AVT is unclear; more is known regarding its function. Human fetal ependymal cells release an active principle in tissue culture possessing antidiuretic, uterotonic, and hydro-osmotic properties similar to AVT.[72] AVT slows water movement from the maternal to the fetal side of the guinea pig amnion in vitro.[113] In the chronically catheterized ovine fetus, AVT decreases lung fluid production, elevates blood pressure, produces bradycardia, and evokes antidiuresis. Thus fetal AVT may play a potential role in the regulation of water exchange at placental,

TABLE 13–1 Physiologic Stimuli for Neurohypophyseal Hormone Secretion

Maternal
AVP
Hypovolemia
Hyperosmolality
Hypotension
OT
Nipple stimulation
Cervical/vaginal dilation
AVT
No evidence of secretion
Fetal
AVP
Hypovolemia
Hyperosmolality
Hypotension
Hypoxia
Acidosis
Labor
Furosemide
Epinephrine
AVT
No stimulus identified to date
Newborn
AVP
Hypovolemia
Hyperosmolality
Hypoxia
OT
Unknown
AVT
No stimulus identified to date

lung, or renal sites. Similar to AVP, AVT may influence cardiovascular adaptation as well. AVT in newborn and adult cats suppresses active sleep and promotes quiet sleep.[73] Thus AVT may play a hypnogenic role in some species.

Arginine Vasopressin

AVP acts on the kidney by binding to receptors in collecting duct cell membranes and activating adenylate cyclase. This, in turn, results in the conversion of adenosine triphosphate (ATP) to cyclic adenosine monophosphate (cAMP). By mechanisms as yet undelineated, increased cAMP ultimately results in the insertion of preformed membrane pockets or pores that produce increased permeability of the luminal membrane to water and facilitate increased reabsorption of free water from the collecting duct. In the adult human, AVP also plays a role in blood pressure regulation, corticotropin releasing factor–like activity, prostaglandin synthesis, platelet aggregation, hepatic glycogenolysis, and perhaps memory consolidation.

AVP secretion is mainly determined by changes in plasma osmolality, as detected by osmosensitive cells in the anterior hypothalamus. AVP secretion is also affected by changes in blood pressure and extracellular volume, detected by high and low pressure volume receptors found in the carotid sinus, along the aortic arch, and in the left atrium. There are parallel effects on the thirst mechanism and on AVP secretion following changes in osmolality. AVP secretion is also affected by carotid chemoreceptors;[37, 38, 74] the renin-angiotensin system;[10] other hormones, including thyroxine, cortisol, and prostaglandins;[21] thermoreceptors;[34, 35, 37, 48, 97] nausea; surgery;[67] hypoglycemia; and pain and emotional influences associated with psychosis or severe pain.[45, 55]

Drugs stimulating AVP secretion include clofibrate, cyclophosphamide, vincristine, carbamazepine, chlorpropamide, cholinergic agents, nicotine, morphine, and barbiturates. Diphenylhydantoin, alcohol, and clonidine appear to inhibit secretion.[68]

Oxytocin

OT plays a major role in milk ejection during lactation. OT binds to receptors on myoepithelial cells of the mammary gland and produces contraction of the mammary smooth muscle. Myoepithelial cells are arranged longitudinally on the lactiferous ducts and around the alveoli. With contraction, there is widening and shortening of the passage from the milk-containing alveoli to the mammary sinuses leading to the mammary ducts.

OT secretion occurs following stimulation of nerve endings in the nipple responsive to pressure and temperature. Afferent fibers from these receptors traverse to the lateral funiculi and spinocervicothalamic and spinoreticular system via the spinal cord.[26] The suckling reflex also involves the reticular formation and midbrain.[108]

Uterine smooth muscle contraction occurs in response to OT following actin-myosin interaction triggered by calcium-dependent phosphorylation of thick filament myosin. Phosphoinositides act as the second messenger for myometrial contraction.[12] The effect of OT on uterine contractility may be a direct one, although an indirect effect mediated by increased synthesis of prostaglandins by endometrial cells has been described.[81] When prostaglandins and OT are administered together, lower doses of each result in uterine activity.[80] In addition, OT is released by infused prostaglandin.[41] Ovarian steroids modulate the OT-stimulated production of prostaglandin F_2 in the isolated ovine endometrium.[82] Progesterone antagonizes the effect of estrogen on the enhancement of OT-induced prostaglandin synthesis.[77, 78, 83, 84]

Uterine responsiveness to OT increases markedly from 20 to 36 weeks' gestation. This is thought to be due to an increase in myometrial OT receptors secondary to an enhanced effect of estrogen in the face of a waning influence of progesterone. Increasing sensitivity to OT as term approaches appears to be confined to the uterus. A comparison of intramammary pressure responses during OT administration to pregnant women from 12 weeks' gestation to 1 week postpartum shows that the patterns of myoepithelial contractile response, threshold intensity, threshold lag period, and spontaneous and mechanically induced activity are not significantly changed with increasing gestational age.[116]

ROLE OF MATERNAL NEUROHYPOPHYSEAL HORMONES IN PARTURITION

Basal plasma AVP levels remain unchanged from prepregnancy levels during pregnancy. The AVP osmostat is reset, however, beginning in the first 2 months of pregnancy, producing plasma osmolalities 5 to 10 mOsm below that of nonpregnant women and lowering the osmotic threshold for thirst.[19] The reset of the osmostat may be under the influence of chorionic gonadotropin.[19] Because maternal plasma AVP levels do not change during labor, AVP does not appear to play a role in human parturition.

Before delivery, basal plasma OT levels in plasma of pregnant women are similar to that of nonpregnant and male subjects. Although several studies using OT radioimmunoassays have shown increasing concentrations of maternal OT as pregnancy progressed, with exceedingly high OT concentrations during labor,[112] these results have not been confirmed by bioassay or by other studies using sensitive radioimmunoassays.[3, 7, 13, 20, 106] OT levels measured by bioassay in plasma of maternal cows, horses, sheep, goats, and rabbits generally show no increase before or during the first stage of labor and increased levels only during fetal expulsion. Circulating OT levels measured by radioimmunoassay in the same species and in the pig also show increased maternal OT levels only during birth itself. Exogenous OT infusion produces uterine contractions in women at term as well as in rats, pigs, mares, and guinea pigs when administered within a few hours of the onset of spontaneous labor; OT infusions do not always produce human labor, however. Moreover, hypophysectomy involving the hypothalamus and pituitary may delay but does not prevent parturition.[33, 70]

Several studies have examined the possibility that the endogenous release of maternal or fetal OT initiates labor. OT content in the fetal pituitary decreases during birth in rats and guinea pigs. Gibbens and Chard[40] identified small spurts of OT release in the first stage of human labor but were unable to detect concentrations between spurts. The frequency of spurt release increased as labor progressed, reaching the maximum at the end of the second stage. Alcohol infusion suppressed these OT spurts, but uterine contractions continued. Boyd and Chard[11] failed to demonstrate a rise in urinary OT during labor. Cobo[16] showed that no rise in intramammary pressure occurs during spontaneous labor, whereas one can be demonstrated with an injection of exceedingly small quantities (2 mU) of OT. Leake et al.[59, 62] found that plasma OT concentrations in human pregnancy do not differ from concentrations in nonpregnant women and men. Mechanical breast pump stimulation during the second or third trimesters or during early labor also failed to increase plasma OT concentrations.[58, 92] In labor even with the crowning of the fetal head, plasma OT levels were not significantly elevated relative to those in nonpregnant women. The stimulus of delivery of the fetal head, however, resulted in a significant elevation of plasma OT in the maternal circulation.[62] This may represent a response to cervical dilation, as suggested by Ferguson.[32] OT hypersecretion appears to continue in the first minutes after delivery, perhaps leading to further uterine contractions that facilitate placental expulsion. Even low levels of circulating OT might play a facilitative role[105] in labor because increased numbers of OT receptors appear before labor, and myometrial gap junctions increase as well.

Human and ovine pregnancy plasma also contains OT-gly,[4–6] a novel material that migrates similarly but not identically to OT on HPLC. As outlined earlier, the nonapeptide, OT, is linked to its neurophysin in the prohormone by a tripeptide bridge consisting of glycine, lysine, and arginine; OT-gly presumably arises as a partially processed form of the OT prohormone. Low levels of OT-gly also are present in plasma of nonpregnant women and sheep as well as in both sheep and human cord blood. Plasma OT-gly concentrations are elevated in estrogen-enriched states including human pregnancy, in males given a single dose of estrogen, and in human newborns. The function of OT-gly remains unclear. The presence of circulating OT-gly explains high levels of OT in pregnancy plasma measured by some antibodies as well as the increase in estrogen-stimulated neurophysin in women receiving oral contraceptives.

MATERNAL HORMONAL ADAPTATION IN THE POSTPARTUM PERIOD

Breast-feeding in the first 2 to 3 days postpartum is associated with secretion of OT in the maternal circulation to a level comparable to that of the late second stage of labor.[115] There is no concomitant secretion of AVP. OT release during nursing does not appear to be modulated by opioid peptides.[52] Long-term nursing (up to 1 year postdelivery) continues to evoke an OT plasma response.[59] The effect of OT on nursing appears to vary somewhat in different species. In the cat, dog, rabbit, and rat, OT is released and milk ejection subsequently occurs owing to contraction of the mammary myoepithelium. Milk yield continues in the absence of OT release in the cow and occurs despite denervation of the goat udder.[15]

Interestingly, there appear to be times in the reproductive cycle of the sheep, goat, and human when OT secretion is suppressed in response to stimuli that would otherwise result in increased plasma OT.[57, 58, 62, 69, 77–79, 83, 84] Roberts and Share demonstrated a marked increase in OT levels during uterine massage in lactating and cycling ewes but no response in the pregnant ewe.[83] Estrogen increased OT release in cycling ewes, and progesterone inhibited OT secretion. In the human reproductive cycle, mechanical (breast pump) stimulation produces a significant increase in plasma OT levels during the luteal but not the follicular phase of the menstrual cycle.[57] Neither manual nor mechanical breast stimulation evokes increased plasma OT levels during pregnancy,[58, 92] although both produce a vigorous response following delivery. These differing responses during various times may be due to changes in steroid production (during estrus, for example) which are known to influence firing of the magnocellular neurons controlling OT release.

PLACENTAL TRANSFER OF NEUROHYPOPHYSEAL HORMONES

Little evidence exists to suggest that either AVP or OT crosses the placenta.[71] Infusion of 25 μg of synthetic AVP in the fetal sheep, for example, failed to alter basal concentrations in the maternal circulation.[60] Exogenous OT infused to the fetus or maternal ewe failed to produce changes in OT levels on the opposite side of the placenta.[43] Further, several studies have demonstrated concentration gradients for both AVP and OT in fetal sheep compared with maternal sheep[36, 42, 60, 114] and for maternal and cord concentrations in the human.[20, 46, 50, 56]

NEUROHYPOPHYSEAL EMBRYOGENESIS AND FETAL NEUROHYPOPHYSEAL PEPTIDE CONTENT

The human posterior pituitary develops from the infundibular process of the third ventricle by the fifth week after conception. By 12 weeks, the first hypothalamic nuclei and supraoptic tract fibers can be identified histologically,[66] and by 16 weeks the hypothalamus contains measurable AVP and OT. By 16 weeks' gestation, the median eminence and remainder of the hypothalamic nuclei can be distinguished. Similar development of the posterior pituitary occurs in the sheep fetus by 50 days.[100] The pituitary portal vascular system progresses simultaneously, being largely complete by 30 to 35 weeks' gestation. Blood is carried directly by this capillary network from the ventral hypothalamus to the anterior pituitary. The hypothalamic neurosecretory nuclei may play a regulatory role in anterior pituitary function because the pituitary portal vascular system transports neurohypophyseal hormone in concentrations 20,000 times greater than that of the general circulation.[44, 118]

AVP is detectable after 10 to 12 weeks' gestation in the human fetal neurohypophysis.[100] By 16 weeks' gestation, neurosecretory granules are present in the hypothalamic nuclei.[76] By 40 weeks' gestation, fetal posterior pituitary

AVP content is 20% that of adult humans;[49] 0.9 to 1.0 μg of AVP is present in the entire gland at birth. AVP is found after 50 days in the fetal lamb pituitary, doubling in concentration between 90 days and term.[100]

There is OT in the human fetal pituitary by 11 to 15 weeks' gestation. Concentrations of AVP initially exceed those of OT, but as pregnancy progresses the AVP to OT ratio falls. OT is detected in the fetal sheep pituitary by 80 to 90 days, also increasing relative to AVP as pregnancy progresses.[100]

MATURATION OF FETAL SECRETION AND ORGAN RESPONSE

Plasma AVP levels in the human fetus remain unknown. In the chronically catheterized sheep, baseline fetal osmolality is dependent on maternal osmolality owing to transplacental water and solute transfer; fetal plasma AVP levels under basal conditions reflect maternal levels, approximating 2.5 pg/mL.[1]

From midgestation onward, the sheep fetus responds to osmolar and volume stimuli with increased AVP secretion. Hemorrhage,[87] hypertonic saline,[114] furosemide, and epinephrine[28] infusion result in increased fetal secretion of AVP. There is a clear maturation of the AVP responses to an osmolar stimulus (hypertonic saline), furosemide infusion, and dehydration between 100 days and term. During hemorrhage, plasma AVP levels correlate with the volume of blood removed, rather than with transient decreases in blood pressure. After withdrawal of approximately 13% of the fetal blood volume, the fetal plasma AVP threshold is exceeded.[89]

Hypertonic saline infused in the maternal ewe produces significant, sustained increases in fetal AVP concentrations greater than those following direct fetal infusion of hypertonic saline.[60] This suggests that a rapid fetal to maternal transfer of water produces a combined volume and osmolar stimulus of fetal AVP secretion.

Fetal hypoxia evokes AVP secretion,[93] more so for acute than chronic hypoxia.[94] Hypoxia produced by exposure of the maternal ewe to 11% oxygen for 30 minutes evokes AVP secretory responses greater in older (>130 days' gestation) than younger fetuses (<130 days' gestation).[102] There is a highly significant correlation between the (log) fetal AVP concentration and both the duration of hypoxia and the (log) fetal PO_2 values; the AVP response in the adult ewe is negligible.[102] The combination of hypoxia, metabolic acidosis, and hypercapnia evokes a fetal AVP response markedly greater than that of hypoxia alone.[22, 30] Interestingly, fetal urinary and amniotic fluid levels of AVP also increase following fetal hypoxia,[86] the latter probably secondary to contribution of AVP from the fetal urine. Ovine fetal urine output decreases by approximately half, urinary osmolality doubles, and urinary AVP levels and excretion rates increase markedly with this stimulus. Amniotic fluid AVP does not appear to influence amniotic to maternal water transfer[90] (as does prolactin, for example), but because of its prolonged half-life (8 hours), amniotic fluid AVP may prove a marker for fetal hypoxia.

Basal ovine fetal urine is hypotonic throughout gestation,[53, 86, 117] compared with fetal plasma or adult urine despite vigorous AVP secretory capability and the presence of AVP renal receptors.[88] Fetal sheep respond to AVP infusion with an increase in urine osmolality and a decrease in urine flow and free water clearance; the responsiveness of the system increases with advancing gestational age in response to both exogenous and endogenous AVP.[9] In the sheep, as little as 10 pg/mL AVP produces maximal antidiuresis.

Human fetal plasma OT concentrations before delivery are not known. Basal ovine fetal OT concentrations measured by radioimmunoassay are 3.0 ± 0.4 pg/mL between 124 and 140 days' gestation. The onset of ovine labor is not associated with an increase in plasma OT levels; however, during delivery, maternal OT levels increase to levels significantly greater than prelabor levels or that of fetal lambs.[42]

ROLE OF FETAL NEUROHYPOPHYSEAL HORMONES IN PARTURITION

Umbilical arterial and venous AVP concentrations in infants delivered by cesarean section without previous labor or after a short period of labor are only minimally elevated relative to baseline levels in healthy adults; following active labor, significant elevations in cord blood plasma AVP are observed. Umbilical arterial AVP concentrations exceed umbilical venous levels, suggesting fetal AVP production. Cord blood AVP levels approximate 250 pg/mL in umbilical arterial plasma. These levels exceed those producing maximal antidiuresis (10 pg/mL) and evoking fetal bradycardia and increased blood pressure (20 to 40 pg/mL) in the ovine fetus. Umbilical arterial AVP concentrations correlate with the length of labor (r = 0.8). In deliveries by cesarean section after some time of labor, umbilical artery concentrations are proportional to the degree of cervical dilation at delivery (r = 0.9). Fetal AVP hypersecretion during delivery may represent compression of the fetal head because AVP hypersecretion is produced by acutely elevating intracranial pressure. In monkeys, elevation of intracranial pressure produced by expanding balloons leads to increased AVP secretion.[39] Intermittent elevations of fetal intracranial pressure may be a stimulus to AVP hypersecretion in human labor. Fetal cord blood AVP levels reflect the effects of hypoxia, hypercarbia, acidosis, and hypotension as well.[30, 93]

Increased secretion of AVP may play a role in fetal adaptation to birth. Endogenous or exogenous AVP decreases fetal lung fluid production, and as shown in acutely exteriorized goats and chronically catheterized sheep, net lung water absorption occurs.[91] Catecholamines and cortisol produce the same effect. These hormones working in concert may aid in removal of lung fluid at birth.

OT is also significantly elevated in cord blood following labor,[14] with an umbilical arteriovenous relationship in human newborns similar to AVP, suggesting fetal secretion of OT.[56] Newborn OT concentrations drop rapidly over the first 30 minutes after delivery but remain elevated for the first 5 days compared with basal OT values in the human adult.[61] The stimulus for this continued secretion remains unclear. The significance of neonatal OT secretion during labor and in the postdelivery period remains unknown.

NEUROHYPOPHYSEAL HORMONES IN ADAPTATION TO EXTRAUTERINE LIFE

It was previously believed that the human newborn was incapable of AVP secretion. Bioassay and indirect evidence later demonstrated an AVP response following stimulation by asphyxia,[31] surgery,[50] furosemide,[98] or hypertonic saline.[35, 98] Using sensitive, specific radioimmunoassays, we and others[23] have demonstrated that newborn AVP concentrations in both preterm and term newborns fall progressively after birth from umbilical arterial AVP concentrations (following labor) of 198 ± 33 pg/mL (mean ± SEM) to peripheral plasma venous levels of 12.1 ± 1.9 by 30 minutes and 2.86 ± 0.4 by 2 hours.[46] By 24 hours of age, concentrations are less than 2.2 pg/mL and equivalent to adult levels. Elevated cord blood AVP levels may play a role in blood flow redistribution associated with birth by means of increased placental, myocardial, and cerebral blood flow in conjunction with reduced gastrointestinal and peripheral blood flow.[51] Additionally, umbilical artery AVP levels reflect acute asphyxia; plasma AVP levels, however, do not aid in defining the source of the asphyxia or quantifying its severity.

Responses in ovine newborns following osmotic and volume stimuli have been compared with those of the adult sheep. Infusion of hypertonic saline, water restriction, water loading, furosemide administration, and hemorrhage were performed in 2- to 49-day-old lambs.[63] Peak responses in plasma AVP concentrations were prompt (varying from 3 minutes posthemorrhage to 30 minutes following hypertonic saline infusion) and appropriate during the period studied. Dehydration produced the greatest plasma AVP rise (when compared with change in osmolality), demonstrating a combined response to volume and osmolar stimulation. Hypertonic saline produced elevations in plasma AVP (per milliosmole change in osmolality) identical to that produced in the maternal ewe with a similar stimulus. Water loading produced a plasma AVP response identical to that following maternal or newborn hypertonic saline although opposite in direction. The furosemide response appears to represent angiotensin II release because it can be blocked by nephrectomy or angiotensin II antagonists. The furosemide response is augmented in the fetus and newborn compared with the adult perhaps because of the highly stimulated renin-angiotensin levels during this period.[99] These studies taken in sum demonstrate that the osmolar and volume control of AVP secretion is fully mature in the newborn lamb.

The human newborn's inability to concentrate urine to adult levels does not appear to be due to lack of AVP but rather may indicate decreased sensitivity of receptors in the renal collecting ducts, diminished cAMP generation, or inability to maintain a hypertonic medullary interstitium, with resultant decreased effective countercurrent mechanism. In the rat, AVP receptors have been demonstrated 2 to 46 days after birth.[75] In the newborn piglet and rat, there is a reduced level of responsiveness of the cAMP system to AVP.[96]

AVT levels in umbilical arterial and venous blood samples approximate 5 pg/mL. The stimuli leading to AVT secretion and its possible function in the newborn period remain unclear. It is known that AVT administered into the lateral ventricle of newborn cats increases quiet sleep and decreases active sleep, whereas AVT antiserum produces opposite effects. AVT, AVP, and OT are present in neonatal cerebrospinal fluid; concentrations approximate 8, 6, and 23 pg/mL in newborns undergoing a sepsis workup and subsequently shown to be healthy.

SUMMARY

NHP hormones are found in the fetal pituitary early in gestation, and there is evidence that AVP can be released by qualitatively similar stimuli in both the fetus and the adult. Osmoreceptor and volume receptor–mediated responses are present from midtrimester on in fetal sheep. The responses mature with advancing gestation and become similar to adult responses by the neonatal period. Interestingly, the fetal and newborn response to hypoxia is vigorous, whereas the adult response is markedly obtunded. Fetal AVP secretion may play a role in fetal water conservation, amniotic fluid volume (by means of effects on fetal lung and urine volumes), fetal responses to hypoxia and volume loss, and transition to extrauterine life. There is no evidence of transplacental transfer of NHP hormones. Fetal AVP or OT secretion does not play a role in the initiation and maintenance of labor. Circulating OT in the maternal circulation may play a permissive role in the onset of labor, but there do not appear to be surges of OT secretion initiating labor. Release of OT in the second stage of labor, however, may augment uterine contractions and play a secondary role in delivery itself.

REFERENCES

1. Alexander DP, Bashore RA, Britton HG, Forsling ML. Maternal and fetal arginine vasopressin in the chronically catheterized sheep. Biol Neonate 1974;25:242.
2. Alexander DP, Bashore RA, Britton HG, Forsling ML. Antidiuretic hormone and oxytocin release and antidiuretic hormone turnover in the fetus lamb and ewe. Biol Neonate 1976;30:80.
3. Allen WE, Chard T, Forsling ML. Peripheral plasma levels of oxytocin and vasopressin in the mare during parturition. J Endocrinol 1973;57:175.
4. Amico JA, Ervin MG, Finn FN, et al. The plasma of pregnant women contains a novel oxytocin-vasotocin-like peptide. Metabolism 1986;35:596.
5. Amico JA, Ervin MG, Leake RD, et al. A novel oxytocin-like and vasotocin-like peptide in human plasma after administration of estrogen. J Clin Endocrinol Metab 1985;60:5.
6. Amico JA, Hempel I. A glycine extended form of oxytocin circulation in the plasma of individuals administered estrogen. Neuroendocrinology 1989;51:437.
7. Amico JA, Seitchik J, Robinson AG. Studies of oxytocin in plasma of women during hypocontractile labor. J Clin Endocrinol Metab 1984;58:274.
8. Artman HG, Leake RD, Weitzman RE, et al. Radioimmunoassay of arginine vasotocin and other neurohypophyseal peptides in human neonatal CSF and amniotic fluid. Dev Pharmacol Ther 1984;7:39.
9. Bell RJ, Congiu M, Hardy KJ, Wintour EM. Gestation-dependent aspects of the response of the ovine fetus to the osmotic stress induced by maternal water deprivation. Q J Exp Physiol 1984;69:187.
10. Bonjour JP, Malvin RL. Stimulation of ADH release by the renin-angiotensin system. Am J Physiol 1970;218:1555.
11. Boyd NRH, Chard T. Human urine oxytocin levels during pregnancy and labor. Am J Obstet Gynecol 1973;115:827.
12. Carsten ME, Miller JD. A new look at uterine muscle contraction. Am Obstet Gynecol. 1987;157:1303.
13. Chard T, Boyd NRH, Forsling MD, et al. The development of a radioimmunoassay for oxytocin: the extraction of oxytocin from plasma, and its measurements during parturition in human and goat blood. J Endocrinol 1970;48:223.
14. Chard T, Edwards CRW, Boyd NRH, Hudson CN.

Release of oxytocin and vasopressin by the human foetus during labor. Nature 1971;234:352.

15. Cleverley JD, Folley SJ. The blood levels of oxytocin during machine milking in cows with some observations on its half-life in the circulation. J Endocrinol 1970;46:347.

16. Cobo E. Uterine and milk-ejecting activities during human labor. J Appl Physiol 1978;24:317.

17. Daniel SS, Stark RI, Husain MK, et al. Excretion of vasopressin in the hypoxic lamb: comparison between fetus and newborn. Pediatr Res 1984;18:227.

18. Davison JM, Sheills EA, Barron WM, et al. Changes in metabolic clearance of vasopressin and in plasma vasopressinase throughout human pregnancy. J Clin Invest 1989;83:1313.

19. Davison JM, Shiells EA, Philips PR, Lindheimer MD. Influence of humoral and volume factors on altered osmoregulation of normal human pregnancy. Am J Physiol 1990;258:F900.

20. Dawood MY, Raghakan KS, Poclask C. Radioimmunoassay of oxytocin. J Endocrinol 1978;76:261.

21. DeRubertis FR, Michelis MF, Bloom ME, et al. Impaired water excretion in myxedema. Am J Med 1971;51:41.

22. DeVane GW, Naden RP, Porter JC. Mechanism of arginine vasopressin release in the sheep fetus. Pediatrics 1982;16:504.

23. DeVane GW, Porter JC. An apparent stress-induced release of arginine vasopressin by human neonates. J Clin Endocrinol Metab 1980;51:1412.

24. Dogterom J, Van Wimersma Greidanus TB, Swaab DF. Evidence for the release of vasopressin and oxytocin into cerebrospinal fluid: measurements in plasma and CSF of intact and hypophysectomized rats. Neuroendocrinology 1977;24:108.

25. Douglas WW. How do neurones secrete peptides? Exocytosis and its consequences, including "synaptic vesicle" formation, in the hypothalamo-neurohypophyseal system. Prog Brain Res 1973;39:21.

26. Eayrs JT, Baddeley RM. Neural pathways in lactation. J Anat 1956;90:161.

27. Ervin MG, Amico JA, Leake RD, et al. Arginine vasotocin and a novel oxytocin-vasotocin like material in plasma of humans. Biol Neonate 1988;53:17.

28. Ervin MG, Castro R, Sherman DJ, et al. Ovine fetal renal and hormonal responses to changes in plasma epinephrine. Am J Physiol 1991; 260:R82.

29. Fabian MI, Forsling ML, Jones JJ, Pryor JS. The clearance and antidiuretic potency of neurohypophyseal hormones in man and their plasma binding and stability. J Physiol 1969;264:653.

30. Faucher DJ, Lowe TW, Magness RR, et al. Vasopressin and catecholamine secretion during metabolic acidemia in the ovine fetus. Pediatr Res 1987;21:38.

31. Feldman W, Drummond KN, Klein M. Hyponatremia following asphyxia neonatorum. Acta Paediatr Scand 1970;59:52.

32. Ferguson JKW. A study of the mobility of the intact uterus at term. Surg Obstet Gynecol 1941;73:359.

33. Fisher C, Magoun HW, Ranson SW. Dystocia in diabetes insipidus. Am J Obstet Gynecol 1938;36:1.

34. Fisher DA. Cold diuresis in the newborn. Pediatrics 1967;40:636.

35. Fisher DA, Pyle HR, Porter JC, et al. Studies of control of water balance in the newborn. Am J Dis Child 1963;106:137.

36. Forsling M, Jack PMB, Nathanielsz PW. Plasma oxytocin concentrations in the foetal sheep. Horm Metab Res 1975;7:197.

37. Forsling ML, Rees M. Effects of hypoxia and hypercapnia on plasma vasopressin concentration. J Endocrinol 1975;67:62P.

38. Forsling ML, Ullmann E. Release of vasopressin during hypoxia. J Physiol (Lond) 1974;241:35P.

39. Gaufin L, Skowsky WR, Goodman SJ. Release of antidiuretic hormone during mass-induced elevation of intracranial pressure. J Neurosurg 1977;46:627.

40. Gibbens GLD, Chard T. Observations on maternal oxytocin release during human labor and the effect of intravenous alcohol administration. Am J Gynecol 1976;126:243.

41. Gillespie A, Brummer HC, Chard T. Oxytocin release by infused prostaglandin. BMJ 1972;1:543.

42. Glatz TH, Weitzman R, Eliot RJ, et al. Ovine maternal and fetal plasma oxytocin concentrations before and during parturition. Endocrinology 1981;108:1328.

43. Glatz TH, Weitzman RE, Nathanielsz PW, Fisher DA. Metabolic clearance rate of oxytocin in maternal and fetal sheep. Pediatr Res 1978;12:413.

44. Goldman H, Linder L. Antidiuretic hormone concentrations in blood perfusing the adenohypophysis. Experientia 1962;18:279.

45. Gullick HD, Raisz LG. Changes in renal concentrating ability associated with major surgical procedures. N Engl J Med 1960;262:1309.

46. Hadeed AJ, Leake RD, Weitzman RE, Fisher DA. Possible mechanisms of high blood levels of vasopressin during the neonatal period. J Pediatr 1979;94:805.

47. Hayward JN. Neurohumoral regulation of neuroendocrine cells in the hypothalamus. In: Lederis K, Cooper KB, eds. Recent studies of hypothalamic function. International Symposium, Calgary, 1973. Basel: Karger, 1974:166.

48. Hayward JN, Baker MA. Diuretic and thermoregulatory responses to preoptic cooling in the monkey. Am J Physiol 1968;214:843.

49. Heller H, Zaimis EJ. The antidiuretic and oxytocin hormones in the posterior pituitary glands of newborn infants and adults. J Physiol 1949;109:162.

50. Hoppenstein JM, Miltenberger FW, Moran WH. The increase in blood levels of vasopressin in infants during birth and surgical procedures. Surg Gynecol Obstet 1968;127:966.

51. Iwamoto HS, Rudolph AM, Keil LC, Heymann MA. Hemodynamic responses of the sheep fetus to vasopressin infusion. Circ Res 1979;44:430.

52. Johnson MR, Andrews MN, Seckl JR, Lightman SL. Effect of naloxone on neurohypophyseal peptide responses to breast feeding and breast stimulation in man. Clin Endocrinol 1990;33:81.

53. Jones CT, Rolph TP. Metabolism during fetal life: a functional assessment of metabolic development. Physiol Rev 1985;65:357.

54. Kelley RT, Rose JC, Meis PJ, et al. Vasopressin is important for restoring cardiovascular homeostasis in fetal lambs subjected to hemorrhage. Am J Obstet Gynecol 1983;146:807.

55. Kendler KS, Weitzman RE, Fisher DA. The effect of pain on plasma arginine vasopressin concentrations in man. Clin Endocrinol 1978;8:89.

56. Kumaresan P, Anandarangam PB, Dianzon W, Vasicka A. Plasma oxytocin levels during human pregnancy and labor as determined by radioimmunoassay. Am J Obstet Gynecol 1974;119:215.

57. Leake RD, Buster JE, Fisher DA. The oxytocin secretory response to breast stimulation in women during the menstrual cycle. Am J Obstet Gynecol 1984;148:457.

58. Leake RD, Fisher DA, Ross MG, Buster JE. Oxytocin secretory response to breast stimulation in pregnant women. Am J Obstet Gynecol 1984;148:259.

59. Leake RD, Waters CB, Rubin RT, et al. Oxytocin and prolactin responses in long term breast feeding. Obstet Gynecol 1983;62:565.

60. Leake RD, Weitzman RE, Effros RM, et al. Maternal fetal osmolar homeostasis: fetal posterior pituitary autonomy. Pediatr Res 1977;11:408.

61. Leake RD, Weitzman RE, Fisher DA. Oxytocin concentrations during the neonatal period. Biol Neonate 1981;39:127.

62. Leake RD, Weitzman RE, Glatz T, Fisher DA. Plasma oxytocin concentrations in men, nonpregnant women and pregnant women before and during spontaneous labor. J Clin Endocrinol Metab 1981;53:730.

63. Leake RD, Weitzman RE, Weinberg JA, Fisher DA. Control of vasopressin secretion in the lamb. Clin Res 1977;25:189A.

64. Lederis K. Neurosecretion and the functional structure of the neurohypophysis. In: Greep RO, Astwood EB, eds. Handbook of physiology. Section 7, Endocrinology. Vol IV, The pituitary gland and its neuroendocrine control. Part I. Washington, DC: American Physiological Society, 1974:81.

65. Legros JJ, Louis F, Demoulin A, Franchimont P. Immunoreactive neurophysins and vasotocin in human foetal pineal glands. J Endocrinol 1976;69:289.

66. Levina SE. Endocrine features in development of human hypothalamus, hypophysis and placenta. Gen Comp Endocrinol 1968;11:151.

67. Moran WH Jr, Miltenberger FW, Shuayb WA, et al. The relationship of antidiuretic hormone secretion to surgical stress. Surgery 1964;56:99.

68. Moses AM, Miller M. Drug induced dilutional hyponatremia. N Engl J Med 1974;291:1234.

69. Negoro H, Visessuwan S, Holland RC. Reflex activation of paraventricular nucleus units during the reproductive cycle in ovariectomized rats treated with estrogen or progesterone. J Endocrinol 1972;59:559.

70. Nibbelink KDW. Paraventricular nuclei, neurohypophysis and parturition. Am J Physiol 1901;200:1229.

71. Noodle BA. Pharmacology transfer of oxytocin from the maternal to the foetal circulation in the ewe. Nature 1964;203:414.

72. Pavel S. Vasotocin biosynthesis by neurohypophyseal cells from human fetuses. Evidence for its ependymal origin. Neuroendocrinology 1975;19:150.

73. Pavel S, Addrien J. Vasotocin increases quiet sleep and suppresses active sleep in newborn cats. Opposite effects after vasotocin immunoneutralization. Brain Res Bull 1989;23:463.

74. Pluss RG, Anderson RJ, Schrier RW. Effect of hypoxia on renal water excretion. Clin Res 1977;25:139A.

75. Rajerison RM, Butlen D, Jard S. Ontogenic development of antidiuretic hormone receptors in the rat kidney: comparison of hormonal binding and adenylate cyclase activation. J Mole Cell Endocrinol 1976;4:271.

76. Rinne UK, Kivalo E, Talanti S. Maturation of human hypothalamic neurosecretion. Biol Neonate 1982;4:351.

77. Roberts JS. Seasonal variations in the reflexive release of oxytocin and in the effect of estradiol on the reflex in goats. Endocrinology 1971;89:1029.

78. Roberts JS. Functional integrity of the oxytocin-releasing reflex in goats: Dependence on estrogen. Endocrinology 1973;93:1309.

79. Roberts JS. Cyclical fluctuations in reflexive oxytocin release during the estrous cycle of the goat. Biol Reprod 1975;13:214.

80. Roberts JS, ed. Oxytocin. Vol 1. Quebec: Eden Press, 1977:44.

81. Roberts JS, Barcikowski B, Wilson L, et al. Hormonal and related factors affecting the release of prostaglandin $F_{2\alpha}$ from the uterus. J Steroid Biochem 1975;6:1091.

82. Roberts JS, McCracken JA, Gavagan JE, Soloff MS. Oxytocin stimulated release of prostaglandin $F_{2\alpha}$ from ovine endometria in vitro: correlation with estrous cycle and oxytocin-receptor binding. Endocrinology 1976;99:1107.

83. Roberts JS, Share L. Effects of progesterone and estrogen on blood levels of oxytocin during vaginal distention. Endocrinology 1969;84:1706.

84. Roberts JS, Share L. Inhibition by progesterone of oxytocin secretion during vaginal stimulation. Endocrinology 1970;87:812.

85. Robillard JE, Weitzman RE, Brumeister L, Smith FG Jr. Development aspects of the renal response to hypoxia in the lamb fetus. Circ Res 1981;48:128.

86. Robillard JE, Weitzman RE, Fisher DA, Smith FG Jr. The dynamics of vasopressin release and blood volume regulation during fetal hemorrhage in the lamb fetus. Pediatr Res 1979;13:606.

87. Robillard JE, Weitzman RD, Smith FG Jr. Presence of functioning vasopressin receptors in the fetal kidney. Proceedings VII International Congress of Nephrology, Montreal, 1978.

88. Rosenbloom AA, Sack J, Fisher DA. The circulating vasopressinase of pregnancy: species comparison using radioimmunoassay. Am J Obstet Gynecol 1975;121:316.

89. Ross MG, Ervin MG, Humme JA, Fisher DA. Continuous ovine fetal hemorrhage: sensitivity of plasma and urine arginine vasopressin response. Am J Physiol 1986;251 (Endocrinol Metab 14):E464.

90. Ross MG, Ervin MG, Leake RD, et al. Bulk flow of amniotic fluid water in response to maternal osmotic challenge. Am J Obstet Gynecol 1983;147:697.

91. Ross MG, Ervin MG, Leake RD, et al. Fetal lung liquid regulation by neuropeptides. Am J Obstet Gynecol 1984;150:421.

92. Ross MG, Ervin MG, Leake RD. Breast stimulation contraction stress test: uterine contractions in the absence of oxytocin release. Am J Perinatology 1986;3:35.

93. Rurak DW. Plasma vasopressin levels during hypoxemia and the cardiovascular effects of exogenous vasopressin in foetal and adult sheep. J Physiol (Lond) 1978;277:342.

94. Ruth V, Fyhrquist F, Clemons G, Raivio KO. Cord plasma vasopressin, erythropoietin, and hypoxanthine as indices of asphyxia at birth. Pediatr Res 1988;24:490.

95. Sawyer WH. Neurohypophyseal principles of vertebrates. In: Harris GW, Donovan BT, eds. The pituitary gland. Vol 3. London: Butterworth, 1966:307.

96. Schlondorff D, Weber H, Trizna W, Fine LG. Vasopressin responsiveness of renal adenylate cyclase in newborn rats and rabbits. Am J Physiol 1978;234:F16.

97. Segar WE, Moore WW. The regulation of antidiuretic hormone release in man. Effects of change in position and ambient temperature on blood ADH levels. J Clin Invest 1968;47:2143.

98. Siegel SR, Leake RD, Weitzman RE, et al. Effects of furosemide and acute salt loading on vasopressin and renin secretion in the fetal lamb. Pediatr Res 1980;14:869.

99. Siegel SR, Weitzman RE, Fisher DA. Endogenous angiotensin stimulation of vasopressin in the newborn lamb. J Clin Invest 1979;63:287.

100. Skowsky WR, Fisher DA. Fetal neurohypophyseal arginine vasotocin in man and sheep. Pediatr Res 1977;11:627.

101. Stark RI, Wardlow SL, Daniel SS, et al. Vasopressin secretion induced by hypoxia in sheep: developmental changes and relationship to B endorphin release. Am J Obstet Gynecol 1982;143:204.

102. Stegner H, Artman HG, Leake RD, et al. The effect of hypoxia on neurohypophyseal hormone release in fetal and maternal sheep. Pediatr Res 1984;18:188.

103. Stegner H, Leake RD, Palmer SM, et al. Arginine vasopressin metabolic clearance and production rates in fetal sheep, lambs, maternal and nonpregnant adult sheep. Dev Pharmacol Ther 1984;7:87.

104. Sterba G. Ascending neurosecretory pathways of the peptidergic type. In: Knowles F, Vollrath F, eds. Neurosecretion: the final neuroendocrine pathway. New York: Springer Verlag, 1974:38.

105. Theobald GW. Oxytocin reassessed. Obstet Gynecol Surg 1968;23:109.

106. Thornton S, Davison JM, Baylis PH. The progress of labour is not dependent upon plasma oxytocin. In: Eicosanoids and fatty acids. Vienna: Facultas, 1988:149.

107. Thornton S, Davison JM, Baylis PH. Effect of human pregnancy on metabolic clearance rate of oxytocin. J Physiol 1990;259:F21.

108. Tindall JS, Knaggs GS. Further studies on the afferent path of the milk-ejection reflex in the brain stem of the rabbit. J Endocrinol 1975;66:107.

109. Tuppy H. The influence of enzymes on neurohypophyseal hormones and similar peptides. Hdbk Exp Pharmacol 1969;23:67.

110. Uyehara CFT, Claybaugh JR. Vasopressin metabolism in the amniotic sac of the fetal guinea pig. Endocrinology 1988;123:2040.

111. Vandesande F, Dierickx K, de Mey J. Identification of vasopressin-neurophysin II and oxytocin-neurophysin I producing cells in the brain and hypothalamus. Cell Tissue Res 1975;156:189.

112. Vasicka A, Kumaresan P, Han GS, Kumaresan M. Plasma oxytocin in initiation of labor. Am J Obstet Gynecol 1978;130:263.

113. Vizsolyi E, Perks AM. The effect of arginine vasotocin on the isolated amniotic membrane of the guinea pig. Can J Zool 1974;52:371.

114. Weitzman RE, Fisher DA, Robillard J, et al. Arginine vasopressin response to an osmotic stimulus in the fetal sheep. Pediatr Res 1978;12:35.

115. Weitzman RE, Leake RD, Rubin RT, Fisher DA. The effect of nursing on neurohypophyseal hormones and prolactin in human subjects. J Clin Endocrinol 1980;51:836.

116. Wiederman J, Feund M, Stone ML. The human breast and uterus: a comparison of sensitivity of oxytocin during gestation. Obstet Gynecol 1963;21:272.

117. Wintour EM, Congiu M, Hardy KJ, Hennessy DP. Regulation of urine osmolality in fetal sheep. Q J Exp Physiol 1982;67:427.

118. Zimmerman EA, Carmel PW, Husain MK, et al. Vasopressin and neurophysin: high concentrations in monkey hypophyseal portal blood. Science 1973;182:925.

The Fetal Adrenal

Beverley E. Pearson Murphy

Charlotte Laplante Branchaud

The human fetal adrenal differs from that of other species by virtue of its enormous size relative to that of the adult organ (Fig. 14–1). At 12 weeks' gestational age, it is approximately the same size as the fetal kidney, but although the kidney alters from 0.6% body weight in the fetus to 0.2% in the adult, the adrenal falls to 0.02%, at least a 20-fold difference. The fetal adrenal also differs from the adult in its cellular structure (Fig. 14–2), having a large zone, the *fetal zone,* which takes up the bulk of the fetal gland but which is lost soon after birth. This zone is present only in primates,[7, 52, 71, 72, 77, 119] in whom, apart from the human, it has been little studied, and it has no exact parallel in any nonprimate species. Lack of a suitable animal model has been one reason why many basic questions concerning the human fetal adrenal remain unanswered. Even among primates there is considerable variation[8, 27, 62]; in the macaque, the fetal zone involutes before birth, whereas in the Congo potto and marmoset,[74] it involutes postnatally, as in the human. The function of the large fetal adrenal is still a matter of speculation, as it has been for the last hundred years or more.

EMBRYOLOGY AND DEVELOPMENT

The parenchymal cells of the adrenal cortex are derived from the coelomic mesothelium, whereas those of the medulla are derived from the neural crest. The adrenal primordium forms early in development, being first discernible in the 5- to 6-mm embryo (4 weeks' postconception).[27, 98] The primitive adrenocor-

FETUS   **ADULT**

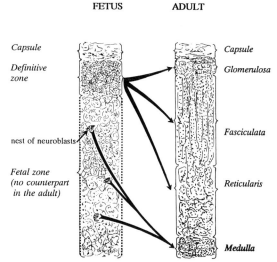

FIGURE 14–2. Histologic zones of the adrenal in fetus and adult.

tical cells proliferate rapidly and organize into two zones, the outer *permanent* cortex and the inner *fetal* zone (see Fig. 14–2). The cells of the narrow outer cortex first appear as distinct from the inner fetal zone cells in the 14-mm fetus, i.e., at 7 weeks' fetal age (9 weeks' gestational age).* The cortex continues to grow rapidly, mitotic activity occurring mainly in the outer cortical zone. Cells formed in the periphery migrate to the central fetal zone, which constitutes more than 80% of the gland at term.

Neural elements, some of which differentiate into chromaffin cells, migrate into the primordium at 4 to 5 weeks' fetal age.[27, 51] The neural elements and chromaffin cells are distributed throughout the cortex, often in association with vascular sinusoids. Concomitant with the rapid degeneration of the fetal zone postnatally, the neural elements and chromaffin cells come to lie in the center of the gland, forming a "true" medulla.

The adrenal gland is supplied by multiple arteries arising from the inferior phrenic artery, aorta, and renal artery.[98] These vessels

---

*Fetal age is expressed in a variety of ways, and care must be taken when interpreting the literature. *Fetal* age refers to time postconception and should be distinguished from *gestational* age, which dates from the onset of the mother's last normal menstrual period. The gestational period of approximately 9 calendar months is sometimes divided into 10 lunar (4 week) months. Unfortunately, occasionally it is impossible to be certain of the author's usage.

FETUS   **ADULT**

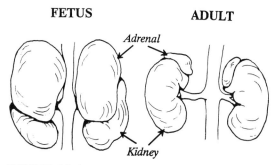

FIGURE 14–1. Relative size of the fetal adrenal and kidney at 13 weeks' gestation (11 weeks' fetal age) and in the adult.

anastomose over the surface of the gland, dividing into 50 to 60 smaller arterial vessels that enter the capsule. The effluent blood emerges in a single central vein; the shorter right adrenal vein enters the aorta, and the longer left vein joins the left inferior phrenic or left renal vein.

The pattern of fetal adrenal growth relative to total body weight[19, 61, 109, 115, 152] is shown in Figure 14–3. The weight of the adrenals increases most rapidly toward the end of the first trimester, when they reach a combined weight of approximately 80 mg, about 0.6% of body weight. After 24 weeks, there is a decline to a plateau by 30 weeks, with a small rise at 39 weeks.

The fetal zone degenerates rapidly after birth; by 1 week after birth, adrenal size has decreased to 40% of that at birth.[95] Concomitant with the disappearance of the fetal zone, the permanent cortex proliferates rapidly, and the medullary cells previously mixed with the fetal cortex now collect at the center of the gland to form the medulla.

HISTOLOGY

The cellular features of the two zones of the fetal adrenal are shown in Figure 14–2. They

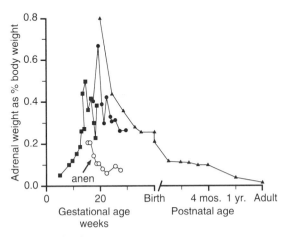

FIGURE 14–3. Ontogeny of relative adrenal weight (percent total body weight) according to various authors, calculated using the body weights of Potter and Craig.[109] ▲-▲ Data of Schulz et al.[115] ■-■ Data of Carr and Casey.[19] ●-● Data of Young et al. ○-○ Data of Young et al[152] for anencephalics (anen). (From Branchaud CL, Murphy BEP. Physiopathology of the fetal adrenal. In: Pasqualini J, Scholler R, eds. Hormones and Fetal Physiology. New York: Marcel Dekker, 1992:53–85. With permission.)

are quite distinct, the fetal zone comprising large eosinophilic cells with abundant cytoplasm and pale-staining nuclei,[98] whereas the cells of the permanent or definitive zone are smaller, with little cytoplasm and more darkly staining nuclei.

The ultrastructural differences have been described in detail.[63, 98] In the first trimester, the definitive zone has features characteristic of those of a germinative zone: There is active protein synthesis as indicated by numerous free ribosomes and glycogen particles; the fetal zone has the characteristics of steroid-producing tissues, i.e., prominent smooth endoplasmic reticulum (SER) and Golgi apparatus and numerous large mitochondria. The definitive zone acquires the latter features toward the end of the second trimester and the early third trimester and increases in width during the last trimester; however, it continues to appear less differentiated than the fetal zone. There is also evidence of a transitional zone consisting of cells with the features of both zones.

In the adult, the adrenal cortex comprises three distinct zones: the zona glomerulosa, zona fasciculata, and zona reticularis. These lie in concentric layers beneath the capsule with the medulla in the center of the gland.

The zona glomerulosa is a thin layer of cells arranged in clusters immediately beneath the capsule. These cells are the only source of aldosterone; they are small round cells with little cytoplasm and dense nuclei. Ultrastructurally they exhibit abundant elongated mitochondria, a prominent Golgi apparatus, and scanty SER.[98]

The zona fasciculata composes the major portion of the adult cortex and consists of long cords of cells extending from the glomerulosa to the zona reticularis. These are large cells with abundant cytoplasm and round dense nuclei. The ultrastructural characteristics vary; cells bordering on the glomerulosa have scanty SER, small ovoid mitochondria with few vesicles, and abundant liposomes, and cells closer to the reticularis have increased SER and larger spherical mitochondria with many vesicles.

The zona reticularis occupies the inner 25 to 30% of the cortex. Its cells are intermediate in size between those of the glomerulosa and fasciculata. These "compact" cells have a granular eosinophilic cytoplasm, densely packed SER, and little lipid.

Thus the narrow, relatively undifferentiated "permanent" zone of the fetal adrenal gives rise to the characteristic three zones of the adult cortex; the large, well-differentiated fetal zone disappears completely soon after birth.

FUNCTIONS

In 1940, Uotila[134] commented: "Observations that the fetal cortex forms the bulk of the fetal adrenal, is highly vascular, persists as a well-developed organ throughout intrauterine life, but degenerates soon after birth suggest strongly that it serves some important function in the physiology of the embryo and fetus, and is not a mere phylogenetic relic." Despite great increases in knowledge over the past 50 years, this comment is still valid; the true role of the fetal adrenal in embryonic life remains speculative.

Steroidogenesis

Fetal Zone

In 1956, Bloch et al.[11] showed that the human fetal adrenal contains considerable amounts of C19 and C21 steroids, and they hypothesized that the fetal zone was the site of adrenal androgen production. This hypothesis was supported by subsequent perfusion studies of previable fetuses,[31, 126] by short-term incubation of tissue slices or homogenates, and by organ and monolayer cultures of fetal zone tissue. These studies showed that the major steroid produced by the fetal zone is dehydroisoandrosterone (DHA) (Fig. 14–4), mainly in the sulfoconjugated form (DHAS). Much of the DHA and DHAS are hydroxylated at C16 in the fetal adrenal and liver.[139] Consequently plasma DHAS[33, 76] and 16OH-DHAS[76] levels are very high in the fetal arterial blood (Table 14–1). The shunting of the steroid pathway to DHAS appears to be due to a lack of 3β-hydroxysteroid dehydrogenase isomerase (3β-HSD) activity. It has been suggested that this lack is due to an inhibition of activity of the enzyme by the high circulating levels of pro-

gesterone and estrogens during fetal life[17, 141]; however, studies suggest that 3β-HSD activity is low because the enzyme, and indeed the 3β-HSD gene itself, is minimally expressed in the fetal zone.[32, 140] Cholesterol derived from de novo synthesis and from circulating low-density lipoprotein (LDL) cholesterol provides the substrate for DHAS production.[24]

Deficient 3β-HSD activity appears to account for the low production of cortisol by the fetal zone. This tissue, however, is able to convert labeled progesterone to cortisol in vitro and in vivo.[126, 137] Explant cultures of the fetal zone are better able than the definitive zone or adult adrenocortical tissue to use progesterone for cortisol production.[15] Thus there is high activity of enzymes required to synthesize DHAS and except for 3β-HSD to synthesize cortisol (i.e., 17-, 21-, and 11-hydroxylases). Fetal plasma levels of progesterone are several times higher than maternal levels[2, 76, 84, 132] (see Table 14–1), and there is a large arteriovenous difference in both early[84] and late[2] pregnancy, with higher levels on the venous side indicating that the fetus metabolizes large amounts of progesterone; however, the exact quantitative contribution of progesterone to cortisol synthesis remains unknown. mRNA for 17- and 21-hydroxylases have been demonstrated by 13 weeks' gestation[30, 143] and are quantitatively similar up to 20 weeks.[83]

Definitive Zone

In contrast to the fetal zone, somewhat higher 3β-HSD activity relative to that of other steroidogenic enzymes is present in the definitive zone, which produces more cortisol than DHAS in vitro.[13, 23, 124] The definitive zone has fewer LDL-binding sites, makes less cholesterol de novo, and is less able to use progesterone for cortisol synthesis than the fetal zone.[14] It also contains less sulfokinase activity.[67] Mineralocorticoid secretion is low, suggesting that 18-hydroxylase is lacking as well.[97]

Medulla

Although chromaffin tissue does not form a "true" medulla until after birth, the nests of chromaffin cells scattered throughout the fetal zone stain positively for catecholamines as well

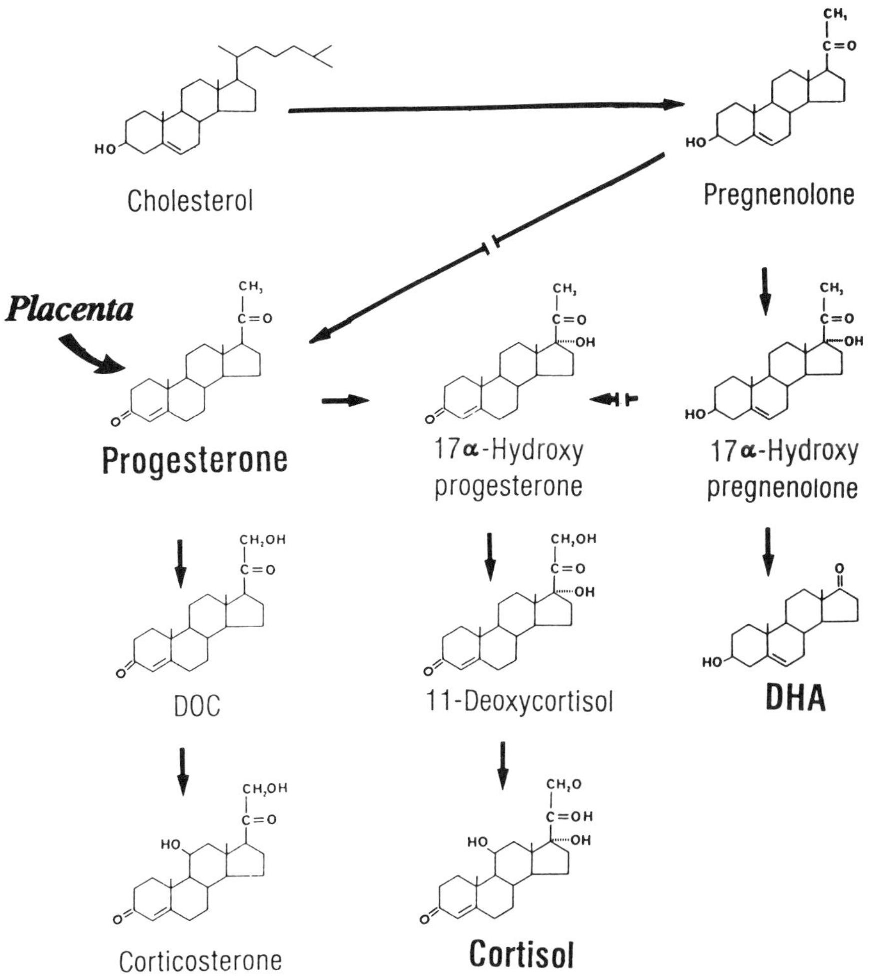

FIGURE 14–4. Steroidogenic pathways in the fetal adrenal.

TABLE 14–1. Steroid Levels in Fetal and Maternal Serum (Mean ± SEM ng/mL)

| Steroid | Reference | Gestational Age | Fetal | | Maternal |
			Venous	Arterial	Venous
DHAS	33	Term delivery	1300 ± 59	1620 ± 62	1000 ± 52
"	76	Term delivery	1640 ± 110	2330 ± 180	1010 ± 150
"	29	Term delivery	1337 ± 117 (female)		
			1334 ± 94 (male)		
"	105	Term delivery	2463 ± 250		
"	105	33–34 wk delivery	1238 ± 114		
"	105	18–22 wk delivery	1256 ± 181		
"	96	21–30 wk cordocentesis	763 (310–1370)*		
16OH-DHAS	33	Term delivery	870 (310–1480)*	1100 (350–2500)*	≤100
Progesterone	2	Term delivery	633 ± 59	362 ± 33	
"	76	Term delivery	1020 ± 100	500 ± 80	170 ± 15
"	132	Term elective CS	440 ± 69	318 ± 39	174 ± 39
"	84	12–20 wk	≥268	106 ± 35	

*Range.

as the catecholamine-synthesizing enzymes dopamine β-hydroxylase and phenylethanolamine N-methyltransferase as early as the latter part of the first trimester.[51, 148] Leu- and met-enkephalin, which in the adult are cosecreted with catecholamines in response to stress, have also been demonstrated immunocytochemically, colocated in the catecholamine synthesizing cells.[148] Both norepinephrine and epinephrine have been measured in equal amounts in adrenal extracts from 11 weeks, and their concentrations increase substantially after 20 weeks.[149] Adrenal content of met-enkephalin shows a different ontogenic pattern, being higher between 15 and 20 weeks than at 20 to 25 weeks.[149] The precise role of these medullary factors during fetal development has not been defined. Their presence in the gland, however, as well as the fact that mature innervation of the developing medulla is observed after the third month, suggests that they could be of biologic importance.

Interaction with Placenta (Fetoplacental Unit)

The original observations of Frandsen and Stakemann[42, 43] in the early 1960s that estriol levels were low in anencephalic pregnancies, in which the adrenals in the third trimester are small, led to the recognition that the fetus provided the major portion of the precursor of estriol (see section on pathology). The fetal adrenal is unable to hydrolyze steroid sulfates or aromatize androgens. Although the adrenal fetal zone lacks the 3β-HSD necessary to convert DHA to an aromatizable substrate, the placenta is well supplied with this enzyme. Although the fetal adrenal is adept at making large amounts of DHA, much of it sulfated, the placenta lacks the 17-hydroxylase necessary to convert pregnenolone and progesterone to androgens. Thus the placenta is able to convert the large amounts of DHA and DHAS and their 16-hydroxylated derivatives reaching it from the fetal circulation (100 to 200 μg/dL; 200 to 400 μm/L)[68] to estrone, estradiol, and estriol. Conversely, the adrenal is able to use the large amounts of progesterone supplied by the placenta to make cortisol. This selective distribution of enzymes in the fetal adrenal

and placenta has given rise to the concept of the *fetoplacental unit*. In anencephaly, in which the fetal zone is small in the third trimester, the estriol levels are low, although they overlap with the widely varying normal levels.[42, 43]

Fetal Metabolism of Cortisol

Another source of cortisol in the fetus is conversion of cortisone in amniotic fluid to cortisol by the choriodecidua.[8, 87] Because the fetus swallows considerable amounts of amniotic fluid, this cortisol would be absorbed and contribute to the cortisol pool.[90] Virtually all fetal tissues contain large amounts of C_{11}-hydroxysteroid dehydrogenase, the enzyme that converts biologically active cortisol to inactive cortisone, a mechanism that may protect the fetus against inappropriately early fetal maturation.[89]

Maternal-Fetal Relationships

Although some maternal cortisol crosses the placenta, about 85% of it is inactivated by conversion to cortisone, a process that is active in placental tissue[6, 85] and in almost all fetal tissues.[88, 89] A positive arteriovenous difference, with higher levels in the arteries (i.e., coming from the fetus), has been demonstrated in both early[84] and late[73, 91] gestation, the difference presumably being due mainly to conversion of progesterone to cortisol by the fetal zone in early gestation. At birth, the fetal cortisol level is only about one third or less that of the mother[18]; this difference is largely accounted for by the increased levels of corticosteroid-binding globulin (CBG, transcortin) in the mother, and the decreased (relative to the adult) CBG levels in the fetus. Because even the fetal adrenal contains 11β-HSD, it also secretes cortisone.

Although the maternal contribution of cortisol is inadequate to prevent the adrenocorticotropic hormone (ACTH) rise responsible for the increased androgens leading to virilization in congenital adrenal hyperplasia, it appears to be sufficient to allow relatively normal development to occur in infants with adrenal hypoplasia or aplasia.

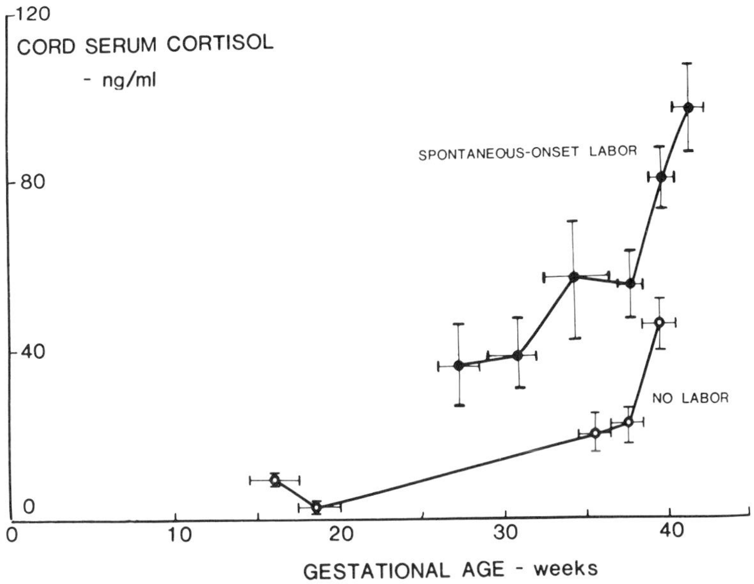

FIGURE 14–5. Levels of cortisol in cord serum (mean ± SE) after the spontaneous onset of labor (●) and in the absence of labor (○). (From Murphy BEP. Human fetal serum cortisol levels related to gestational age; evidence of a midgestational fall and a steep late gestational rise, independent of sex or mode of delivery. Am J Obstet Gynecol 1982;144:276–282. With permission.)

Fetal Dehydroepiandrosterone Sulfate Levels

The circulating DHAS of both mother and fetus provides substrate for estrogen production by the placenta; the placenta is able to convert DHAS and its 16-hydroxylated derivative to DHA by virtue of its abundant sulfatase. Because 16-hydroxy-DHAS is derived almost exclusively from the fetus, as evidenced by the blood levels (see Table 14–1),[76] the bulk of estriol is derived from the fetus. Fetal DHAS levels also exceed maternal levels, so the greater portions of estrone and estradiol are derived from the fetus, although the contribution of the mother is considerable. Nahoul et al.[96] found that levels of DHAS ranged from 310 to 1370 ng/mL over the period from 21 to 30 weeks' gestation as determined by withdrawing blood (mainly venous) from the cord in utero. The values in the fetuses were about 25% higher than those of their mothers. These levels are lower than those of nonpregnant adults (1380 ± 512 ng/mL in women; 2240 ± 93 in men), presumably because of the rapid metabolism of DHAS in the placenta. Parker et al.[105] obtained a mean value of 1250 ng/mL in infants delivered after the spontaneous onset of labor at 18 to 34 weeks' gestation; the mean level rose to 2463 ng/mL by 39

to 40 weeks. Lower values (a mean of 1335 ng/mL) were obtained at normal term delivery by De Peretti and Forest[29] using the same method; no differences were observed between males and females. The latter group showed that the levels of DHAS at delivery fell in newborns to an average of 10 ± 12 ng/mL by 1 month of age and remained low until the onset of puberty.

Fetal Cortisol Levels

The cortisol level is made up of that bound to CBG and albumin and an unbound or free portion. CBG binding is tight (i.e., high affinity), whereas that to albumin is much looser (low affinity). The unbound portion and much of that bound to albumin are able to diffuse readily into the tissues, whereas that bound to CBG is largely held in the circulation. The measurement of cortisol in fetal blood is difficult, owing to the very large amounts of many steroids not present in the adult. Thus assays validated for adult blood are not suitable for fetal blood, a fact that has given rise to many erroneous data in the literature.[92]

The levels of total fetal cortisol are depicted in Figure 14–5. They remain low (5 to 12 ng/mL or 14 to 33 nm/L) from 15 to 30 weeks,[91, 96] then rise to 20 ± 10 ng/mL (56 ± 28 nm/L) by 37 to 38 weeks and to 45 ng/mL (125 nm/L) at term in the absence of labor.[91] The diffusible (i.e., unbound plus albumin-bound) level is about 4 ng/mL (11 nm/L) at 15 to 20 weeks' gestation, rising to about 31 ng/mL (86 nm/L) at term, a level comparable to that of the nonpregnant adult.[18]

The total levels approximately double in association with labor,[91] rise further in the first hour or two following delivery,[60] and then fall to levels averaging 15 to 80 ng/mL during the first week of life.[66, 125] Premature infants born with the respiratory distress syndrome have lower levels than normal infants but are able to increase their cortisol levels promptly in response to stress.[85, 86]

A factor that affects the *effective* cortisol level reaching the tissues is the extremely high progesterone level[2, 76, 84, 132] because progesterone competes strongly for sites on the cortisol receptor but does not act as a glucocorticoid. This thus provides another mechanism for keeping the effective cortisol level low in rapidly growing tissues. Large doses of glucocorticoids given to pregnant rats and mice early in pregnancy cause cleft palate and other birth defects, and treatment doses administered to children cause stunted growth.

Maturation of Enzyme Systems

Although growth is retarded by excessive cortisol, a sufficient amount of cortisol appears to be necessary in late gestation to effect maturation of various enzymes, some of which are essential for extrauterine survival.[75] Such processes affect glycogen accumulation in liver; development of pancreatic β cells; development of the adrenal medulla; and differentiation of type II alveolar lung cells and pulmonary surfactant production, epithelial maturation, and alkaline phosphatase activity of the small intestine and levels of thyroid hormones.[75, 100] Cortisol is probably important in fetal lung maturation (see Chapter 19).

Influence on Gestation Length

The length of normal human pregnancy with spontaneous onset of delivery as estimated from the first day of the last normal menstrual period is 281 ± 12 (SD) days.[34] In anencephaly (see also section on pathology), in which pituitary and hypothalamus are essentially lacking and the adrenals are small, the standard deviation is much greater. In a group of 22 cases with anencephalic fetuses, in which there were minimal or no complications, the duration of pregnancy was prolonged to 311 days (range, 283 to 349).[82] In a group with complications such as hydramnios or toxemia, it was shortened to an average of 253 days. Other authors[54] have found a similar distribution, although they concluded that some of the uncomplicated cases also delivered prematurely.

No alteration in pregnancy duration was found in a group of 38 infants with congenital adrenal hyperplasia.[110] Although the data are sparse, no obvious change in gestation length was noted in cases of adrenal hypoplasia.

Role of the Fetal Adrenal in Parturition

Although a role for the fetal adrenal in rats[131] and sheep[75] has been clearly demonstrated, such a role has not been apparent for the human species. In contrast to nonprimate mammals, administration of cortisol or estrogen to the fetus does not initiate labor, there is no convincing fall in progesterone or rise in estrogens in association with labor, and progesterone administration does not prevent the onset of labor. The cortisol level in the absence of labor rises as term approaches[91] (see Fig. 14–5), but there is no premature rise in most premature infants, many of whom have low cortisol levels at birth (before the initiation of normal and premature labor).

REGULATION

Because fetal adrenal steroids may play an important role in fetal development, it is important to understand the factors controlling the growth and steroid production of the fetal adrenal. Many studies have been designed to clarify this issue, and have been reviewed.[24, 62, 98, 108, 149]

Growth

In early studies, steroidogenesis was used as an end point to assess regulatory factors; more recently, however, it has been realized that factors that stimulate steroidogenesis do not necessarily stimulate growth. A number of studies have examined the effects of hormones and growth factors on monolayer cultures of fetal adrenal cells.[1, 26, 56, 98, 113, 124]

The small adrenals present at birth in anencephalic infants provide an indication that fetal adrenal growth is at least to some extent dependent on pituitary factors. The fetal gland, however, develops apparently normally up to about 14 weeks' gestational age,[48] suggesting that other factors must be involved, at least in early gestation.

In a study of 102 normal and 38 anencephalic fetuses in midgestation, Young et al.[152] found that the adrenal weights in anencephalics were lower than normal after 17 weeks' gestation. Their observations were interpreted as indicating that the fetal pituitary controls adrenal growth, mainly through ACTH. As noted later, Kuhnle et al.[70] found a virilized infant with 21-hydroxylase deficiency who had adrenals of normal size at 20 weeks' gestation, suggesting that in the first half of gestation, ACTH does not stimulate growth. Indeed, under culture conditions, ACTH has been shown to be antimitogenic at the same time that it stimulated steroidogenesis.[1, 26, 124]

There seems to be no doubt that the anencephalic adrenal develops normally in early gestation. What factor stimulates growth at this time? It seems likely that some factor other than ACTH is involved. The presence of such a factor is also suggested by the profound changes that occur in the adrenal following birth, despite apparently normal pituitary function. The large fetal zone degenerates, largely by 1 week, then more gradually thereafter, whereas the definitive zone cells multiply to form the adult type of cortical tissue. Over the first month, DHAS falls 20-fold to 30-fold.[29] Such dramatic changes suggest a dependence of the fetal adrenal at least in part on maternal or placental factors.

Among the placental hormones, human chorionic gonadotropin (hCG) has appeared to be the most likely candidate for a fetal adrenal growth factor. A purified preparation of hCG, however, did not stimulate growth of fetal adrenal cells in monolayer culture.[1] Placental lactogen, another proposed fetal growth factor, was also without effect.[113] Estrogens and progesterone had no effect at physiologic concentrations and inhibited cell growth at higher concentrations.[113]

In recent years, a great number of growth factors have been isolated from human placental tissue, including the transforming growth factors α[130] and β[44] (TGF-α and TGF-β). TGF-α binds to the epidermal growth factor (EGF) receptor, shares significant homology with EGF, and may be an embryonic form of EGF. TGF-β binds to its own receptor and stimulates or inhibits cell growth, depending on the cell type concerned and the presence or absence of other growth factors. Other placental growth factors include nerve growth factor[45] (NGF), fibroblast growth factor[46] (FGF), platelet-derived growth factor[47] (PDGF), insulin-like growth factors 1 (IGF-1) and 2[38] (IGF-2), and a 34-kd growth factor different antigenically from these known growth factors.[116, 117]

In vitro conditioned medium from both early and term placenta (PM) greatly increases growth of fetal zone adrenal cells.[113] As well, extracts of early placental homogenates increase the number of definitive zone cells up to eightfold.[123] Of the aforementioned placental factors, EGF and FGF[26, 113, 124] as well as TGF-α (Branchaud et al., unpublished observations) stimulate growth of cultured fetal adrenal cells (Table 14–2). Maximum stimulation by these growth factors, however, is twofold to 2.5-fold as compared with threefold to 10-fold by PM. In addition, the stimulatory effect of EGF and FGF is dependent on the presence of serum,[26] whereas that of PM is not.[113] Further, ACTH, antimitogenic by itself, reverses the growth stimulating effect of EGF,[113] FGF,[113] and TGF-α (Branchaud et al., unpublished observations) but not that of PM.[113] TGF-β[112] and activin A[128] are growth inhibitory, whereas NGF, PDGF, IGF-1, IGF-2, and growth hormone are without effect.[113] Thus PM appears to be more effective than any of the individual factors tested to date. It is possible that the effect of PM is due to combined growth factor effects that may or may not include a hitherto undefined growth factor. Enhanced mitogenic responses to combinations of growth factors have been de-

TABLE 14–2. Effects of Growth Factors on Growth and Function of the Human Fetal Adrenal Cortex

Growth Factor	Cell Type	Mitogenic Effect	Steroidogenic Effect*
FGF	FZ	Stimulatory × 2[26, 113]	No effect (F,DHAS)[26, 113]
	DZ	Stimulatory × 4[23]	
EGF	FZ	Stimulatory × 2[26, 113]	No effect (F,DHAS)[26, 113]
TGFα	FZ	Stimulatory × 2†	No effect†
TGFβ	FZ	Inhibitory[112, 128]	No effect DHAS[112]
			?Stimulatory F[112]
	DZ	Inhibitory[128]	Inhibitory F,DHAS[21]
Activin A	FZ	Inhibitory[128]	
IGF I	FZ	No effect[81, 113]	Stimulatory (F)[16]
IGF I plus EGF	FZ	Stimulatory 1.5 × EGF alone[81]	
IGF II	FZ	No effect†, [81]	No effect(F)†
IGF II plus insulin	FZ	Stimulatory × 2–3[81]	
IGF II plus insulin plus EGF plus FGF	FZ	Stimulatory × 3–4[81]	
NGF	FZ	No effect[113]	No effect[113]
PDGF	FZ	No effect[113]	No effect[113]
TNFα	FZ	No effect[60]	Inhibitory F × 1/7[60]
			Inhibitory DHAS × 2/3[59, 60]
			Increases DHAS/F[59, 60]
Placental medium	FZ	Stimulatory × 3–10[118]	Inhibitory F × 1/1[113]
			Inhibitory DHAS × 1/2[113]
			Increases DHAS/F[113]
PDMF‡	DZ	Stimulatory × 7[123]	

DZ = Definitive zone; FZ = fetal zone; F = cortisol.
*ACTH-stimulated steroidogenesis.
†Branchaud et al., unpublished observations.
‡Placental-derived mitogenic factor.

scribed.[81] In addition, the role of ACTH in adrenal growth may be manifested through stimulation of growth factor production in the adrenal itself. ACTH has been shown to enhance IGF-2 mRNA accumulation[143, 144] and IGF-2[80, 81] and bFGF[79, 80] gene expression.

Proopiomelanocortin (POMC)-related peptides other than ACTH, which have been identified in the fetal pituitary,[120] have also been proposed to account for early fetal adrenal growth. In contrast to the adult gland, the human fetal pituitary has an intermediate lobe that regresses at birth. In the intermediate lobe, ACTH is further processed to give α-melanocyte-stimulating hormone (α-MSH)(ACTH 1-13) and corticotropin-like intermediate lobe peptide (CLIP)(ACTH 18-39),[121] and β-lipotropin (β-LPH) gives rise to β-endorphin.[69] None of these peptides has so far been shown to be mitogenic for fetal zone adrenal cells in vitro. Although ACTH itself is antimitogenic in culture conditions, ACTH augments bFGF and IGF-2 mRNAs, and it has been postulated that a growth stimulatory effect of ACTH in vivo could be brought about via locally produced growth factors.[79, 142]

Steroidogenesis

To date, only ACTH has been shown to stimulate steroidogenesis in vitro. Studies of ACTH regulatory effects in the steroidogenic pathway, however, have demonstrated not only that ACTH acts at many levels, but also that other factors, growth factors included, can influence steroidogenesis (see Table 14–2). An extensive review of developments in the area has been published.[108]

Substrates for Steroidogenesis

LDL cholesterol, derived from the fetal liver, has been shown to be the major substrate for steroid synthesis in the fetal adrenal.[20, 22, 24] ACTH increases the number of LDL receptors on the adrenal cell surface, permitting more LDL cholesterol to be internalized and degraded, releasing active cholesterol for steroid synthesis.

Provided that ACTH is present, however, the human fetal adrenal can also synthesize cholesterol from acetate[20, 24] and may account for up to 30% of DHAS and cortisol produced by cultured fetal adrenal tissue; the rate-limiting step is 3-hydroxy-3-methylglutaryl coenzyme A (HMG-CoA) reductase, whose activity depends on ACTH.

Steroidogenic Enzymes

Production of DHAS and cortisol from cholesterol is catalyzed by a number of enzymes, including the cytochrome P450 oxidases:[83, 98] the cholesterol side-chain cleavage enzyme (P450scc), 17α-hydroxylase and 17,20-lyase (P450c17), 21-hydroxylase (P450c21), and 11-hydroxylase (P450c11). 3β-HSD is required to convert pregnenolone and 17-hydroxypregnenolone, both of which have a 5-ene configuration, to the 4-ene steroids progesterone and 17-hydroxyprogesterone; hydroxysteroidsulfotransferase is necessary for sulfation of the steroid products. Adrenodoxin and adrenodoxin reductase form an electron transport system for the hydroxylation of steroids. The cytochrome P450 oxidases are present in the fetal adrenal in large amounts as judged by their activities[14, 55] and their mRNAs.[142] Adrenodoxin mRNA has been shown to be present in the fetal adrenal in early gestation.[144]

Maintenance of the activity and the mRNAs of the cytochrome P450 enzymes in cultured fetal adrenal cells requires ACTH,[30, 55, 146] as does the accumulation of adrenodoxin mRNA.[146] ACTH also induces 3β-HSD activity[124] as well as its mRNA[139] in cultured fetal adrenal cells (see also section on peptide growth factors next); however, it does not seem to be required for expression of P450 hydroxylases because the mRNA content of all hydroxylases and adrenodoxin was comparable in adrenal tissue from both anencephalic and normal fetuses; the concentrations of P450scc, P450c17, and adrenodoxin protein were also similar.[64] Thus it appears that in the fetal adrenal, the expression of these steroidogenic enzymes must depend on factors other than ACTH.

Peptide Growth Factors

It is becoming evident that peptide growth factors influence the differentiated function of many steroid-producing cells as well as affecting their growth. Their effect appears to vary between tissues as well as species. For instance, TGF-β inhibits ACTH-stimulated cortisol secretion by adult ovine[111] and bovine[39, 57] adrenocortical cells. TGF-β is without effect on DHAS and slightly enhances cortisol production by human fetal zone adrenal cells.[112]

The differentiative role of IGF-1 in steroidogenic tissues has received much attention recently. In cultured bovine adult[107] and ovine fetal[94] adrenocortical cells, IGF-1 enhances both ACTH-stimulated and angiotensin II–stimulated corticosteroid production. As well, nanomolar concentrations of IGF-1 increase ACTH-stimulated cortisol production by cultured human fetal zone adrenal cells.[16] At least one of the mechanisms by which IGF-1 exerts this effect is by an enhancement of 3β-HSD activity.[16]

It is clear that ACTH induces fetal adrenal 3β-HSD in vitro; 3β-HSD mRNA,[138] immunoreactive 3β-HSD,[32] and cortisol production[122, 124] increase in response to ACTH in adrenal cell cultures. It has also been hypothesized that induction of 3β-HSD in vitro occurs because the tissue is no longer exposed to circulating placental estrogens, which inhibit fetal adrenal 3β-HSD in utero.[17, 140, 141]

It is difficult to assess the possible interaction of ACTH, IGF-1, and estrogens in regulating 3β-HSD in vivo. Significant levels of ACTH circulate in the fetus, but 3β-HSD remains low. Also, in vitro studies of ACTH induction of 3β-HSD have been performed in the presence of serum that contains significant amounts of IGF-1. ACTH has been shown to increase IGF-2 mRNA in the fetal adrenal,[143] and one could speculate that IGF-1 might be regulated by ACTH as well. Indeed, high levels of IGF-1 mRNA have been demonstrated in the parenchymal elements of the fetal adrenal.[49] Fetal adrenal 3β-HSD activity is inhibited by high concentrations of estrogens in vitro[17, 141]; however, it remains to be demonstrated that the 3β-HSD gene can be inhibited by estrogens. Certainly many questions regarding 3β-HSD regulation are still to be answered.

Interesting findings that could shed some light on the reason for the distinctive steroidogenic pathway in the fetal zone have been reported recently.[59, 60] Tumor necrosis factor α (TNF-α), a cytokine with many different biologic effects, has been shown to suppress fetal adrenal cortisol production markedly while having much less effect on DHA or DHAS production. Thus TNF-α in effect mediates a shift toward the fetal zone pattern of mainly androgen synthesis. This has been observed in both explant and primary monolayer cultures of human fetal zone adrenal tissues.[59, 60]

TNF-α[59, 60] had no effect on cell number,[60] nor was it cytotoxic.[59] It is intriguing that TNF-α has been detected immunologically in fetal but not adult adrenal extracts. TNF-α is also measurable in fetal adrenal culture medium.[114]

TNF-α was shown to inhibit mRNAs for all adrenal cytochrome P450 oxidases, P450scc, P450c11, P450c17, and P450c21.[60] The authors speculate, however, that the TNF-α-mediated shift from glucocorticoids to androgens may be due to a more potent inhibition of P450c11. TNF-α did not appear to affect 3β-HSD activity greatly and thus did not reproduce the complete in vivo fetal zone pattern. Further investigation of this peptide, however, is warranted.

In light of these findings, it is pertinent that conditioned PM also markedly inhibits steroid production by cultured fetal zone cells.[113] The PM effect on cortisol production is much more pronounced (one-tenth of control) than that on DHAS production (one-half of control), greatly increasing the DHAS to F (cortisol) ratio. These findings are consistent with a placental contribution to the maintenance of the fetal zone steroidogenic pattern. TNF-α has been identified in placental extracts,[114] but whether the steroid inhibitory effect of PM is due to its content of TNF-α remains to be determined.

PATHOLOGY

Congenital Anomalies of the Adrenal Gland

Adrenal rests and accessory adrenal glands are common and are not strictly pathologic.[98] This material probably becomes separated from the gland proper before encapsulation occurs, at the time that the neural elements destined to become the medulla invade the adrenal primordium. Although usually found in the abdomen or pelvis, they may occasionally be found in almost any other tissue, including lung and even brain. They may contain both cortex and medulla but more commonly one or the other. Rarely the adrenal is embedded in the kidney or liver.

Occasionally ectopic elements, usually ovarian, may be present within the adrenals. Adrenal cysts occur rarely, although they may develop later in life.

Rh-incompatibility may be associated with adrenal cytomegaly, cytoplasmic vacuolation of the fetal zone, and intra-adrenal hematopoietic foci. Hereditary xanthomatosis may be associated with enlarged adrenals containing large amounts of cholesterol and triglycerides owing to acid esterase deficiency.

Congenital Adrenal Hyperplasia (Genetic Defects in Cortisol Synthesis)

Hyperplasia of the adrenal is much more common than hypoplasia and is due to genetic defects in adrenal steroid production.[98] Most defects result in adrenal hyperplasia because low cortisol production stimulates increased ACTH production. When the syndrome of masculinization of female fetuses associated with enlarged adrenal glands was first recognized, it was called the *adrenogenital syndrome.* These steroidogenetic defects may be only partial, so there are no obvious abnormalities at birth, but the disease becomes apparent in adulthood, usually because of hirsutism in the female. The same enzyme defects occur in the gonads. Steroidogenic enzymes common to both adrenals and gonads are affected in both tissues.

The hyperplasia probably occurs only in the latter half of pregnancy because ACTH does not appear to affect the growth of the adrenal appreciably in the first half of pregnancy (see section on regulation). In three of these defects, virilization occurs because although the mineralocorticoid and glucocorticoid pathways are blocked, the androgen pathway is not and is therefore stimulated excessively by ACTH. Virilization, however, may occur in the absence of hyperplasia at 20 weeks.[70]

The blocks resulting from these enzyme defects are depicted in Figure 14–6. All are autosomal recessive.

Cholesterol Desmolase Deficiency

The earliest block in the pathway is that of cholesterol desmolase, which accomplishes the conversion of cholesterol to pregnenolone by hydroxylation at C20 and cleavage of the C20-22 side chain. This is an essential step in the formation of all steroids, and this defect is virtually always fatal. The adrenals are very large and contain excessive amounts of cholesterol.[98]

3 β-Hydroxysteroid Dehydrogenase/Isomerase Deficiency

The next step along the pathway to cortisol requires 3β-HSD to form progesterone by shifting the double bond from C5 to C4, necessary for the formation of gonadal steroids and mineralocorticoids as well as glucocorticoids. This rare defect results in the production of large amounts of DHA. Genitalia may be ambiguous in both sexes because of the partial masculinizing effects of large amounts of DHA in the female and the lack of testosterone in the male. Clinically these defects are manifested at birth by ambiguous genitalia, vomiting, failure to thrive, or death due to vascular collapse. Partial deficiency of this enzyme has been suggested as a cause of hirsutism in peripubertal and adult women.[103] This enzyme is essentially lacking in the fetal zone of the fetal adrenal (see section on embryology and development).

17-Hydroxylase Deficiency

In 17-hydroxylase deficiency, neither pregnenolone nor progesterone is hydroxylated, preventing the production of cortisol and also of androgens and estrogens but leaving the mineralocorticoid pathway intact. Therefore males fail to develop masculine external genitalia, and females fail to develop secondary sex characteristics at puberty. Hypertension may occur. Therapy consists of glucocorticoid replacement and estrogen or androgen administration at puberty.

21-Hydroxylase Deficiency

By far the most common defect is 21-hydroxylase deficiency, which accounts for about 95% of all cases of adrenal hyperplasia. The estimated frequency in the general population is 1:15,000 to 1:40,000, with a heterozygote frequency of 1:100 to 1:50. In southwestern Alaska, however, among the Yupik Eskimos, the incidence is 1:500 births, with a heterozygotic frequency of 1:11.[53] An extensive study relating hormonal data to genotype has been made by New et al.[99]

Clinically affected infants are virilized and in the more severe or salt-losing form develop hyponatremia, hyperkalemia, acidosis, and dehydration, which may lead to vascular collapse. A mild form may be diagnosed only after puberty in women complaining of hirsutism.[103]

Because of the high incidence in Alaska, a newborn screening program was set up.[104] Neonatal blood samples were collected 2 to 14 days after birth on filter paper and assayed for 17-hydroxyprogesterone. Normal infants had values ranging up to 40 pg/disc, whereas those in infants with congenital adrenal hyperplasia varied from 57 to 980 pg/disc. Of approximately 20,000 births, 16 had high values, and 4 cases (3 of 1131 Yupik Eskimos and 1 of 13,733 Caucasians) were subsequently confirmed.

A trial screening program for congenital adrenal hyperplasia was also conducted on the 5th to 10th day after birth in 100,000 newborns in Portugal,[136] where the incidence was found to be 1:1430 (7 of the 21 initially categorized as positive).

Prenatal diagnosis has been made by finding elevated levels of amniotic fluid 17α-hydroxyprogesterone in second-trimester pregnancies known to be at risk[58] and more recently at 8 to 10 weeks' gestation using molecular genetic techniques combined with chorionic villus sampling.[40, 127] Provided that treatment is begun early (7 weeks, i.e., before definitive diagnosis), the virilization can probably be prevented[40] (see also section on glucocorticoid therapy). If the infant is male or heterozygous, the treatment can be discontinued. Replacement is accomplished using dexamethasone (about 20 μg/kg prepregnancy weight) because cortisol and prednisolone are largely

20-Desmolase deficiency

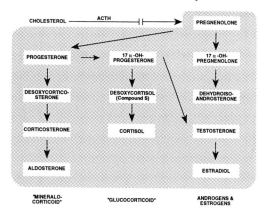

3β-Hydroxysteroid Dehydrogenase deficiency

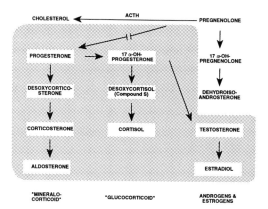

17α-Hydroxylase deficiency

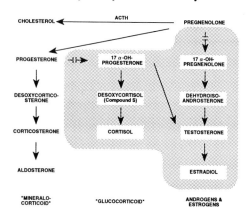

21-Hydroxylase deficiency

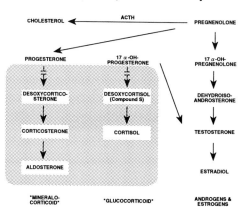

11β-Hydroxylase deficiency

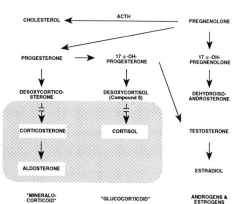

18-Hydroxysteroid deficiency

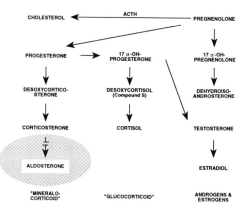

FIGURE 14–6. Congenital defects in steroid biosynthesis. Shaded areas indicate the pathways blocked. (Modified after Liddle GW. The adrenals. In: Williams RH, ed. Textbook of Endocrinology. Philadelphia: WB Saunders, 1981:286–288. With permission.)

metabolized by the placenta and therefore do not reach the fetus in an active form.[10, 93] Such a low dose of dexamethasone does not appear to be associated with other abnormalities in pregnancy.

Partial 21-hydroxylase deficiency resulting from an allelic mutation at the 21-hydroxylase locus may be manifested as hirsutism at puberty or even later.[103]

11β-Hydroxylase Deficiency

Hydroxylation at the C11 position is required to make cortisol and corticosterone. Lack of this hydroxylase results in an excess of 11-desoxysteroids (including 11-desoxycorticosterone) and androgens, leading to hypertension and virilization. The diagnosis can be made by the high plasma 11-desoxycortisol levels. The hypertension responds promptly to replacement therapy.

The possibility of partial acquired deficiency was explored in 260 hirsute women by measuring 11-desoxycortisol levels before and after ACTH stimulation.[3] Two women had a net increment greater than threefold the upper 95th percentile of 41 control subjects, an incidence of 0.8%, and were presumed to suffer from the late-onset form of 11β-hydroxylase deficiency.

Other Congenital Defects in Steroidogenesis

17,20-Desmolase Deficiency

This defect is rare[41] and gives rise to excessive amounts of 17-hydroxylated progesterone and pregnenolone and low DHA, androstenedione, and DHAS. Ambiguous genitalia in the male result because the same defect is present in the testis. Combined 17α-hydroxylase/17,20-lyase deficiency has been reported.[151]

18-Hydroxysteroid Dehydrogenase Deficiency

Lack of 18-hydroxysteroid dehydrogenase, which occurs rarely, leads to decreased aldosterone production, which is associated with sodium depletion, potassium retention, hypotension, dehydration, and increased plasma renin.[133] It is corrected by mineralocorticoid replacement therapy, usually 9α-fluorohydrocortisone.

Congenital Adrenal Hypoplasia

Primary adrenal hypoplasia is rare and may be inherited as a sex-linked or autosomal trait. Unless diagnosed prenatally or soon after birth, it is likely to be fatal.[102, 129] Adrenal hypoplasia may also be secondary to pituitary aplasia or hypoplasia or rarely to hypothalamic abnormalities (see also following discussion of anencephaly). It is noteworthy that absence or hypoplasia of the adrenals does not give rise to any obvious developmental defects of the fetus, possibly because maternal cortisol provides a sufficient amount of cortisol for survival provided that treatment is given promptly after birth. So far this condition has been diagnosed usually only after birth; occasionally the diagnosis has been suspected owing to death of a sibling. With currently available ultrasound technology, the diagnosis can now be made in utero.[50]

Anencephaly

Anencephalic infants lack a properly developed forebrain and have no functional cerebral cortex but only a fibrotic mass of neurons and glia with variable presence of other neural tissues; they lack bone and skin over the residual brain elements.[135] Cleft palate is commonly associated.

Usually the cause is not apparent and is considered to be multifactorial.[78] Some anencephalics may have chromosomal abnormalities, whereas in others anencephaly may be due to mechanical factors. Geographic variations occur, an incidence of 2 to 4:1000 live births occurring in Ireland and Scotland,[36] compared with an overall worldwide incidence of about 0.3:1000. The sex incidence favors females to males 2.3:1. The pituitary is absent in about half, and the adrenals are always hypoplastic at birth. About one-third have other, nonneural congenital anomalies.

Although the absence of the brain is apparent within the first few weeks, the fetal adrenals grow relatively normally during the early weeks of gestation (see Fig. 14–4). Decreased volume of the fetal zone after 14 weeks' gestation (the time of maximal relative adrenal weight), however, has been documented,[48] so that at 17 weeks, the fetal zone formed $58 \pm 3\%$ of the gland compared with $77 \pm 2\%$ in the normal controls. The weight of the fetal adrenals in anencephalics changes little from 15 to 20 weeks onward,[65] and at birth the combined weight is usually 1 g or less compared with about 8 g in the normal infant; at this time, the fetal zone constitutes about 25% of the volume in the anencephalic, whereas it normally is 75%.[7, 137]

Young et al.[152] have also compared the adrenals of normal and anencephalic fetuses as well as three fetuses with congenital adrenal hyperplasia. Unfortunately, because they have few data at the critical time of 14 weeks' gestation, their conclusion that fetal adrenal growth is dependent entirely on pituitary function can apply only from about 17 weeks onward. Because they talk about *fetal gestational age,* it is not entirely clear whether they are dating their fetuses from the date of the last menstrual period (gestational age) or 2 weeks later (fetal age), although the latter seems more likely.

GLUCOCORTICOID THERAPY

Glucocorticoids may be given to pregnant women for a number of reasons: to treat the mother for various diseases, to prevent the respiratory distress syndrome in the newborn, and, more recently, to treat the fetus in utero.

The purpose of the treatment determines the particular steroid used. Cortisone and prednisone, which have a C11-ketone, depend for their effectiveness on their hepatic conversion to the C11-hydroxy forms, cortisol (hydrocortisone) and prednisolone. This conversion is almost absent in the fetus.[89] The usual treatment doses of cortisol or cortisone and prednisone or prednisolone have little effect on the fetus because of the very active 11β-HSD present in the placenta, which converts about 85% of the cortisol to biologically inactive cortisone and prednisolone to its inactive analog prednisone.[93] In addition, the fetus also rap-

idly degrades these compounds in the same way. Beitins et al.[5] found that the fetal plasma concentration of prednisolone was 10% that of the mother. Thus these agents are useful in treating the mother, while having no adverse effects on the fetus.

Some synthetic steroids, such as dexamethasone and to a lesser extent betamethasone, cross the placenta essentially unchanged[10] and are therefore effective in treating the fetus. After prenatal betamethasone therapy to prevent respiratory distress syndrome (12 mg intramuscularly), Ballard et al.[4] found a level of betamethasone in cord blood approximately one-third that of the maternal level; however, following 8 mg dexamethasone, Osathanondh et al.[101] found the fetal plasma concentration to be approximately equal to that of the mother.

Dexamethasone, in essentially replacement doses (1 mg/day) that do not harm the mother, has been used effectively in early pregnancy to prevent virilization of the female fetus affected with 21-hydroxylase deficiency (see section on pathology).

SIGNIFICANCE OF THE FETOPLACENTAL UNIT

The concept of the fetus and placenta together forming a unit that converts fetal adrenal DHA to estrogens has been accepted for more than 2 decades. The functional significance of such a unit is questionable, however, because development appears to proceed relatively normally in its absence, i.e., in congenital absence of the adrenals and in placental sulfatase deficiency as well as in the anencephalic, where adrenal function is decreased and estrogen production is low.

Such a fetoplacental steroidogenic unit is lacking in most other species, although in evolutionary terms, important functions tend to be conserved. Possibly the peculiarities of the fetal zone are really only secondary to the effects of the high concentrations of steroids coming from the placenta.[98, 150] If so, the roles of the fetal adrenal may be essentially similar to those of the adult adrenal, i.e., to secrete adequate amounts of cortisol and aldosterone to permit survival after birth. In vitro high concentrations of estrogens inhibit 3β-HSD activity.[12, 35, 118, 138, 141] Thus fetal ACTH levels may be increased to compensate for these low levels and also for the rapid conversion of cortisol to cortisone, which occurs in virtually all fetal tissues.[88, 89, 106] Thus according to some workers, the characteristic morphology of the fetal cortex may be due to these high ACTH levels.[65, 150]

It seems clear that ACTH is important in regulation of the fetal adrenal in the second half of pregnancy and almost certainly accounts for the hypertrophy that occurs in congenital adrenal hyperplasia (see section on pathology) and for adrenal hypertrophy in postnatal life; however, it does not appear to account for the rapid growth of the adrenal that takes place in the first trimester (Fig. 14–2), the time of maximum growth relative to body weight. This rapid growth occurs equally in the anencephalic, where the pituitary is often lacking or atrophic, and continues up to about 17 weeks' gestation. Even at 17½ weeks' gestational age, the fetal zone is largely retained (57% of the gland compared with 77% in the normal).[48] Thus we are forced to postulate the presence of some factor other than ACTH that causes the initial growth spurt of the fetal adrenal. The evidence available suggests that this factor(s) is derived from the placenta.

REFERENCES

1. Abu-Hakima M, Branchaud CL, Goodyer CG, Murphy BEP. The effects of human chorionic gonadotropin on growth and steroidogenesis of the human fetal adrenal gland in vitro. Am J Obstet Gynecol 1987;156:681.
2. Antonpillai I, Murphy BEP. Serum oestrogens and progesterone in mother and infant at delivery. Br J Obstet Gynaecol 1977;84:179.
3. Azziz R, Bradley E, Boots LR, et al. 11β-Hydroxylase deficiency in hyperandrogenism. Fertil Steril 1991;55:733.
4. Ballard PL, Granberg P, Ballard RA. Glucocorticoid levels in maternal and cord serum after prenatal betamethasone therapy to prevent respiratory distress syndrome. J Clin Invest 1975;56:1548.
5. Beitins IZ, Bayard F, Ances IG, et al. The transplacental passage of prednisone and prednisolone in pregnancy near term. J Pediatr 1972;81:936.
6. Beitins IZ, Kowarski A, Shermeta DW, et al. The metabolic clearance rate, blood production, interconversion and transplacental passage of cortisol and cortisone in pregnancy near term. Pediatr Res 1973;7:509.
7. Benirschke K. Adrenals in anencephaly and hydrocephaly. Obstet Gynecol 1956;8:412.
8. Benirschke K, Richart R. Observations on the fetal adrenals of marmoset monkeys. Endocrinology 1964;74:382.
9. Bernal AL, Flint APF, Anderson ABM, Turnbull AC. 11β-Hydroxysteroid dehydrogenase activity (E.C. 1.1.1.146) in human placenta and decidua. J Steroid Biochem 1980;13:1081.
10. Blanford AT, Murphy BEP. In vitro metabolism of prednisolone, dexamethasone, betamethasone and cortisol by the human placenta. Am J Obstet Gynecol 1977;127:264.
11. Bloch E, Benirschke K, Rosemberg E. C19 steroids, 17α-hydroxycorticosterone and a sodium retaining factor in human fetal adrenal glands. Endocrinology 1956;58:626.
12. Bongiovanni AM, Eberlein WR, Goldman AS, New M. Disorders of adrenal steroid biogenesis. Rec Prog Horm Res 1967;23:375.
13. Branchaud CT, Goodyer CG, Hall C St. G, et al. Steroidogenic activity of hACTH and related peptides on the human neocortex and fetal adrenal cortex in organ culture. Steroids 1978;31:557.
14. Branchaud CL, Goodyer CG, Shore P, et al. Functional zonation of the midgestation human fetal adrenal cortex: fetal versus definitive zone use of progesterone for cortisol synthesis. Am J Obstet Gynecol 1985;151:271.
15. Branchaud CL, Lipowski L, Dhanani B, et al. Contribution of exogenous progesterone to human adrenal cortisol synthesis in vitro: a comparison of early gestation fetal and adult tissues. Steroids 1986;47:269.
16. Branchaud CL, Murphy BEP. Physiopathology of the fetal adrenal. In: Pasqualini JR, Scholler R, eds. Hormones and fetal pathophysiology. New York: Marcel Dekker; 1992:53.
17. Byrne GC, Perry YS, Winter JSD. Steroid inhibitory effects upon human adrenal 3β-hydroxysteroid dehydrogenase activity. J Clin Endocrinol Metab 1986;62:413.
18. Campbell AL, Murphy BEP. The maternal-fetal cortisol gradient during pregnancy and at delivery. J Clin Endocrinol Metab 1977;45:435.
19. Carr BR, Casey ML. Growth of the adrenal gland of the normal human fetus during early gestation. Early Human Dev 1982;6:121.
20. Carr BR, MacDonald PC, Simpson ER. The regulation of de novo synthesis of cholesterol in the human fetal adrenal gland by low density lipoprotein and adrenocorticotrophin. Endocrinology 1980;107:1000.
21. Carr BR, McAllister JM, Byrd EW, Rainey WE. Transforming growth factor beta inhibits human fetal adrenal cell steroidogenesis (abstr). Proceedings of Annual Meeting Endocrine Society, Washington, 1991.
22. Carr BR, Ohashi M, MacDonald PC, Simpson ER. Human anencephalic adrenal tissue; low density lipoprotein metabolism and cholesterol synthesis. J Clin Endocrinol Metab 1981;53:406.
23. Carr BR, Parker CR Jr, Milewich L, et al. Steroid secretion by ACTH-stimulated human adrenal tissue during the first week in organ culture. Steroids 1980;36:563.
24. Carr BR, Simpson ER. Lipoprotein utilization and cholesterol synthesis by the human fetal adrenal gland. Endocr Rev 1981;2:306.
25. Carr BR, Simpson ER. Synthesis of cholesterol in the human fetus: 3-hydroxy-3-methylglutaryl coenzyme A reductase activity of liver microsomes. J Clin Endocrinol Metab 1981;53:810.

26. Crickard K, Ill CR, Jaffe RB. Control of proliferation of human fetal adrenal cells in vitro. J Clin Endocrinol Metab 1981;53:790.

27. Crowder RE. The development of the adrenal gland in man, with special reference to origin and ultimate location of cell types and evidence in favor of the 'cell migration' theory. Contrib Embryol (Carnegie Inst) 1957;36:195.

28. David M, Forest MG. Prenatal treatment of congenital adrenal hyperplasia resulting from 21-hydroxylase deficiency. J Pediatr 1984;105:799.

29. DePeretti E, Forest MG. Pattern of plasma dehydroepiandrosterone sulfate levels in human from birth to adulthood: evidence for testicular production. J Clin Endocrinol Metab 1978;47:572.

30. DiBlasio AM, Voutilainen R, Jaffe RB, Miller WL. Hormonal regulation of messenger ribonucleic acids for P450scc (cholesterol side-chain cleavage enzyme) and P450c17 (17α-hydroxylase/17,20-lyase) in cultured human fetal adrenal cells. J Clin Endocrinol Metab 1987;65:170.

31. Diczfalusy E. Steroid metabolism in the feto-placental unit. In: Pecile A, Finzi C, eds. The Foeto-Placental Unit. Amsterdam: Excerpta Medica Foundation, 1969:65.

32. Doody KM, Carr BR, Rainey WE, et al. 3β-Hydroxysteroid dehydrogenase/isomerase in the fetal zone and neocortex of the human fetal adrenal gland. Endocrinology 1990;126:2487.

33. Easterling WE Jr, Simmer HH, Dignam WF, et al. Neutral C_{19}-steroids and steroid sulfates in human pregnancy. II. Dehydroepiandrosterone sulfate, 16α-hydroxydehydroepiandrosterone, and 16α-hydroxydehydroepiandrosterone sulfate in maternal and fetal blood of pregnancies with anencephalic and normal fetuses. Steroids 1966;8:157.

34. Eastman NJ. Maternal physiology in pregnancy. In: Eastman NJ, Hellman LM, eds. Williams obstetrics, ed 13. New York: Appleton-Century-Crofts, 1966:218.

35. Eberlein WR. Steroids and sterols in umbilical cord blood. J Clin Endocrinol Metab 1965;25:1101.

36. Elwood JH. Anencephalus in the British Isles. Dev Med Child Neurol 1970;12:582.

37. Facchinetti F, Storchi AR, Furani S, et al. Pituitary changes of desacetyl-α-melanocyte-stimulating hormone throughout development. Biol Neonate 1988;54:86.

38. Fant M, Munro H, Moses AC. An auto-crine/paracrine role for insulin-like growth factors in the regulation of human placental growth. J Clin Endocrinol Metab 1986;63:499.

39. Feige JJ, Cochet C, Chambaz EM. Type β transforming growth factor is a potent modulator of differentiated adrenocortical cell functions. Biochem Biophys Res Comm 1986;139:693.

40. Forest MG, Betuel H, David M. Prenatal treatment in congenital adrenal hyperplasia due to 21-hydroxylase deficiency: up-date 88 of the French multicentric study. Endocr Res 1989;15:277.

41. Forest MG, Lecornu M, dePeretti E. Familial male pseudohermaphroditism due to 17-20-desmolase deficiency. I. In vivo endocrine studies. J Clin Endocrinol Metab 1980;50:826.

42. Frandsen VA, Stakemann G. The site of production of oestrogenic hormones in human pregnancy. Hormone excretion in pregnancy with anencephalic foetus. Acta Endocrinol 1961;38:383.

43. Frandsen VA, Stakemann G. The site of production of oestrogenic hormones in human pregnancy. III. Further observations on the hormone excretion in pregnancy with anencephalic fetuses. Acta Endocrinol 1964;47:265.

44. Frolik CA, Dart LL, Meyers CA, et al. Purification and initial characterization of a type β transforming factor from human placenta. Proc Nat Acad Sci USA 1983;80:3676.

45. Goldstein LD, Reynolds CP, Perez-Polo JR. Isolation of human nerve growth factor from placental tissue. Neurochem Res 1978;3:175.

46. Gospodarowicz D, Cheng J, Lui G-M, et al. Fibroblast growth factor in the human placenta. Biochem Biophys Res Comm 1985;128:554.

47. Goustin AS, Betsholz C, Pfeifer-Ohlsson S, et al. Co-expression of the sis- and myc- proto-oncogenes in developing human placenta suggests autocrine control of trophoblast growth. Cell 1985;41:301.

48. Gray ES, Abramovich DR. Morphologic features of the anencephalic adrenal gland in early pregnancy. Am J Obstet Gynecol 1980;137:491.

49. Han VKM, Lung PK, Lee DC, D'Ercole AS. Expression of somatomedin/insulin-like growth factor messenger ribonucleic acids in the human fetus: identification, characterization and tissue distribution. J Clin Endocrinol Metab 1988;66:422.

50. Hata K, Hata T, Kitao M. Ultrasonographic identification and measurement of the human fetal adrenal gland in utero. Int J Gynaecol Obstet 1985;23:355.

51. Hervonen A. Development of catecholamine-storing cells in human fetal paraganglia and adrenal medulla. Acta Physiol Scand 1971;368(Suppl):1.

52. Hill WCD. Observations on the growth of the suprarenal cortex. J Anat 1930;64:479.

53. Hirschfeld AJ, Fleshman JK. An unusually high incidence of salt-losing congenital adrenal hyperplasia in the Alaskan Eskimo. J Pediatr 1969;75:492.

54. Honnebier WJ, Swaab DF. The influence of anencephaly upon intrauterine growth of fetus and placenta and upon gestation length. J Obstet Gynaecol Br Commonw 1973;80:577.

55. Hornsby PJ, Aldern KA. Steroidogenic enzyme activities in cultured human definitive zone adrenocortical cells: comparison with bovine adrenocortical cells and resultant differences in adrenal androgen synthesis. J Clin Endocrinol Metab 1984;58:121.

56. Hornsby PJ, Sturek M, Harris SE, Simonian MH. Serum and growth factor requirements for proliferation of human adrenocortical cells in culture: comparison with bovine adrenocortical cells. In Vitro 1983;19:863.

57. Hotta M, Baird A. The inhibition of low density lipoprotein metabolism by transforming growth factor-β mediates its effects on steroidogenesis in bovine adrenocortical cells in vitro. Endocrinology 1987;121:150.

58. Hughes IA, Dyas J, Laurence KM. Amniotic fluid steroid levels and fetal adrenal weight in congenital adrenal hyperplasia. Horm Res 1987;28:20.

59. Jaattela M, Carpén O, Stenman U-H, Saksela E. Regulation of ACTH-induced steroidogenesis in human fetal adrenals by rTNF-α. Mol Cell Endocrinol 1990;68:R31.

60. Jaattela M, Ilvesmaki V, Voutilainen R, et al. Tumor necrosis factor as a potent inhibitor of adrenocorticotropin-induced cortisol production and steroidogenic P450 enzyme gene expression in cultured human fetal adrenal cells. Endocrinology 1991;128:623.

61. Jackson CM. On the prenatal growth of the human body and the relative growth of the various organs and parts. Am J Anat 1909;9:119.

62. Jaffe RB, Seron-Ferré M, Crickard K, et al. Regulation and function of the primate fetal adrenal gland and gonad. Rec Prog Horm Res 1981;37:41.

63. Johannisson E. The fetal adrenal cortex in the human. Its ultrastructure at different stages of development and in different functional states. Acta Endocrinol (Copenh) 1968;130(Suppl):1.

64. John ME, Simpson ER, Carr BR, et al. Ontogeny of adrenal steroid hydroxylases: evidence for cAMP-independent gene expression. Mol Cell Endocrinol 1987;50:263.

65. Jost A. The fetal adrenal cortex. In: Greep RO, Astwood EB, eds. Handbook of physiology. Vol VI. Adrenal gland. Washington: American Physiological Society, 1975:107.

66. Kauppila A, Koivisto M, Pukka M, Tuimala R. Umbilical cord and neonatal cortisol levels: effect of gestational and neonatal factors. Obstet Gynecol 1978;52:666.

67. Korte K, Hemsell PG, Mason JI. Sterol sulfate metabolism in the adrenals of the human fetus, anencephalic newborn, and adult. J Clin Endocrinol Metab 1982;55:671.

68. Korth-Schutz S, Levine LS, New MI. Dehydroepiandrosterone sulfate (DS) levels, a rapid test for abnormal adrenal androgen secretion. J Clin Endocrinol Metab 1976;42:1005.

69. Krieger DT. Placenta as a source of 'brain' and 'pituitary' hormones. Biol Reprod 1982;26:55.

70. Kuhnle U, Bohm N, Wolff G, et al. Virilization without adrenal hyperplasia in 21-hydroxylase deficiency during fetal life. J Clin Endocrinol Metab 1984;58:574.

71. Lanman JT. The fetal zone of the adrenal gland. Medicine 1953;32:389.

72. Lanman JT. The adrenal fetal zone: its occurrence in primates and a possible relationship to chorionic gonadotropin. Endocrinology 1957;61:684.

73. Leong MKH, Murphy BEP. Cortisol levels in maternal venous and umbilical cord arterial and venous serum at vaginal delivery. Am J Obstet Gynecol 1976;124:471.

74. Levine J, Wolfe LG, Schiebinger RJ, et al. Rapid regression of fetal adrenal zone and absence of adrenal reticular zone in the marmoset. Endocrinology 1982;111:1797.

75. Liggins GC. Adrenocortical-related maturational events in the fetus. Am J Obstet Gynecol 1976;26:931.

76. Mathur RS, Landgrebe S, Moody LO, et al. Plasma steroid concentrations in maternal and umbilical circulation after spontaneous onset of labor. J Clin Endocrinol Metab 1980;51:1235.

77. McNulty WP, Novy MJ, Walsh SW. Fetal and postnatal development of the adrenal glands in Macac mulatta. Biol Reprod 1981;25:1079.

78. Medical Task Force on Anencephaly. The infant with anencephaly. N Engl J Med 1990;322:609.

79. Mesiano S, Mellon SH, Gospodarowicz D, et al. Basic fibroblast growth factor expression is regulated by corticotropin in the human fetal adrenal: a model for adrenal growth regulation. Proc Natl Acad Sci USA 1991;88:5428.

80. Mesiano S, Mellon SH, DiBlasio AM, et al. Both FGF and IGF-II expression are regulated by ACTH in the human fetal adrenal: a model for adrenal gland growth (abstr). Proceedings, 72nd Annual Meeting Endocrine Society, Atlanta, 1990:30.

81. Mesiano S, Okumura S, Jaffe RB. Interacting roles of IGF-II, bFGF and EGF in the regulation of fetal adrenal growth (abstr). Proceedings, 73rd Annual Meeting of Endocrine Society, Washington, 1991.

82. Milic AB, Adamsons K. The relationship between anencephaly and prolonged pregnancy. J Obstet Gynaecol Br Commonw 1969;76:102.

83. Miller WL. Molecular biology of steroid hormone synthesis. Endocr Rev 1988;9:295.

84. Murphy BEP. Steroid arteriovenous differences in umbilical cord plasma: evidence of cortisol production by the human fetus in early gestation. J Clin Endocrinol Metab 1973;36:1037.

85. Murphy BEP. Evidence of cortisol deficiency at birth in infants with the respiratory distress syndrome. J Clin Endocrinol Metab 1974;38:158.

86. Murphy BEP. Cortisol and cortisone levels in the cord blood at delivery of premature infants with and without the respiratory distress syndrome. Am J Obstet Gynecol 1974;119:1111.

87. Murphy BEP. The chorionic membrane as a source of fetal cortisol in human amniotic fluid. Nature 1977;266:179.

88. Murphy BEP. Cortisol and cortisone in human fetal development. J Steroid Biochem 1979;11:509.

89. Murphy BEP. Ontogeny of cortisol-cortisone interconversion in human tissues; a role for cortisol in human fetal development. J Steroid Biochem 1981;14:811.

90. Murphy BEP. The absorption by the human fetus of intra-amniotically injected cortisol. J Steroid Biochem 1982;16:415.

91. Murphy BEP. Human fetal serum cortisol levels related to gestational age; evidence of a midgestational fall and a steep late gestational rise, independent of sex or mode of delivery. Am J Obstet Gynecol 1982;144:276.

92. Murphy BEP. Human fetal serum cortisol levels: a review. Endocr Rev 1983;4:150.

93. Murphy BEP, Clark SJ, Donald IR, et al. Conversion of maternal cortisol to cortisone during placental transfer to the human fetus. Am J Obstet Gynecol 1974;118:2.

94. Naaman E, Chatelain P, Saez JM, Durand P. In vitro effect of insulin and insulin-like growth factor I on cell multiplication and adrenocorticotrophin responsiveness of fetal adrenal cells. Biol Reprod 1989;40:570.

95. Nagata H, Hata K, Hata T, et al. Ultrasonographic measurements of fetal and neonatal adrenal glands. Acta Obstet Gynaecol Jpn 1987;30:486.

96. Nahoul K, Daffos F, Forestier F, Scholler R. Cortisol, cortisone and dehydroepiandrosterone sulfate levels in umbilical cord and maternal plasma between 21 and 30 weeks of pregnancy. J Steroid Biochem 1985;23:445.

97. Nelson HP, Kuhn RW, Deyman ME, Jaffe RB. Human fetal adrenal definitive and fetal zone metabolism of pregnenolone and corticosterone: alternate biosynthetic pathways and absence of detectable aldosterone biosynthesis. J Clin Endocrinol Metab 1990;70:693.

98. Neville AM, O'Hare MJ. The human adrenal cortex. Berlin: Springer-Verlag, 1982.

99. New MI, Lorenzen F, Lerner AJ, et al. Genotyping steroid 21-hydroxylase deficiency: hormonal reference data. J Clin Endocrinol Metab 1983;57:320.

100. Osathanondh R, Chopra IJ, Tulchinsky D. Effects of dexamethasone on fetal and maternal thyroxine, triiodothyronine, reverse triiodothyronine and thyrotropin levels. J Clin Endocrinol Metab 1978;47:1236.

101. Osathanondh R, Tulchinsky D, Kamali H, et al. Dexamethasone levels in treated pregnant women and newborn infants. J Pediatr 1977;90:617.

102. Pakravan P, Kenny FM, Depp R, Allen AC. Familial congenital absence of adrenal glands; evaluation of glucocorticoid, mineralocorticoid, and estrogen metabolism in the perinatal period. J Pediatr 1974;84:74.

103. Pang S, Lerner AJ, Stoner E, et al. Late-onset adrenal steroid 3β-hydroxysteroid dehydrogenase deficiency. I. A cause of hirsutism in pubertal and postpubertal women. J Clin Endocrinol Metab 1985;60:428.

104. Pang S, Murphey W, Levine LS, et al. A pilot newborn screening for congenital adrenal hyperplasia in Alaska. J Clin Endocrinol Metab 1982;55:413.

105. Parker CR Jr, Leveno K, Carr BR, et al. Umbilical cord plasma levels of dehydroepiandrosterone sulfate during human gestation. J Clin Endocrinol Metab 1982;54:1216.

106. Pasqualini JR, Nguyen BL, Uhrich F, et al. Cortisol and cortisone metabolism in the human foeto-placental unit at midgestation. J Steroid Biochem 1970;1:209.

107. Penhoat A, Chatelain PG, Jaillard C, Saez JM. Characterization of insulin-like growth factor I and insulin receptors on cultured bovine adrenal fasciculata cells. Role of these peptides on adrenal cell function. Endocrinology 1988;122:2518.

108. Pepe GJ, Albrecht ED. Regulation of the primate fetal adrenal cortex. Endocr Rev 1990;11:151.

109. Potter EL, Craig JM. Pathology of the fetus and infant, ed 3. Chicago: Year Book Medical Publications, 1975:15.

110. Price HV, Cone BA, Keogh M. Length of gestation in congenital adrenal hyperplasia. J Obstet Gynaecol Br Commonw 1971;78:430.

111. Rainey WE, Baird I, Mason JI, et al. Effects of transforming growth factor beta on ovine adrenocortical cells. Mol Cell Endocrinol 1988;60:189.

112. Riopel L, Branchaud CL, Goodyer CG, et al. Growth-inhibitory effect of TGF-β on human fetal adrenal cells in primary monolayer culture. J Cell Physiol 1989;140:233.

113. Riopel L, Branchaud CL, Goodyer CG, et al. Effect of placental factors on growth and function of the human fetal adrenal in vitro. Biol Reprod 1989;41:779.

114. Saksela E, Jaattela M. Tumor necrosis factor in the human fetoplacentary unit. Int J Dev Biol 1989;33:173.

115. Schulz DM, Giodano DA, Schulz DH. Weights of organs of fetuses and infants. Arch Pathol 1962;74:244.

116. Sen-Majumdar A, Murthy U, Das M. A new trophoblast-derived growth factor from human placenta. Purification and receptor identification. Biochemistry 1986;25:627.

117. Sen-Majumdar A, Murthy U, Dianese D, Das M. A specific antibody to a new peptide growth factor from human placenta: immunocytochemical studies on its location and biosynthesis. Biochemistry 1986;25:634.

118. Serra GB, Pérez-Palacios G, Jaffe RB. Enhancement of 3β-hydroxysteroid dehydrogenase-isomerase in the human fetal adrenal by removal of the soluble cell fraction. Biochem Biophys Acta 1971;244:186.

119. Serron-Ferre M, Hess DL, Lindholm U, Jaffe RB. Persistence of fetal zone function in the infant rhesus monkey adrenal gland. J Clin Endocrinol Metab 1986;62:460.

120. Silman RE, Chard T, Lowry PJ, et al. Human

121. Silman RE, Chard T, Lowry PJ, et al. Human fetal corticotrophin and related pituitary peptides. J Steroid Biochem 1977;8:553.

122. Simonian MH, Capp MW. Characterization of steroidogenesis in cell cultures of the human fetal adrenal cortex: comparison of definitive zone and fetal zone cells. J Clin Endocrinol Metab 1984;59:643.

123. Simonian MH, Capp MW, Templeman MC, Chang EC. Placental-derived mitogenic factor for human fetal adrenocortical cell cultures. In Vitro Cell Dev Biol 1987;23:57.

124. Simonian MH, Gill GN. Regulation of the fetal human adrenal cortex: effects of adrenocorticotropin on growth and function of monolayer cultures of fetal and definitive zone cells. Endocrinology 1981;108:1769.

125. Sippell WG, Becker H, Versmold HT, et al. Longitudinal studies of plasma aldosterone, corticosterone, deoxycorticosterone, progesterone, 17-hydroxyprogesterone, cortisol, and cortisone determined simultaneously in mother and child at birth and during the early neonatal period. I. Spontaneous delivery. J Clin Endocrinol Metab 1978;46:971.

126. Solomon S, Bird CE, Ling W, et al. Formation and metabolism of steroids in the fetus and placenta. Rec Prog Horm Res 1967;23:297.

127. Speiser PW, Laforgia N, Kato K, et al. First trimester prenatal treatment and molecular genetic diagnosis of congenital adrenal hyperplasia (21-hydroxylase deficiency). J Clin Endocrinol Metab 1990;70:838.

128. Spencer SJ, Rabinovici J, Jaffe RB. Human recombinant activin-A inhibits proliferation of human fetal adrenal cells in vitro. J Clin Endocrinol Metab 1990;71:1678.

129. Sperling MA, Wolfsen AR, Fisher DA. Congenital adrenal hypoplasia: an isolated defect of organogenesis. J Pediatr 1973;82:444.

130. Stromberg K, Pigott DA, Ranchalis JE, Twardzik DR. Human term placenta contains transforming growth factors. Biochem Biophys Res Comm 1982;106:354.

131. Thorburn GC. Hormonal control of parturition in the sheep and goat. Sem Perinatol 1978;2:235.

132. Tulchinsky D, Okada DM. Hormones in human pregnancy. IV. Plasma progesterone. Am J Obstet Gynecol 1975;121:293.

133. Ulick S, Eberlein WR, Bliffeld AR, et al. Evidence for an aldosterone biosynthetic defect in congenital adrenal hyperplasia. J Clin Endocrinol Metab 1980;51:1346.

134. Uotila UU. The early embryological development of the fetal and permanent adrenal cortex in man. Anat Rec 1940;76:183.

135. Van Hale HM, Turkel SB. Neuroblastoma and adrenal morphologic features in anencephalic infants. Arch Pathol Lab Med 1979;103:119.

136. Vaz Osorio R, Vilarinho L. Assessment of a trial screening program for congenital adrenal hyperplasia in Portugal based on an antibody-coated tube RIA for 17α-OH-progesterone. Clin Chem 1989;35:2338.

137. Villee DB. Effects of progesterone on enzyme activity of adrenals in organ culture. Adv Enz Reg 1966;4:269.

138. Villee DB. The development of steroidogenesis. Am J Med 1972;53:533.

139. Villee DB, Engel LL, Loring JM, Villee CA. Steroid hydroxylation in human fetal adrenal: formation of 16α-hydroxyprogesterone, 17-hydroxyprogesterone

foetal pituitary peptides and parturition. Nature 1976;260:716.

and deoxycorticosterone. Endocrinology 1961;69: 354.

140. Voutilainen R, Ilvesmaki V, Miettinen PJ. Low expression of 3β-hydroxy-5-ene steroid dehydrogenase gene in human fetal adrenals in vivo; adrenocorticotropin and protein kinase C-dependent regulation in adrenocortical cultures. J Clin Endocrinol Metab 1991;72:761.

141. Voutilainen R, Kahri AI. Placental origin of the suppression of 3β-hydroxysteroid dehydrogenase in the fetal zone cells of human fetal adrenals. J Steroid Biochem 1980;13:39.

142. Voutilainen R, Kahri AI, Salmenpera M. The effects of progesterone, pregnenolone, estriol, ACTH and hCG on steroid secretion of cultured human fetal adrenals. J Steroid Biochem 1979;10:695.

143. Voutilainen R, Miller WL. Developmental expression of genes for the steroidogenic enzymes P450scc (20,22-desmolase), P450c17 (17α-hydroxylase/17,20-lyase), and P450c21 (21-hydroxylase) in the human fetus. J Clin Endocrinol Metab 1986;63:1145.

144. Voutilainen R, Miller WL. Coordinate tropic hormone regulation of mRNAs for insulin-like growth factor II and the cholesterol side-chain-cleavage enzyme, P450ssc, in human steroidogenic tissues. Proc Nat Acad Sci USA 1987;84:1519.

145. Voutilainen R, Miller WL. Developmental and hormonal regulation of mRNAs for insulin-like growth factor II and steroidogenic enzymes in human fetal adrenals and gonads. DNA 1988;7:9.

146. Voutilainen R, Picado-Leonard J, DiBlasio AM, Miller WL. Hormonal and developmental regulation of adrenodoxin messenger ribonucleic acid in steroidogenic tissues. J Clin Endocrinol Metab 1988;66:383.

147. Waterman MR, Simpson ER. Regulation of the biosynthesis of cytochromes P450 involved in steroid hormone synthesis. Mol Cell Endocrinol 1985;39:81.

148. Wilburn LA, Goldsmith PC, Chang K-J, Jaffe RB. Ontogeny of enkephalin and catecholamine-synthesizing enzymes in the primate fetal adrenal medulla. J Clin Endocr Metab 1986;63:974.

149. Wilburn LA, Jaffe RB. Quantitative assessment of the ontogeny of met-enkephalin, norepinephrine and epinephrine in the human fetal adrenal medulla. Acta Endocrinol (Copenh) 1988;118:453.

150. Winter JSD. The adrenal cortex in the fetus and neonate. In: Anderson DC, Winter JSD, eds. The adrenal cortex. London: Butterworths, 1985:32.

151. Yanase T, Sanders D, Shibata A, et al. Combined 17α-hydroxylase/17,20-lyase deficiency due to a 7-base pair duplication in the N-terminal region of the cytochrome P450_{17α} (CYP17) gene. J Clin Endocrinol Metab 1990;70:1325.

152. Young MC, Laurence KM, Hughes IA. Relationship between fetal adrenal morphology and anterior pituitary function. Horm Res 1989;32:130.

CHAPTER 15

The Fetal Gonad and Sexual Differentiation

Lauri J. Pelliniemi

Martin Dym

The development of the genital system differs from that of other organs in that it has a duplicate regulatory system. Superimposed on the general temporally correlated differentiation are the separate mechanisms of sexual dimorphism (Fig. 15–1). In principle, the sex differentiation factors modify the basic processes and organize the development from a common and sexually indifferent primordium into two different organ systems, which in developmental disorders may manifest with different combinations of intermediate features.

The present state of research in sexual differentiation can be compared to a tunnel-digging project, in which geneticists and molecular biologists proceed in the analysis of the regulatory genes at one end, and embryologists and cell biologists at the other end describe the events of cell and tissue differentiation down to the macromolecular level. Considerable progress has been made in the characterization of genes for testicular differentiation.[45, 71, 77, 126] The gene for the testicular regulatory substance responsible for the regression of the paramesonephric (müllerian) ducts in the male has also been cloned and expressed.[15, 46, 54, 115] On the basis of the thoroughly covered morphologic and endocrinologic differentiation of the genital system,[7, 13, 26, 41, 85, 108, 114, 120, 142] cellular differentiation mechanisms are currently studied by analysis of cytoskeletal components and extracellular matrix[28, 91, 94, 95, 97, 111] with their connections and other cell adhesion systems, in the hope of eventually coordinating with the effects of the genetic regulatory factors approaching from the other end of the still incomplete tunnel.

DEVELOPMENT OF SEXUAL DIFFERENCES

Outline of Sexual Differentiation

Sexual differentiation is accomplished by the development of the reproductive system and sex-related organs from common indifferent primordia into different directions in males and females. The currently available information indicates that the female pattern is the basic type in mammalian sexual differentiation.[66] A male phenotype develops only on the additional effects of male organizing factors.

The sexual characteristics of a mature individual are a result of a series of successive developmental events that occur mainly in the prenatal period (Fig. 15–2). The gene guiding the gonadal sex differentiation into the male direction is most probably located in the Y chromosome.[77] The gene becomes activated in medullary cells of the male indifferent gonads, and consecutive biochemical and morphologic changes lead to differentiation of the testis. After gonadal differentiation in the male has taken place, the testicular hormones and effector substances regulate the subsequent steps of the sexual differentiation. Shortly after testicular differentiation, the Leydig cells appear and start androgen secretion, which induces the male type of differentiation in the mesonephric duct, the accessory sex glands, the external genitalia, and the neuroendocrine system. The female gonad lacking the male determining gene remains undifferentiated longer and then develops into an ovary under the control of female genes. The female genital tract, external genitalia, and neuroendocrine system differentiate according to the genetic sex without any known hormonal control from the ovary (see Figs. 15–1 and 15–2). The mesonephric duct in the female degenerates in the absence of testosterone. Another difference between the two sexes is in the initiation of meiosis, which in the ovary starts in the fourth fetal month and in the testis at puberty.

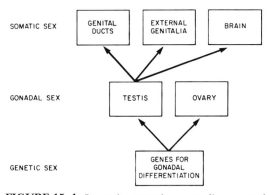

FIGURE 15–1. Successive stages in mammalian prenatal sex differentiation. The regulatory relationships are indicated by arrows. Note that testicular factors are responsible for male somatic differentiation, whereas the ovary has no known regulatory role.

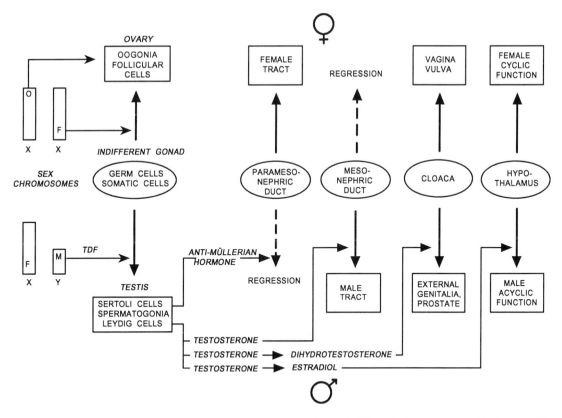

FIGURE 15–2. The proposed regulatory mechanisms in prenatal sexual differentiation as presented in the text. The indifferent stages are in the middle oval blocks. Female structures differentiate upward (thick arrows) and male structures downward (thick arrows). Regulatory factors and their source and target are indicated by thin arrows. Regression is indicated by dashed thick arrows. F-Gene for ovarian differentiation; M-gene for testicular differentiation; O-gene for further ovarian development; TDF-testis-determining factor.

Definition of Sex at Various Developmental Stages

In normal clinical practice, the sex of an individual is identified in the newborn according to the anatomy of the external genitalia. The neonate, however, already has developed through four different ontogenic stages of sex (see Fig. 15–1): (1) the genetic sex consisting of the genic sex as defined by the sex-determining genes and the chromosomal sex as defined by the sex chromosome complement; (2) the gonadal sex as defined by the structure and function of the gonads; (3) the somatic sex as defined by genital organs other than the gonads; and (4) the central nervous or neuroendocrine sex as defined by the cyclic or constant release of gonadotropin-releasing hormones, which in the human is most probably determined before birth (Table 15–1). In normal individuals, all four stages are of the same sex.

After birth, the sexual differentiation continues, and new stages appear, including (1) social sex, representing the way of rearing; (2) psychologic sex as expressed by the individual's own sex identity; (3) secondary sex characteristics developing at puberty; and (4) legal (official) sex. Thus a mature human has proceeded through at least eight stages of sex differentiation. Therefore in developmental disorders, the term *sex* should always be used in reference to a particular stage, e.g., gonadal sex, social sex.

GENETIC SEX

The genetic material of an individual is established by union of the haploid genomes of the ovum and the spermatozoon into a diploid ge-

TABLE 15–1. Definitions of Sex at Successive Prenatal and Perinatal Stages

Stage of Sex Differentiation	Definition of Sex	
	Male	*Female*
1. Genetic sex		
Chromosomal sex	XY sex chromosomes	XX sex chromosomes
Genic sex	TDF: regulatory gene for testicular differentiation in Y chromosome*	Postulated gene for ovarian differentiation*
2. Gonadal sex	Testis with testicular cords and interstitium	Ovary with follicles and primordial germ cells
3. Somatic sex		
Ducts and glands	Ductuli efferentes, epididymis, ductus deferens, vesicula seminalis, prostate	Oviduct, uterus, vagina
External genitalia	Penis and scrotum	Vulva
4. Neuroendocrine sex	Acyclic release of gonadotropins	Cyclic release of gonadotropins

A hypothesis is not yet fully established.

nome of the zygote. Because the oocyte always has an X chromosome, the sex of the zygote is determined by the male gamete bearing either an X or a Y chromosome. The genetic material guiding the sexual differentiation in the male direction is located in the Y chromosome. Before gonadal sex differentiation in the seventh week, the sex chromosomes and their sex-determining genes provide the only criterion for sex identification, and they are collectively referred to as *genetic sex*. Routine clinical laboratory methods are currently available for the identification of sex chromosomes but not for sex-determining genes. The genetic sex can be investigated by DNA hybridization and nucleotide sequence analysis in some research laboratories.

Chromosomal Sex

There are two different methods of identifying the chromosomal sex. Counting of X and Y chromatin bodies in interphase cell nuclei provides a fast and inexpensive means of preliminary screening for sex chromosome anomalies. Complete chromosome analysis is the second and more accurate method in which the actual mitotic metaphase chromosomes are visualized, allowing a detailed morphologic analysis of the whole chromosomal complement down to specific regions of the sex chromosomes.

X Chromatin

The inactive X chromosome[87] is attached to the inner surface of the nuclear envelope as a heterochromatic body,[4] also known as the Barr body or sex chromatin body. This structure can be visualized in many somatic interphase cells; counting of these bodies has been widely used to determine the number of X chromosomes in various cells.

Y Chromatin

The Y chromosome in interphase cells does not bind the ordinary sex chromatin stains. Caspersson et al.[14] developed the binding technique using quinacrine fluorescence, which binds actively to the long arm of the Y chromosome. When applied to human interphase leukocytes, an intense fluorescent spot (Y body, F body) representing the Y chromosome was noted in the male cells.[99] The number of Y chromatin bodies matches the number of Y chromosomes in the cell. Because the method of analyzing the sex chromosomal status of a human patient by counting nuclear chromatin bodies has several inherent pitfalls, however,[89, 134] the results should always be confirmed by a complete chromosome analysis.

Chromosome Analysis

A direct and accurate method of identifying the chromosomal sex is through a complete analysis of metaphase chromosomes from cultured leukocytes or fibroblasts. If fetal tissue is available, a direct method not requiring culture for trapping cells at mitotic metaphase can be used.[112] The main indications for chromosome analysis are antenatal sex identification and postnatal diagnosis of disorders of sex differentiation.

Sex-Determining Genes

Genes for Testicular Differentiation

The genetic factor guiding sexual differentiation into the male direction is located in the Y chromosome.[140] Considering the complexity of the sex differentiation process, it is evident that several genes located in different chromosomes are involved[105] (Table 15–2). The present information suggests that the testis-organizing gene is located in the short arm of the Y chromosome and codes a DNA-binding protein, which works as a transcription factor for other genes involved.[77] The X chromosome probably contains the genes for ovarian differentiation and further development (see Fig. 15–2).

The search for the testis-determining factor (TDF) has proceeded through the histocompatibility-Y (H-Y) antigen and a zinc finger protein down to a 35-kb sequence, which is the most promising candidate for the TDF.[77, 79] The first experimental proof is male development of chromosomally female mice made transgenic for DNA from the TDF region.[71] The nature and location of other possible genes for gonadal sex differentiation remain to be determined. New regulators may be found from the mechanisms of parental genomic imprinting, which theoretically would be suitable for the regulation of sexual differences at all developmental stages.[82, 133]

The disorders resulting in the failure of the testicular differentiation genes to act in the proper place and at the proper time are characterized by differentiation of the gonads in the female direction.[55, 56] The resulting lack of testicular androgens and antimüllerian hormone allows other genital organs and sex-related structures and functions to develop as in the female.

Gene for Testosterone Receptor

A second gene involved in male sexual differentiation codes the receptor for testosterone (see Table 15–2). Mutation of this gene to an inactive form causes the testicular feminization (TF) syndrome. It is therefore referred to as the TF gene. It is located in the X chromosome and is transmitted through heterozygous mothers to half of the 46,XY offspring.[80]

A third group of genes that code for the enzymes involved in the sex steroid synthesis pathway becomes activated after gonadal differentiation (see Table 15–2). Mutations in the genes for these enzymes may cause excessive androgen production in the female or deficient androgen production in the male and result in respective anomalies in sexual differentiation, as is discussed later. Several other unidentified genes are involved in various stages of sexual differentiation, as demonstrated by the great variety of disorders of which the cause still remains unknown.

Direct methods for analyzing sex differentiation–linked genes are now available.[56, 90]

INDIFFERENT STAGES OF GONADS

The mammalian gonad is composed of two original components: the primordial germ cells and the somatic cells of the anterior part of the mesonephros (see Fig. 15–2; Fig. 15–3). The primordial germ cells are first seen in the yolk sac wall, and in the fourth week, they start their migration into the gonadal ridge via the hindgut mesentery.[144] They move actively with pseudopods and divide mitotically during the migration. They contain alkaline phosphatase that has been used as a histochemical marker enzyme for their identification. Individual cells take different routes and are possibly guided by a substance emitted from the gonadal ridge. Some primordial germ cells migrate away from the gonads, and they are regarded as possible origins of germinal neoplasms in different parts of the body.[27]

The gonadal ridge is a derivative of the splanchnic mesoderm of the anterior mesonephric surface. The first sign of gonadal development is columnar elongation of the superficial cells in the fifth week. Concomitantly the subjacent mesenchyme condenses, and as a result the early gonadal primordium becomes evident as a longitudinal thickening on the mesonephros (see Fig. 15–3). The superficial as well as the mesenchymal cells prolifer-

TABLE 15–2. Genes Apparently Involved in Prenatal Sexual Differentiation

Gene(s) for	Probable Location in Chromosomes	Site of Expression	Target of Product	Action of Product	Proposed Regulator (R) or Inducer (I) of Gene(s)
TDF	Y chromosome short arm	Male gonadal cells	Regulatory elements of male structural genes	Transcription factor for testicular cord formation genes	—
		Female cells in general	Male and female cells in general	H–Y antigen among other proteins	
Steroid synthesis enzymes	—*	Testicular Leydig cells, ovarian cells	Steroid synthesis	Steroid synthesis	hCG (R)
Testosterone receptor	X chromosome	Testosterone target tissues	Testosterone	Binding to testosterone and then to regulatory elements of genes	—
5α-reductase	—	Dihydrotestosterone target tissues	Testosterone	Conversion of testosterone to dihydrotestosterone	—
hCG	—	Placental trophoblast	Testicular Leydig cells	Stimulation of androgen synthesis	—
			Gubernaculum testis	Testicular descent	—
hCG receptor	—	Testicular Leydig cells	Membrane of testicular Leydig cells	Signal initiation by binding of hCG into receptor membrane	—
		Gubernaculum testis	—	—	—
Initial ovarian differentiation	X chromosome	Ovarian cells	Ovarian cells	Ovarian cord, cluster, and follicle formation	—
Further ovarian development	X chromosome	Ovarian cells	Follicles	Follicle maintenance and growth	—
Antimüllerian hormone	Chromosome 19 short arm	Testicular Sertoli cells	Male paramesonephric duct	Regression of the duct	—
Meiosis-preventing substance	—	Testicular Sertoli cells	Spermatogonia	Inhibition of meiosis	—
Meiosis-inducing substance	—	Ovarian rete cells	Oogonia	Initiation of meiosis	—

No data available.

ate actively and via epithelial differentiation organize as the surface epithelium and the primitive gonadal cords.[28, 101]

The primordial germ cells arrive in the gonadal ridge in the sixth week and migrate into the epithelial cords and into the surface epithelium.[103] The mechanism of recognition between the germ and epithelial cells is not known. Apparently specific cell surface components are responsible for guiding the migration and for identifying the final goal. The gonadal ridge grows rapidly in thickness and becomes roughly spherical in cross section. The growing primitive cords provide the interior of the gonad with unorganized cells that form a dense cellular mass called *gonadal blastema* when mixed with mesenchymal cells and primordial germ cells. Basement membrane starts to form around the cords, and concomitant changes take place in the cytoskeletal organization of their cytoplasm as shown in rats.[28] The indifferent gonad immediately be-fore its differentiation into testis or ovary is composed of three histologic components: the surface epithelium, the primitive cords continuous with the epithelium, and the gonadal blastema (see Fig. 15–3).

TESTIS

Histologic Differentiation

Sexual differentiation of the male gonad starts in the seventh week by organization of the gonadal blastema into the testicular cords and interstitium.[57, 136, 142] The process involves embedding the primordial germ cells into the prospective testicular cords and the completion of the synthesis and apposition of a basal lamina to surround the developing testicular cords (see Fig. 15–3), as studied by immunocytochemistry in rats.[28, 97, 111] The early interstitium contains loosely packed, undifferentiated

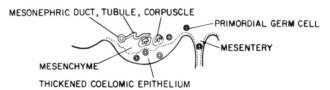

GONADAL RIDGE 5 WEEKS

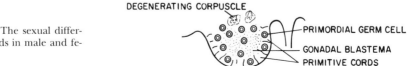

INDIFFERENT GONAD 6 WEEKS

FIGURE 15–3. The sexual differentiation of gonads in male and female. See text.

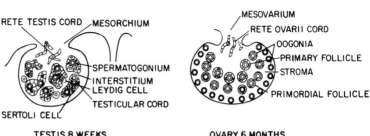

TESTIS 8 WEEKS

OVARY 6 MONTHS

mesenchymal cells and blood vessels[102, 110] embedded in a matrix containing types I and III collagen as shown in rats.[91] The connections between the columnar surface epithelium and the gonadal cords disappear, and mesenchyme underlying the surface epithelium differentiates into fibroblasts to form the tunica albuginea. The testicular cords are composed of primitive Sertoli cells and spermatogonia.[100] The shape of the cords is irregular, and they are randomly organized in the early testis. The fetal Sertoli cells contain both cytokeratin and vimentin intermediate filaments as shown in men[128] and rats.[28, 95]

Regulation of Testicular Differentiation

The process of reorganization of gonadal cell components is the first and decisive step in the male differentiation of the embryonic gonad and is most probably regulated by the sex-determining genes associated in mammals with the Y chromosome (see Table 15–2; Table 15–3). Several hypotheses about the regulatory

mechanisms have been proposed in the past, as reviewed by Jost and associates.[63–66] A model based on cattle gonads was presented by Ohno[86] involving the formation of indifferent common blastema that organized into testicular or ovarian components. This model fits fairly well with the observations in humans, as described, and basically also with pigs.[104]

The role of the primordial germ cells in the regulation of gonadal differentiation has been a matter of controversy. Experimental evidence in mutant mice suggests strongly that the primordial germ cells do not have a regulatory role.[78, 86] The best candidate for the TDF is the as yet uncharacterized protein coded by the sex-determining region of the Y chromosome (SRY), as described earlier.[77, 79]

Development of Interstitium

The second step in testicular differentiation is the appearance of the Leydig cells by the end of the eighth week (see Fig. 15–3 and Table 15–3). They contain 3β-hydroxysteroid dehydrogenase,[84] and ultrastructurally they

TABLE 15–3. Gonadal Sex Differentiation: Appearance of Sexual Differences in Prenatal Male and Female Gonads

Male	Proposed Regulator	Age	Female	Proposed Regulator
Organization of testicular cords and interstitium	TDF	6 wk		
Appearance of Leydig cells	—*	7 wk	Organization of medullary cords	—
Appearance of enzymes for steroid synthesis	—		Appearance of enzymes for steroid synthesis†	—
Appearance of hCG receptors	—			
Initiation of androgen secretion and elevation of serum levels	—		Initiation of estrogen synthesis but no elevated serum levels†	—
Initiation of antimüllerian hormone secretion by Sertoli cells	—	8 wk	Ability to convert androgens to estrogens	—
Cessation of spermatogonial mitoses and no initiation of meiosis	Meiosis-preventing substance	12 wk	Initiation of oogonial meiosis	Meiosis-inducing substance
			Medullary cords degenerated	
			Appearance of interstitial cells	
		4 mo	Appearance of primordial follicles	—
Testicular descent starts	hCG	6 mo	Appearance of primary follicles	—
		8 mo	All oogonia differentiated into primary oocytes in resting dictyotene stage of meiotic division	
Testes descended into inguinal canal or into scrotum	hCG	9 mo		

No data available.
†Results in rabbits, as mentioned in text.

have the characteristics of steroid-secreting cells with extensive agranular endoplasmic reticulum.[106, 110] The Leydig cells start almost immediately to synthesize androgens,[121, 124] and the concentrations of testosterone in testicular tissue,[50, 130] in blood, and in the amniotic fluid begin to rise, reaching a maximum of 3 μg/L

in fetal serum by the 15th to 18th week (Fig. 15–4). The rise in testosterone synthesis results from an increase in the amount of Leydig cells, from undetectable numbers at 7 weeks to 50% of the relative tissue area at 14 weeks.[84] During subsequent weeks, the number of Leydig cells decreases, and only a few are seen at

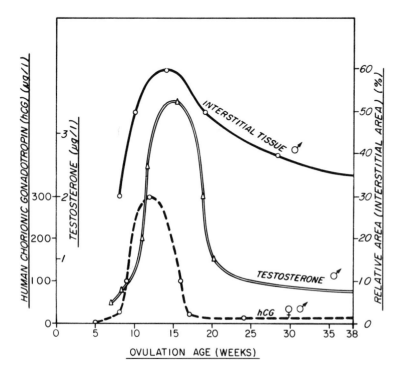

FIGURE 15–4. Summary of hormone concentrations in serum and histologic development of interstitial tissue in the testis. The left ordinate shows testosterone in male fetuses, and hCG, which is similar in both sexes, according to Clements et al[18] and Winter et al.[143] The right ordinate shows the relative area occupied by interstitial tissue when measured on tissue sections as percent of the total tissue area.[84]

birth. Concomitantly the testosterone levels decrease to about 0.7 μg/L in serum at birth.[67] A clinically interesting feature is that the difference in testosterone levels in serum and amniotic fluid between male and female fetuses persists until birth[24] and can therefore be used for fetal sex identification.

Regulation of Leydig Cell Differentiation

The Leydig cells probably originate from the undifferentiated mesenchymal cells in the interstitium.[17, 110] The mechanism of their differentiation is not known, but the rise in human chorionic gonadotropin (hCG) preceding the first appearance of the Leydig cells (see Fig. 15–4) and the later decrease of hCG, which is followed by involution of Leydig cells, suggest that hCG is the hormone that triggers the differentiation of the mesenchymal cells into Leydig cells.[110] Moreover, the presence of hCG in testis[52] and hCG receptor in fetal Leydig cells supports a proposed regulatory role for this hormone.[16, 51] Experimental evidence of adenylate cyclase activity suggests that the onset of testosterone production is independent of gonadotropin control.[145] In rabbit Leydig cells, the enzymatic activities necessary for testosterone synthesis appear before the responsiveness to hCG stimulation becomes established.[30] This suggests that the initiation of androgen synthesis, at least in the rabbit, is independent of extragonadal hormone stimulation. The regulatory mechanism for the initiation of androgen synthesis is not yet known. After its initiation, testosterone synthesis is apparently regulated by hCG.[51] Luteinizing hormone (LH) is unlikely to play a major role because LH and follicle-stimulating hormone (FSH) are not detectable in blood before the 10th week.[67]

Development of Testicular Cords

In the fetal period, the testicular cords grow in length and become circular in cross section. In the fourth month of fetal life, the convoluted cords are organized into anastomosing loops, the ends joining the rete cords and the arch facing toward the testicular surface. The cords remain without a lumen throughout the fetal period.

The fetal Sertoli cells multiply during growth of the cords until they constitute the majority of the cord cells. The cells contacting the basal lamina are columnar, whereas those in the middle of the cord are spherical or irregular in shape. The nucleus is irregular or elongated, sometimes indented, and contains one to three small nucleoli. In contrast to the spermatogonia, the Sertoli cells are rich in organelles. They contain elongated mitochondria with transverse cristae, free ribosomes, and granular endoplasmic reticulum. Agranular reticulum typical for steroid-secreting cells has not been found in fetal Sertoli cells.[100] Cytoskeletal organization follows the histologic changes as shown in rats.[95]

There has been only sparse information about the functions of Sertoli cells in the prenatal period. The observation of Picon[116] that testicular tissue in organ culture induces the physiologic degeneration of the paramesonephric (müllerian) ducts has predicated an important regulatory role for the fetal Sertoli cell.[54, 62, 66] The Sertoli cells secrete a substance called *antimüllerian hormone* or *müllerian inhibiting substance*. This constitutes the third major difference between the two sexes in gonadal differentiation (see Table 15–3).

Biochemical characterization of bovine antimüllerian hormone indicates that it is a glycoprotein; a molecular weight of 140 k was obtained by gel electrophoresis for unreduced and that of 70 k for reduced protein.[54] The human protein has not yet been purified. The hormone appears at 7 weeks and is also present in postnatal testis and ovary. The genes of human and bovine hormone have been cloned and sequenced. The human gene is translated as a precursor of 560 amino acids with a calculated molecular weight of 57 k.[54] The human gene has been localized in the tip of the short arm of chromosome 19.[62] The transcription of the human gene in fetal testis is greatly stimulated by cyclic adenosine monophosphate (cAMP) but not with gonadotropins, whereas that in adult granulosa cells was stimulated by cAMP and hCG, but not by FSH.[137] Ultrastructurally the fetal Sertoli cells have all the protein synthesis organelles, but presence of secretory granules has not been reported.[34, 100]

Sertoli cells apparently have a supporting function for the maintenance and development of the spermatogonia because the germ cells that remain outside the testicular cords degenerate rapidly. Ultrastructurally the Sertoli cells show evidence of phagocytic activity and are probably responsible for clearing the cords of degenerated germ cells.[39] It is also suggested that the Sertoli cells inhibit the onset of meiosis of the spermatogonia in the fetal testis.[65] These data suggest that fetal Sertoli cells probably have several important functions that are not yet fully understood.

The fetal spermatogonia are located in the cords among the fetal Sertoli cells (see Fig. 15–3). Some of them settle on the basal lamina at 14 weeks. The germ cells have been called gonocytes before entering the periphery of the cord and prespermatogonia when in the periphery resting on the basal lamina.[29, 34] The fetal spermatogonia are large and roughly spherical cells with a round nucleus and a prominent nucleolus.[25, 100] The cytoplasm appears pale owing to the scarcity of organelles. Some spherical mitochondria, free polysomes, granular endoplasmic reticulum, and a Golgi complex, however, can be found. Intercellular bridges between pairs of peripheral spermatogonia are seen at 12 weeks.[139] A portion of the spermatogonia undergoes degeneration during the fetal period, and these are phagocytosed by Sertoli cells.[39]

A remarkable feature of the male fetal germ cells is that they do not start their meiotic division before puberty, whereas in the female germ cells, meiosis starts in the fourth fetal month. In addition to the histologic organization of cords and interstitium, steroid synthesis, and antimüllerian hormone synthesis, the onset of meiosis is the fourth major difference between the two sexes in gonadal differentiation (see Table 15–3). Because the female developmental pattern is dominant in mammalian sex differentiation, there apparently must be a mechanism preventing the male germ cells from initiating meiosis.[63] Experimental evidence in mice suggests that the rete testis secretes a meiosis-inducing substance, and the other part of the testis, probably Sertoli cells,[65]

secretes a meiosis-preventing substance.[11, 12] Human spermatogonia cease their mitotic activity at approximately the same time as the oogonia enter the meiotic prophase.[39] This could indicate that the inhibitory mechanism would prevent any type of prophase in spermatogonia.[132] Steroid hormones may also have a role in the prevention of germ cell meiosis.[12]

Growth and Descent of Testis

After sexual differentiation, the fetal testis acquires the shape of an adult testis and grows from about 20 mg at 14 weeks[136] to about 850 mg at birth.[1] The testicles start to descend into the inguinal canal at 6 months, followed by the epididymis and the adjacent ductus deferens (see Table 15–3). They enter the scrotal swellings shortly before birth. On the basis of observations in human patients and animal experiments, there are different interpretations that gonadotropin, luteinizing hormone–releasing hormone (LH-RH), Leydig cells, and antimüllerian hormone regulate the testicular descent.[49, 53, 141] Treatment with chorionic gonadotropin or LH-RH has been successful in bringing about testicular descent.

OVARY

Histologic Differentiation

The indifferent gonadal stage persists longer in the female than in the male (see Table 15–3). The spade-shaped cross section and crenated surface are characteristic of the ovary in the seventh week.[136] The medullary gonadal blastema begins to differentiate into medullary cords and interstitium in the eighth week.[58, 114] Primordial germ cells stay with the cord cells and are thereafter called *oogonia*. The medullary cords are actually irregular groups of cells that subsequently degenerate, leaving scattered groups of cells in the hilar region representing the prospective rete ovarii. By the end of the 12th week, the medulla consists predominantly of connective tissue.

The cortical layers of the early ovary consist of surface epithelium with individual small oogonia; by the 11th week, clusters of large, mitotically dividing oogonia surrounded by cord cells appear deeper in the cortex.[38] Thin incomplete septa of interstitial connective tissue intervene among the epithelial clusters.

Regulation of Ovarian Differentiation

Theories about gonadal sex differentiation propose that the X chromosome carries a gene for ovarian differentiation. It is somehow linked to the testis-organizing gene, so the ovary gene can act only if the testis gene is not active. For the primary differentiation of the ovary, only one gene and one X chromosome are necessary in humans (see Fig. 15–2). The ovary of 45,X individuals, however, degenerates before birth, indicating that a second gene and X chromosome are necessary for further development. It is of interest that 39,X female mice are fertile, which demonstrates a great variability in the regulatory mechanism. Information about the nature of this gene and its regulation, products, and site of action is not available.

Development of Follicles and Ova

The ovarian cortex begins to thicken at 3 months as a result of increased mitotic activity of the primitive granulosa cells and of the oogonia.[117] Simultaneously the large oogonia in the deepest layer of the cortex enter the prophase of their first meiotic division (see Table 15–3).[114] Both X chromosomes are apparently active in the germ cells before entering meiosis.[81] Maturation proceeds gradually toward the superficial layers. After the diplotene stage, the first meiotic division stops, and the chromosomes enter a resting dictyotene stage. The first meiotic division that started in the fetus is continued and completed just before ovulation in the adult.[87] All oogonia enter the dictyotene stage and become primary oocytes by the ninth fetal month. A considerable number of germ cells degenerates during the maturation period, reaching a peak between 16 and 20 weeks.[38] The remains of the degenerated cells undergo phagocytosis by the granulosa cells.

Primordial follicles appear in the fifth month. They are composed of one oocyte surrounded by a single layer of squamous epithelial cells. In the seventh month, the follicular epithelium in the deep cortical layer becomes cuboidal, and stroma-derived cells make up the theca layer around the primary follicle (see Fig. 15–3). At birth, the superficial cortical layer still contains many primordial follicles, and occasional atretic follicles are encountered in the medulla.

Regulation of Meiosis

The initiation of meiosis in female fetuses is the fourth major sexual difference in fetal gonads, as noted (see Table 15–3). Experimental evidence in mice suggests that the rete tissue in the hilar region of the ovary secretes a meiosis-inducing substance that is responsible for the initiation of oogonial meiosis.[11] This substance is also believed to induce male germ cells to enter meiosis in vitro. The inducing substance is thought to be produced in the rete region by cells derived from the mesonephros.[12] These results also suggest that the meiosis-inducing effect is independent of steroid hormones. An understanding of the mechanisms regulating meiotic divisions in both sexes could provide effective reversible and physiologic methods for fertility control, especially for the male, whose germ cells undergo meiosis in every spermatogenic cycle. Human studies are not yet available, and much more experimental work remains to be done before practical applications become feasible.

Development of Stroma

The connective tissue of the medulla is contiguous with the interstitial tissue of the cortex (see Table 15–3).[91] Together they are referred to as ovarian stroma. By the end of the third month, the stromal development starts at sites below the surface epithelium. Epitheliocortical connections are maintained between the stromal areas throughout the fetal period, and the proper ovarian tunica albuginea develops in the perinatal period.

From the fetal age of 3 months, the stroma

contains solitary interstitial cells that have abundant agranular endoplasmic reticulum and are ultrastructurally similar to the testicular Leydig cells.[23, 40] Their significance is not known. The fetal ovary is not able to synthesize testosterone during the first half of pregnancy,[124] therefore the testis is the only significant source for androgens during sexual differentiation of the genital organs. Human ovaries are able to convert androgens to estrogens from the fetal age of 8 weeks.[32] Estrogen formation was undetectable in testes at all stages. Estrogen content of the rabbit ovary started to rise at the same time as testosterone did in the testis.[31] In contrast to testosterone, however, elevated serum estrogen levels were not observed. This suggests that the estrogens may act locally within the gonad, stimulating follicle development.

The shape of the ovary remains elongated, and the cross section is spade shaped throughout the whole fetal period. The ovary weighs about 16 mg at 14 weeks[136] and grows to about 330 mg at birth. Ovaries descend during the 12th week into the minor pelvis and occupy a transverse position. Various aspects of ovarian development have been covered in several books and review articles.[35, 48, 59, 83, 113, 114]

GONADAL DUCTS

In the sequence of sexual differentiation, the gonadal ducts represent a part of the somatic sex (see Fig. 15–1). The female ducts differentiate autonomously without any known gonadal or other regulatory factors (see Fig. 15–2). In contrast, the male differentiation of the ducts is regulated by testicular androgens and antimüllerian hormone.

Differentiation of Mesonephric (Wolffian) Ducts

The uropoietic system provides the male gonad with the excurrent ducts and associated glands. Above the testis, the mesonephric duct and tubules degenerate. In the sixth week, the testicular rete cords and adjacent mesonephric tubules grow together, and the tubuli become the ductuli efferentes. The testicular end of the mesonephric duct differentiates into the epididymis,[107, 109] and the rest becomes ductus deferens. Seminal vesicles develop as buds from the distal part of the mesonephric duct, and the end becomes the ejaculatory duct.

Extensive experimental evidence (Fig. 15–5) shows that testosterone from the fetal testis is the factor inducing the development of male derivatives of the mesonephric duct.[66, 109, 124] Without proper exposure to testosterone, the mesonephric duct, even if genetically male, degenerates by the end of the fourth month (see Fig. 15–2) as it normally does in the female. Cytologic details of these processes in humans are unknown, but in the rat the changes in the extracellular matrix, basement membrane, and cytoskeletal elements have been studied by immunocytochemistry and electron microscopy.[92, 93, 96, 98]

Differentiation of Paramesonephric (Müllerian) Ducts

The paramesonephric duct is a derivative of the coelomic splanchnopleure adjacent and lateral to the mesonephric duct. In the female, it becomes the genital tract: the oviduct, uterus, and proximal vagina. In the male, the duct degenerates by the end of the second month.[72, 119, 129]

The bulk of the present information about regulation of the paramesonephric duct comes from the laboratories of Jost,[66] Josso et al.,[62] and Hutson et al.[54] The normal differentiation in the female is independent of the gonads and steroid hormones and apparently autonomous (see Fig. 15–5). The regression in the male is induced by the Sertoli cell–secreted glycoprotein called antimüllerian hormone,[62] or müllerian inhibiting substance.[119] The genetically female duct reacts to the hormone in the same way as does the male. The hormone is apparently transmitted through diffusion because it affects only the ipsilateral duct. The duct is responsive to the antimüllerian hormone only during a short period before 8 weeks. The mechanism of action of the hormone is not yet fully understood. Present evidence suggests that antimüllerian hormone acts by blocking phosphorylation of tyrosine

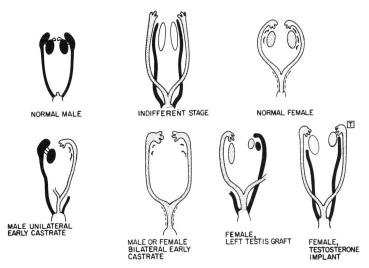

FIGURE 15–5. Relationships of the testis (black) and ovary (stippled) to the differentiation of the mesonephric (black) and paramesonephric (stippled) ducts in normal and experimental conditions, according to Jost.[63] Unilateral early castration in the male demonstrates that on the contralateral side the testicular testosterone has a partial effect in preserving the mesonephric duct, whereas the contralateral paramesonephric duct remains uninhibited. Early bilateral castration in either sex results in female differentiation of the genital organs. A testis grafted into the female tract causes local inhibition of the paramesonephric duct and persistence of the mesonephric duct. Unilateral implantation of a testosterone crystal (T) into the female tract causes almost complete persistence of the mesonephric ducts but has no effect on the paramesonephric ducts.

on membrane proteins.[54] The high molecular weight of approximately 140 k suggests a mechanism in which the effect is mediated through a receptor on the cell membrane of the duct epithelial cells.

UROGENITAL SINUS AND EXTERNAL GENITALIA

The distal parts of the genital tract in both sexes differentiate from the same primordia as do the urinary organs. Again, female differentiation occurs in both genetically male or female organs, regardless of the presence of ovary, as long as testosterone is not present (see Fig. 15–2). Under the influence of testosterone,[69] the prostate gland differentiates as a derivative of the vesicourethral canal, starting with the differentiation of the periurethral mesenchyme in the ninth week.[68, 69] The fusion of the urogenital folds and growth of the genital tubercle complete the male differentiation of the urogenital tract (Fig. 15–6). Testosterone is readily converted into 5α-dihydrotestosterone by the cells of the differentiating urogenital sinus, suggesting that dihydrotestosterone is the effective intracellular androgen.

The sex of the newborn is identified according to the appearance of the external genitalia. Any abnormality in the anatomy of the external genitalia is an indication for complete investigation of the status of all genital organs and analysis of the genetic sex. Early diagnosis can often prevent problems that would otherwise arise at a later stage of development. A summary of the male and female derivatives in the genital system is presented in Table 15–4.

CENTRAL NERVOUS SYSTEM

The irreversible inhibition of cyclic hypothalamic control of gonadotropin release in female rats by testosterone administration in the early postnatal period indicates that androgens are also responsible for sexual differentiation of the central nervous system.[75] It has been shown that the hypothalamus of human fetuses and several animal species is capable of aromatizing androgens to estrogens.[64] Estrogens are even more potent than testosterone in masculinizing the brain. In the female rat, the circulating estrogens have a high affinity for α-fetoprotein in blood,[75] and this may be a general mechanism to render the hormones ineffective. It has been suggested that estro-

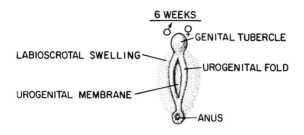

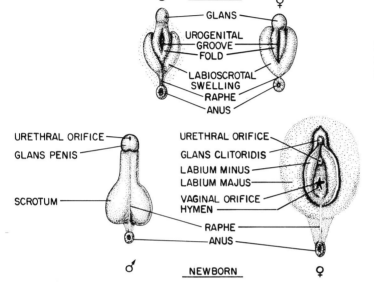

FIGURE 15–6. Development and differentiation of male and female external genitalia.

TABLE 15–4. Developmental Derivatives of the Indifferent Primordia of the Genital System in Male and Female

Male	Indifferent Stage	Female
Testis	Indifferent gonad	Ovary
Spermatogonia	Primordial germ cells	Oogonia
Sertoli cells	Gonadal blastema	Follicular cells
Leydig cells		Theca cells
Rete testis	Gonadal blastema and/or mesonephric tubules	Rete ovarii
Tunica albuginea	Coelomic epithelium	Surface epithelium
Ductuli efferentes	Mesonephric tubules	Epoophoron*
Ductuli aberrantes*		Paroophoron*
Paradidymis*		
Appendix of epididymis*	Mesonephric duct (wolffian)	Vesicular appendage*
Epididymis		Duct of epoophoron*
Ductus deferens		Gartner duct*
Seminal vesicle		
Ejaculatory duct		
Appendage testis*	Paramesonephric duct (müllerian)	Oviduct
Utriculus prostaticus?*		Uterus
		Proximal vagina
Penis	Genital tubercle and urogenital folds	Clitoris
		Labia minora
Scrotum	Labioscrotal swellings	Labia majora
Urethra (in part)	Urogenital sinus	Distal vagina
Prostate		Vestibule

Vestigial structures.

gens in the rat would have an effect on the patterning of critical neuronal circuitry in the developing brain.[76] The synaptic connections established in the presence of estrogens would then be responsible for the acyclic mode of gonadotropin release in the male. Apparently these mechanisms are functional also in humans, in whom masculinization of the brain seems to take place before birth, and behavioral and temperamental sex differences appear to be modified by prenatal sex hormones.[22] The importance of the preterm hormonal activities is supported by high serum FSH and LH in premature girls and high serum testosterone in premature boys.[131]

DISORDERS OF SEXUAL DIFFERENTIATION

A cause for a disorder in sexual differentiation can often be traced to the gene level. A specific gene can be absent, multiple, modified functionally, or translocated, and the type of the gene's abnormality determines where and when primary phenotypic disorders manifest. The primary disorder may cause secondary disorders if it affects a regulatory function at a later differentiation stage.

Chromosome analysis with various banding techniques to reveal structural aberrations is the basic tool for the identification of the genetic sex. At present, several individual genes can be analyzed by methods of gene technology, and the diagnosis is based on disorders in the gene, the RNA, and the protein at the posttranslational level. The presence of the apparent testis-determining gene can be shown by DNA-hybridization tests.[5, 56, 90]

An extragenital hormone is present in several enzyme defects of the adrenal cells and in some hormone-producing tumors. The developing organism may also be exposed to teratogenic drugs[3, 129] given to the mother or to radiation during the critical period, resulting in developmental defects in the fetus.

The patients and their detailed medical records are indispensable for research into the mechanisms of human development. Disorders of human sexual differentiation (Table 15–5) can be classified and presented in var-

ious ways, as indicated in the literature.[36, 37, 41, 43, 60, 118, 125] We emphasize the regulatory relationships and advances in our understanding of the complex malformation syndromes.

Gonadal Agenesis

Total absence of one or both gonads is a rare anomaly, usually combined with the absence of the renal system on the affected side that suggests a major defect in the early development of the nephrogenic mesenchyme.[122] The gonadal ducts and external genitalia are rudimentary.[125] Either the gonads have never developed, or they may have degenerated at an early stage, as suggested by some variation in the degree of differentiation of the external genitalia. The cause is unknown, but a polygenic defect or a teratologic agent are the most plausible explanations.

Gonadal Dysgenesis with Normal Karyotype

Streak gonads, containing only fibrous stromal tissue, and a female hypoplastic genital system are sometimes associated with 46,XX or 46,XY karyotype in persons having no other Turner stigmata.[138] It is of interest that a patient with XY gonadal dysgenesis has now been found to have a frame shift mutation in the candidate testis-determining gene.[56] She had a streak with no signs of malignancy. The most plausible explanation is that the modified gene was not able to organize a testis and that more than one gene is required for a complete morphogenesis. Unfortunately, data of the gonadal differentiation in the embryonic period are not available. Therefore the possibility of proper initial differentiation and subsequent degeneration of the gonads at a later stage, which happens in the 45,X females, cannot be ruled out.

Chromosomal Abnormalities

46,XX Males

Phenotypically male individuals with a female chromosome complement are rare, and the reported cases deal mainly with adults. These

TABLE 15–5. Comparative Summary of Disorders of Sexual Differentiation

Disorder	Chromosomes	Genes	Gonads	Ducts	External Genitalia	Hormones	Cause
Gonadal agenesis	Majority 46,XY	—*	Absent	Rudimentary; ambiguous	Small; ambiguous	—	Polygenic defect or teratogen†
Gonadal dysgenesis with normal karyotype	46,XY	TDF mutation in one patient	Streak, or degenerated testis, tumors	Immature female	Female, may be clitoral enlargement	Elevated gonadotropins	Mutant gene, frame shift in one patient†
	46,XX	—	Streak	Immature female	Female	Elevated gonadotropins	Mutant gene†
46,XX males	46,XX	TDF translocated from Y	Small testes	Male	Male, but small	Testosterone low, gonadotropins normal or elevated	Gene translocation, mutation, mosaicism, or chimerism†
Turner's syndrome	45,X	Deficiency of gene for further ovarian development†	Streak	Hypoplastic female	Female, but small	Estrogens low, androgens low, gonadotropins elevated	Nondisjunction in prenatal gametogenesis or in early embryo†
Klinefelter's syndrome	47,XXY	—	Testes, germinal epithelium degenerates	Male	Male	Testosterone low, gonadotropins elevated	Nondisjunction in gametogenesis or in early embryo†
True hermaphroditism	46,XX	H–Y antigen positive in some cases	Testicular and ovarian tissue	Female and male, variable	Ambiguous or predominantly male	FSH normal	Translocation of testicle differentiating gene, mutant gene, or mosaicism†
	46,XY	—	Testicular and ovarian tissue	Female and male	Male	FSH normal	Translocation of ovary-differentiating gene, mutant gene, or mosaicism†
	46,XX/46,XY	—	Testicular and ovarian tissue	Female and male	Ambiguous, or male	FSH normal	Union of two zygotes†
Male pseudohermaphroditism Sex chromosomal mosaicism	45,X/46,XY or other with at least one Y	—	Streak or dysgenetic testis, tumors	Female and/or male	Female, ambiguous, or male	—	Pathologic mitosis in early zygote†

Deficiency of antimüllerian hormone	46,XY	Deficiency of an X chromosomal gene for antimüllerian hormone†	Testis	Female and male	Male, often cryptorchid	Amount varies, may involve peripheral insensitivity	X chromosomal recessive gene mutation†
Deficiency of an enzyme in steroid synthesis	46,XY	Defective gene for one of the steroid synthesis enzymes	Testis, cryptorchid-like	Male	Ambiguous	Testosterone low	Probably autosomal recessive gene mutation†
5α-reductase deficiency	46,XY	Deficiency of an autosomal gene for 5α-reductase	Testis, cryptorchid-like	Male	Ambiguous	Testosterone and gonadotropins normal	Probably autosomal recessive gene mutation†
Complete testicular feminization	46,XY	Deficiency of an X-chromosomal gene for testosterone receptor	Testes	Rudimentary male	Infantile female	Testosterone normal or high, gonadotropins elevated	X chromosomal recessive mutation of the gene for testosterone receptor
Incomplete testicular feminization	46,XY	Partial deficiency of X chromosomal gene for testosterone receptor	Testes	Rudimentary or male	Ambiguous	Testosterone normal or high, gonadotropins elevated	Probably X chromosomal recessive mutant alleles of the gene for testosterone receptor
Female pseudohermaphroditism							
Adrenogenital syndromes	46,XX	Deficiency of gene(s) for adrenal steroid synthesis enzymes	Ovary	Female	Masculinized	Androgens elevated (intermediates from adrenal)	Autosomal recessive mutation of gene(s) for adrenal steroid synthesis enzymes
Nonadrenal masculinization	46,XX	—	Ovary	Female	Clitoral hypertrophy	—	Gene mutation†
Exogenous teratogens	46,XX	—	Ovary	Female	Masculinized	Androgens may be elevated	Aminoglutethimide; inhibits 3β-hydroxysteroid dehydrogenase Androgens from maternal tumors or medication

*No data available.
†The information is not yet established.

patients, however, are interesting in terms of the mechanism for regulating testicular differentiation. During the prenatal and also the prepubertal period, their sexual differentiation proceeds normally.[19] The external genitalia and testes are small in size, hair growth is decreased, and the pubic hair sometimes shows a female pattern. The adult testis contains fewer seminiferous tubules; they are smaller in diameter and usually, but not always, devoid of germ cells. The Leydig cells are hyperplastic, and the interstitium is fibrotic. Plasma testosterone is lower, or approximately half that of a normal male, and urinary gonadotropins are normal or elevated.

The mechanism of testicular development in the absence of Y chromosome is explained by translocation of the testis-determining gene into an autosome or into an X chromosome.[90] The inability of germ cells to undergo spermatogenesis could be due to the presence of the second X chromosome or due to the lack of appropriate Y chromosomal genes.

Turner's Syndrome (45,X)

Lack of one X chromosome is usually associated with female phenotype, sexual infantilism, short stature, webbing of the neck, and other anomalies, known collectively as Turner's syndrome.[73] The gonadal differentiation in the embryo proceeds normally to the stage of primordial follicles. Thereafter the oogonia and follicular epithelium start to degenerate, and the result is a streak gonad composed of fibrous stroma. The genital tract and external genitalia are female but underdeveloped in the adult.

Similar genital status has been detected in association with other abnormalities of X chromosome, mosaicism 45,X/46,XX, and deletions of the short or long arm of the X chromosome. These clinical data suggest that the X chromosome carries at least one gene in each arm governing the differentiation of the female gonad (see Fig. 15–2).

Klinefelter's Syndrome (47,XXY)

The phenotype of taller than normal males with additional typical characteristics as described by Klinefelter[123] is usually associated with a 47,XXY chromosomal complement. Patients with more than two X chromosomes and at least one Y chromosome have basically similar status.

The external genitalia and the reproductive tract are well differentiated. Except for a decreased number of spermatogonia,[21] the testes are approximately normal until puberty. After puberty, the tubular epithelium degenerates into hyaline material. The Leydig cells are morphologically and functionally abnormal with a decreased testosterone secretion. Occasional spermatozoa are detected.[127]

Prenatal sexual differentiation in these patients with one or more extra X chromosomes is apparently not impaired. This suggests that the extra genes in the X chromosome are inactive and do not interfere with the normal intrauterine sexual development. It also indicates that germ cells do not have a regulatory role in genital differentiation because they seem to be behaving abnormally at puberty.

True Hermaphroditism

By definition, an individual having both ovarian and testicular tissue is called a true hermaphrodite. Approximately two-thirds of the reported patients have a normal female (46,XX) and about one-eighth a normal male (46,XY) karyotype. The remaining one-fifth are variable cases of chimerism and mosaicism.[135]

In most cases, the testicular tissue of 46,XX individuals is in the right gonad. The seminiferous tubules are small and hyalinized, and usually no spermatozoa are present. The ovarian follicles are often fairly normal. In an ovotestis, the two tissues are almost always located one in each end of the gonad. The amount of testicular tissues seems to be directly proportional to the degree of descent of the ovotestis, suggesting normal endocrinologic function. Uterus and tubes are usually present. The male duct derivatives, when present, are on the same side as testicular tissue. This suggests that the testicular antimüllerian hormone functions normally. The cause of this intersex state is unknown. The possibilities include translocation of testicular differentiation genes to the X chromosome or to an autosome, a mutant gene, or undetected XY cells in the gonad—maybe only in the prenatal period. DNA probes for specific genes may become an important test in the differential diagnostics of intersex patients.

True hermaphrodites with 46,XY karyotype usually have phenotypically male external genitalia. In almost all cases, a uterus is present, and the gonadal histology is similar to that of the other true hermaphrodites. The cause is unknown, but cells with functioning ovary-organizing genes must have been present in the gonad, at least in the prenatal period. A small number of 46,XX cells in the gonad would easily go undetected in the ordinary chromosome analysis in leukocytes or in fibroblasts. Another possibility is a proper translocation or mutation of the gonadal differentiation genes suppressing the expression of the male and allowing that of the female genes. The presence of a uterus and tubes indicates a defective function of the antimüllerian hormone.

The third cytogenetic group of true hermaphrodites is 46,XX/46,XY chimeras, in which the two cell lines derive from different zygotes. The testicular histology shows usually hyalinized tubules with only Sertoli cells and occasional spermatozoa. The number of Leydig cells is sometimes increased. The ovarian tissue contains morphologically normal stages of follicles and also corpora lutea as an indication of ovulation. A uterus and tube on the ovarian side and male duct derivatives on the testicular side are usually present. The external genitalia are variably ambiguous but are generally more of the male type. The cause involves the union of two zygotes of different genetic sex, and each of the two cell lines develops normally according to the limits determined by their topographic distribution during early ontogeny.

Male Pseudohermaphroditism

Individuals having testes and features of the opposite sex in the gonadal duct system or in the external genitalia are called male pseudohermaphrodites.[125] In this terminology, the sex of the individual is the sex of the gonad. The pseudohermaphrodites are etiologically a mixed population, and in the literature there is considerable variation in what is included under this title.

Sex Chromosomal Mosaicism

Ambiguous genitalia are sometimes seen in individuals with 45,X/46,XY karyotypes or other mosaics with at least one Y chromosome. The internal and external genital phenotypes vary from an almost male to an almost female pattern. In many cases, one testis is dysgenetic, and the patient also falls into the category of mixed gonadal dysgenesis. Streak gonads of sex chromosome mosaic patients have a tendency to undergo neoplastic transformation and are therefore usually removed. The abnormalities result from varying degrees of impaired androgen or antimüllerian hormone secretion or both. The cause is most probably a pathologic mitosis in the early zygote.

Deficiency of Antimüllerian Hormone

The presence of a uterus and tubes in otherwise normally differentiated males is usually detected in connection with an inguinal herniation of the uterus. Cryptorchidism is often associated in this state with occasional neoplastic conversion.[9] The familial occurrence suggests that the cause is an X chromosomal regressive gene encoding the antimüllerian hormone or some factor in the target organ.[47]

Leydig Cell Agenesis

Testes with hyalinized tubuli and morphologically normal Sertoli cells but no Leydig cells are sometimes found in association with a 46,XY karyotype and normal male internal genitalia.[6] Serum testosterone is low, LH is high, and FSH is normal. The absence of paramesonephric derivatives and an increase in FSH after castration suggest that the antimüllerian hormone and inhibin production by Sertoli cells is normal. The testosterone present in plasma is apparently from the adrenal glands because it responds to dexamethasone suppression and ACTH stimulation. Functional Leydig cells may have been present in the fetal stages because the male gonadal ducts are normally differentiated. The mechanism of the Leydig cell inhibition remains to be clarified.

Enzyme Deficiency in Testosterone Synthesis

The defects proximal to the pregnenolone synthesis result usually from the lack of 20,22-desmolase or 20α-hydroxylase.[125] Cholesterol then accumulates in the adrenal cells, a state known as congenital adrenal lipoid hyperplasia. Other defects causing impaired testosterone synthesis are lack of 17,20-desmolase, 17-ketosteroid reductase, and 17α-hydroxylase. In these disorders, chromosomally normal males have cryptorchid-like testes and male gonadal ducts, but cloacal derivatives and external genitalia are more or less feminized (depending on the extent of the enzymatic block), as one would expect in the absence of the male regulator. The cause seems to be an autosomal recessive defective gene.

Enzyme Deficiency of Dihydrotestosterone Formation

The external genitalia of these individuals are feminized in a standard way, as described by the descriptive clinical diagnosis of pseudovaginal perineoscrotal hypospadias.[37] The male mesonephric duct derivatives are present, and cryptorchid-like testes[88] are in the inguinal canal or labia, whereas tissues derived from the urogenital sinus and from the anlage of the external genitalia are female in character. In contrast to the previous group of enzymatic defects, these patients virilize at puberty and usually assume a male gender; they should therefore be raised as males. They may have normal spermatogenesis, and their testosterone and gonadotropins are within normal limits. The cause most probably is an autosomal recessive defect in the gene encoding the enzyme 5α-reductase, which in the target tissue converts testosterone into dihydrotestosterone, which induces masculinization of the external genitalia.

Target Organ Androgen Insensitivity

COMPLETE TESTICULAR FEMINIZATION SYNDROME. As a result of defective testosterone utilization by the target tissues, all the structures requiring testosterone or dihydrotestosterone (see Fig. 15–2) for male differentiation are female in these patients. This includes the infantile external genitalia; a short, blindly ending vagina; and, at puberty, the development of breasts and female fat distribution. Chromosomal sex is normal male, and the gonads are definitive testes although often cryptorchid. Seminiferous tubules consist mainly of Sertoli cells and spermatogonia. Leydig cells are often in prominent clumps and hyperplastic. The male tract is rudimentary, but the paramesonephric ducts have regressed normally. Plasma FSH is normal; LH is normal or above normal and not suppressed, apparently because there are no testosterone receptors in the hypothalamus.

The mechanism for the androgen insensitivity is the lack of testosterone receptor protein, which after coupling with testosterone is capable of binding to DNA—a step indispensable for testosterone action.[42] The cause most probably is a mutation of an X-linked recessive or sex-limited gene encoding the receptor protein.

INCOMPLETE TESTICULAR FEMINIZATION SYNDROMES. The term *incomplete* refers to the external genitalia, which in these patients show a variable degree of ambiguity instead of full feminization as in the previous group.[42] This abnormality is due to weakened androgen action rather than decreased androgen synthesis, and the clinical manifestations are related to the degree of androgen insensitivity. The clinical spectrum of abnormalities may include defects of mesonephric duct differentiation; abnormal virilization of the urogenital sinus and external genitalia with phallic enlargement and testicular abnormalities, such as cryptorchidism and sterility; and, at puberty, incomplete development of the secondary sex characteristics and gynecomastia. Paramesonephric duct regression is consistently normal. Affinity of the receptor protein to bind dihydrotestosterone is normal or partially deficient, and the turnover of the protein is within the normal range.[2] This suggests that the mutations in these disorders affect the DNA-binding or transportation properties of the receptor protein. The family history suggests an X-linked recessive trait, and the different phenotypes could represent different alleles of the same locus or genes at different loci.

Female Pseudohermaphroditism

Genetic Etiology

ADRENOGENITAL SYNDROMES. Normal female karyotype, ovaries, and female internal genitalia but external genitalia masculinized to a varying degree are characteristics of a female who has been exposed to androgens during the critical period in sex differentiation. The source of androgens is the adrenal glands. Lack of 21-hydroxylase, 11α-hydroxylase, or 3β-hydroxysteroid dehydrogenase enzymes results in the accumulation and secretion of intermediate steroid metabolites, including androgens. Internal ducts are not masculinized because adrenal activity starts at a later stage of development. All these enzyme defects are probably autosomal recessive traits (For further details, see Chapters 14 and 22.)

NONADRENAL MASCULINIZATION. Clitoral hypertrophy is sometimes seen without any apparent cause, in association with multiple skeletal anomalies. The occurrence in sibs suggests a genetic cause.[125]

Exogenous Teratologic Agents

Androgens and related progestins given to the mother as well as various other compounds (aminoglutethimide) may cause masculinization of the external genitalia. It is of interest that they have never been seen to affect the internal genitalia, even if the exposure happened during the critical period. The androgens can also be derived from maternal tumors such as arrhenoblastoma or pregnancy luteoma.

REFERENCES

1. Altman PL, Dittmer DS, eds. Growth. Washington DC: Federation of American Societies for Experimental Biology, 1962:347.
2. Amrhein JA, Klingesmith GJ, Walsh PC, et al. Partial androgen insensitivity. The Reifenstein syndrome revisited. N Engl J Med 1977;297:350.
3. Bardin CW, Taketo T, Gunsalus GL, et al. The detection of agents that have toxic effects on the testis and male reproductive tract. In: Banbury Report 11. New York: Cold Spring Harbor Laboratory, 1982:337.
4. Barr ML. Sex chromatin techniques. In: Yunis JJ, ed. Human chromosome methodology. New York: Academic Press, 1965:1.
5. Berta P, Hawkins JR, Sinclair AH, et al. Genetic evidence equating SRY and the testis-determining factor. Nature 1990;348:448.
6. Berthezene F, Forest MG, Grimaud JA, et al. Leydig-cell agenesis. A cause of male pseudohermaphroditism. N Engl J Med 1976;295:969.
7. Blandau RJ, Bergsma D, eds. Morphogenesis and malformation of the genital system. Birth defects original article series, vol XIII. No. 2. New York: Alan R. Liss, 1977.
8. Boczkowski K. Sex determination and gonadal differentiation in man. A unifying concept of normal and abnormal sex development. Clin Genet 1971;2:379.
9. Brook CGD, Wagner H, Zachmann M, et al. Familial occurrence of persistent müllerian structures in otherwise normal males. BMJ 1973;1:771.
10. Byskov AG. Does the rete ovarii act as a trigger for the onset of meiosis? Nature 1974;252:396.
11. Byskov AG. The meiosis-inducing interaction between germ cells and rete cells in the fetal mouse gonad. Ann Biol Anim Biochem Biophys 1978;18(2B):327.
12. Byskov AG. Regulation of initiation of meiosis in fetal gonads. Int J Androl 1978;2(suppl):29.
13. Byskov AG. Differentiation of mammalian embryonic gonad. Physiol Rev 1986;66:71.
14. Caspersson T, Zech L, Johansson C, Modest EJ. Identification of human chromosomes by DNA-binding fluorescent agents. Chromosoma 1970;30:215.
15. Cate RL, Mattaliano RJ, Hession C, et al. Isolation of the bovine and human genes for Müllerian inhibiting substance and expression of the human gene in animal cells. Cell 1986;45:685.
16. Childs GV, Hon C, Russel LR, Gardner PJ. Subcellular localization of gonadotropins and testosterone in the developing fetal rat testis. J Histochem Cytochem 1978;26:545.
17. Christensen AK. Leydig cells. In: Hamilton DW, Greep RO, eds. Handbook of physiology. Section 7, Endocrinology. Vol 5, Male reproductive system. Washington DC: American Physiological Society, 1975:57.
18. Clements JA, Reyes FI, Winter JSD, Faiman C. Studies on human sexual development. III. Fetal pituitary and serum, and amniotic fluid concentrations of LH, CG, and FSH. J Clin Endocrinol Metab 1976;42:9.
19. De la Chapelle A. Analytic review: nature and origin of males with XX sex chromosomes. Am J Hum Genet 1972;24:71.
20. Dosik H, Wachtel SS, Khan F, et al. Y-chromosomal genes in a phenotypic male with a 46,XX karyotype. JAMA 1976;236:2505.
21. Edlow JB, Shapiro LR, Hsu LYF, Hirschhorn K. Neonatal Klinefelter's syndrome. Am J Dis Child 1969;118:788.
22. Ehrhardt AA, Meyer-Bahlburg HFL. Effects of prenatal sex hormones on gender-related behavior. Science 1981;211:1312.
23. Erickson GF, Magoffin DA, Dyer CA, Hofeditz C. The ovarian androgen producing cells: a review of structure/function relationships. Endocr Rev 1985;6:371.
24. Forest MG, Cathiard AM. Pattern of plasma testosterone and Δ4-androstenedione in normal newborns:

evidence for testicular activity at birth. J Clin Endocrinol Metab 1975;41:977.

25. Francavilla S, Concordia N, De Martino C. Ultrastructure of human germ cells in sex-indifferent gonad, in early fetal testis or ovary and in testicular cancers. In: Developments in ultrastructure of reproduction. New York: Alan R. Liss, 1989:31.

26. Fraser BA, Sato AG. Morphological sex differentiation in the human embryo: a light and scanning electron microscopic study. J Anat 1989;165:61.

27. Friedman NB, Van de Velde RL. Germ cell tumors in man, pleiotropic mice, and continuity of germplasm and somatoplasm. Hum Pathol 1981;12:772.

28. Fröjdman K, Paranko J, Kuopio T, Pelliniemi LJ. Structural proteins in sexual differentiation of embryonic gonads. Int J Dev Biol 1989;33:99.

29. Fukuda T, Hedinger C, Groscurth P. Ultrastructure of developing germ cells in the fetal human testis. Cell Tiss Res 1975;161:55.

30. George FW, Catt KJ, Neaves WB, Wilson JD. Studies on the regulation of testosterone synthesis in the fetal rabbit testis. Endocrinology 1978;102:665.

31. George FW, Milewich L, Wilson JD. Estrogen content of the embryonic rabbit ovary. Nature 1978;274:172.

32. George FW, Wilson JD. Conversion of androgen to estrogen by the human fetal ovary. J Clin Endocrinol Metab 1978;47:550.

33. Gillman J. The development of the gonads in man, with a consideration of the role of fetal endocrines and the histogenesis of ovarian tumors. Contrib Embryol Carnegie Inst 1948;32:81.

34. Gondos B. Testicular development. In: Johnson AD, Gomes WR, eds. The testis. Vol 4. New York: Academic Press, 1977:1.

35. Gondos B. Oogonia and oocytes in mammals. In: Jones RE, ed. The vertebrate ovary; comparative biology and evolution. New York: Plenum Publishing, 1978:83.

36. Gondos B. Diagnosis of abnormalities in gonadal development. Ann Clin Lab Sci 1982;12:276.

37. Gondos B. Gonadal disorders in infancy and early childhood. Ann Clin Lab Sci 1991;21:62.

38. Gondos B, Bhiraleus P, Hobel CJ. Ultrastructural observations on germ cells in human fetal ovaries. Am J Obstet Gynecol 1971;110:644.

39. Gondos B, Hobel CJ. Ultrastructure of germ cell development in the human fetal testis. Z Zellforsch 1971;119:1.

40. Gondos B, Hobel CV. Interstitial cells in the human fetal ovary. Endocrinology 1973;93:736.

41. Gray SW, Skandalakis JE. Embryology for surgeons: the embryological basis for the treatment of congenital defects. Philadelphia: WB Saunders, 1972.

42. Griffin JE, Wilson JD. Disorders of androgen receptor function. Ann NY Acad Sci 1984;438:61.

43. Grumbach MM, van Wyk JJ. Disorders of sex differentiation. In: Williams RH, ed. Textbook of endocrinology, ed 5. Philadelphia: WB Saunders, 1974:423.

44. Grund SK, Pelliniemi LJ. Reaggregation cultures as a model of gonadal differentiation in vitro. In: Parvinen M, Huhtaniemi I, Pelliniemi LJ, eds. Development and function of the reproductive organs, vol II. Serono Symposia Review No. 14. Rome: Ares-Serono Symposia, 1988:71.

45. Gubbay J, Collignon J, Koopman P, et al. A gene mapping to the sex-determining region of the mouse Y chromosome is a member of a novel family of embryonically expressed genes. Nature 1990;346:245.

46. Guerrier D, Boussin L, Mader S, et al. Expression of the gene for anti-Müllerian hormone. J Reprod Fertil 1990;88:695.

47. Guerrier D, Tran D, Vanderwinden JM, et al. The persistent Müllerian duct syndrome: A molecular approach. J Clin Endocrinol Metab 1989;68:46.

48. Guraya SS. Recent advances in the morphology, histochemistry, and biochemistry of the developing mammalian ovary. Int Rev Cytol 1977;51:49.

49. Hadziselimovic F, Girard J. Pathogenesis of cryptorchidism. Horm Res 1977;8:76.

50. Huhtaniemi I, Ikonen M, Vihko R. Presence of testosterone and other neutral steroids in human fetal testis. Biochem Biophys Res Commun 1970;38:715.

51. Huhtaniemi IT, Korenbrot CC, Jaffe RB. hCG binding and stimulation of testosterone biosynthesis in the human fetal testis. J Clin Endocrinol Metab 1977;44:963.

52. Huhtaniemi IT, Korenbrot CC, Jaffe RB. Content of chorionic gonadotropin in human fetal tissues. J Clin Endocrinol Metab 1978;46:994.

53. Hutson JM, Donahoe PK. The hormonal control of testicular descent. Endocr Rev 1986;7:270.

54. Hutson JM, Metcalfe SA, MacLaughlin DT, et al. Müllerian inhibiting substance. In: Burger H, de Kretser D, eds. The testis. New York: Raven Press, 1989:143.

55. Jacobs PA, Ross A. Structural abnormalities of the Y chromosome in man. Nature 1966;210:352.

56. Jäger RJ, Anvret M, Hall K, Scherer G. A human XY female with a frame shift mutation in the candidate testis-determining gene SRY. Nature 1990;348:452.

57. Jirasek JE. Development of the genital system and male pseudohermaphroditism. Baltimore: Johns Hopkins University Press, 1971.

58. Jirasek JE. Principles of reproductive embryology. In: Simpson JL, ed. Disorders of sexual differentiation. New York: Academic Press, 1976:51.

59. Jones RE, ed. The vertebrate ovary. Comparative biology and evolution. New York: Plenum Publishing, 1978.

60. Josso N, ed. Intersex child. Pediatric and adolescent endocrinology, vol 8. Basel: S Karger, 1981.

61. Josso N, Picard JY, Tran D. The antimüllerian hormone. Rec Prog Horm Res 1977;33:117.

62. Josso N, Vigier B, Picard JY. Anti-müllerian hormone: recent developments. In: Parvinen M, Huhtaniemi I, Pelliniemi LJ, eds. Development and function of the reproductive organs, vol II. Serono Symposia Review No. 14. Rome: Ares-Serono Symposia, 1988:29.

63. Jost A. Hormonal factors in the sex differentiation of the mammalian foetus. Phil Trans Roy Soc Lond (B) 1970;259:119.

64. Jost A. Genetic and hormonal factors in sex differentiation of the brain. Psychoneuroendocrinology 1983;8:183.

65. Jost A, Magre S, Cressent M, Perlman S. Sertoli cells and early testicular differentiation. In: Mancini RE, Martini L, eds. Male fertility and sterility. London: Academic Press, 1974:1.

66. Jost A, Vigier B, Prepin J, Perchellet JP. Studies on sex differentiation in mammals. Rec Prog Horm Res 1973;29:1.

67. Kaplan SL, Grumbach MM, Aubert ML. The ontogenesis of pituitary hormones and hypothalamic factors in the human fetus: maturation of central nervous system regulation of anterior pituitary function. Rec Prog Horm Res 1976;32:161.

68. Kellokumpu-Lehtinen PL, Santti R, Pelliniemi LJ. Early cytodifferentiation of human prostatic urethra and Leydig cells. Anat Rec 1979;194:429.

69. Kellokumpu-Lehtinen PL, Santti R, Pelliniemi LJ. Correlation of early cytodifferentiation of the human fetal prostate and Leydig cells. Anat Rec 1980;196:263.

70. Kellokumpu-Lehtinen P, Santti RS, Pelliniemi LJ. Development of human fetal prostate in culture. Urol Res 1981;9:89.

71. Koopman P, Gubbay J, Vivian N, et al. Male development of chromosomally female mice transgenic for Sry. Nature 1991;351:117.

72. Lauteala L, Kellokumpu-Lehtinen PL, Pelliniemi LJ. Regression of müllerian ducts in pig and human embryos. Proceedings of Annual Meeting of Scandinavian Society for Electron Microscopy, Tampere, Finland, 1978:24.

73. Lippe B. Turner syndrome. Endocrinol Metab Clin North Am 1991;20:121.

74. Lyon MF. Genetic activity of sex chromosomes in somatic cells of mammals. Phil Trans Roy Soc Lond (B) 1970;259:41.

75. MacLusky NJ, Naftolin F. Sexual differentiation of the central nervous system. Science 1981;211:1294.

76. McEwen BS. Neural gonadal steroid actions. Science 1981;211:1303.

77. McLaren A. What makes a man a man? Nature 1990;346:216.

78. McLaren A. Development of the mammalian gonad: the fate of the supporting cell lineage. BioEssays 1991;13:151.

79. McLaren A. The making of male mice. Nature 1991;351:96.

80. Meyer WJ III, Migeon BR, Migeon CJ. Locus on human X chromosome for dihydrotestosterone receptor and androgen insensitivity. Proc Nat Acad Sci USA 1975;72:1469.

81. Migeon BR, Jelalian K. Evidence for two active X chromosomes in germ cells of female before meiotic entry. Nature 1977;269:242.

82. Moore T, Haig D. Genomic imprinting in mammalian development: a parental tug-of-war. Trends Genet 1991;7:45.

83. Mossman HW, Duke KL. Comparative morphology of the mammalian ovary. Madison: University of Wisconsin Press, 1973:53.

84. Niemi M, Ikonen M, Hervonen A. Histochemistry and fine structure of the interstitial tissue in the human foetal testis. In: Wolstenholme GEW, O'Connor M, eds. Ciba Foundation colloquia on endocrinology: endocrinology of the testis. Vol 16. London: J & A Churchill, 1967:31.

85. O'Rahilly R. The timing and sequence of events in the development of the human reproductive system during the embryonic period proper. Anat Embryol 1983;166:247.

86. Ohno S. Sex chromosomes and sex-linked genes. Berlin: Springer Verlag, 1967.

87. Ohno S, Klinger HP, Atkin NB. Human oogenesis. Cytogenetics 1962;1:42.

88. Okon E, Livni N, Rösler A, et al. Male pseudohermaphroditism due to 5α-reductase deficiency. Arch Pathol Lab Med 1980;104:363.

89. Olson C, Prescott GH, Pernoll ML, Hecht F. Dangers in nuclear-sexing the fetus. Lancet 1974;2:226.

90. Page DC, de la Chapelle A, Weissenbach J. Chromosome Y-specific DNA in related human XX males. Nature 1985;315:224.

91. Paranko J. Expression of type I and III collagen during morphogenesis of fetal rat testis and ovary. Anat Rec 1987;219:91.

92. Paranko J, Foidart J-M, Pelliniemi LJ. Basement membrane in differentiating mesonephric and paramesonephric ducts of male and female rat fetuses. Differentiation 1985;29:39.

93. Paranko J, Foidart J-M, Pelliniemi LJ. Developmental changes in interstitial collagens of fetal rat genital ducts. Dev Biol 1986;113:364.

94. Paranko J, Fröjdman K, Grund SK, Pelliniemi LJ. Differentiation of epithelial cords in the fetal testis. In: Parvinen M, Huhtaniemi I, Pelliniemi LJ, eds. Development and function of the reproductive organs, vol II. Serono Symposia Review No. 14. Rome: Ares-Serono Symposia, 1988:21.

95. Paranko J, Kallajoki M, Pelliniemi LJ, et al. Transient coexpression of cytokeratin and vimentin in differentiating rat Sertoli cells. Dev Biol 1986;117:35.

96. Paranko J, Pelliniemi LJ, Foidart J-M. Epithelio-mesenchymal interface and fibronectin in the differentiation of the rat mesonephric and paramesonephric ducts. Differentiation 1984;27:196.

97. Paranko J, Pelliniemi LJ, Vaheri A, et al. Morphogenesis and fibronectin in sexual differentiation of rat embryonic gonads. Differentiation 1983;23(suppl): S72.

98. Paranko J, Virtanen I. Epithelial and mesenchymal cell differentiation in the fetal rat genital ducts: changes in the expression of cytokeratin and vimentin type of intermediate filaments and desmosomal plaque proteins. Dev Biol 1986;117:135.

99. Pearson PL, Bobrow M, Vosa CG. Technique for identifying Y-chromosomes in human interphase nuclei. Nature 1970;226:78.

100. Pelliniemi LJ. Fine structure of germ cords in human fetal testis. In: Horstmann E, Holstein AF, eds. Morphological aspects of andrology. Vol 1. Berlin: Grosse Verlag, 1970:5.

101. Pelliniemi LJ. Ultrastructure of gonadal ridge in male and female pig embryos. Anat Embryol 1975;147:19.

102. Pelliniemi LJ. Ultrastructure of the early ovary and testis in pig embryos. Am J Anat 1975;144:89.

103. Pelliniemi LJ. Human primordial germ cells during migration and entrance to the gonadal ridge. J Cell Biol 1976;70:226a.

104. Pelliniemi LJ. Ultrastructure of the indifferent gonad in male and female pig embryos. Tissue Cell 1976;8:163.

105. Pelliniemi LJ, Dym M. The fetal gonad and sexual differentiation. In: Tulchinsky D, Ryan KJ, eds. Maternal-fetal endocrinology, ed 1. Philadelphia: WB Saunders, 1980:252.

106. Pelliniemi LJ, Dym M, Crigler JF, et al. Development of Leydig cells in human fetuses and in patients with androgen insensitivity. In: Steinberger A, Steinberger E, eds. Testicular development, structure, and function. New York: Raven Press, 1980:49.

107. Pelliniemi LJ, Kellokumpu-Lehtinen P, Hoffer AP. Glycogen accumulations in differentiating mesonephric ducts and tubuli in male human embryos. Anat Embryol 1983;168:445.

108. Pelliniemi LJ, Kellokumpu-Lehtinen P-L, Lauteala L. Development of sexual differences in the embryonic genitals. Ann Biol Anim Biochem Biophys 1979;19:1211.

109. Pelliniemi LJ, Kellokumpu-Lehtinen P, Tapanainen J, et al. Ultrastructural and hormonal differentiation of the human prenatal testis and the mesonephric duct. In: Byskov AG, Peters H, eds. International Congress Series No. 559. Development and function

of reproductive organs. Amsterdam: Excerpta Medica, 1981:61.

110. Pelliniemi LJ, Niemi M. Fine structure of the human foetal testis. I. The interstitial tissue. Z Zellforsch Mikrosk Anat 1969;99:507.

111. Pelliniemi LJ, Paranko J, Grund SK, et al. Extracellular matrix in testicular differentiation. Ann NY Acad Sci 1984;438:405.

112. Pelliniemi LJ, Salonius A-L. Cytological identification of sex in pig embryos at indifferent gonadal stages. Acta Anat 1976;95:558.

113. Peters H, ed. The development and maturation of the ovary and its functions. Amsterdam: Excerpta Medica, 1973.

114. Peters H, McNatty KP. The ovary. London: Granada Publishing, 1980.

115. Picard J-Y, Benarous R, Guerrier D, et al. Cloning and expression of cDNA for anti-Müllerian hormone. Proc Natl Acad Sci USA 1986;83:5464.

116. Picon R. Action du testicule foetal sur le developpement in vitro des canaux de Müller chez le rat. Arch Anat Microsc Morphol Exp 1969;58:1.

117. Pinkerton JHM, McKay DG, Adams EC, Hertig AT. Development of the human ovary—a study using histochemical techniques. Obstet Gynecol 1961;18:152.

118. Pinsky L. Human male sexual maldevelopment: teratogenetic classification of monogenic forms. Teratology 1974;10:193.

119. Price MJ, Donahoe PK, Ito Y, Hendren WH III. Programmed cell death in the müllerian duct induced by müllerian-inhibiting substance. Am J Anat 1977;149:353.

120. Rabinovici J, Jaffe RB. Development and regulation of growth and differentiated function in human and subhuman primate fetal gonads. Endocr Rev 1990;11:532.

121. Reyes FI, Winter JSD, Faiman C. Endocrinology of the fetal testis. In: Burger H, de Kretser D, eds. The testis. New York: Raven Press, 1989:119.

122. Sarto GE, Opitz JM. The XY gonadal agenesis syndrome. J Med Genet 1973;10:288.

123. Schwartz ID, Root AW. The Klinefelter syndrome of testicular dysgenesis. Endocrinol Metab Clin North Am 1991;20:153.

124. Siiteri PK, Wilson JD. Testosterone formation and metabolism during male sexual differentiation in the human embryo. J Clin Endocrinol Metab 1974;38:113.

125. Simpson JL. Abnormal sexual differentiation in humans. Ann Rev Genet 1982;16:193.

126. Sinclair AH, Berta P, Palmer MS, et al. A gene from the human sex-determining region encodes a protein with homology to a conserved DNA-binding motif. Nature 1990;346:240.

127. Steinberger E, Smith KD, Perloff WH. Spermatogenesis in Klinefelter's syndrome. J Clin Endocrinol Metab 1965;25:1325.

128. Stosiek P, Kasper M, Karsten U. Expression of cytokeratins 8 and 18 in human Sertoli cells of immature and atrophic seminiferous tubules. Differentiation 1990;43:66.

129. Taguchi O, Cunha GR, Robboy SJ. Experimental study of the effect of diethylstilbestrol on the devel-

opment of the human female reproductive tract. Biol Res Pregn 1983;4:56.

130. Tapanainen J, Kellokumpu-Lehtinen P, Pelliniemi L, Huhtaniemi I. Age-related changes in endogenous steroids of human fetal testis during early and mid-pregnancy. J Clin Endocrinol Metab 1981;52:98.

131. Tapanainen J, Koivisto M, Vihko R, Huhtaniemi I. Enhanced activity of the pituitary-gonadal axis in premature human infants. J Clin Endocrinol Metab 1981;52:235.

132. Tarkowski AK. Are the genetic factors controlling sexual differentiation of somatic and germinal tissues of a mammalian gonad stable or labile? In: Kretchmer N, Walcher DN, eds. Environmental influences on genetic expression; biological and behavioral aspects of sexual differentiation. Fogarty International Center Proceedings, No. 2. Washington DC: US Government Printing Office, 1969:49.

133. Thomas BJ, Rothstein R. Sex, maps, and imprinting. Cell 1991;64:1.

134. Vakil DV, Lewin PK, Conen PE. Value of fluorescent Y chromosome and sex chromatin tests. Acta Cytol 1973;17:220.

135. van Niekerk WA. True hermaphroditism: clinical, morphologic and cytogenetic aspects. New York: Harper & Row, 1974.

136. van Wagenen G, Simpson ME. Embryology of the ovary and testis: *Homo sapiens* and *Macaca mulatta*. New Haven, CT: Yale University Press, 1965.

137. Voutilainen R, Miller WL. Human Müllerian inhibitory factor messenger ribonucleic acid is hormonally regulated in the fetal testis and in adult granulosa cells. Mol Endocrinol 1987;1:604.

138. Warner BA, Monsaert RP, Stumpf PG, et al. 46,XY dysgenesis: is oncogenesis related to H-Y phenotype or breast development? Hum Genet 1985;69:79.

139. Wartenberg H, Holstein A-F, Vossmayer J. Zur Cytologie der pränatalen Gonadenentwicklung beim Menschen. II. Elektronenmikroskopische Untersuchungen über die Cytogenese von Gonocyten und fetalen Spermatogonien im Hoden. Z Anat Entwickl-Gesch 1971;134:165.

140. Welshons WJ, Russell LB. The Y-chromosome as the bearer of male determining factors in the mouse. Proc Nat Acad Sci USA 1959;45:560.

141. Wensing CJG. The embryology of testicular descent. Horm Res 1988;30:144.

142. Wilson JD. Sexual differentiation. Ann Rev Physiol 1978;40:279.

143. Winter JSD, Faiman C, Reyes FI. Sex steroid production by the human fetus: its role in morphogenesis and control by gonadotropins. In: Blandau RJ, Bergsma D, eds. Morphogenesis and malformation of the genital system. Birth defects original article series. Vol 13, No. 2. New York: Alan R. Liss, 1977:41.

144. Witschi E. Migration of the germ cells of human embryos from the yolk sac to the primitive gonadal folds. Contr Embryol Carneg Inst 1948;32:67.

145. Word RA, George FW, Wilson JD, Carr BR. Testosterone synthesis and adenylate cyclase activity in the early human fetal testis appear to be independent of human chorionic gonadotropin control. J Clin Endocrinol Metab 1989;69:204.

The Ontogenesis of Thyroid Function and Actions

Delbert A. Fisher

Daniel H. Polk

PLACENTAL INFLUENCES ON FETAL THYROID DEVELOPMENT

Mammalian fetal development critically depends on placental regulation of substrate supply, water balance, and excretory capacity. The placenta also provides important influences on fetal endocrine development, acting as a source for many polypeptide hormones as well as actively metabolizing hormonal substrates derived from both fetal and maternal compartments. With regard to thyroid function, the placenta allows for fetal thyroid system maturation largely independent of maternal influence. The placental permeability to various thyroid system–related substances is summarized in Figure 16–1. Although glycosylation and relatively large molecular mass preclude placental transfer of maternal thyrotropin (thyroid-stimulating hormone [TSH]), the placenta does produce large amounts of chorionic gonadotropin (CG), which has TSH-like

bioactivity. The α subunits of hCG and TSH are identical, and the β subunits of hCG and TSH share structural homology. The thyrotropin-like bioactivity of hCG, however, is only about 0.01% of that of native TSH. Additional chorionic TSH-like proteins have been proposed but inadequately characterized.[21] Placental hCG is secreted predominantly into maternal blood, and levels peak at the end of the first trimester. Because of the large amount of hCG produced by the placenta and the high maternal blood levels, there is a transient effect of hCG on maternal thyroid function at this time.[22] There is little influence, however, on fetal thyroid function.

The tripeptide thyrotropin-releasing hormone (TRH) readily crosses the placenta in humans and several animal species; maternally administered exogenous TRH increases fetal levels of TSH and thyroid hormones.[25, 44] This observation is currently being exploited clinically in human pregnancies in an attempt to accelerate fetal pulmonary maturation in preterm infants at risk for premature delivery and subsequent respiratory failure.[42] The low circulating levels of maternal serum TRH preclude significant maternal to fetal transfer. The high levels of circulating TRH characteristic of the fetus are due in part to low TRH degrading activity in fetal plasma.[45] In addition, the placenta and gut tissues contribute to circulating fetal TRH levels via active synthesis.[55] The function of placentally derived TRH in fetal thyroid system maturation remains unclear.

The placental transfer of thyroid hormones is dependent on fetal thyroid status and the species being studied. Most of the data regarding placental triiodothyronine (T_3) and thyroxine (T_4) transfer are derived from studies in rats and sheep; human studies are limited.[43] Most studies support a relative impermeability of the placenta to maternally derived iodothyronines, with permeability decreasing among species in the order rat > human > sheep. The placental barrier is due in part to the presence of a placental iodothyronine inner ring monodeiodinase, which deiodinates T_4 to the inactive metabolite reverse T_3 (rT_3) and inactivates T_3 by conversion to diiodothyronine (T_2). The best evidence for human maternal to fetal thyroid hormone transfer was de-

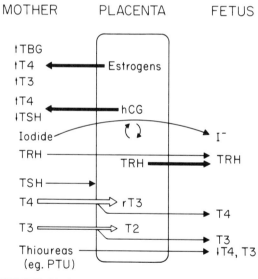

FIGURE 16–1. Placental role in maternal and fetal thyroid function. Heavy arrows indicate placental production of estrogens and hCG predominantly into maternal blood and TRH into fetal blood. Iodide is actively transported from the maternal to fetal direction. The placenta is impermeable to TSH in either direction. Transfer of the iodothyronines, T_4 and T_3, is limited by inherent placental barriers and by type III iodothyronine deiodinase, which converts T_4 to rT_3 and T_3 to T_2. Small amounts of active hormone appear to be transported. The relatively free transfer of antithyroid drugs (propylthiouracil [PTU] and methimazole) can inhibit fetal thyroid T_4 and T_3 production.

rived by Vulsma et al.[68] in pregnancies associated with fetal thyroid agenesis or the total inability of the fetus to synthesize iodothyronines. In these pregnancies, the average umbilical cord blood total T_4 level in the neonates approximated 4 μg/dL (50 nmol/L) and ranged from 30 to 70 mmol/L in contrast to a normal level of 11 μg/dL (140 nmol/L).[68] This T_4 was considered to be of maternal origin, and it has been suggested that during fetal hypothyroidism, this maternal source of thyroid hormones might be important for normal development of fetal organs that are particularly thyroid hormone sensitive. Although placental transfer of maternal thyroid hormone is demonstrable in the hypothyroid fetus, however, the fetal levels of thyroid hormones are not adequate to suppress the elevated thyrotropin levels associated with these syndromes.

The placenta also is permeable to iodide, and the fetal thyroid is particularly sensitive to the inhibitory effects of iodine on thyroid function. In the adult, thyroid autoregulation of iodide transport into the follicular cell protects against iodine overload or deficiency.[26] The capacity of the fetal thyroid to autoregulate iodide transport in response to increased circulating iodine levels does not develop until near term.[8] Maternally derived immunoglobulins of the IgG subclass are actively transported across the placenta in the maternal to fetal direction during the last trimester. Thus maternal autoantibodies directed against the TSH receptor may affect fetal thyroid function; both TSH-receptor stimulating and blocking antibodies have been described.[73] Finally, the thiourea class of antithyroid drugs (e.g., propylthiouracil) crosses the placenta and may compromise fetal thyroid hormone synthesis.[40]

Placental permeability to maternally derived thyroid-related molecules may affect fetal thyroid function, particularly in selected pathophysiologic states (autoimmune thyroid disease, acute iodide administration, pharmacotherapy of thyrotoxicosis). The fetal pituitary-thyroid axis, however, normally develops independently of maternal influences. In the normal human fetus, the extent and significance of maternal to fetal iodothyronine transfer remain unclear.

FETAL THYROID SYSTEM MATURATION

Maturation of the thyroid axis in humans begins during the first trimester and continues through the first weeks after birth. This process requires a coordinated series of complex processes involving the hypothalamus, the pituitary and thyroid glands, and most peripheral tissues. Generally maturation of thyroid function involves embryogenesis of relevant structures, maturation of hypothalamic-pituitary regulation of thyroid secretion, and maturation of peripheral thyroid hormone metabolic systems, ultimately culminating in thyroid-dependent actions in a myriad of tissue sites.

Embryogenesis

The process begins with the embryogenesis of the fetal thyroid and pituitary glands and the hypothalamus.

Thyroid Gland

The human thyroid gland is a derivative of the primitive buccopharyngeal cavity. It develops from contributions of two endodermal analogs: (1) a midline thickening of the pharyngeal floor (median anlage) and (2) paired ultimobranchial bodies derived from the fourth pharyngobranchial pouch (lateral anlagen).[11, 53] The lateral anlagen are the source of the calcitonin-producing perifollicular cells.[53] Both median and lateral anlagen are discernible by day 17 of gestation; by 24 days' gestation, the median anlage has developed a thin, flask-like diverticulum extending from the floor of the buccal cavity down to the fourth branchial arch. At 40 days' gestation, median and lateral anlagen have fused, and by 50 days' gestation, the buccal stalk has ruptured and the thyroid gland migrates caudally to its definitive location in the anterior neck, helped in part by its relationship with developing cardiac structures. Histologically further thyroid gland maturation proceeds in three phases: precolloid, beginning colloid, and follicular growth phases. It is during the final period of follicular growth, by 70 to 80 days' gestation, that both iodide uptake and thyroid hormone synthesis occur.[63]

Pituitary Gland

The anterior pituitary gland is derived from dorsal buccal-pharyngeal endoderm. By 5 weeks' gestation, this derivative, known as Rathke's pouch, encounters a ventral diverticulum from the third cerebral ventricle destined to become the posterior pituitary gland or neurohypophysis. The developing sphenoid bone disrupts the buccal connection to Rathke's pouch, and by 12 weeks' gestation, the anterior and posterior components of the pituitary gland are partially encapsulated within the sella turcica. By this time during development, anterior pituitary thyrotrophs and thyrotropin (TSH) are evident.[13]

Hypothalamus

By 5 weeks' gestation, the third cerebral ventricle and neurohypophysial primordia are present. The first hypothalamic nuclei and the supraoptic tract are demonstrable by 12 weeks' gestation, with the remainder of the hypothalamic nuclei and median eminence developing by 16 weeks' gestation. TRH is demonstrable in hypothalamic extracts by 10 weeks' gestation.[69] Although a superficial plexus of capillaries known as the supratuberal plexus develops in association with Rathke's pouch, the tufted capillaries characteristic of the hypothalamic plexus of the portal vascular system are first discernible by 16 weeks' gestation.[58] Histologic maturation of the hypothalamic-pituitary portal system is largely completed by 30 to 35 weeks' gestation.

Thyroid Hormone Synthesis and Metabolism

Circulating thyroid hormones are derived from thyroidal secretion of T_4 and T_3 as well as peripheral tissue conversion of T_4 to T_3. Although thyroid secretion is the only source of T_4, monodeiodination of T_4 in peripheral tissues is the predominant source of circulating T_3. In the thyroid gland, circulating plasma iodide enters the follicular cells and is organified through a series of enzyme-catalyzed steps to form T_4 and T_3. The major events culminating in thyroid hormone synthesis include (1) active transport of inorganic iodide from plasma into the thyroid cell; (2) synthesis of thyroglobulin, which is rich in tyrosine residues that serve as iodine acceptors; (3) organification of sequestered iodide as thyroglobulin-bound iodotyrosines; (4) coupling of monoiodotyrosines (MIT) and diiodotyrosines (DIT) to form the iodothyronines, T_3 and T_4, with storage of the iodinated thyroglobulin in follicular colloid; (5) endocytosis and proteolysis of colloid thyroglobulin to release MIT, DIT, T_3, and T_4; and (6) deiodination of released iodotyrosines within the thyroid cell with iodine reutilization. Various defects in these processes have been described leading to varying degrees of clinical hypothyroidism.

Deiodination of thyroxine is a major route of metabolism; monodeiodination may occur either at the outer (β) ring or inner (α) ring of the iodothyronine molecule (Fig. 16–2). Outer ring monodeiodination of T_4 produces T_3, the active form of thyroid hormone with the greatest affinity for the thyroid hormone receptor. Inner ring monodeiodination of T_4 produces rT_3 (3,3',5'-triiodothyronine), an inactive metabolite. In mature humans, most of the circulating T_3 (70 to 90%) is derived from peripheral monodeiodination of T_4; only 10 to 30% arises from direct glandular secretion. Nearly all the circulating rT_3 is derived from peripheral conversion, with only 2 to 3% coming directly from the thyroid gland. T_3 and rT_3 are progressively metabolized to diiodinated, monoiodinated, and noniodinated forms of thyronine, none of which possesses biologic activity. The iodothyronines can be glucuronide or sulfate conjugated, and both conjugates have been isolated. Conjugated iodothyronines also are biologically inactive; however, studies in rats suggest that sulfation facilitates deiodination.[38] In adults, very little of the circulating iodothyronine is conjugated. Our preliminary studies in fetal sheep, however, document high levels of circulating T_4 and T_3 sulfates, suggesting that sulfation is a major route of iodothyronine metabolism in the mammalian fetus.[72]

Two types of outer-ring iodothyronine monodeiodinase (5'-MDI) have been described. Type I 5'-MDI, predominantly expressed in liver and kidney, is a high Km enzyme, inhibited by propylthiouracil, and its activity is induced by thyroid hormone. Type

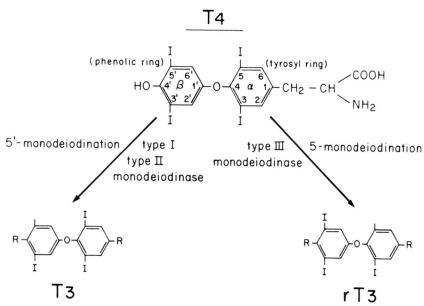

FIGURE 16–2. Pathways of T_4 monodeiodination. Iodination occurring at the 5' position of the beta ring produces T_3, whereas position 5' deiodination of the alpha ring produces rT_3. See text for details.

II 5'-MDI, predominantly located in brain, pituitary, and brown adipose tissues, is a low Km enzyme insensitive to propylthiouracil, and its activity is inhibited by thyroid hormone.[59] In adults, type I 5'-MDI activity in liver (and perhaps kidney and muscle) probably accounts for most of the peripheral deiodination of T_4. The type II 5'-MDI acts primarily to increase local intracellular levels of T_3 in the brain and pituitary and is important to brown adipose tissue function during development. The outer-ring iodothyronine deiodinase also deiodinates rT_3 to diiodothyronine. Ontogeny of these deiodinases, studied in sheep, differs; the type II enzyme activity in brain appears by midgestation, whereas the hepatic type I activity is low at midgestation, increasing only near term.[70] Both types of enzyme activity are responsive to fetal thyroid status. Hepatic type I 5'-MDI activity, however, becomes thyroid hormone responsive (i.e., activity decreases with hypothyroidism) only during the final weeks of gestation.[57] Brain type II activity, in contrast, is responsive (increases with hypothyroidism) throughout the final third of gestation. It is proposed that the type II deiodinase, particularly in the hypothyroid fetus, plays an important role to provide a source of intracellular T_3 to those tissues (such as pituitary and, in some

species, brown fat and brain) that are dependent on T_3 during fetal life.[43, 50]

An inner (α) ring iodothyronine monodeiodinase (type III 5-MDI) has been characterized in most fetal tissues, including the placenta.[70] This enzyme system catalyzes the conversion to T_4 to rT_3 and T_3 to diiodothyronine. Fetal thyroid hormone metabolism is characterized by a predominance of type III enzyme activity, particularly in liver, kidney, and placenta, and this activity is believed to account for the increased circulating levels of rT_3 and probably rT_3 sulfate observed in the fetus. Placental type III deiodinase contributes to amniotic fluid rT_3 levels and presumably also contributes to circulating fetal rT_3. The persistence of high circulating rT_3 levels for several weeks in the newborn, however, indicates that type III 5'-MDI activities expressed in nonplacental tissues are also important to the maintenance of high circulating rT_3 levels.

Both T_3 and T_4 in blood are associated with various plasma proteins, including thyroxine-binding globulin (TBG), thyroxine binding prealbumin (TBPA), and albumin. TBG serves as the primary transport protein for both T_4 and T_3; about 70% of the total T_4 and 40 to 60% of total T_3 are bound to TBG. The rest of the thyroid hormones are distributed about equally between TBPA and albumin. The binding affinities of these proteins are such that adult free T_4 and T_3 concentrations are about 0.03 and 0.3% of the total hormone concentrations. TBG, TBPA, and albumin are produced by the liver, and fetal production of these proteins increases progressively during the final half of gestation.

Maturation of Thyroid Hormone Production

The pattern of perinatal thyroid hormone secretion in the human is shown in Figure 16–3. Maturation of thyroid system control can be considered to occur in three phases: hypothalamic, pituitary, and thyroidal. Changes in these systems are complex and superimposed on both the increasing production of serum TBG and changes in fetal tissue 5'-MDI activities. Although the fetal thyroid gland is able to concentrate iodide and synthesize thyroglobulin at 70 to 80 days' gestation, little thyroid hormone secretion occurs until after 18 weeks' gestation. At 17 to 19 weeks, thyroid follicular cell iodine uptake increases, and T_4 becomes measurable in the serum. Both total and free T_4 concentrations then increase steadily until

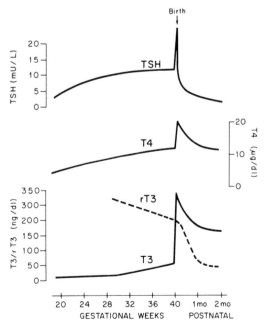

FIGURE 16–3. Patterns of TSH, T_4, T_3 and rT_3 secretion in the developing human. See text for details.

the final weeks of pregnancy.[12] This pattern differs from the pattern of development of serum T_3 levels in the fetus. The fetal T_3 concentration is low (<15 ng/dL, then 0.23 nmol/L) until 30 weeks and increases slowly in two distinct phases, a prenatal and postnatal phase. Prenatally serum T_3 increases slowly after 30 weeks' gestation to reach a level of approximately 50 ng/dL (0.77 nmol/L) in term cord serum. The prenatal increase in serum T_3 seems to be largely due to progressive maturation of hepatic type I (outer ring) iodothyronine deiodinase activity and increasing hepatic conversion of T_4 to T_3, although other tissue sources of deiodinase such as brown fat and kidney may be involved.

Fetal serum TSH increases rapidly from a low level (2 to 4 mU/L, 2 to 4 µU/mL) at 18 to 20 weeks to a relatively high value (8 to 12 mU/L) at term. Earlier data from cord blood of premature infants suggested a rapid increase in fetal serum TSH between 20 and 24 weeks to 15 to 20 mU/L (15 to 20 µU/mL) followed by a slow decline to about 10 mU/L (10 µU/mL) at term.[13] Data derived from in utero cord blood sampling indicate a progressive increase in TSH levels between midgestation and parturition.[67] The earlier data probably reflected the stress of delivery including neonatal cooling before the time of cord sampling. In either case, fetal thyroid gland function matures under the influence of a moderately elevated TSH level during the last half of gestation, suggesting that changes in both thyroid follicular cell sensitivity to TSH and pituitary thyrotroph sensitivity to the negative feedback effect of thyroid hormones occur during this period. The pituitary gland contains a type II 5' iodothyronine deiodinase that converts T_4 to active T_3; activity of this enzyme, similar to the type II monodeiodinase activity in brain, appears to mature during the second trimester of gestation. It is likely that the circulating T_4 level is most important in TSH control via the intrapituitary conversion to T_3. Thus even when the circulating T_3 level is low (as in midgestation), there is significant negative feedback control (by T_4) of pituitary TSH secretion.

The ontogeny of TRH secretion and function in the human fetus remain somewhat obscure. TRH immunoactivity is detectable in the hypothalamus by midgestation, increasing markedly in the third trimester as the serum TSH level increases. The premature infant (before 30 to 32 weeks) is characterized by low levels of T_4 and free T_4, a normal or low serum TSH value, and a normal or prolonged TSH response to TRH, indicating a state of physiologic TRH deficiency. This physiologic hypothyroid state spontaneously resolves during the early weeks of postnatal life and appears to mirror the intrauterine maturative state. The full-term human fetus, however, responds to pharmacologic maternal doses of TRH with a somewhat prolonged increase in TSH, suggesting a residual degree of relative hypothalamic (tertiary) hypothyroidism even at term.[61] Nonhypothalamic fetal sources of TRH (placental and pancreas) contribute to the elevated circulating levels of fetal and cord blood TRH. The significance of ectopic fetal TRH to the development of thyroid system control, however, remains to be clarified. There also appears to be a progressive maturation of the thyroidal follicular cell response to TSH. Studies in fetal sheep during the last third of gestation have shown a progressive increase in the T_4 to TSH ratio response to exogenous TRH.[28] Whether this is due to an increase in follicular cell TSH receptor number or maturation of TSH postreceptor responsiveness is not known. Similar data are not available in the human fetus.

Parturition is associated with profound changes in the hypothalamic-pituitary-thyroidal axis and in the iodothyronine metabolic pathways in a variety of tissues. Birth in the full-term infant is accompanied by an acute increase in pituitary TSH secretion, which, in turn, stimulates thyroid function, including iodine uptake and release of thyroidal T_4 and T_3. Peak neonatal TSH levels are reached by 30 minutes after birth, then gradually decline during the next few days of life, reaching values comparable to those in the adult by 3 to 4 weeks of age.[13] Serum T_3 and T_4 values mirror this TSH surge, peaking at 36 to 48 hours and decreasing to adult values by 4 to 5 weeks of life. The major physiologic stimulus for the acute postnatal TSH peak appears to be the cooling of the infant in the extrauterine environment.[13] The relative contributions of TRH or the sympathoadrenal system in regulating the TSH response to hypothermia are unknown.

In addition to the acute neonatal TSH effects on thyroidal hormone secretion, there are changes in thyroid hormone metabolism during the early neonatal period. In the sheep, in addition to the early (1 to 6 hours) newborn surge in circulating T_3 derived from thyroidal secretion, there is a progressive increase in T_4 to T_3 conversion in hepatic and, to a lesser extent, renal and brown adipose tissues; increased 5′-MDI activities can be demonstrated in these tissues.[56, 57, 71] The TSH surge is transient, whereas the increase in T_4 to T_3 conversion is permanent and accounts for the dramatic transition from low circulating T_3 levels in the fetus to the much higher values characteristic of infants and children. Studies in neonatal sheep also show a rapid fall in the circulating levels of sulfated iodothyronines, suggesting important adaptive changes in sulfation pathway metabolism in the neonatal period.[72]

The control of fetal thyroid hormone secretion can be characterized as a balance among increasing hypothalamic TRH secretion, increasing thyroid follicular cell sensitivity to TSH, and increasing pituitary sensitivity to thyroid hormone inhibition of TSH release. The fetus progresses from a state of combined primary (thyroidal) and tertiary (hypothalamic) hypothyroidism during the first half of gestation, through a state of tertiary hypothyroidism in the third trimester, to fully mature thyroid function in the perinatal period.

THYROID HORMONES AND NEONATAL THERMOGENESIS

The physiologic significance of the marked neonatal changes in circulatory thyroid hormone levels remains the focus of many investigators. Because of the major role of thyroid hormone in maintaining basal respiration in adult tissues[10, 20] and the importance of establishing autonomous thermogenesis in the newborn, it is tempting to link the perinatal changes in thyroid function with influences on neonatal thermogenesis. To understand the possible roles of thyroid hormone on neonatal thermogenesis, a review of those processes responsible for autonomous heat production in the newborn is presented.

Brown Adipose Tissue Thermogenesis

In the human newborn, oxygen consumption can double or triple during cold stress.[1] The two principal contributors to thermogenesis are shivering in skeletal muscle and nonshivering (chemical) thermogenesis in a variety of tissues. The relative contributions of these two systems to thermogenesis in the human newborn are unknown. In most large experimental neonatal mammals, however, nonshivering thermogenesis is the primary mechanism of heat production immediately postpartum, and most mammalian species are provided with a specialized brown adipose tissue that plays a critical role in the newborn thermogenic response. In newborn humans, brown adipose tissue constitutes about 1.4% of body weight,[41] and its anatomic distribution is important to its function. By far, the largest mass of brown adipose tissue envelops the kidneys and adrenal glands, with smaller masses present around the great vessels extending into the neck and out of the thoracic cavity into the axillae and under the clavicles.[27] The proximity of brown adipose tissue to these large blood vessels and vital vascular organs provides for the rapid transfer of heat to the circulation.

Additional anatomic studies reveal the rich adrenergic innervation of brown adipose tissue, which is critical to its thermogenic function. Thermogenesis is stimulated by norepinephrine binding to brown adipocyte membrane β-adrenergic receptors. Ultrastructurally, brown adipocytes demonstrate complex mitochondria, with sparse endoplasmic reticulum and few free ribosomes, consistent with the largely catabolic and oxidative functions of these cells. Chemically, in addition to large amounts of triglycerides and other lipids, brown adipose tissue contains an abundance of electron transport compounds: flavoproteins, heme-sulfur compounds, and the cytochromes as well as a great deal of cytochrome oxidase activity. The characteristic color of brown adipose tissue undoubtedly arises as a result of these compounds.

The unique structure and chemical makeup of these adipocytes provide the ability to generate more power, approximately 350 to 500 watt/kg, than any other tissue.[47] This is accomplished via several mechanisms. The oxidative degradation of substrates (largely lipids) coupled with the production of high-energy phosphate bonds, conserved in purine nucleotides, provides substantial energy that is ultimately expressed as heat. In brown adipose tissue mitochondria, the coupling of oxidation and phosphorylation is modulated via a unique 32,000 molecular weight guanidine diphosphate binding protein (uncoupling protein or thermogenin) first isolated by Ricquier et al.[60] Thermogenin uncouples phosphorylation, allowing for more energy dissipation as heat, thus providing the brown adipocyte a unique thermogenic mechanism.[48] That brown adipose tissue serves as the primary site for nonshivering thermogenesis in the newborn is supported by several observations. Cold stress in newborn rabbits results in an increase in temperature over sites of brown adipose tissue as well as release into the circulation of glycerol and free fatty acids.[24, 66] Extirpation of the brown fat in these animals decreases these responses nearly 80%. Moreover, in the human, the amount of brown fat decreases markedly with postnatal age.[2]

Thyroid Hormone Effects on Brown Fat

Several possible sites of thyroid hormone influence on thermogenesis in brown adipose tissue are depicted in Figure 16–4. The major effects are to increase brown adipose tissue 5'-MDI activity and increase the level of uncoupling protein.[16] Brown adipose tissue is a rich source of 5'-MDI. Both type I and type II 5' monodeiodinase activities are present in brown adipose tissue.[37, 71] In the rat, in vivo pulse labeling demonstrates that the major source of brown adipocyte T_3 is the intracellular deiodination of T_4, rather than uptake of serum T_3.[4] In this and other species, the type II 5' monodeiodinase activity in brown fat increases severalfold in response to hypothyroidism, thus tending to preserve intracellular T_3 levels and thermogenesis despite reduced cir-

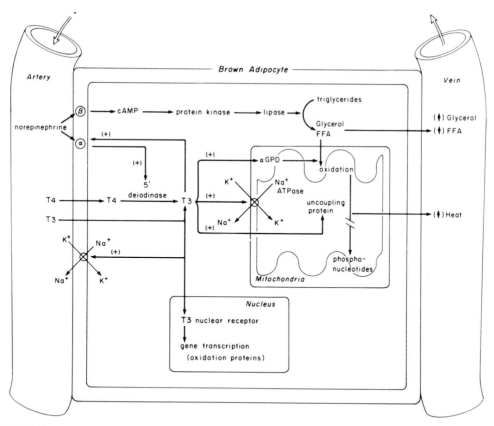

FIGURE 16–4. Thyroid hormone effects on brown adipocyte thermogenesis. See text for abbreviations and details.

culating T_4 levels.[4, 37, 71] The low level of uncoupling protein characteristic of brown adipocyte mitochondria from genetically obese (ob/ob) mice increases after thyroid hormone administration.[23] Moreover, in hypothyroid rats, the dose of exogenously administered T_3 required to restore normal uncoupling protein activity results in hypertriiodothyronemia, whereas a single replacement dose of T_4 normalizes uncoupling protein activity despite continued low serum thyroid hormone levels in T_4-treated animals.[5] These data support the view that local T_3 production via monodeiodination of intracellular T_4 to T_3 is critical to the optimal thermogenic function of brown adipose tissue.

Similar events probably are occurring in neonatal animals. Hypothyroidism in neonatal rat pups prevents the nearly 10-fold rise in thermogenin mRNA that occurs at the time of parturition.[49] Hypothyroidism induced by thyroidectomy 2 weeks before birth in the newborn lamb is associated with marked hypother-

mia, decreased circulating free fatty acid levels, and decreased oxygen consumption by brown adipocytes.[54] Thyroidectomy in fetal sheep 1 hour before birth, however, obtunds the neonatal increase in circulating T_3 levels but does not alter the thermogenic response; the 24-hour half-life for circulating T_4 probably allows continued in situ conversion of T_4 to T_3 in brown fat.[56] In contrast, thyroidectomy 2 weeks before delivery at term causes low levels of both serum T_3 and T_4 and markedly obtunds thermogenesis.

In addition to the actions on thermogenin levels and on T_4 to T_3 conversion, thyroid hormones may stimulate thermogenesis in brown adipocytes via effects on cell growth, lipid composition, or both. Hyperthyroid rat pups demonstrate hypertrophy and increased lipid content of brown adipocytes; hypothyroidism is associated with altered lipid composition and depletion. Although we have demonstrated that cell size and lipid content are important determinants of brown adipose tissue, we were unable to demonstrate changes in cell size or lipid content with altered thyroid status in developing sheep or rabbits.[29, 30, 54] It has also been suggested that thyroid hormones exert direct effects on brown adipose tissue metabolism via effects on mitochondrial enzyme activities. The glycerol phosphate shunt controls ion transport between cytosolic nicotinamide adenosine dehydrogenase (NAD) and mitochondrial cytochromes through a key enzyme, α glycerophosphate dehydrogenase. Activity of α glycerophosphate dehydrogenase doubles during the perinatal period[30] and increases after thyroid hormone administration to euthyroid neonatal rabbits.[29] We have not been able, however, to demonstrate an effect of hypothyroidism on glycerophosphate dehydrogenase activity in fetal sheep,[30] suggesting the effect may be species specific.[32]

$NA^+ - K^+$ ATPase may provide another level for thyroid hormone regulation of brown fat thermogenesis. This enzyme controls ion transport across both cell and mitochondrial membranes, thus maintaining ion gradients crucial to the coupling of oxidative phosphorylation in several tissues.[20] Hepatic $Na^+ - K^+$ ATPase activity increases after T_3 treatment of hypothyroid neonatal rabbits.[29] We have been unable to demonstrate an effect of thyroid hormone, however, on neonatal brown adipocyte levels of $NA^+ - K^+$ ATPase.[31]

Finally, thyroid hormones modulate brown fat thermogenesis through an effect on the sympathoadrenal system. The sympathetic nervous system plays a crucial role in the regulation of brown adipose tissue metabolism. Stimulation of adrenergic pathways innervating brown adipose tissue leads to increased heat production, an effect mimicked by β-adrenergic receptor agonist administration.[24, 35] Infusion of norepinephrine increases oxygen consumption and heat production in newborn rabbits; this effect is abolished by removing the brown fat in these animals.[48] Normal brown adipose tissue uncoupling protein expression is dependent on both adrenergic receptor activity and thyroid hormone levels.[64] In addition, α-adrenergically mediated sympathetic stimulation of 5′ monodeiodinase activity in brown adipose tissue also occurs.[65] In turn, thyroid status has been shown to influence circulating catecholamine levels,[9] adrenergic receptor binding characteristics,[6, 52] and adrenergic postreceptor adenyl cyclase activity.[33] Newborn animals are particularly dependent on circulating catecholamines for sympathoadrenal function.[51] Studies in newborn rats suggest that hypothyroidism decreases the thermogenic response associated with exogenously administered norepinephrine.[64] As previously stated, however, obtundation of the postnatal T_3 surge by acute thyroidectomy in term fetal lambs is not associated with major thermogenic effects or alterations in oxygen consumption.[7] This observation is supported by data in congenitally hypothyroid infants who manifest only subtle physical signs and are not usually hypothermic in the first few days of life. Thus, although the importance of both the thyroidal and the sympathoadrenal system integrity in the thermogenic response in newborns is clear, further studies are required to document the interplay of these two important systems.

MATURATION OF OTHER THYROID HORMONE EFFECTS

In addition to the influence of thyroid hormone on brown adipose tissue and tissue thermogenesis, there are important maturational effects on metabolism and development. The extent of these effects depends on the timing of appearance of thyroid hormone receptors as well as postreceptor events. Although plasma membrane and mitochondrial receptors for thyroid hormones have been described, the putative receptors from these sites have not been characterized, and their significance remains unclear. It is likely that the most important mediators of thyroid hormone action are the 50 kilodalton nuclear receptors, which function as gene transcription factors and are members of the superfamily of DNA-binding, thyroid-steroid hormone receptors.[36]

There are two nuclear thyroid hormone receptor genes in humans, one on chromosome 3 and one on chromosome 17. These are referred to as α and β, and each can be transcribed and translated into several mRNA products and several protein receptors, which have variable T_3-binding capacities.[36] Moreover, these receptors appear to bind to specific DNA thyroid response elements within thyroid-responsive genes. The capacity of thyroid hormone receptors to modulate responsive gene transcription appears to depend on their capacity to bind T_3, to dimerize, and to bind to DNA. Nuclear thyroid hormone receptors have been demonstrated by receptor binding studies in brain, liver, heart, and lung tissues of 10- to 19-week-old human fetuses.[3, 19] Other tissues were not studied, and there are no data regarding receptor mRNA levels during human development.

The pattern of ontogenesis of thyroid hormone effects in the human fetus and newborn are summarized in Figure 16–5. The TSH response to hypothyroxinemia is observed near midgestation and relates temporally to the increase in serum TSH observed in the normal fetus.[15] Bone maturation is responsive to thyroid hormone in utero in some human fetuses: one-third to one-half of athyroid human fetuses are born with a modest retardation of epiphyseal maturation.[34, 39] Quantitatively this may amount to 4 to 12 weeks and is corrected with early treatment. There also may be some delay in cerebral fontanelle closure. Birth length and weight of the athyroid fetus are normal, but linear bone growth and weight gain become thyroid responsive soon after birth, and by 6 weeks of age, significant reduction in growth can be detected in athyroid infants.[39] The striking observation, however, is that athyroid infants generally show few if any metabolic signs of hypothyroidism at birth. A few manifest prolonged hyperbilirubinemia, transient mild hypothermia, or both, but only

about 5% of infants with congenital hypothyroidism are detected by clinical signs or symptoms before the chemical diagnosis is reported.[15, 34, 39] Moreover, IQ values in such infants treated shortly after birth and tested at 5 to 8 years of age are similar to values in sibling and social status–matched controls.[18, 46]

There are reports that infants with very low T_4 levels and retarded bone maturation at birth have significantly lower IQ values at 5 to 7 years of age.[17, 62] This has not been a consistent observation, however, and data to support early adequate treatment of these infants are not available.[14] It has been proposed on the basis of data in fetal rats that transplacental passage of maternal T_4 in the athyrotic human fetus protects the brain from the effects of hypothyroidism.[43, 50, 68] A dependency on thyroid hormone during the early months of extrauterine life and extending to 2 to 3 years is clear. Whether T_4 has a role in human fetal brain maturation in utero, however, is not clear.

In addition to effects on thermogenesis and brain maturation, there are other important effects of thyroid hormones on metabolic and developmental events in human infants. These include hepatic function and hepatic enzyme activities, β-adrenergic receptor binding in a variety of tissues, carcass and muscle growth, skeletal maturation, skin maturation, growth hormone secretion and action, and epidermal growth factor metabolism.[15] Deficiency of thyroid hormones during the early months of life leads to the progressive accumulation of signs and symptoms during this period, and classic cretinism usually is manifest by 5 to 6 months of age in such infants.

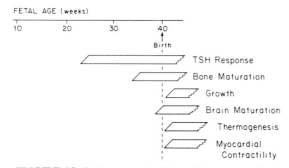

FETAL AGE (weeks)

FIGURE 16–5. Ontogenesis of thyroid hormone effects in the developing human. The left edge of the bar indicates the approximate time of onset of the specified effect. See text for details.

REFERENCES

1. Adamson SK Jr, Gandry GM, James LS. The influence of thermal factors upon oxygen consumption of the newborn infant. J Pediatr 1965;66:495.
2. Aherne W, Hull D. Brown adipose tissue and heat production in the newborn infant. J Pathol 1966;91:223.
3. Bernal J, Pekonen F. Ontogenesis of nuclear 3,5,3′ triiodothyronine receptor in human fetal brain. Endocrinology 1984;114:677.
4. Bianco AC, Silva JE. Nuclear 3,5,3′ triiodothyronine (T_3) in brown adipose tissue: receptor occupancy and sources of T_3 as determined by in-vivo techniques. Endocrinology 1984;114:1513.

5. Bianco AC, Silva JE. Intracellular conversion of thyroxine to triiodothyronine is required for the optimal thermogenic function of brown adipose tissue. J Clin Invest 1987;79:295.

6. Bilezikan JP, Loeb J. The influence of hyperthyroidism on the beta and alpha adrenergic receptor systems and adrenergic responsiveness. Endocr Rev 1983;4:378.

7. Breall SA, Rudolph AM, Heymann MA. Role of thyroid hormone in postnatal and metabolic adjustments. J Clin Invest 1984;73:1418.

8. Castaign H, Fournet JP, Leger FA, et al. Thyroid of the newborn and postnatal iodine overload. Arch Franc Pediat 1979;36:356.

9. Coulombe P, Dussault JH, Walter P. Plasma catecholamine concentrations in hyperthyroidism and hypothyroidism. Metabolism 1976;23:973.

10. Dauncey MJ. Thyroid hormones and thermogenesis. Proc Nutr Soc 1990;49:203.

11. Erickson LE, Fredriksson G. Phylogeny and ontogeny of the thyroid gland. In: Greer ME, ed. The thyroid gland (comprehensive endocrinology). New York: Raven Press, 1990:1.

12. Fisher DA. Thyroid hormone and thyroglobulin synthesis and secretion. In: Delange F, Fisher DA, Malvaux P, eds. Pediatric thyroidology. Basel: Karger, 1985:44.

13. Fisher DA, Dussault JH, Sack J, Chopra IJ. Ontogenesis of hypothalamic-pituitary-thyroid function and metabolism in man, sheep and rat. Recent Prog Horm Res 1977;33:59.

14. Fisher DA, Foley B. Early treatment of congenital hypothyroidism. Pediatrics 1989;83:785.

15. Fisher DA, Polk DH. Maturation of thyroid hormone actions. In: Delange F, Fisher DA, Glinoer D, eds. Research in congenital hypothyroidism. NATO ASI Series, New York: Plenum Press, 1988:61.

16. Freake HC, Schwartz HL, Oppenheimer JH. The regulation of lipogenesis by thyroid hormone and its contribution to thermogenesis. Endocrinology 1989;125:2868.

17. Glorieux J, Desjardins M, Dussault JH. Useful parameters to predict the eventual mental outcome of hypothyroid children. Pediatr Res 1988;24:6.

18. Glorieux J, Dussault JH, Morissette J, et al. Follow up at ages 5 and 7 years on mental development in children with hypothyroidism detected by Quebec screening program. J Pediatr 1985;107:913.

19. Gonzales LW, Ballard PL. Identification and characterization of nuclear 3,5,3′ triiodothyronine binding sites in fetal human lung. J Clin Endocrinol Metab 1981;53:21.

20. Guernsey DL, Edelman IS. Regulation of thermogenesis by thyroid hormones. In: Oppenheimer JH, Samuels NH, eds. Molecular basis of thyroid hormone action. New York: Academic Press, 1983:293.

21. Harada A, Hershman JM. Extraction of human chorionic thyrotropin from term placentas: failure to recover thyrotropic activity. J Clin Endocrinol Metab 1978;47:681.

22. Harada A, Hershman JM, Reed AW, et al. Comparison of thyroid simulators and thyroid hormone concentrations in the sera of pregnant women. J Clin Endocrinol Metab 1979;48:793.

23. Hogan S, Hims-Hagen J. Abnormal brown adipose tissue in genetically obese mice (ob/ob): effects of thyroxine. Am J Physiol 1981;241:436.

24. Hull D, Segall MM. The effects of sympathetic denervation and stimulation on brown adipose tissue in the newborn rabbit. J Physiol (Lond) 1965;177:63.

25. Ikegami M, Polk D, Tabor B, et al. Corticosteroid and thyrotropin releasing hormone effects on preterm lung function. J Appl Physiol 1991;70:2268.

26. Ingbar SH. Effects of iodine: autoregulation of the thyroid. In: Werner SC, Ingbar SH, eds. The thyroid. Hagerstown, MD: Harper & Row, 1978:206.

27. Itoh S, Kuroshima A. Distribution of brown adipose tissue in Japanese newborn infants. J Physiol Soc Jpn 1967;29:660.

28. Klein AH, Fisher DA. TRH stimulated pituitary and thyroid gland responsiveness and T₃ suppression in fetal and neonatal lambs. Endocrinology 1980;106:697.

29. Klein AH, Jenkins JJ, Reviczky A, et al. Thyroid hormone sensitive brown adipose tissue respiration in the newborn rabbit. Am J Physiol 1981;241:449.

30. Klein AH, Reviczky A, Chou P, et al. Development of brown adipose tissue thermogenesis in the ovine fetus and newborn. Endocrinology 1983;112:1162.

31. Klein AH, Reviczky A, Padbury JF, et al. Effect of changes in thyroid status on tissue respiration in fetal and newborn sheep. Am J Physiol 1983;244:603.

32. Kleitke B, Heitz G, Wollenberger A. Influence of thyroxine treatment on the activity of mitochondrial α glycerolphosphate dehydrogenase in liver, heart and skeletal muscle of several mammalian species. Biochim Biophys Acta 1966;130:270.

33. Krishna G, Hymie S, Brodie BB. Effects of thyroid hormones on adenyl cyclase in adipose tissue and on free fatty acid mobilization. Proc Natl Acad Sci USA 1968;59:884.

34. LaFranchi SH, Hanna CE, Krantz PL, et al. Screening for congenital hypothyroidism with specimen collection at two time periods: results of Northwest Regional Screening Program. Pediatrics 1985;76:734.

35. Landsberg L, Saville ME, Young JE. Sympathoadrenal system and regulation of thermogenesis. Am J Physiol 1984;247:181.

36. Lazar MA, Chin WW. Nuclear thyroid hormone receptors. J Clin Invest 1990;86:1777.

37. Leonard JL, Milley SA, Larsen PR. Thyroxine 5′ deiodinase activity in brown adipose tissue. Endocrinology 1983;112:1153.

38. Leonard JL, Visser TJ. Biochemistry of deiodination. In: Henneman NG, ed. Thyroid hormone metabolism. New York: Marcel Dekker, 1986:189.

39. Letarte J, LaFranchi SL. Clinical features of congenital hypothyroidism. In: Dussault JH, Walker PW, eds. Congenital hypothyroidism. New York: Marcel Dekker, 1983:351.

40. Marchant B, Brownlie BEW, Hant DM, et al. The placental transfer of propylthiouracil, methimazole and carbimazole. J Clin Endocrinol Metab 1977;45:1187.

41. Merklin RJ. Growth and distribution of fetal brown fat. Anat Rec 1974;178:637.

42. Morales WJ, O'Brien WF, Angel JF, et al. Fetal lung maturation: the combined use of corticosteroids and thyrotropin releasing hormone. Obstet Gynecol 1989;73:11.

43. Morreale de Escobar G, Obregon MJ, Escobar del Rey F. Transfer of thyroid hormones from the mother to the fetus. In: Delange F, Fisher DA, Glinoer D, eds. Research in congenital hypothyroidism. New York: Plenum Press, 1988:15.

44. Moya F, Mena P, Hensser F, et al. Response of the maternal, fetal and neonatal pituitary thyroid axis

to thyrotropin-releasing hormone. Pediatr Res 1986;20:982.

45. Neary JT, Nakamura C, Davies IJ, et al. Lower levels of thyrotropin releasing hormone degrading enzyme activity in human cord and maternal sera than in the serum of euthyroid, nonpregnant adults. J Clin Invest 1978;62:1.

46. New England Congenital Hypothyroid Collaborative. Neonatal screening: status of patients at 6 years of age. J Pediatr 1985;107:915.

47. Nicholls DG, Locke RM. Cellular mechanisms of heat dissipation. In: Girardier L, Stock MJ, eds. Mammalian thermogenesis. New York: Chapman & Hall, 1983:8.

48. Nicholls DG, Locke RM. Thermogenic mechanisms in brown fat. Physiol Rev 1984;64:1.

49. Obregon MJ, Pitamber R, Jacobsson A, et al. Euthyroid status is essential for the perinatal increase in thermogenic m-RNA in brown adipose tissue of rat pups. Biochem Biophys Res Comm 1987;148:9.

50. Obregon MJ, Ruiz deOna C, Escobar del Rey F, Morreale de Escobar G. Regulation of intracellular thyroid hormone concentration in the fetus. In: Delange F, Fisher DA, Glinoer D, eds. Research in congenital hypothyroidism. New York: Plenum Press, 1988:79.

51. Padbury JF, Agata Y, Ludlow J, et al. Effect of fetal adrenalectomy on catecholamine release and physiologic adaptation at birth in sheep. J Clin Invest 1987;80:1096.

52. Padbury JF, Klein AH, Lam RW, et al. The effect of thyroid status on lung and heart beta adrenergic receptors in fetal and newborn sheep. Dev Pharmacol Ther 1986;9:44.

53. Pearse AGE, Carvalheira AF. Cytochemical evidence for an ultimobranchial origin of rodent thyroid C cells. Nature 1967;214:929.

54. Polk DH, Callegari CC, Newnham J, et al. Effect of fetal thyroidectomy on newborn thermogenesis in lambs. Pediatr Res 1987;21:453.

55. Polk DH, Reviczky A, Lam RW, Fisher DA. Thyrotropin releasing hormone in the ovine fetus: ontogeny and effect of thyroid hormone. Am J Physiol 1991;260:E53.

56. Polk DH, Wu SY, Fisher DA. Serum thyroid hormones and tissue 5' monodeiodinase activity in acutely thyroidectomized newborn lambs. Am J Physiol 1986;251:151.

57. Polk DH, Wu SY, Wright C, et al. Ontogeny of thyroid hormone effects on 5' monodeiodinase activity in fetal sheep. Am J Physiol 1988;254:337.

58. Raiha N, Hjelt L. The correlation between the development of the hypophyseal portal system and the onset of neurosecretory activity in the human fetus and infant. Acta Pediatr 1957;46(suppl):610.

59. Refetoff S, Larsen PR. Transport, cellular uptake and

metabolism of thyroid hormone. In: De Groot LJ, Besser M, Burger H, et al, eds. Endocrinology. Philadelphia: WB Saunders, 1989:541.

60. Ricquier D, Lin CS, Kingenberg M. Isolation of the GDP binding protein from brown adipose tissue mitochondria of several animals and amino acid composition study in rat. Biochem Biophys Res Commun 1982;106:582.

61. Roti E, Ghudi A, Braverman L, et al. Human cord blood concentrations of thyrotropin, thyroglobulin and iodothyronines after maternal administration of thyrotropin-releasing hormone. J Clin Endocrinol Metab 1981;53:813.

62. Rovet J, Ehrlich R, Sorbara D. Intellectual outcome in children with fetal hypothyroidism. J Pediatr 1987;110:700.

63. Shepard TH. Onset of function in the human fetal thyroid: biochemical and radioautographic studies from organ culture. J Clin Endocrinol 1967;27:945.

64. Silva JE. Full expression of uncoupling protein gene requires the concurrence of norepinephrine and triiodothyronine. Mol Endocrinol 1988;2:706.

65. Silva JE, Larsen PR. Adrenergic activation of T_3 production in BAT. Nature 1983;305:712.

66. Smith PE, Horwitz BA. Brown fat and thermogenesis. Physiol Rev 1969;49:330.

67. Thorpe-Beeston JG, Nicolaides KH, Felton CV, et al. Maturation of the secretion of thyroid hormone and thyroid stimulating hormone in the fetus. N Engl J Med 1991;324:532.

68. Vulsma T, Gons MH, DeVijlder JJM. Maternal-fetal transfer of thyroxine in congenital hypothyroidism due to a total organification defect or thyroid agenesis. N Engl J Med 1989;321:13.

69. Winters AJ, Eskay RL, Porter JD. Concentration and distribution of TRH and LRH in the human fetal brain. J Clin Endocrinol Metab 1974;39:960.

70. Wu SY, Fisher DA, Polk DH, Chopra I. Maturation of thyroid hormone metabolism. In: Wu SY, ed. Thyroid hormone metabolism. Boston: Blackwell Scientific Publications, 1990:293.

71. Wu SY, Merryfield ML, Polk DH, Fisher DA. Two pathways for thyroxine 5' monodeiodination in brown adipose tissue in fetal sheep: ontogenesis and divergent responses to hypothyroidism and 3,5,3' triiodothyronine replacement. Endocrinology 1990;126:1950.

72. Wu SY, Polk DH, Elbanna IM, et al. Is triiodothyronine sulfate (T_3s) the hidden metabolite of thryroxine (T_4) metabolism in fetal sheep? (abstr). Proceedings of the Endocrinology Society, 1991:1261.

73. Zakarija M, McKenzie JM. Pregnancy-associated changes in the thyroid stimulating antibody of Graves disease and the relationship to neonatal hyperthyroidism. J Clin Endocrinol Metab 1983;57:1036.

Endocrinology of Implantation*

Koji Yoshinaga

---

*All material in this chapter is in the public domain, with the exception of any borrowed figures or tables.

The current concept of endocrinology cannot be discussed without including the paracrine and autocrine mechanisms of signal transduction. The classic endocrine mechanism deals with a signal transduction from the endocrine gland to the target tissues. The signal (hormone) that is produced in the endocrine gland is secreted into the blood stream, and the hormone exerts its action on being transported by the blood stream to the target tissue distant from the site of hormone production. The paracrine mechanism is a signal transduction between adjacent cells that does not need blood-borne transportation of the signal(s). Modification of the epithelial cells by the underlying stromal cells by means of growth factors is considered as an example of the paracrine mechanism.[15] The autocrine mechanism is a signal transduction directed to the cell itself that produces the signal. The self-promoting tumor growth by growth factors produced and secreted by breast cancer cells themselves is an example of the autocrine mechanism. The phenomenon of blastocyst implantation is a series of local interactions between trophoblast cells and the endometrial cells or extracellular matrix components. Because the process of implantation is limited locally in a small portion of the endometrium, it is reasonable to assume that the implantation process involves the paracrine or autocrine mechanisms (or both) at some stages in the whole process of blastocyst implantation.

In the first section of this chapter, we consider the classic hormone profiles and hormonal requirement for blastocyst implantation. Following, preparation for implantation is considered regarding the endometrial preparation and blastocyst maturation. The concept of uterine receptivity is presented in this section. In the next section, a possible sequence of events during blastocyst implantation is described. Cell to cell interactions are considered with reference to possible paracrine or autocrine mechanisms involved in a series of steps of the implantation process. The scarcity of human or nonhuman primate data is supplemented by suggestions by extrapolating available animal data and by the analogy of tumor cell invasion. The final section considers some clinical aspects related to implantation, i.e., implantation of the transferred embryos fertilized in vitro and ectopic pregnancy.

HORMONE LEVELS AND HORMONAL REQUIREMENT FOR IMPLANTATION

Hormone Levels

The precise cyclic patterns and changes of the pituitary and ovarian hormone levels in peripheral blood or plasma became available with increasing precision of radioimmunoassay methods. In the ovary, selected follicles grow under the influence of gonadotropins and presumably of local agents, such as growth factors. Among these selected follicles, only one attains the graafian follicle stage. The estrogen level rapidly increases during the last 5 days before ovulation. After ovulation, the ruptured follicle luteinizes, and the resulting corpus luteum secretes progesterone and estrogen. Estrogen secretion is increased during the luteal phase, corresponding with the increase in progesterone. The magnitude of the estrogen secretion increase during the luteal phase, however, is not as prominent as seen during the follicular phase. In response to the cyclic ovarian steroid hormone secretion, the uterine endometrium exhibits morphologic and functional changes characteristic of the proliferative and secretory phases. For useful information on human pituitary and ovarian hormones in implantation and early pregnancy, the readers are referred to a concise review by Lenton.[37]

Daily mean plasma hormone concentrations measured by Lenton et al.[38] are shown in Figure 17–1. The data presented depict the hormone profiles during nonconception cycles and those of conception cycles. They indicate that the progesterone concentrations in the conception cycle are significantly higher than those in the nonconception cycle during the preimplantation period. These workers consider the higher progesterone concentration a manifestation of the maternal recognition of pregnancy in women.

The higher progesterone concentrations during the preimplantation period in the conception cycle is likely due to some factors associated with the presence of early conceptus other than human chorionic gonadotropin (hCG). Involvement of hCG in the luteotropic complex during such an early stage of pregnancy appears unlikely because hCG becomes

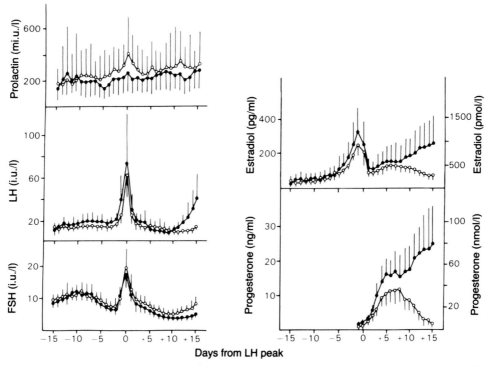

FIGURE 17–1. Mean (± SD) log hormone concentrations in plasma during the nonconception cycles (○–○) and conception cycles (●–●) in women. (From Lenton EA, Sulaiman K, Sabowale O, Cooke ID. The human menstrual cycle: Plasma concentrations of prolactin, LH, FSH, oestradiol and progesterone in conceiving and non-conceiving women. J Reprod Fertil 1982;65:131. With permission.)

detectable only after embryos fertilized in vitro attain the blastocyst stage and hatch out of the zonae pellucidae, and hCG becomes detectable only after implantation in vivo. The significantly higher progesterone levels during the preimplantation period in pregnancy than in pseudopregnancy have also been observed in the rat.[11]

The influence of the conceptus on the maternal endocrine system varies among different species. The variation is due to the functional difference in the trophoblastic cells. For example, the two different functions are observed when comparison is made between the human and the sheep. In the human and other primates, the syncytiotrophoblast cells secrete CG (a luteinizing hormone [LH]–like heterodimer), which acts on the corpus luteum and prolongs its ephemeral life span, to elevate progesterone secretion until such time that the placental progesterone secretion can take over that of the corpus luteum. In sheep, the hormone secreted by the trophoblastic cells is not a gonadotropin but an antiluteoly-

sin (ovine trophoblast protein-1 [oTP-1]). The chemical nature of this antiluteolysin is an interferon of the α family, and it acts on the uterine endometrial epithelial cells to prevent the release of prostaglandin $F_{2\alpha}$.[57] Although rodent chorion-derived protein hormones have luteotropic activity, their molecules are prolactin-like single-chain proteins and thus called (placental) luteotropin and are distinguished from CGs.

It is not known whether the maintenance of the luteal function is actually carried out by both the gonadotropin and the antiluteolysin of trophoblast origin in any mammalian species. The findings of interferons in human and laboratory animal placentae, however, suggest that placental interferons may have physiologic or immunologic roles to facilitate establishment and maintenance of pregnancy. The antiviral activity of murine conceptus and placental tissue has been shown to be classic interferon α or β. The production rate of interferons by sheep conceptuses is, however, much greater than nonruminant conceptuses or placental tissues. In the human, we do not have convincing evidence that substances such as prostaglandins exert a luteolytic effect. Thus the antiluteolytic activity in primates appears to be minimal, if any. Antiviral activity of the placental interferons is considered by itself useful to protect the developing embryos and fetuses. Besides the antiviral activity, interferons may play a role in immunologic protection. A possible mechanism postulated is that interferon α acts as an autocrine signal on the trophoblast cells to stimulate the production of cell surface antigens that make the invading trophoblast "nonforeign."[66] Clarification of the immunologic role of trophoblast interferon is awaited.

Although their physiologic roles are less defined than hCG and ruminant conceptus-derived interferons, other factors have been reported to influence the successful establishment of pregnancy. Early pregnancy factor is a glycoprotein with a molecular weight of approximately 20 kD and is found in mammalian serum and urine in the very early stage of pregnancy even before implantation.[63] Platelet activating factor is a phosphocholine and has been shown to be released by preimplantation mice and human embryos within hours of fertilization—this was correlated with their ability to implant.[22, 49] The roles of pregnancy-specific β_1 glycoprotein 1, human placental lactogen, pregnancy-associated plasma protein-A, and other proteins in implantation remain to be investigated.

Hormonal Requirement

It is well established that progesterone is essential to prepare the uterine endometrium for blastocyst implantation. Abolition of the ovaries soon after fertilization and replacement therapy with progesterone clearly provide the evidence that progesterone is indispensable for implantation. Progesterone alone is reported to be sufficient for implantation in the rhesus monkey because pregnancy was successfully maintained in the rhesus monkeys that were ovariectomized soon after fertilization and treated only with progesterone.[44] Even if an artificial treatment can mimic the ovarian function during early pregnancy, it does not

necessarily mean that the ovarian function during early pregnancy is progesterone secretion only. Administration of antiestrogen before implantation in monkeys interferes with the establishment of pregnancy.[46] Ovariectomized monkeys treated with ovarian steroids by placing Silastic tubings of progesterone and estrogen for scheduled periods display cyclic activity of the uterus mimicking the menstrual cycle. The embryos transferred into the fallopian tubes or the uteri of such monkeys resulted in the establishment of pregnancy.[28] The essential role of estrogen in inducing implantation in the uterus preexposed to progesterone has been clearly shown in laboratory rodents because implantation cannot be induced in these species of animals with progesterone alone. Implantation can be induced in progesterone-treated rats or mice with much smaller doses of estrogen than those that cause estrous behavior. Estrogen exerts its action locally on the uterus or blastocyst in synergizing with progesterone. Studies[17, 50] suggest that estrogen action is mediated by growth factors at the local sites.

Because estrogen secretion is increased in parallel with progesterone during the luteal phase, the preimplantation rise in estrogen in humans is likely to be important for successful implantation. Too much estrogen, however, has adverse effects on the endometrium. When the estrogen to progesterone ratio is high, the pregnancy outcome after embryo transfer is poor,[36] and controlled ovarian hyperstimulation has been reported to inhibit embryo implantation after in vitro fertilization (IVF) by decreasing endometrial receptivity.[54]

PREPARATION FOR BLASTOCYST IMPLANTATION

Preparation of the Uterus for Implantation

The cyclic changes in ovarian steroid levels are reflected on the cyclic changes of the endometrial structure and function. After menstruation, the endometrium is thin, and its glands are sparse, narrow, and straight. The epithelial cells of the uterine glands are cuboidal to columnar. Under the influence of the increasing level of estrogen, the endometrium increases its thickness, the growth of glandular epithelial cells exceeds that of the stromal tissue, and the mitotic activity of the epithelial cells increases, resulting in tortuous appearance of uterine glands. The luminal and glandular epithelial cells increase their height to be tall columnar. The stroma becomes edematous. The stromal cells are spindle shaped and scattered in edematous stromal tissue. The cytoplasm is scanty. At the end of the proliferative phase, the edema regresses; thus the endometrium temporarily reduces its thickness, and thus the uterine glands become more tortuous. The daily morphologic changes of the endometrium are described in detail.[16, 21, 62]

The mitogenic action of estrogen and progesterone on the endometrial cells is clearly tissue specific; i.e., estrogen stimulates mitosis of the epithelial cells, whereas progesterone stimulates stromal cell mitosis.[41] The results obtained on the primate uterus suggest that estrogen acts directly on the stromal cells that contain estrogen receptors, and stromal cell–originated growth factor(s) stimulate proliferation of epithelial cells.[9] Thus quantitation and localization of steroid hormone receptors in the endometrial tissues do not provide sufficient information to understand the steroid hormone action. One report indicates that insulin-like growth factor-1 is predominantly synthesized in the glandular and luminal epithelium on days 1 to 2, in stromal cells on days 3 to 4, and in decidual cells on days 5 to 6 in pregnant mice.[32] These results indicate that it is important to investigate the steroid hormone action on the uterine tissues in terms of the localization and activity of steroid receptors and the production and action site of the second message (e.g., growth factor) that is produced as a result of the binding of the steroid-receptor complex to the DNA.

During the secretory phase of the cycle, the human uterine endometrium exhibits special ultrastructural features under the influence of increasing progesterone and estrogen. The morphologic features of the glandular epithelial cells are subnuclear glycogenization, nucleolar channel system, and subsequent glycoprotein secretion. The active glandular secretion reaches its maximum level around the time of blastocyst implantation (on cycle days 21 to

23), and the stromal tissue becomes edematous.

Receptivity of the Uterus for Blastocyst Implantation

Embryo transfer and transplantation studies in experimental animals indicate that the uterus is usually not an accommodating organ to a blastocyst. When blastocysts are removed from the uterus before implantation and are transplanted into ectopic sites, most of the transplanted blastocysts initiate invasion of the recipient tissues. The blastocysts transferred into the lumen of the uterus outside of the receptive phase are either expelled out of the uterus, or, if the expulsion is prevented by ligation of the cervical end of the uterus, the blastocysts degenerate. It is only a brief period of time, termed the *receptive phase*, that a mature blastocyst is permitted to implant into the endometrium. The uterus that has already experienced the receptive phase automatically enters into the refractory phase. This transition takes place regardless of the occurrence of implantation during the receptive phase.

In natural pregnancy, the timing of ovulation, fertilization, subsequent development of the preimplantation embryo, and transportation of the embryo to the site of attachment to the surface of the endometrium coincide with the preparation of the uterus for receiving the mature blastocyst. The importance of the synchrony between the embryonic development and the uterine preparation has been clearly shown as pregnancy failure in a number of different conditions. Preimplantation embryos transferred asynchronously in laboratory and domestic animals have been shown to fail establishing pregnancy[1]; implantation is delayed by lactation concurrent with early pregnancy in small rodents[35]; and exposure of early pregnant mice to the odor of males of different strains of mice, upsetting the endocrine balance, terminates pregnancy.[8, 51]

Duration of the Receptive Phase

Lenton,[37] using an ultrasensitive assay, determined that hCG becomes first detectable on the days 8, 9, or 10 after the LH surge. Therefore the receptive phase in the human is considered to start around or a little earlier than 8 days after the LH surge. It is controversial, however, how long the uterus remains receptive to a mature blastocyst.

The receptive phase lasts for a short period of time; it is less than 24 hours in the rat. In castrated monkeys treated with a sequential estrogen-progesterone therapy, Hodgen[28] demonstrated that embryos transferred into the fallopian tube implanted in the uterus, and the surrogate mothers became pregnant. Analysis of the time of embryo transfer during the hormone treatment and the stage of the transferred embryos that resulted in successful pregnancy led Hodgen to the assumption that the receptive phase in the rhesus monkey is as long as 3 days. In the human, the results of IVF and embryo transfer studies indicate that successful pregnancies are obtained only in the patients in whom implantation takes place 5 to 7 days after the LH surge.[36] Salat-Baroux et al.[58] also examined the duration of the receptive phase (implantation window) by analyzing the data obtained in their studies on the pregnancy outcome after transfer of frozen-thawed embryos in the cycle following the stimulated cycle when the oocytes were recovered. Based on the results obtained, these researchers consider the *implantation window* is wider than the reported assumption between the 17th and 19th day of the menstrual cycle. Navot et al.[47] studied the window of implantation in ovarian failure patients who have been treated with estrogen and progesterone in the protocol to mimic closely the natural 28-day cycle. Two-cell to 12-cell stage embryos, 42 to 48 hours after insemination, were transferred onto endometria chronologically and histologically dated to days 16 through 24 of a 28-day cycle. Successful embryo implantation occurred only with embryo transfers between days 16 and 19 of the cycle. These results indicate that the receptive phase may last for 4 days in the human.

Characteristics of the Receptive Uterus

The endometrium of the rhesus monkey at the time of implantation is generally moderately edematous and vascular; both the luminal and the glandular epithelium of relatively superficial zones have scattered ciliated cells and more ubiquitous secretory cells with the subsurface accumulation of secretory vesicles.[20] Ultrastructural studies indicate that new epithelial surface structures, pinopods, appear as the uterus enters into the receptive phase (Fig. 17–2). These bulbous cytoplasmic protrusions appear to persist only during the receptive phase.[40, 64] Although their function has not clearly been defined, the pinopods appear to facilitate attachment of the overlying blastocyst to the surface of the epithelium by means of endocytosis[64, 52] (Fig. 17–3).

An ultrastructural study on the human epithelial cells reports that the receptive endometrial epithelial cells contain giant mitochondria surrounded by rough endoplasmic reticulum, a typical nuclear channel system, and loose interdigitation of the membranes in the middle and basal part of the lateral wall.[36] Thick, negatively charged glycoproteins coat the endometrial epithelial surface. Before or at the time of implantation, luminal surface negativity is reduced, and glycocalyx morphology is altered.[45] In the rabbit, certain proteins, including a protein with a molecular weight of 42 kD on the epithelial surface, appear coincidentally with the receptive phase.[30] A similar observation has been made in the monkey uterus.[4] In the human endometrial stroma, fibroblast-like stromal cells enlarge to plump, spherical *predecidual cells* with vesicular nuclei and abundant clear cytoplasm. Another major population of cells—large granular lymphocytes—was formerly called *endometrial granulocytes*.[16] Their function remains to be clarified. The stromal extracellular matrix also changes under the influence of ovarian hormones. Further studies are needed as to what biochemical and structural changes are indeed made to prepare the stromal tissue for accepting the implanting blastocyst.

Maturation of Blastocyst

Human blastocyst implantation takes place at the fundus of the uterus during its seventh day of development.[27] In parallel with the endometrial preparation for implantation, the blas-

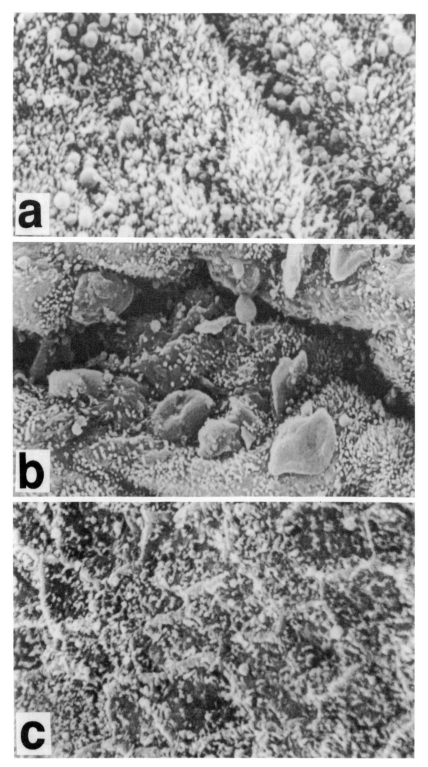

FIGURE 17–2. Scanning electron micrographs of the rat uterine epithelial surface: *A*, The prereceptive phase; *B*, the receptive phase; and *C*, the refractory phase. The epithelial surface in the receptive phase is characterized by the appearance of the pinopods, the bulbous cytoplasmic protrusions. (From Martel D, Frydman K, Sarantis L, et al. Scanning electron microscopy of the uterine luminal epithelium as a marker of the implantation window. In: Yoshinaga K, ed. Blastocyst Implantation. Boston: Adams Publishing Group [Serono Symposia USA], 1989:225–230. With permission.)

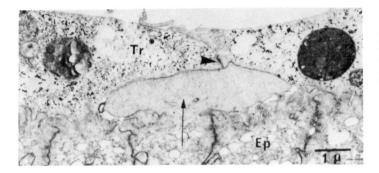

FIGURE 17–3. Rat trophoblast cells attached to a pinopod of an epithelial cell. Tr = Trophoblast cell; arrow = pinopod; arrow head = tight junction. (From Tachi S, Tachi C, Lindner HR. Ultrastructural features of blastocyst attachment and trophoblastic invasion in the rat. J Reprod Fertil 1970;21:37. With permission.)

tocyst achieves its final stage of preimplantation development. The morula stage embryo initiates tissue differentiation, and as a fluid-accumulating cavity is being formed, blastomeres differentiate into the trophectoderm and inner cell mass cells. Following the cavity formation, the blastocyst exhibits a number of maturational morphologic changes in cellular organelles, trophoblast cell junctions, and basal lamina formation.[18] These morphologic maturational changes are considered to be regulated both endogenously and exogenously by autocrine or paracrine mechanisms. When a mouse preimplantation embryo is cultured by itself, the embryonic development is poor. When 5 or 10 embryos are cultured together, however, they develop better than a singly cultured embryo. Addition of epidermal growth factor (EGF) or transforming growth factors also improves the development of embryos into the blastocyst stage.[50] Production of fibroblast growth factor–like (FGF-like) growth factors[56] and EGF and EGF receptor[17] by preimplantation embryos also supports the notion that the embryonic maturation before implantation is regulated by autocrine or paracrine mechanisms.

The mature blastocyst "hatches" out of the zona pellucida before implantation into the uterine endometrium. Hatching can be observed in vitro. Empty zonae pellucidae, together with hatched blastocysts, may be occasionally observed in the flushings of the rodent uteri before implantation. Although the precise mechanism of the zona shedding is not clear, involvement of prostaglandins and enzymes of trophoblast and of uterine origin have been suggested. Deprivation of estrogen or inhibition of prostaglandin synthesis results in a delay in hatching. EGF and EGF receptors

were localized in the blastocyst.[17, 50] Although the mechanism of the zona hatching remains to be clarified, these results lead to a hypothetical mechanism by which estrogen stimulates the zona hatching: It may be speculated that estrogen acts on the blastocyst to increase the production of EGF receptor on trophoblast cell surface as well as the production of EGF in the blastocyst itself and the uterine epithelium. In the trophoblast cells, the produced EGF binds the EGF receptor of its own or neighboring trophoblast cells, by the paracrine or autocrine mechanism. This results in secretion of prostaglandins, which, in turn, stimulates proteinase activity. The increase in the enzyme activity of the trophoblast cells results in digestion of the zona pellucida.

PROCESS OF BLASTOCYST IMPLANTATION

Site of Implantation

The process of implantation may be considered to be divided into three successive steps: apposition, adhesion, and invasion. In the youngest known human blastocyst specimen, the blastocyst has penetrated the uterine epithelium. The epithelial tissue has disappeared at the site of blastocyst invasion, and this site has been closed by a coagulum of fibrin. Thus we do not know how the site of blastocyst attachment is chosen. In polytocous animals, blastocysts are rather evenly distributed along the tubal uterine horns. Muscle contractions are considered to play a major role in the even distribution of multiple blastocysts along the uterine horns. Even when the number of blastocysts is increased by transferring a large number of blastocysts, most of them are able to implant, although many of them cannot survive.[42] Thus it is conceivable that there are many sites in the endometrium where a blastocyst can implant, but the blastocyst that happens to be carried to a site on the midline by muscle movements implants when the uterus becomes receptive. Apposition of the blastocyst is to situate itself against the uterine epithelium, and this results in interdigitation of the microvilli of the trophoblast and luminal epithelial cells.

In many mammalian species, the blastocyst implants on the antimesometrial side of the tubal uterine horn. In the primate, the first attachment is on the dorsal or ventral uterine wall midline because this position corresponds to the antimesometrial side of a bicornuate uterus. In some other species, the implantation takes place on the mesometrial side. As to the orientation of the embryonic disc, or the inner cell mass, within the blastocyst in relation to the uterus, it may be mesometrial (as seen in small rodents), antimesometrial (the primate), or lateral. The factors that determine the site of the uterus and the orientation of the blastocyst are considered to be localized expressions of the membrane constituents that are involved in the initial attachment (carbohydrate moieties, glycoproteins, ligands, and their receptors) on both the trophoblast and uterine epithelial cell membranes.

There has been an intriguing hypothesis that the site of trophoblast attachment and invasion through uterine epithelium was on the location of underlying endometrial blood vessels.[7] Hoffman and Winfrey[29] reexamined the Boving hypothesis by analyzing their own morphologic data in the rabbit. Their survey suggests that initial attachment of trophoblast is somewhat more random than implied by previous reports, and preferential attachment over either crypts (gland openings) or to epivascular epithelium was not apparent. Further studies, however, appear to be needed to negate this theory conclusively.

Adhesion Proteins

The initial adhesion step involves glycocalyces on the cell surfaces. In general, there are a number of glycoproteins that serve the cell-cell adhesion. According to the structure of the molecule, cell adhesion molecules are classified into two groups: (1) The members of the first group have structural features similar to those found in antibodies (immunoglobulins); (2) the members of the second group are those molecules that require calcium for their activity.[14] Further, cell adhesion molecules, substrate adhesion molecules, and cell junctional molecules play important roles in the regulation of morphologic changes, cell adhesion, and migration.

The first step of cell to cell adhesion appears to concern the cell adhesion molecules. Hoffman et al.[30] identified such a glycoprotein with a molecular weight of 42 kD that appears coincidental with the period during which the uterus is receptive for blastocyst implantation in the rabbit. In the human, such a glycoprotein has not yet been identified.

The initial site of invasion by trophoblast of the uterine epithelium is between the epithelial cells. This initial invasion site is observed in guinea pigs, rhesus monkeys, and humans where implantation is intrusive (Fig. 17–4). The initial interepithelial cell invasion is also observed in rats.[33] Because the epithelial cells are joined together by tight junctions (zonulae occludentes), trophoblast cells must interact with these junctional complexes during the interepithelial cell penetration. The tight junction contains specific protein, ZO-1,[3] and cingulin.[12] At the lateral-basal aspects of epithelial cells, E-cadherin, or uvomorulin (one type of calcium-dependent cell adhesion molecule), serves as a cell to cell adhesion molecule. E-cadherin is produced by epithelial cells and localized between the polarized uterine epithelial cells in vitro.[24]

The fact that the initial site of the trophoblast invasion of the epithelium is the junctional complex nearest to the surface suggests that the trophoblast cells appear to have affinity to these junctional complex components. As is described for the basal lamina invasion by trophoblast cells, the trophoblast cell surface may have either ligands or receptors to the uterine cell surface components, particularly to the components of the cell to cell junctional complexes. Although there is no direct evidence that indicates the trophoblast cells

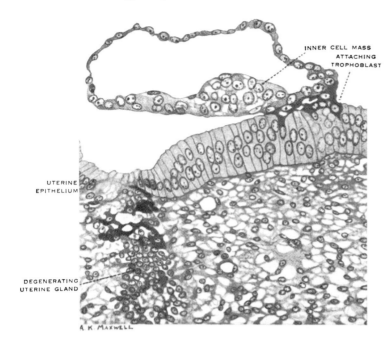

INNER CELL MASS

ATTACHING
TROPHOBLAST

UTERINE
EPITHELIUM

DEGENERATING
UTERINE GLAND

A K MAXWELL

FIGURE 17–4. The early attachment stage of the trophoblast to the uterine epithelium in the monkey. (From Hamilton WJ, Boyd JD, Mossman HW. The implantation of the blastocyst and the development of the fetal membranes, placenta and decidua. In: Human Embryology. Baltimore: Williams & Wilkins, 1972;83:131. With permission. [After Wislocki and Streeter.[65]])

contain receptors to ZO-1 or other junction-specific proteins, the invading trophoblast cell surface may have a special affinity to the cell junction-specific proteins. Babalola et al.[6] proposed that cytotrophoblast cells aggregate via the intermediacy of cell surface proteins and that E-cadherin is one protein that participates in this process. After aggregation, E-cadherin becomes undetectable in the resulting syncytiotrophoblast cell. Thus the invading syncytiotrophoblast cells are capable of digesting E-cadherin. Once the invading trophoblast uncouples the tight junction, the lateral adhesion proteins, E-cadherin and others, are considered to be easily digested by the trophoblast cells.

Formation of Junctions Between Trophoblast and Uterine Cells

The electron microscopic studies of cell to cell attachment at the early stages of implantation clearly indicate the establishment of junctional complexes between the trophoblast cell and the uterine epithelial cell. These junctional complexes established between the trophoblastic cell membrane and that of the maternal cell are tight junctions[64] and desmosomes[13, 19] (Fig. 17–5). The desmosome is a complex disc-shaped structure at the surface of one cell that is matched with an identical structure at the surface of another cell. The cell membranes are flat, and some material is often present in the intercellular space. Inside the membrane of each cell is a circular plaque, and groups of intermediate filaments of the cytokeratin variety are inserted into the plaque or make a hairpin turn to the cytoplasm. The function of the desmosome is to provide firm attachment between the cells. Because the formation of junctions is considered to require a prior cell adhesion molecule-mediated event,[43] it is quite likely that the initial attachment of the trophoblast cell membrane and the uterine epithelial cell membrane involves cell adhesion proteins.

Although the process of the establishment of junctions between the trophoblastic cells and the uterine luminal epithelial cells has not as yet been clarified, it may be postulated that trophoblast and epithelial cells bind each other by means of carbohydrate linkage and a ligand-receptor binding mechanism. Many membrane receptors have been shown to be coupled to G proteins, and the binding of ligand to its receptor results in activation of G protein as a means of signal transduction. The assembly of cytoskeleton components, such as actin and tubulin, has been shown to be controlled by G proteins,[10] and the ligand binding results in rearrangement of cytoskeletal elements. The ligand-receptor bindings also cause lateral movement of the bound receptors in the plasma membrane, resulting in clustering, patching, and capping of the receptors.[2] This lateral movement of bound receptors in the membrane is regulated by cytoskeletal tubules and microfilaments. It may be thus considered that the formation of desmosomes is a result of ligand-receptor binding. The desmosome formation between the trophoblast and the uterine cells is an important process for firm attachment and further penetration of the entire blastocyst into the stroma and for the establishment of placental blood circulation.

Penetration of the Basal Lamina by Blastocyst

It has been observed in the implantation of rat blastocyst that the trophoblast pauses at the residual basal lamina after penetration through and removal of the uterine luminal epithelium, before progressing into the endometrial stroma.[59] As has been suggested by Liotta et al.[39] for the cellular mechanism of cancer cell invasion of the basal lamina, attachment of the trophoblast cells to the basal lamina appears to be mediated by the receptors on the invading cell surface to their ligands in the basal lamina. Mouse blastocysts attach in vitro to various components of the extracellular matrix, including laminin, type IV collagen, and fibronectin, by a ligand-receptor binding mechanism. If we apply the cancer cell invasion hypothesis to the blastocyst invasion of the basal lamina, the trophoblast on the basal lamina attaches itself by means of receptors, such as receptors for laminin, and anchors itself to the membrane. The trophoblast next secretes proteases to break down the type IV collagen, which is one of the major components of the basal lamina. The trophoblast cell then penetrates the basal lamina. In the case of the rat, the cells that penetrate the basal lamina are not trophoblast cells but the decidualized stromal cells[19] (Fig. 17–6). This may be explained by a hypothesis that prostaglandins produced by trophoblast cells penetrate the basal lamina and act on decidualized stromal cells and stimulate the activity of type IV colla-

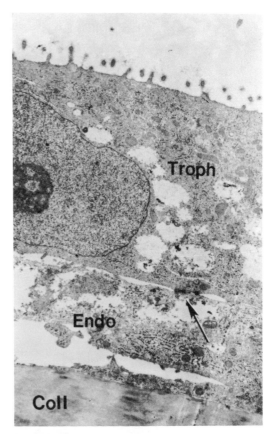

FIGURE 17–5. Transmission electron micrograph of trophoblast (Troph) on a confluent epithelial endometrial cell layer (Endo) cultured on a collagen membrane (Coll). Desmosomes are present at points of contact of trophoblasts with the endometrial cells (arrow). (Courtesy of Dr. C. Coutifaris, University of Pennsylvania, Philadelphia, Pennsylvania.)

genase. Type IV collagenase breaks the basal lamina from the stromal side. Prostaglandin production by blastocysts[26, 53] and prostaglandin activation of type IV collagenase in different cell types[55] have been shown in experimental animals.

Interactions Between Trophoblast Cells and Uterine Stromal Components

In the stroma, trophoblast cells have direct contact with decidual cells and other components of the stroma. In the rat, stromal cells decidualize even before invasion of the epithelium is initiated. The decidual cells immedi-

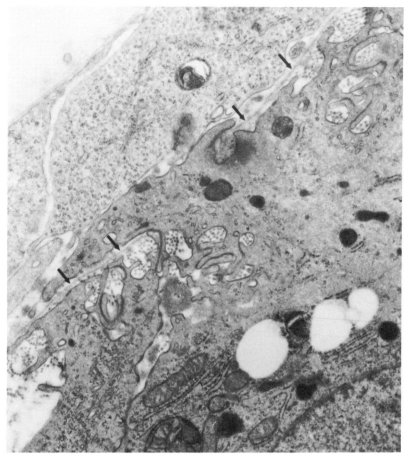

FIGURE 17–6. Penetration of the basal lamina by a decidual cell: Electron micrograph of a rat implantation site, day 7, 2 PM. In the center of the micrograph, a large decidual cell process has penetrated the residual basal lamina (arrows) of the uterine luminal epithelium and spread in contact with the trophoblast. Processes from decidual cells surround clusters of collagen fibrils (cut in cross-section). (Magnification ×23,200.) (Courtesy of Dr. A. O. Welsh, University of California, Davis, California.)

ately under the basal lamina are packed so tightly that molecules such as albumin cannot reach the embryo through this decidual zone (the primary decidual zone). These decidual cells degenerate apoptotically, and trophoblast cells phagocytose them. In the human, degeneration of decidual cells also appears to involve apoptosis and phagocytosis because trophoblast cells do not appear to "attack" maternal cells, and degeneration of maternal cells appears to be a result of blocking oxygen supply caused by invading cells.[34] Invasion of the endometrial stroma by trophoblast cells may also be considered to involve ligand-receptor binding for anchoring themselves to the surrounding cells.

Decidual cells have been shown to produce laminin. One component of the dense granular material in the decidual cell secretory body is heparan sulfate proteoglycan—another component of the basal lamina. Thus penetration of decidual tissue by trophoblast cells appears to use the same mechanism as it does for the basal lamina penetration. As the trophoblast cells penetrate the stromal tissue, capillaries adjacent to the trophoblast become congested and become intercommunicating sinusoids. Invading syncytia tap these sinusoids and maternal blood flow into the developing trophoblast lacunae. When the trophoblastic lacunae are in direct communication with arterioles and venules, the difference in blood pressure induces directional flow of maternal blood, establishing the interlacunar circulation and leading to formation of future placenta.[25]

CLINICAL ASPECTS OF IMPLANTATION

Transfer of Embryos Fertilized In Vitro

As described in the foregoing sections in this chapter, the time period of the receptive phase, the so-called implantation window, is limited. If and when embryos are transferred into the uterus outside of the receptive phase, particularly after the receptive phase is over and the uterus is in the refractory phase, there is little chance for the embryo to establish normal pregnancy even if the transferred embryos are healthy and mature blastocysts. It has been reported that the transferred embryos fail to implant in the patients whose blood level of estrogen to progesterone ratios is high.[36] This result, however, has not been confirmed by Forman et al.[23] Because the steroid hormone action on the endometrium is mediated at first by the corresponding steroid receptors and then by the gene products in response to the binding of the steroid-receptor complex to the steroid response element of the gene, mere measurements of peripheral level of steroids may not provide clear-cut information as to the receptivity of the endometrium. In view of the involvement of a host of growth factors in steroid hormone action on the endometrium, finding of useful assayable marker(s) for the receptive state of the endometrium is urgently needed.

In the investigation of the time period of the implantation window in the human, it is essential to consider the developmental stage of the embryo at the time of transfer as well as the condition of the uterus. Some ambiguous presentations of these two crucial items of information appear to confuse the issue of the implantation window. The term *embryo transfer* should be used to signify the placement of the embryo in the lumen of the genital tract. *Transplantation* or *implantation* should not be used in place of *transfer*.

Ectopic Pregnancy

Compared with other mammalian species, the human suffers a relatively high risk of ectopic pregnancy. When the blastocyst attaches to and implants into a tissue outside of the uterine cavity, it is important to know whether it is in the same way the blastocyst attaches and implants into the endometrium. If animal blastocysts are transplanted in ectopic sites such as the anterior chamber of the eye, the testis, under the kidney capsule, and the lung, the transplanted blastocyst invades the neighboring tissues. This type of study provides information that the trophoblastic cells become invasive at the ectopic sites. In the uterine cavity, the endometrium is protected against the invasive trophoblast except for the receptive period. This view may be supported by the results of an intrauterine inoculation of carcinosarcoma cells under various hormonal conditions.[60] In this study, the inoculated tumor cells proliferated in the uterus only under the hormonal condition that rendered the uterus receptive. It is possible to assume that these ectopic sites are vulnerable to the invasive trophoblast cells because the ectopic sites where transplanted blastocysts developed do not respond to steroid hormones, and no protective mechanism (similar to the refractory state of the uterus) has been developed under the influence of the steroid hormones.

In this sense, one must be cautious in extrapolating the blastocyst adhesion on different substrates in vitro. Adhesion of trophoblast cells to a substrate indicates that the trophoblast cells may contain the receptor for the substrate if the adhesion is due to a ligand-receptor binding. It does not necessarily mean, however, that binding always happens in the uterus because either the receptor or the ligand may not be available in the uterus.

Endocrine parameters (hCG and ovarian steroids) have been reported to be useful to detect ectopic pregnancy. The slope of hCG increases during a unit time period is significantly lower in ectopic patients.[31] Depressed hCG secretion has been confirmed in a large-scale study.[48] Detailed methods are discussed by Stabile et al.[61]

REFERENCES

1. Adams CE. Mammalian egg transfer. Boca Raton, FL: CRC Press, 1982.
2. Albertini DF, Anderson E. Microtubule and microfilament rearrangements during capping of concanavalin

A receptors on cultured ovarian granulosa cells. J Cell Biol 1977;73:111.

3. Anderson JM, Stevenson BR, Jesaitis LA, et al. Characterization of ZO-1, a protein component of the tight junction from the mouse liver and Madin-Darby canine kidney cells. J Cell Biol 1988;106:1141.

4. Anderson TL. Biomolecular markers for the window of uterine receptivity. In: Yoshinaga K, ed. Blastocyst implantation. Boston: Adams Publishing Group (Serono Symposia USA), 1989:219.

5. Anderson TL, Hoffman LH. Alterations in the epithelial glycocalyx of rabbit uteri during early pseudopregnancy and pregnancy, and following ovariectomy. Am J Anat 1984;171:321.

6. Babalola GO, Yamamoto R, Kao L-C, et al. Morphogenesis of human placenta: aggregation and fusion of cytotrophoblast cells. In: Moudgal RN, Yoshinaga K, Rao AJ, Adiga PR, eds. Perspectives in primate reproductive biology. New Delhi: Wiley Eastern, 1991:105.

7. Boving BG. Implantation mechanisms. In Hartman CG, ed. Mechanisms concerned with contraception. New York: Pergamon Press, 1963:321.

8. Brennan P, Kaba H, Keverne EB. Olfactory recognition: a simple memory system. Science 1990;250:1223.

9. Brenner RM, West NB, McClellan MC. Estrogen and progestin receptors in the reproductive tract of male and female primates. Biol Reprod 1990;42:11.

10. Casey PJ, Gilman AG. G protein involvement in receptor-effector coupling. J Biol Chem 1988;263:2577.

11. Chatterton RT, Macdonald GJ, Ward DA. Effects of blastocysts on rat ovarian steroidogenesis in early pregnancy. Biol Reprod 1975;13:77.

12. Citi S, Sabanay H, Jakes R, et al. Cingulin, a new peripheral component of tight junctions. Nature 1988;333:272.

13. Coutifaris C, Babalola GO, Abisogun AO, et al. In vitro systems for the study of human trophoblast implantation. Ann NY Acad Sci 1991;622:191.

14. Cunningham BA. Cell adhesion molecules and the regulation of development. Am J Obstet Gynecol 1990;164:939.

15. Cunha GR, Higgins SJ, Donjacour AA, et al. The role of stromal-epithelial interactions in the regulation of growth and differentiation in adult epithelial cells. In: Krey LC, Gulyas BJ, McCracken JA, eds. Autocrine and paracrine mechanisms in reproductive endocrinology. New York: Plenum Press, 1989:67.

16. Dallenbach-Hellweg G. Histopathology of the endometrium. New York: Springer-Verlag, 1977.

17. Dey SK, Paria BC, Andrews GK. Uterine EGF ligand-receptor circuitry and its role in embryo-uterine interactions during implantation in the mouse. In Strauss JF, Lyttle CR, eds. Uterine and embryonic factors in early pregnancy. New York: Plenum Press, 1991:51.

18. Enders AC. Morphological manifestations of maturation of the blastocyst. In: Yoshinaga K, Mori T, eds. Development of preimplantation embryos and their environment. New York: Alan R. Liss, 1989:211.

19. Enders AC, Schlafke S. Comparative aspects of blastocyst-endometrial interactions at implantation. In: Maternal recognition of pregnancy. Ciba Foundation Series 64 (new series). Amsterdam: Excerpta Medica, 1979:3.

20. Enders AC, Welsh AO, Schlafke S. Implantation in the rhesus monkey: endometrial responses. Am J Anat 1985;173:147.

21. Ferenczy A, Bergeron C. Histology of the human endometrium: from birth to senescence. Ann NY Acad Sci 1991;622:6.

22. Fleming S, O'Neill C, Collier M, et al. The role of embryonic signals in the control of blastocyst implantation. In: Yoshinaga K, ed. Blastocyst implantation. Boston: Adams Publishing Group (Serono Symposia USA), 1989:17.

23. Forman R, Fries N, Testar J, et al. Evidence for an adverse effect of elevated serum estradiol concentration on embryo implantation. Fertil Steril 1988;49:118.

24. Glasser SR, Julian JA, Decker GL, et al. Development of morphological and functional polarity in primary cultures of immature rat uterine epithelial cells. J Cell Biol 1988;107:2409.

25. Hamilton WJ, Boyd JD, Mossman HW. The implantation of the blastocyst and the development of the fetal membranes, placenta and decidua. In: Human Embryology. Baltimore: Williams & Wilkins, 1972:83.

26. Harper MJK, Jones MA, Norris CJ, Woodard DS. Prostaglandin synthesis by Day-6 rabbit blastocysts in vitro. J Reprod Fertil 1989;86:315.

27. Hertig AT. Implantation of the human ovum: the histogenesis of some aspects of spontaneous abortion. In: Behrman SJ, Kistner RW, eds. Progress in infertility, ed 2. Boston: Little, Brown, 1975:411.

28. Hodgen GD. Surrogate embryo transfer combined with estrogen-progesterone therapy in monkeys. Implantation, gestation, and delivery without ovaries. JAMA 1983;250:2167.

29. Hoffman LH, Winfrey VP. Is trophoblastic invasion hemotropic in the rabbit? In: Yoshinaga K, ed. Blastocyst implantation. Boston: Adams Publishing Group (Serono Symposia USA), 1989:95.

30. Hoffman LH, Winfrey VP, Anderson TL, Olson GE. Uterine receptivity to implantation in the rabbit: evidence for a 42 kDa glycoprotein as a marker of receptivity. In: Denker H-W, Aplin JD, eds. Trophoblast research, Vol 4. New York: Plenum Publishing, 1990:243.

31. Kadar N, Caldwell BV, Romero R. A method of screening for ectopic pregnancy and its indications. Obstet Gynecol 1981;58:162.

32. Kapur S, Tamada H, Dey SK, Andrews GK. Expression of insulin-like growth factor-I (IGF-I) and its receptor in the peri-implantation mouse uterus, and cell-specific regulation of IGF-I gene expression by estradiol and progesterone. Biol Reprod 1992;46:208.

33. Kirby DRS. Blastocyst-uterine relationship before and during implantation. In: Blandau RJ, ed. The biology of the blastocyst. Chicago: University of Chicago Press, 1971:393.

34. Larsen JF. Human implantation and clinical aspects. Prog Reprod Biol 1980;7:284.

35. Lataste MF. Des variations de durée de la gestation chez les mammifères et des circonstances qui déterminent ces variations: théorie de la gestation retardée. C R Soc Biol 1891;9:21.

36. Lejeune B, Dehou MF, Leroy F. Tentative extrapolation of animal data to human implantation. Ann NY Acad Sci 1986;476:63.

37. Lenton EA. Pituitary and ovarian hormones in implantation and early pregnancy. In: Chapman M, Grudzinskas G, Chard T, eds. Implantation. Heidelberg: Springer-Verlag, 1988:17.

38. Lenton EA, Sulaiman R, Sobowale O, Cooke ID. The human menstrual cycle: plasma concentrations of prolactin, LH, FSH, oestradiol and progesterone in conceiving and non-conceiving women. J Reprod Fertil 1982;65:131.

39. Liotta LA, Steeg PS, Stetler-Stevenson WG. Cancer metastasis and angiogenesis: an imbalance of positive and negative regulation. Cell 1991;64:327.

40. Martel D, Frydman R, Sarantis L, et al. Scanning electron microscopy of the uterine luminal epithelium as a marker of the implantation window. In: Yoshinaga K, ed. Blastocyst implantation. Boston: Adams Publishing Group (Serono Symposia USA), 1989:225.

41. Martin L, Finn CA. Hormonal regulation of cell division in epithelial and connective tissue of mouse uterus. J Endocrinol 1968;41:363.

42. McLaren A, Michie D. Studies on the transfer of fertilized mouse eggs to uterine foster-mothers. II. The effect of transferring large numbers of eggs. J Exp Biol 1959;36:40.

43. Mege R-M, Matsuzaki F, Gallin WJ, et al. Construction of epithelioid sheets by transfection of mouse sarcoma cells with cDNAs for chicken cell adhesion molecules. Proc Natl Acad Sci USA 1988;85:7274.

44. Meyer RK, Wolf RC, Arslan M. Implantation and maintenance of pregnancy in progesterone-treated ovariectomized monkeys (Macaca mulatta). In: Proceedings of the Second International Congress on Primates, Vol 2. New York: Karger, 1969:30.

45. Morris J, Potter SW. A comparison of developmental changes in surface charge in mouse blastocysts and uterine epithelium using DEAE beads and dextran sulfate. Dev Biol 1984;103:190.

46. Moudgal NR, Ravindranath N. Requirement for estrogen in implantation and post-implantation survival of blastocyst in the bonnet monkey. In: Yoshinaga K, Mori K, eds. Development of preimplantation embryos and their environment. New York: Alan R. Liss, 1989:277.

47. Navot D, Anderson TL, Droesch K, et al. Hormonal manipulation of endometrial maturation. J Clin Endocrinol Metab 1989;68:801.

48. Okamoto SH, Healy DL, Morrow LM, et al. Predictive value of plasma hCG beta-subunit in diagnosing ectopic pregnancy after in vitro fertilisation and embryo transfer. BMJ 1987;294:667.

49. O'Neill C, Spinks N. Embryo-derived platelet activating factor. In: Chapman M, Grudzinskas G, Chard T, eds. Implantation. London: Springer-Verlag, 1988:83.

50. Paria BC, Dey SK. Preimplantation embryo development in vitro: cooperative interactions among embryos and role of growth factors. Proc Natl Acad Sci USA 1990;87:4756.

51. Parkes AS, Bruce HM. Pregnancy-block in female mice placed in boxes soiled by males. J Reprod Fertil 1962;4:303.

52. Parr MB. Endocytosis in the uterine epithelium during early pregnancy. Prog Reprod Biol 1980;7:81.

53. Parr MB, Parr EL, Munaretto K, et al. Immunohistochemical localization of prostaglandin synthase in the rat uterus and embryo during the peri-implantation period. Biol Reprod 1988;38:333.

54. Paulson RJ, Sauer MV, Lobo RA. Embryo implantation after human in vitro fertilization: importance of endometrial receptivity. Fertil Steril 1990;53:870.

55. Reich R, Stradford B, Klein K, et al. Inhibitors of collagenase IV and cell adhesion reduce the invasive activity of malignant tumor cells. In: Metastasis. Ciba Foundation Symposium 141. Chichester: Wiley, 1988:193.

56. Rizzino A, Tiesman J, Hines R, Kelly D. Developmental regulation of the KS-FGF oncogene by embryonal carcinoma cells and early mouse embryos. In: Heyner S, Wiley LM, eds. Early embryo development and paracrine relationships. New York: Wiley-Liss, 1990:53.

57. Roberts RM, Farin CE, Cross JC. Trophoblast proteins and maternal recognition of pregnancy. In: Milligan SR, ed. Oxford Review of Reproductive Biology 12. Oxford: Oxford University Press, 1990:147.

58. Salat-Baroux J, Tibi C, Cornet D, et al. Pregnancies after replacement of frozen-thawed embryos in a donation program. Fertil Steril 1988;49:817.

59. Schlafke S, Welsh AO, Enders AC. Penetration of the basal lamina of the uterine luminal epithelium during implantation in the rat. Anat Rec 1985;212:47.

60. Short RV, Yoshinaga K. Hormonal influence on tumor growth in the uterus of the rat. J Reprod Fertil 1967;14:284.

61. Stabile I, Westergaard JG, Grudzinskas JG. Ectopic pregnancy: diagnostic aspects. In: Chapman M, Grudzinskas G, Chard T, eds. Implantation. London: Springer-Verlag, 1988:229.

62. Strauss JF, Gurpide E. The endometrium: regulation and dysfunction. In: Yen SSC, Jaffe RB, eds. Reproductive endocrinology, ed 3. Philadelphia: WB Saunders, 1991:309.

63. Sueoka K, Kusama T, Baba J, et al. Biochemical consideration of human early pregnancy factor (EPF). In: Yoshinaga K, Mori T, eds. Development of preimplantation embryos and their environment. New York: Alan R. Liss, 1989:317.

64. Tachi S, Tachi C, Lindner HR. Ultrastructural features of blastocyst attachment and trophoblastic invasion in the rat. J Reprod Fertil 1970;21:37.

65. Wislocki GB, Streeter GL. On the placentation of the Macaque (Macaca mulatta), from the time of implantation until the formation of the definitive placenta. Contr Embryol Carneg Instn 1938;27:1.

66. Yoshinaga K. A possible immunological action mechanism of ovine trophoblast protein-1 (oTP-1). In: Yoshinaga K, ed. Blastocyst implantation. Boston: Adams Publishing Group (Serono Symposia USA), 1989:185.

Maintenance of Pregnancy and the Initiation of Normal Labor

Tommaso Falcone

A. Brian Little

The classic physiologic states of the uterus were defined many years ago as facultas retentrix (the cervix) and facultas expultrix (the corpus). The maintenance of pregnancy requires that the uterus grow and expand to accommodate the growing fetus, while the cervix remains closed and the uterine contractions remain minimal. This is followed by a softening and opening of the cervix with a dramatic increase in expulsive contractions. The placenta, which is essentially fetal in origin, provides the hormonal control generally believed to be necessary for the growth of the uterus and maintenance of pregnancy. Estrogen stimulates the growth of the uterus, and progesterone acts to inhibit contraction of the uterus. The myriad of other placental hormones, either peptide or steroid in nature, have not been carefully assessed for their contribution, although relaxin may act synergistically with progesterone,[56] and growth factors augment estrogen action.[12]

The termination of pregnancy requires a complex, carefully timed addition or change of both fetal and maternal factors. These include estrogen and progesterone, prostaglandins, oxytocin, and possibly sympathomimetic amines. Between the two stages of complete quiescence and active labor, there is a long preparatory state during which there is increased activity of the uterus (Braxton Hicks contractions), which can be observed as a changed pattern of contraction and response to oxytocin and a concomitant change in the cervix. The softening and partial or complete effacement of the cervix occurs over variable lengths of time. In some instances, it occurs rapidly, as in precipitate labor or incompetent cervix; in others, it is inordinately delayed, as in postterm pregnancy, and may lead to the necessity for cesarean section.

ENDOCRINE EVENTS THAT SIGNAL PARTURITION

Fetal Cortisol, Progesterone, Estrogens

The role of the fetus in parturition is more clearly defined in sheep as a model than in humans. In sheep, a clear relationship between fetal adrenal events, which includes an increase in fetal adrenal size in late gestation, an increase in fetal adrenal responsiveness to adrenocorticotropic hormone (ACTH), and an increase in cortisol secretion, and the initiation of labor has been described.[54, 57] Ovine placental steroid 17α-hydroxylase and aromatase are regulated by fetal cortisol.[26] The alterations in estrogen and progesterone synthesis by the placenta, initiated by an increase in fetal cortisol and its effect on the aforementioned enzymes, result in a decrease in progesterone and an increase in estrogen production measured by circulating concentrations.[26, 54, 57] These alterations in estrogen and progesterone production result in the molecular events leading to parturition in the sheep. In the human fetus, there is an increase in circulating cortisol with gestational age in late pregnancy, whether or not labor takes place.[70] Adrenalectomy in the rhesus monkey (Macaca mulatta) fetus appears to have little or no effect on the length of gestation.[69] Fetal anencephaly with accompanying fetal adrenal atrophy in the rhesus monkey does not alter the mean length of gestation, although there is a large variation in the length of individual gestation.[72] Anencephalic human infants as well as those with congenital adrenal hyperplasia deliver at a mean gestational age that is not different from controls, but the variation is broad.[60, 80] The fetal adrenal cortisol metabolism does not appear to have a major influence on the length of gestation or the onset of parturition in the human.

Administration of certain glucocorticoids to human results in a decrease in circulating estrogens, without any change in circulating progesterone concentration or the onset of labor.[55] In the baboon, fetectomy results in an 80% decline in serum estradiol and a 70% decrease in serum progesterone, but there is still no resulting uterine contractility or delivery of the placenta. Spontaneous placental expulsion does not occur following fetectomy until the normal length of gestation has passed.[2, 3, 48] There is also no consistent evidence for a decrease in circulating progesterone at term that precedes labor in the human.[47] There is a continuous increase in circulating progesterone concentration to term.[107] Women before labor show no consistent increase or decrease in circulatory levels of estrogens, progesterone, or prolactin.[4, 22]

Although circulating steroids do not appear to change before parturition, local alterations in concentrations of such steroids may trigger parturition. The fetal membranes are capable of synthesizing both estrogens and progesterone. The chorion and decidua have a high level of sulfatase activity;[15] therefore these tissues can regulate free estrogen concentrations locally. At the time of parturition, there is also an increase in the kinetic activity (Vmax) of chorion sulfohydrolase, which may lead to a rise in local free estrogens.[15]

Estrone sulfate is present at high concentration in maternal plasma, fetal plasma, and amniotic fluid. Estrone sulfate can serve as a precursor for local estrogen synthesis by the chorion and decidua.[88] No difference, however, has been observed between tissue concentrations of estrone or estradiol in fetal membranes of the placenta following spontaneous labor and those from the placentas of women who delivered by cesarean section. Local production of progesterone by the decidua and the chorion occurs by interconversion from pregnenolone, pregnenolone sulfate, and 20α-dihydroprogesterone.[61] The amnion uses only 20α-dihydroprogesterone.[61]

The enzyme implicated in these local endocrine alterations is the 17β- and 20α-hydroxysteroid dehydrogenases, which are the same enzyme in the placenta.[61, 101] This enzyme catalyzes the conversion of estrone to the more metabolically active estradiol and progesterone to less metabolically active 20α-dihydroprogesterone.

Estrogens have been shown to inhibit progesterone formation locally.[21, 36, 63] Theoretically the alterations in local estrogens could lead to the equivalent of local progesterone withdrawal. There has been no demonstrable change, however, in amnion, chorion, or decidual progesterone concentrations associated with the timing of the onset of labor.[61]

High levels of catechol estrogens are observed in amniotic fluid and cord blood at term.[8] There is a further increase in patients in labor as compared with patients who deliver vaginally. Because these changes are not found in maternal peripheral blood,[8] a local production may be postulated. Catechol estrogens

can increase the production of prostaglandins.[42]

Concentrations of progesterone, 17α-hydroxyprogesterone, and corticosteroids increase significantly with gestation in human amniotic fluid. Over the last 2 weeks at term, amniotic fluid concentrations of cortisol actually decrease.[98] Patients in premature labor show no systemic changes in progesterone and estrogen concentration.[38, 100]

Although in mammalian species the onset of labor is caused by progesterone to estrogen ratio change resulting from increased fetal cortisol, labor in humans is not associated with any demonstrable change in circulating steroids. Changes at the cellular level, however, such as the placenta, placental membranes, and myometrium, remain a distinct possibility.

Prostaglandins

The final mediator of parturition appears to be related to eicosanoid formation. Prostaglandins (PGs) and the leukotrienes (LTs) are thought to be involved in labor initiation. Arachidonate derived from plasma membrane phospholipids as a result of cleavage by phospholipase A_2 is metabolized to PGs and LTs via the endoperoxide G/H synthase and lipoxygenase enzymes. Free arachidonic acid can also be made available from the action of phospholipase C (PLC) on cell membranes[59] (Fig. 18–1). The enzyme endoperoxide G/H synthase has both cyclooxygenase and peroxidase activities (Fig. 18–1). These enzymes are subject to self-inactivation. Therefore new enzymes must be synthesized to restore prostaglandin forming capacity.[87] As a result of these enzyme activities on arachidonate, PGs D, E, and F; prostacyclin ($PGI_2[PGI_2]$), and thromboxane (TXA_2) are formed. The products of the lipoxygenase pathway are the hydroperoxides and the LTs. Oxygenation of arachidonic acid by 5-lipoxygenase generates 5-hydroperoxyeicosatetraenoic acid (5-HPETE). From this intermediate, the LTs and 5-hydroxyeicosatraenoic acid (5-HETE) are formed. The predominant PG and LT found in each tissue is the result of the differential expression of the enzymes.

The possible sources of PGs in labor include

Membrane Phospholipid

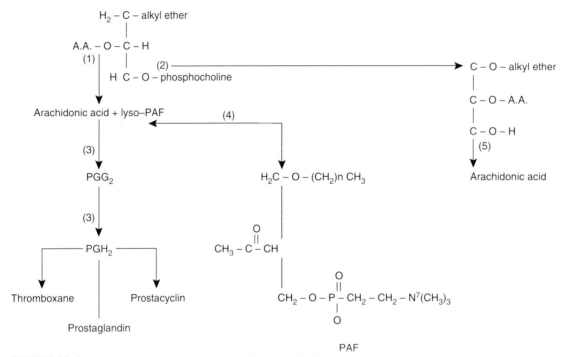

FIGURE 18–1. Prostaglandin synthesis pathway. In the example, the Sn-2 acyl group is A.A. Other membrane phospholipids can be precursors for PAF synthesis. PKC = protein kinase C; A.A. = arachidonic acid; PAF = platelet activating factor. (1) phospholipase A_2; (2) phospholipase C; (3) the PG G/H synthase has both cyclooxygenase and hydroperoxidase activity; (4) acetyl transferase; Ca and protein kinase C–dependent; (5) diacyl glycerol lipase.

the fetal membranes, the decidua, and the myometrium.[41, 112, 113] The amnion produces PGE_2, whereas the decidua produces PGE_2 and $PGF_2\alpha$. The chorion acts principally in the metabolism of PGE_2[73] and does not contribute to its production.[110] It has a high 15-hydroxy PG dehydrogenase and 13,14 PG reductase activity. Quantitatively the decidua contributes more PGE than the amnion.[43]

There is an increase in PG production associated with the onset of labor. The concentration of a metabolite of $PGF_2\alpha$ (13,14 dihydro 15-keto $PGF_2\alpha$:PGFM) increases in the peripheral blood of women at the time of parturition,[35] reaching a maximum at the time of placental separation.[112] There is no definitive evidence of an increase in peripheral blood of PGE_2 or its metabolites.[64] In amniotic fluid, PGE_2, $PGF_2\alpha$, and PGFM increase with gestational age. There is also a dramatic increase in all three with the onset of labor, increasing with cervical dilatation.[9] Further, there is an alteration in the PGE_2 to $PGF_2\alpha$ ratio in am-

niotic fluid, such that $PGF_2\alpha$ is predominant with the progression of labor[24, 96] (Fig. 18–2), and PGI_2 increases minimally. The concentrations of PGE_2, $PGF_2\alpha$, and PGFM are greater in cord blood than in maternal plasma.[13] Higher levels of PGE_2, $PGF_2\alpha$, and PGFM are obtained from cord blood in patients at term in labor rather than from cord blood obtained at cesarean section in nonlaboring patients.[13] It has been suggested that the placenta is the major source of these PGs.[64] In vitro data have shown that fetal membranes and decidua synthesize PGE_2 and $PGF_2\alpha$ at a higher rate when obtained from patients in labor than from nonlaboring patients.[99]

The arachidonic acid content of the amnion and chorion increases during the last trimester.[19] The source of arachidonic acid of the amnion is thought to be the amniotic fluid; the source of the chorion is both the decidua and amnion.[75] PGE_2 is metabolized in the chorion by the enzyme PG dehydrogenase (PGDH) and reductase to inactive metabolites.

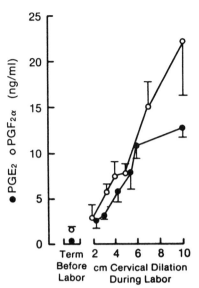

FIGURE 18–2. Concentrations (mean ± SEM) of PGE_2 and $PGF_{2\alpha}$ in amniotic fluid during late pregnancy and labor at term. (From Mitchell MD. Pathways of arachidonic acid metabolism with specific applications to the fetus and mother. Semin Perinatol 10:242–254, 1986.)

It appears, however, that some PGE_2 crosses the chorion unmetabolized to the decidua and myometrium.[71] Little conversion of PGE_2 to $PGF_2\alpha$ appears to occur in the decidua or chorion. Therefore the increase in maternal blood and amniotic fluid $PGF_{2\alpha}$ and its metabolites with labor progression appears to arise principally from the decidua.

Amniotic fluid concentrations of leukotriene B_4 (LTB_4), 12-HETE, and 15-HETE were higher in laboring than in nonlaboring patients.[64] Levels of these leukotrienes were elevated in umbilical plasma samples of all laboring patients but only a minority of nonlaboring patients.[78] The exact role that leukotrienes play in the biochemical event of parturition has yet to be defined, although LTB_4 has been shown to stimulate uterine contractions[11] and, acting as a calcium ionophore, stimulates calcium-dependent phospholipases to release more arachidonic acid.[97] Response to LTB_4 is usually manifested as a contractile response dependent on actomyosin. These responses have been investigated primarily in the airway smooth muscle.[53]

The signals responsible for the increased prostaglandin that mediates the onset of labor are unknown. The general consensus is that the point of control is the release of arachidonic acid, although some have argued that the rate-limiting step in prostanoid formation is at the level of the enzyme endoperoxide synthase.[87] The release of arachidonic acid from phospholipids is mediated through the action of the calcium-dependent enzymes phospholipase A_2 and PLC. There appears to be an increase in the activity of these enzymes throughout gestation but not during labor.[74] Northern blot analysis, however, has revealed a significant increase in phospholipase A_2 gene expression with the onset of labor in the placenta but not in the amnion or chorion.[1] The increased mobilization of arachidonic acid in labor is dependent on the availability of free calcium.[10] Calcium may be acting through intracellular calcium-binding proteins rather than directly on the phospholipases. These include calcium-calmodulin[76] and protein kinase C (PKC). PKC C (a protein serine/threonine kinase that catalyzes phosphorylation of proteins) may also regulate arachidonic acid accumulation by inhibiting acyl transferase, the enzyme responsible for reincorporation of free arachidonic acid in the cell membrane.[29] PKC may be activated by platelet-activating factor (PAF). PAF is an ether-soluble phospholipid formed by the action of phospholipase A_2 on membrane phospholipids. It is present in amniotic fluid, fetal membranes, and decidua.[7] Eicosanoid and PAF metabolism are also linked because the acyl group released by phospholipase A_2 action on its membrane phospholipid precursor may be arachidonic acid (see Fig. 18–1).

Interleukin-1 (IL-1) is one of a group of interleukins that are immunoregulatory polypeptides produced by the decidua,[90] the syncytiotrophoblast, and Hofbauer cells.[104] Two molecules with similar functions have been described: IL-1α and IL-1β. IL-1α has a central role in the acute phase response to infection and tissue injury, including induction of collagenase activity and prostaglandin synthesis. IL-1α is known to stimulate PG synthesis by the amnion and decidua.[89] Although women in active labor are more likely to have detectable IL-1α-like bioactivity and IL-1β immunoreactivity in amniotic fluid than are women at term without labor, there is a significant overlap of values from each group. Therefore IL-1α concentration is not directly associated with labor onset.[91] It may play an important role, however, in labor associated with chorioamnionitis.[104]

The amnion and decidua contain β2-adrenergic receptors, which can be stimulated to increase cyclic adenosine monophosphate (cAMP). An increase in cAMP results in an increase in arachidonic acid release and PGE_2 production. Mechanisms that control the cyclooxygenase enzyme are largely unknown. There is evidence to suggest that a factor in the amnion may have an inhibitory effect on endoperoxide synthase function.[59] The placenta also produces annexins (previously termed *lipocortins*). These calcium-binding proteins may bind arachidonic acid and prevent further metabolism.[109] The role of these proteins in reproductive tissue is controversial.[65] There may exist a variety of inhibitory substances that would trigger arachidonic acid release when their concentrations are reduced.[68, 94, 114] For example, gravidin is a 68-kilodalton protein that limits arachidonic acid release.[114] Its activity decreases after the onset of labor. Chorionic tissue makes a major contribution to the pool of gravidin in amniotic fluid.[114] Although many studies have shown that estrogen stimulates and progesterone inhibits the output of $PGF_{2\alpha}$ from secretory endometrium,[92] the effects of these steroids have not been extensively studied in human pregnancy. PGI_2 relaxes human myometrium in vitro.[77] PGE_2 and $PGF_{2\alpha}$ stimulate the myometrium to contract at all stages of pregnancy.[93]

The action of prostaglandins is mediated through specific receptors. $PGF_{2\alpha}$ receptors are present in the myometrium, decidua, and amnion. PGE_2 receptors are present in myometrium and cervix.[33] In human cervical tissue, PGI_2 appears to be the principal prostaglandin produced.[103] There is no change in receptor number or affinity for either prostaglandin with the onset of labor. Prostaglandins increase intracellular free calcium, which may also be responsible for smooth muscle contraction.

Growth factors, such as epidermal growth factor (EGF) or transforming growth factor-α (TGF-α), that are present in amniotic fluid may influence PG metabolism. They do not affect release of arachidonic acid but may act on the amnion PGF_2 synthase to increase PGI_2 synthesis.[12]

Oxytocin

The most commonly held belief over the years has been that the initiation of labor takes place by increased oxytocin stimulation. Oxytocin's precise role in initiation of labor is, however, unknown. The circulating concentration of oxytocin does not change either immediately before labor or during its first stage.[50] There is no change in the metabolic clearance rate of oxytocin during pregnancy[49] that might affect the circulating concentration. The only demonstrable increase in plasma concentration appears to be in the second stage of labor. It has been shown that there is an increase in myometrial oxytocin receptors with increasing gestation, with an additional increment at the onset of labor.[27, 28] Decidual tissue releases PGE_2 and $PGF_{2\alpha}$ in response to oxytocin stimulation.[14] Oxytocin appears to induce production of PGE_2 in human amnion cells by the activation of PLC. PLC hydrolyzes phosphatidylinositol biphosphate (IP_2) to inositol triphosphate (IP_3) and diacylglycerol (DAG). DAG activates PKC, which is essential for oxytocin-induced PG production.[67] Oxytocin can induce myometrial contraction directly by the same mechanism. Using Northern blot analysis, the mRNA for oxytocin has been detected in the chorion and decidua but not the placenta.[62] The levels of the oxytocin mRNA were higher in tissues obtained following spontaneous labor and delivery as compared with those obtained before the onset of labor.[16] This locally synthesized oxytocin may play a more important role in regulating the timing of human parturition than circulating levels, which mostly are secreted by the pituitary.[62] Biologically active oxytocin is present in the amniotic fluid and umbilical artery, suggesting the fetus itself is another source of oxytocin for labor.[23]

Relaxin

Relaxin is a polypeptide with a similar structure to insulin and insulin-like growth factors 1 and 2. It consists of an A and B chain connected by a C chain in a similar manner as insulin. The largest component of the circulating levels of relaxin in human pregnancy is secreted by the corpus luteum.[111] The decidua and placenta, however, also express the relaxin gene.[95] Specific receptors for relaxin have been identified in the amnion and chorion.[46] Relaxin levels become detectable in early pregnancy and reach a peak in midgestation and remain unchanged to term.[102] Although circulating relaxin is undetectable in nonpregnant women, it may be elevated in women following ovarian stimulation with human menopausal gonadotropins and human chorionic gonadotropin (hCG) for ovulation induction.[81, 105] Multiple gestation produces a significant increase in serum relaxin,[37] whereas ectopic pregnancies are associated with significantly decreased values.[30] Although in some species relaxin produces relaxation of the pubic symphysis with separation, myometrial relaxation, and cervical softening, these have not been clearly identified in the human.[6] There is no change in circulating relaxin concentration before the onset of labor,[82] nor does serum relaxin concentration change in response to prostaglandin induction of labor.[39] Relaxin, however, may increase prostaglandin release by the amnion.[56] Relaxin has been shown to induce cervical dilatation in women when locally applied;[25] it may act on the cervix by stimulating collagenase.[106]

MOLECULAR MECHANISMS OF PARTURITION

Cervical Biochemistry

The cervix is composed of fibrillar collagen, proteoglycans, and smooth muscle. Smooth muscle makes up less than 15% of the cervix. Cervical connective tissue fibers consist of collagen and elastin (less than 1.5%).[20, 52] Thirteen different types of collagen have been identified based on their constituent polypeptide chains. Each molecule of collagen is composed of three chains, termed α *chains*, wound in a triple helix. Each chain has a unique sequence of three amino acids. The α chains associate intracellularly. They are synthesized as a precursor protein called *procollagen*. The carboxyl and amino terminal extensions are removed extracellularly. The cervix is composed mostly of type I (two-thirds) but also type III (one-third) collagen.[45] The rate-limiting step of collagen degradation in the extracellular matrix is the catalytic cleavage of collagen triple helix by interstitial collagenase under physiologic conditions. In infectious and inflammatory conditions, leukocyte, macrophage, and bacterial collagenases and leukocyte elastase are capable of degrading collagen.[40]

There is a decrease in the concentration of collagen with progression of gestation.[25, 41, 44, 108] At the same time, there is an increase in collagenase activity with advancing gestation[86] and in labor.[83, 84] Collagenase is produced in a latent form called *procollagenase*. Further, active collagenase is inhibited by tissue inhibition of metalloproteinase. Signals that lead to an increase in active collagenase in humans (and therefore cervical dilatation) are largely unknown.[85] In the guinea pig, however, increased collagenase is stimulated by 17β-estradiol, human recombinant interleukin 1β, $PGF_{2\alpha}$, and PGE_2.[85] The concentration was equivalent in women with "favorable cervices" and women in spontaneous labor. Women with unfavorable cervices given 0.5 mg PGE_2 gel intracervically had a collagen content that was lower and a collagenolytic activity that was higher than those patients with unfavorable cervices and spontaneous labor.[25] The mechanism by which PGs regulate the expression of collagenase is unknown. Uterine myometrial contractions appear to play an indirect role in causing the changes in cervical compliance associated with delivery; cervical softening is the result of biochemical changes intrinsic to the cervix.[51]

Remodeling of connective tissue is not limited to the cervix. There is a large decrease in collagen concentration in the corpus uteri at term.[34] This is associated with an increase in collagenolytic activity.[34] The concentration of sulfated glycosaminoglycans is lower in the corpus uteri of pregnant women than nonpregnant women.[34] No significant difference in either tensile strength or collagen content of amniotic membranes was found with advancing gestational age.[58] In the cervix, however, there is a marked change in both of these parameters with advancing gestational age.[5]

The amorphorus ground substance of the cervix contains glycosaminoglycans, a long chain of repeating disaccharides each containing uronic acid (glucuronic acid or iduronic acid) linked to a hexosamine (glucosamine or galactosamine). Hyaluronic acid is the principal unsulfated glycosaminoglycan present. Sulfated glycosaminoglycans, such as heparan sul-

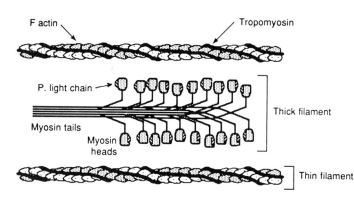

FIGURE 18–3. Schematic diagram of smooth muscle actin thin filaments and myosin thick filaments. The actin filaments show the helical arrangement of the globular actin molecules and the rod-shaped tropomyosin lying in the long pitched grooves on either side. The myosin molecules aggregate by means of their tail regions, with their heads projecting toward the actin filaments. (From Nuwayhid B, Rajasi M. Beta-sympathetic agents. Use in perinatal obstetrics. Clin Perinatol 14:757–782, 1987.)

fate and dermatan sulfate, also occur in the connective tissue matrix.

Formation of Gap Junctions

Cell to cell interaction is important for the unified process of parturition. These interactions between cells can occur via cellular junctions of which there are three forms: the tight junctions, the adhering junctions, and the gap junctions. Formation of cellular junctions requires the presence of morphoregulatory molecules, such as the connexins. Gap junctions provide for the cell to cell communication that must occur in labor. These junctions are present between contiguous cell membranes whereby channels of direct communication exist between the interiors. These channels allow for the free flow of ions (and therefore electrical signals) and small molecules, including steroids and cAMP.[18] Control of the permeability of these junctions is related to the intracellular concentration of free calcium. Gap junctions are low or absent throughout pregnancy until term.[31] The appearance of gap junctions is believed to be the result of stimulation by estrogens and prostaglandins; it is inhibited by progesterone.[32] It has been shown in the rat model that a specific myometrial gap junction protein, connexin 43, is increased during labor. It is regulated positively by estrogen and negatively by progesterone.[79]

Myometrial Contractions

Contraction of smooth muscle cells is a result of interaction between the contractile proteins actin and myosin filaments present in the cy-toplasm. Each myosin molecule is composed of two units: Each consists of two globular heads and a tail (Fig. 18–3). Myosin aggregates to form large thick filaments. Each globular head contains ATPase activity, an actin binding site, and the P light chain. The light chain contains a calcium and magnesium binding site and a phosphorylation site. Actin is a globular protein. The globular actin monomers polymerize in the presence of magnesium. A long tropomyosin molecule then is wound around the helical structure formed by the globular actin (see Fig. 18–3). Tropomyosin blocks the active sites on the actin molecules. Actin binds to myosin and activates the ATPase of myosin. Contraction is regulated by phosphorylation of the myosin light chain (MLC) by a specific kinase called *MLC kinase.* Phosphorylation of the light chain is the pivotal step for uterine contraction (Fig. 18–4). Activation of MLC kinase is mediated by the calcium-binding protein calmodulin. An increase in intracellular calcium forms calcium calmodulin complexes that activate MLC kinase. An increase in intracellular calcium can be the result of oxytocin activation of a cell membrane receptor. Subsequently there is activation of PLC, which acts on phosphatidylinositol bisphosphate. Receptor-stimulated PLC activity is mediated through a G protein (guanosine triphosphate–binding protein).[17] The result is inositol triphosphate (IP_3) and diacylglycerol (DAG). IP_3 mobilizes intracellular calcium. DAG activates PKC in the presence of calcium. PGs appear to act primarily by promoting extracellular calcium entry.[66]

Relaxation of the smooth muscle is a state of electrical polarization achieved by decreasing intracellular calcium or increasing cAMP.

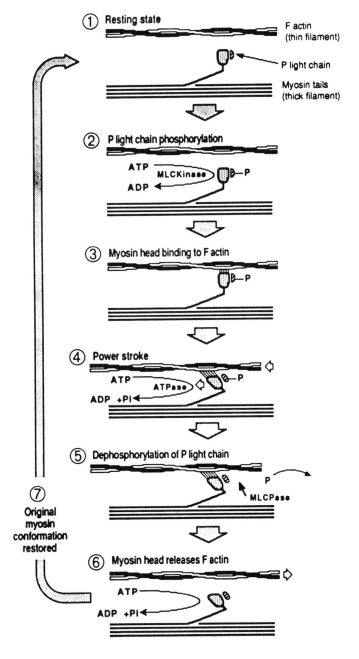

FIGURE 18–4. Diagram illustrating the mechanism of smooth muscle contraction and relaxation. Myosin light-chain kinase, activated by Ca²⁺-calmodulin complex, phosphorylates P-light chain on myosin head (2). This results in activation of binding of myosin head with F-actin (3) and ATP hydrolysis by myosin ATPase. The myosin head undergoes a conformational change while it is bound to the actin filament. Movement of actin filament is powered by ADP release and myosin conformational change (4). Myosin light-chain phosphatase dephosphorylates the P-light chain (5) resulting in inhibition of both myosin head results in restoration of the original conformation of myosin (7), resulting in relaxation.

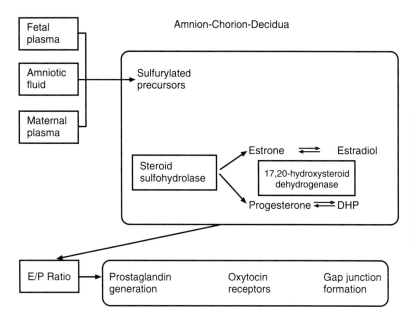

FIGURE 18–5. Proposed mechanism of progesterone and estrogen biosynthesis in human fetal membranes and decidua. (From Mitchell BF, Challis JRG. Estrogen and progesterone metabolism in human fetal membranes. In: Mitchell BF, ed. The Physiology and Biochemistry of Human Fetal Membranes. Ithaca, NY, Perinatology Press, 1988.)

Increase in cAMP can be achieved by activation of β_2 receptors or decreasing the activity of phosphodiesterase. cAMP binds to protein kinase A. Activated protein kinase A phosphorylates MLC kinase and reduces its ability to bind calcium-calmodulin and therefore its ability to phosphorylate MLC, and myometrial relaxation ensues. With a decrease in intracellular calcium, the MLC becomes dephosphorylated, and relaxation occurs.

A complex interaction between changes in local concentrations of steroids and peptides leads to paracrine control of PG generation, changes in oxytocin receptors, and gap junction formation (Fig. 18–5). These events are coordinated with the biomolecular events that occur in the cervix. Integrated into this basic model is a myriad of peptides and steroids that serve as inhibitors or stimulators of the entire process. Labor then ensues.

REFERENCES

1. Aitken MA, Rice GE, Biennecke SP. Gestational tissue phospholipase A_2 messenger RNA content and the onset of spontaneous labour in the human. Reprod Fertil Dev 1990;2:575.
2. Albrecht ED, Haskins AL, Pepe GJ. The influence of fetectomy at mid gestation upon the serum concentrations of progesterone, estrone and estradiol in baboons. Endocrinology 1980;107:766.
3. Albrecht ED, Pepe GJ. Placental steroid hormone biosynthesis in primate pregnancy. Endocr Rev 1990;11:124.
4. Anderman PJB, Hancock KW, Oakey RE. Non-protein-bound oestradiol and progesterone in human peripheral plasma before labour and delivery. J Endocrinol 1985;104:7.
5. Aspden RM. Structural basis of dilatation of the cervix. In: DWL Hukins, ed. Connective tissue matrix. New York, VCH Publishers, 1990:199.
6. Bigazzi M, Nardi E. Prolactin and relaxin: antagonism on the spontaneous motility of the uterus. J Clin Endocrinol Metab 1981;53:665.
7. Billah MM, DiRenzo GC, Ban C, et al. Platelet-activating factor metabolism in human amnion and the responses of this tissue to extracellular platelet activating factor. Prostaglandins 1985;30:841.
8. Biswas A, Choudhury A, Chattoroj S, Dale SL. Do catechol estrogens participate in the initiation of labor. Am J Obstet Gynecol 1991;165:984.
9. Bleasdale JE, Johnston JM. Prostaglandins and human parturition: regulation of arachidonic acid mobilization. Rev Perinatal Med 1985;5:151.
10. Bleasdale JE, Okazaki T, Sagawa N, et al. The mobilization of arachidonic acid for prostaglandin production during parturition. In: MacDonald PC, Porter JC, eds. Initiation of parturition: prevention of prematurity. 4th Ross Conference on Obstetric Research. Columbus, OH, Ross Laboratories, 1983:129.
11. Carraher R, Hahn DW, Ritchie DM, McGuire GL. Involvement of lipoxygenase products in myometrial contractions. Prostaglandins 1983;26:23.
12. Casey ML, Korte K, MacDonald PC. Epidermal growth factor stimulation of prostaglandin E_2 biosynthesis in amnion cells: induction of PGH_2 synthase. J Biol Chem 1988;263:7846.
13. Challis JRG, Osathanondh R, Ryan KJ, Tulchinsky D. Maternal and fetal plasma prostaglandin levels at vaginal delivery and cesarean section. Prostaglandins 1974;6:281.

14. Chan WY, Powell AM, Hruby VJ. Anti-oxytocic and anti-prostaglandin releasing effects of oxytocin antagonists in pregnant rats and pregnant human myometrial strips. Endocrinology 1982;111:48.

15. Chibbar R, Hobbirk R, Mitchell BF. Sulfohydrolase activity for estrone sulfate and dehydroepiandrosterone sulfate in human fetal membranes and decidua around the time of parturition. J Clin Endocrinol Metab 1986;62:90.

16. Chibbar R, Miller F, Mitchell BF. Regulation of oxytocin gene expression in human fetal membranes around the time of parturition (abstr). Presented at 39th Annual Meeting of the Society for Gynecologic Investigation, San Antonio, Texas, 1992:251.

17. Cockcroft S, Gomperts BD. Role of guanine nucleolide-binding protein in the activation of polyphosphoinositide phosphodiesterase. Nature (Lond) 1985;314:534.

18. Cole WC, Garfield RE, Kirkaldy JS. Gap junctions and direct intercellular communication between rat intrauterine smooth muscle cells. Am J Physiol 1985;249:C20.

19. Curbelo V, Bejar R, Benirschke K, Gluck L. Premature labor. I. Prostaglandin precursors in human placental membranes. Obstet Gynecol 1981;57:473.

20. Danforth DN, Veis A, Breen M, et al. The effect of pregnancy and labor on the human cervix: changes in collagen, glycoproteins and glycosaminoglycans. Am J Obstet Gynecol 1974;120:641.

21. Das NP, Khan-Dawood FS, Dawood MY. The effects of steroid hormones and gonadotropins on in vitro placental conversion of pregnenolone to progesterone. J Steroid Biochem 1985;23:517.

22. Davidson BJ, Murray RD, Challis JRG, Valenzuelo GJ. Estrogen, progesterone, prolactin, prostaglandin E_2, prostaglandin $F_{2\alpha}$, 13,14-dihydro-15-keto prostaglandin $F_{2\alpha}$ and 6 keto prostaglandin $F_{1\alpha}$ gradients across the uterus in women in labor and not in labor. Am J Obstet Gynecol 1987;157:54.

23. Dawood MY, Raghavan KS, Pociask C, Fuchs F. Oxytocin in human pregnancy and parturition. Obstet Gynecol 1978;51:138.

24. Dray F, Frydman R. Primary prostaglandins in amniotic fluid in pregnancy and spontaneous labor. Am J Obstet Gynecol 1976;126:13.

25. Evans MI, Dougan MB, Moaund AH, et al. Ripening of the human cervix with porcine ovarian relaxin. Am J Obstet Gynecol 1983;147:410.

26. France JT, Magness RR, Murry BA, et al. The regulation of ovine placental steroid 17α hydroxylase and aromatase by glucocorticoid. Mol Endocrinol 1988;2:193.

27. Fuchs AR, Fuchs F, Husslein P, et al. Oxytocin receptors and human parturition: a dual role for oxytocin in the initiation of labor. Science 1982;215:1396.

28. Fuchs AR, Fuchs F, Husslein P, Soloff MS. Oxytocin receptors in the human uterus during pregnancy and parturition. Am J Obstet Gynecol 1984;150:734.

29. Fuse I, Iwanaga T, Tai HH. Phorbol ester, 1,2-diacylglycerol and collagen induce inhibition of arachidonic acid incorporation into phospholipids in human platelets. J Biol Chem 1989;264:3890.

30. Garcia A, Skurnick JH, Goldsmith LT, et al. Human chorionic gonadotropin and relaxin concentrations in early ectopic and normal pregnancies. Obstet Gynecol 1990;75:779.

31. Garfield RE. Control of myometrial function in preterm versus term labor. Clin Obstet Gynecol 1984;27:572.

32. Garfield RE, Kannun MS, Daniel EE. Gap junction formation in myometrium: control by estrogen, progesterone and prostaglandins. Am J Physiol 1980;238:C81.

33. Giannopoulos G, Jackson K, Kredentsen J, Tulchinsky D. Prostaglandin E and $F_{2\alpha}$ receptors in human myometrium during the menstrual cycle and in pregnancy and labor. Am J Obstet Gynecol 1985;153:904.

34. Granstrom L, Ekman G, Ulmsten U, Malmström A. Changes in the connective tissue of corpus and cervix uteri during ripening and labour in term pregnancy. Br J Obstet Gynecol 1989;96:1198.

35. Green K, Bygdeman M, Toppozada M, Wiqvist N. The role of prostaglandin $F_{2\alpha}$ in human parturition. Endogenous plasma levels of 15-keto-13,14 dihydroprostaglandin $F_{2\alpha}$ during labor. Am J Obstet Gynecol 1974;120:25.

36. Grimshaw RN, Mitchell BF, Challis JRG. Steroid modulation of pregnenolone to progesterone conversion by human placental cells in vitro. Am J Obstet Gynecol 1983;145:234.

37. Haning RV, Steinetz B, Weiss G. Elevated serum relaxin levels in multiple pregnancy after Menotropin treatment. Obstet Gynecol 1985;66:42.

38. Hanssens MCAJA, Selby C, Symonds EM. Sex steroid hormone concentrations in preterm labour and the outcome of treatment with ritodrine. Br J Obstet Gynaecol 1985;92:698.

39. Hochman J, Weiss G, Steinetz BG, O'Byrne EM. Serum relaxin concentrations in prostaglandin and oxytocin-induced labor in women. Am J Obstet Gynecol 1978;130:473.

40. Junqueira LCU, Zugaib M, Montes GS, et al. Morphologic and histochemical evidence for the occurrence of collagenolysis and for the role of neutrophilic polymorphonuclear leukocytes during cervical dilation. Am J Obstet Gynecol 1980;138:273.

41. Keirse MJNC, Turnbull AC. The fetal membranes as a possible source of amniotic fluid prostaglandins. Br J Obstet Gynaecol 1976;83:146.

42. Kelly RW, Abel MH. A comparison of the effects of 4 catechol oestrogens and 2 pyrogallol estrogens in prostaglandin synthesis by the rat and human uterus. J Steroid Biochem 1981;14:787.

43. Khan H, Sullivan MHF, Helmig R, et al. Quantitative production of prostaglandin E_2 and its metabolites by human fetal membranes. Br J Obstet Gynaecol 1991;98:712.

44. Kitamura K, Ito A, Mori Y, Hirakaus S. Changes in the human uterine cervical collagenase with special reference to cervical ripening. Biochem Med 1979;22:332.

45. Kleissel HP, Van der Rest M, Naftolin F, et al. Collagen changes in the human uterine cervix at parturition. Am J Obstet Gynecol 1978;130:748.

46. Koay ESC, Bagnell CA, Bryant-Greenwood GD, et al. Immunocytochemical localization of relaxin in human decidua and placenta. J Clin Endocrinol Metab 1985;60:859.

47. Lanman JT. Parturition in non-human primates. Biol Reprod 1977;16:31.

48. Lanman JT, Thau R, Sundaram K, et al. Ovarian and placental origins of plasma progesterone following fetectomy in monkeys (Macaca mulatta). Endocrinology 1975;96:591.

49. Leake RD, Weitzman RE, Fisher DA. Pharmacokinetics of oxytocin in the human subject. Obstet Gynecol 1980;56:701.

50. Leake RD, Weitzman RE, Glatz TH, Fisher DA.

Plasma oxytocin concentrations in men, nonpregnant women and pregnant women before and during spontaneous labor. J Clin Endocrinol Metab 1981;53:730.

51. Ledger WL, Webster M, Harrison LP, et al. Increase in cervical extensibility during labor induced after isolation of the cervix from the uterus in pregnant ewes. Am J Obstet Gynecol 1985;151:397.

52. Leppert PC, Keller S, Cerretta J, Mandl I. Conclusive evidence for the presence of elastin in human and monkey cervix. Am J Obstet Gynecol 1982;142:179.

53. Lewis RA, Frank Austen K, Soberman RJ. Leukotrienes and other products of the 5-lipoxygenase pathway. N Engl J Med 1991;323:645.

54. Liggins GC, Fairclough RJ, Grieves SA, et al. The mechanism of initiation of parturition in the ewe. Rec Prog Horm Res 1973;29:111.

55. Liggins GC, Fairclough RJ, Grieves SA, et al. Parturition in the sheep. In: Knight J, O'Connor M, eds. The Fetus and Birth. Ciba Foundation Symposium 47. Amsterdam: Elsevier, 1977:5.

56. Lopez-Bernai-A, Bryant-Greenwood GD, Hansell DJ, et al. Effect of relaxin on prostaglandin E production by human amnion: changes in relation to the onset of labour. Br J Obstet Gynaecol 1987;94:1045.

57. Magyar DM, Fridshal D, Elsner CW, et al. Time-trend analysis of plasma cortisol concentrations in the fetal sheep in relation to parturition. Endocrinology 1980;107:155.

58. Manabe Y, Himens N, Fukumoto M. Tensile strength and collagen content of amniotic membrane do not change after the second trimester or during delivery. Obstet Gynecol 1991;78:24.

59. Matsuda T, Imai A, Tamaya T. Phospholipase C activity in human placental membrane. Arch Gynecol Obstet 1989;246:27.

60. Milic AB, Adamsons K. The relationship between anencephaly and prolonged pregnancy. Br J Obstet Gynaecol 1969;76:102.

61. Mitchell BF, Challis JRG, Lukash L. Progesterone synthesis by human amnion, chorion and decidua at term. Am J Obstet Gynecol 1987;157:349.

62. Mitchell BF, Clibban R, Miller FD. (abstr). Presented at the Annual Meeting of the Society of Obstetricians and Gynecologists of Canada (SOGC), 1991.

63. Mitchell BF, Cruikshank B, McLean D, Challis JR. Local modulation of progesterone production in human fetal membranes. J Clin Endocrinol Metab 1982;55:1237.

64. Mitchell MD. Pathways of arachidonic acid metabolism with specific application to the fetus and mother. Semin Perinatol 1986;10:242.

65. Mitchell MD, Lytton FD, Varticovski L. Parodoxical stimulation of both lipocortin and prostaglandin production in human amnion cells by dexamethasone. Biochem Biophys Res Comm 1988;151:137.

66. Molnar M, Hertelendy F. Regulation of intracellular free calcium in human myometrial cells by prostaglandin F_2: comparison with oxytocin. J Clin Endocrinol Metab 1990;71:1243.

67. Moore JJ, Moore RM, Kooy DV. Protein kinase C activation is required for oxytocin induced prostaglandin production in human amnion cells. J Clin Endocrinol Metab 1991;72:1073.

68. Mortimer G, Stimson WH, Hunter IC, Given AD. A role for amniotic epithelium in control of human parturition. Lancet 1985;1:1074.

69. Mueller-Heubach E, Myers RE, Adamsons K. Effects

70. Murphy, BEP. Human fetal serum cortisol levels related to gestational age: evidence of mid gestational fall and a steep late gestational rise, independent of sex or mode of delivery. Am J Obstet Gynecol 1982;144:276.

71. Nakla S, Skinner K, Mitchell BF, Challis JRG. Changes in prostaglandin transfer across human fetal membranes obtained after spontaneous labor. Am J Obstet Gynecol 1986;155:1337.

72. Novy MJ, Walsh SW, Kittinger GW. Experimental fetal anencephaly in the rhesus monkey: effect on gestational length and fetal and maternal plasma steroids. J Clin Endocrinol Metab 1977;45:1031.

73. Okazaki T, Casey ML, Okita JR, et al. Initiation of human parturition. XII. Biosynthesis and metabolism of prostaglandins in human fetal membranes and uterine decidua. Am J Obstet Gynecol 1981;139:373.

74. Okazaki T, Sagawa N, Bleasdale JE, et al. Initiation of human parturition. XIII. Phospholipase C, phospholipase A_2, and diacylglycerol lipase activities in fetal membranes and decidua vera tissues from early and late gestation. Biol Reprod 1981;25:103.

75. Okita JR, Johnston JM, MacDonald PC. Source of prostaglandin precursor in human fetal membranes: arachidonic acid content of amnion and chorion laeve in diamnionic-dichorionic twin placentas. Am J Obstet Gynecol 1983;147:477.

76. Olson DM, Kramar D, Smieja Z. Identification of calmodulin-like activity in term human amnion: effect of calmodulin inhibitors on prostaglandin biosynthesis. J Dev Physiol 1987;9:271.

77. Omini C, Pasargiklian R, Folco GC, et al. Pharmacological activity of PGI_2 and its metabolite 6-oxo-$PGF_{1\alpha}$ on human uterus and fallopian tubes. Prostaglandins 1978;15:1045.

78. Pasetto N, Piccione E, Ticconi C, et al. Leukotrienes in human umbilical plasma at birth. Br J Obstet Gynaecol 1989;96:88.

79. Petrocelli T, Lye SJ. Regulation of the level of the gap junction protein, Connexin 43, in the rat myometrium (abstr). Presented at 39th Annual Meeting of the Society of Gynecologic Investigation, San Antonio, Texas, 1992:225.

80. Price HV, Cone BA, Keogh M. Length of gestation in congenital adrenal hyperplasia. Br J Obstet Gynaecol 1971;78:430.

81. Quagliarello G, Lustig DS, Steinetz B, et al. Absence of a prelabor relaxin surge in women. Biol Reprod 1980;22:202.

82. Quagliarello J, Goldsmith L, Steinetz B, et al. Induction of relaxin secretion in nonpregnant women by human chorionic gonadotropin. J Clin Endocrinol Metab 1980;51:74.

83. Rajabi MR, Dean DD, Beydoun SN, Woessner JF Jr. Elevated tissue levels of collagenase during dilatation of uterine cervix in human parturition. Am J Obstet Gynecol 1988;159:971.

84. Rajabi MR, Dean DD, Woessner JF Jr. Changes in active and latent collagenase in human placenta around the time of parturition. Am J Obstet Gynecol 1990;163:499.

85. Rajabi MR, Solomon S, Poole AR. Hormonal regulation of interstitial collagenase in the uterine cervix of the pregnant guinea pig. Endocrinology 1991;128:863.

86. Rath W, Adelmann-Grill BC, Peiper U, Kukn W. Collagen degradation in pregnant human cervix at term

and after prostaglandin induced cervical ripening. Arch Gynecol 1987;240:177.

87. Rice GE. Labour: a process dependent upon prostaglandin G/H synthase. Reprod Fertil Dev 1990;2:523.

88. Romano WM, Lukash LA, Challis JRG, Mitchell BF. Substrate utilization for estrogen synthesis by human fetal membranes and decidua. Am J Obstet Gynecol 1986;155:1170.

89. Romero R, Durum S, Dinarello CA, et al. Interleukin-1 stimulates prostaglandin biosynthesis by human amnion. Prostaglandins 1989;37:13.

90. Romero R, Wu YK, Brody OT, et al. Human decidua: a source of interleukin-1. Obstet Gynecol 1989;73:31.

91. Romero R, Parrizi ST, Oyarzun E, et al. Amniotic fluid interleukin-1 in spontaneous labor at term. J Reprod Med 1990;35:235.

92. Rueda R, Falcone T, Hemmings R, Tulandi T. Dysfunctional uterine bleeding: a reappraisal. Curr Prob Obstet Gynecol Fertil. 1991;14:71.

93. Rydnert J, Joelsson I. Effect of the naturally occurring prostaglandins E_2 and $F_{2\alpha}$ on the human myometrium in vivo during pregnancy. Acta Obstet Gynecol Scand 1985;64:577.

94. Saeed SA, Strickland DM, Young DC, et al. Inhibition of prostaglandin synthesis by human amniotic fluid obtained during labor. J Clin Endocrinol Metab 1982;55:801.

95. Sakbun V, Ali SM, Greenwood FC, Bryant-Greenwood GD. Human relaxin in the amnion, chorion, decidua parietalis, basal plate, and placental trophoblast by immunocytochemistry and northern analysis. J Clin Endocrinol Metab 1990;70:508.

96. Satoh K, Yasumizu T, Fukuoka H, et al. Prostaglandin $F_{2\alpha}$ metabolite levels in plasma, amniotic fluid and urine during pregnancy and labor. Am J Obstet Gynecol 1979;133:886.

97. Serhan CN, Fridorich J, Goetzl EJ, et al. Leukotriene B4 and phosphatidic acid are calcium ionophores. J Biol Chem 1982;257:4746.

98. Sippell WG, Muller Holve W, Dorr HG, et al. Concentrations of Aldosterone, Corticosterone, 11-deoxycorticosterone, progesterone, 17-hydroxyprogesterone, 71-deoxycortisol, cortisol, and cortisone determined simultaneously in human amniotic fluid throughout gestation. J Clin Endocrinol Metab 1981;52:385.

99. Skinner KA, Challis JRG. Changes in the synthesis and metabolism of prostaglandins by human fetal membranes and decidua at labor. Am J Obstet Gynecol 1985;151:519.

100. Smit DA, Essed GGM, deHaan J. Predictive value of uterine contractility and the serum levels of progesterone and estrogens with regard to preterm labor. Gynecol Obstet Invest 1984;18:252.

101. Strickler RC, Tobias B. Estradiol 17-β-dehydrogenase and 20 α hydroxysteroid dehydrogenase from placental cytosol: one enzyme with two activities? Steroids 1980;36:243.

102. Szlachter BN, Quagliarello J, Jewelewicz R, et al. Relaxin in normal and pathogenic pregnancies. Obstet Gynecol 1982;59:167.

103. Tanaka M, Morita I, Hirakawa S, Murota S. Increased prostacyclin synthesizing activity in human ripening uterine cervix. Prostaglandins 1981;21:83.

104. Taniguchi T, Matsuzaki N, Kameda T, et al. The enhanced production of placental interleukin-1 during labor and intrauterine infection. Am J Obstet Gynecol 1991;165:131.

105. Thomas K, Loumaye E, Ferin J. Relaxin in non-pregnant women during ovarian stimulation. Gynecol Obstet Invest 1980;11:75.

106. Too CKL, Bryant-Greenwood GD, Greenwood FC. Relaxin increases the release of plasminogen activator, collagenase and proteoglycanase from rat granulosa cells in vitro. Endocrinology 1984;115:1043.

107. Tulchinsky D, Hobel CJ, Yeager E, Marshall JR. Plasma estrone, estradiol, estriol, progesterone and 17-hydroxyprogesterone in human pregnancy. I. Normal pregnancy. Am J Obstet Gynecol 1972;112:1095.

108. Uldbjerg N, Ekman G, Malmstrom A, et al. Ripening of the human uterine cervix related to changes in collagen, glycosaminoglycans and collagenolytic activity. Am J Obstet Gynecol 1983;147:662.

109. Wallner BP, Mattaliano RJ, Hession C, et al. Cloning and expression of human lipocortin, a phospholipase A_2 inhibitor with potential anti-inflammatory activity. Nature 1986;320:77.

110. Warrick C, Skinner K, Mitchell BF, Challis JRG. Relation between cyclic adenosine monophosphate and prostaglandin output by dispersed cells from human amnion and decidua. Am J Obstet Gynecol 1985;153:66.

111. Weiss G, O'Byrne EM, Steinetz BG. Relaxin: a product of the human corpus luteum of pregnancy. Science 1976;94:948.

112. Weppelmann B, Hoppen HO, Gethmann U, Schuster E. Plasma levels of prostaglandin metabolites during spontaneous delivery. Adv Prostaglandin Thromboxane Res 1980;8:1409.

113. Willman EA, Collins WP. Distribution of prostaglandins E_2 and $F_2\alpha$ within the fetoplacental unit throughout human pregnancy. J Endocrinol 1976; 69:413.

114. Wilson T. Liggins GC, Joe L. Purification and characterization of a uterine phospholipase inhibitor that loses activity after labor onset in women. Am J Obstet Gynecol 1989;160:602.

The Influence of Hormones on Fetal Lung Development

Barry T. Smith

Martin Post

A number of hormones have been observed to accelerate fetal lung maturation. Indeed the number that can do so probably reflects the critical importance of this process in ontogeny, hence phylogeny. This chapter focuses on those hormones that have been shown to affect the process of fetal lung maturation and on the mechanisms of their action.

GLUCOCORTICOIDS

During early animal studies of hormonal effects on fetal lung maturation, the use of non-injected as well as placebo-injected controls led to the realization that direct intrafetal injection of saline or vehicle can accelerate fetal lung maturation.[139, 142, 148] Other physiologic derangements, such as infection[182] or premature rupture of the membranes,[17] can also lead to precocious lung maturation. That this response might be mediated by endogenous fetal glucocorticoids and that glucocorticoids may play a role in the normal course of lung maturation are suggested by temporal associations between fetal glucocorticoid levels and the process of fetal lung development, endocrine ablation studies, and demonstration of specific glucocorticoid receptors in fetal lung cells and tissue.

With respect to temporal associations between fetal glucocorticoid levels and lung maturity, in fetal rats[155] and rabbits,[107] corticosteroid levels rise when the major upsurge in fetal pulmonary surfactant occurs. In the fetal sheep, Kitterman et al.[82] showed that lung maturation correlates more closely with cortisol levels than with fetal age. Cord blood cortisol levels are lower in premature infants with respiratory distress syndrome than in those with good lung function.[109] The decreased cord blood cortisol levels do not reflect adrenal failure because after onset of the disease, plasma cortisol levels are elevated.[84] Several studies have shown a good correlation between amniotic fluid cortisol levels and lung maturity in humans[47, 52, 154] and in sheep.[166]

Ablation studies at several levels of the pituitary-adrenal axis support a role for adrenal secretions in fetal lung maturation. DeLemos et al.[38] reported that hypophysectomy in the fetal goat delays lung maturation. Decapitation of

fetal rats also delays lung maturation.[20, 21] Chemical adrenalectomy of the fetus with metyrapone (Metopirone) delays maturation in rats,[173] rabbits,[194] and baboons.[85] In the human equivalent of ablation studies, Naeye et al.[110] reported that at autopsy such infants appear to have decreased surfactant stores in their type II cells. Weiss et al.[202] performed serial amniocenteses in anencephalics and observed that the L/S ratio does not reflect maturity as early as expected.

The fetal lung of a number of species contains nuclear and cytosolic glucocorticoid receptors (GR).[8, 9, 53, 55, 56] Their concentration increases with advancing gestational age.[8, 9, 54] There is no apparent change in affinity.[28] Antiglucocorticoids interfere with ligand binding to the GR and block glucocorticoid effects in vitro.[61, 189] The steroid effect can be blocked by inhibitors of protein and RNA synthesis.[61] The antiglucocorticoid RU486 delays fetal lung maturation when administered to the dam.[68, 69] Lung maturation is also delayed in mice with H-2 (HLA) phenotypes that express subnormal amounts of GR.[75] Sweezey et al.[176] studied GR gene expression in the rat fetal lung and found that GR mRNA levels are low on day 18, increase on day 19, and subsequently decline. Binding activity parallels the mRNA levels.[176] Perhaps paradoxically maternal administration of glucocorticoid increases the GR mRNA level.[175] Specific glucocorticoid binding is present in both type II alveolar cells and fetal lung fibroblasts.[9, 14] Although type II cells produce pulmonary surfactant, the presence of GR in fibroblasts may be more significant because this may be the primary glucocorticoid responder, at least with respect to surfactant lipid production (see later). GR transcripts appear in the rat fetal lung fibroblast on day 19, 24 hours before they are seen in type II cells. The appearance in fibroblasts can be advanced by 1 day by exogenous glucocorticoid.[175] Autoradiography shows increased GR amounts in fibroblasts adjacent to type II cells.[18]

Animal studies have clearly demonstrated that glucocorticoid administration to the mother or directly to the fetus accelerates fetal lung maturation. Cortisol as well as a variety of synthetic glucocorticoids has been studied and, when given intrafetally, has relative potencies similar to those seen in other assay systems. Intrafetal administration, however, is complicated by the fact that the injection per se is associated with some maturational response.[11, 142, 148] Thus administration via the maternal compartment provides more clear-cut demonstration of the effect. Maternal cortisol is effective[57, 192] in large doses. Synthetic glucocorticoids, such as betamethasone[26, 130, 143] or dexamethasone,[26, 27] are effective in lower concentrations as in other glucocorticoid target tissues. Adrenocorticotropic hormone (ACTH) also accelerates fetal lung maturation.[139, 195] This effect is indeed due to the fetal adrenal response to ACTH and not to the premature labor that is also induced by this peptide.[196] One potential risk of antenatal steroid administration stems from the observation that treated fetuses have smaller lungs than control littermates,[31, 90, 130, 192] with less protein and DNA,[31, 90, 130] and a lower lung to body weight ratio.[192] Catch-up growth, however, occurs postnatally.[90] Torday et al.[190] observed a similar slowing of lung growth at the time of maximum upsurge in pulmonary maturation in the absence of exogenous hormones.

Human fetal lung cells convert the inactive cortisone to cortisol.[164] Rabbit fetal lung cells also convert cortisone to cortisol.[189] Cortisone action is blocked by 11-oxoprogesterone, which competitively blocks cortisone conversion to cortisol.[189] Cortisone conversion to cortisol occurs in fetal lung fibroblasts.[7, 159] Conversion of cortisone to cortisol increases with advancing gestation.[112, 187] Abramovitz et al.[2] observed cortisone conversion to cortisol in organ cultures of human fetal lung only when fibroblastic outgrowth from the cultures occurred. Although they suggested that human fetal lung probably does not normally convert cortisone to cortisol, these results could also be interpreted as confirming that this activity is resident in fibroblasts.[159] The cortisol to cortisone ratio in amniotic fluid in sheep relates better to lung maturation than do cortisol levels alone.[166] The same phenomenon has been observed in the human fetus.[165] Further, administration of 11-oxoprogesterone blocks cortisone conversion to cortisol and delays lung maturation in the fetal rat.[155] In the fetal sheep, glucocorticoid-dependent foregut derivatives convert cortisone to cortisol and have tissue cortisol levels higher than those in the circulation.[162] Torday et al.[188] found that 11-oxidoreductase is confined to alveolar fibroblasts in keeping with the concept that fibroblasts are the target for glucocorticoids in the fetal lung.

With respect to action on the fetal lung, glucocorticoids increase the amount of surfactant in fetal lung lavage, enhance the incorporation of substrates into surfactant lipids (e.g., phosphatidylcholine) in lung slices and organ explants, increase the content of surfactant proteins, and accelerate the appearance of lamellar bodies.[183] The activities of various enzymes involved in the synthesis of surfactant lipids are increased by glucocorticoid, including choline phosphotransferase,[27, 46, 122] phosphocholine cytidylyltransferase,[122, 142, 143] lysophosphatidylcholine acyltransferase,[122, 130, 142] phosphatidate acid phosphatase,[26, 130, 143] fatty acid synthetase,[97, 128, 141] and glycerophosphate phosphatidyltransferase.[144] Studies with isolated type II cells[133, 134] and mixed fetal lung cells[197] reveal that the effect on phosphatidylcholine synthesis is mediated by activation of phosphocholine cytidylyltransferase. This activation in type II cells is seen in microsomal-associated enzyme and is not accompanied by redistribution of enzyme from cytosol to microsomes.[133, 197]

Glucocorticoids stimulate surfactant synthesis in organ, mixed monolayer, and organotypic cultures of fetal lung tissue, each of which contains both type II cells and fibroblasts. In contrast, the glucocorticoid effect is much less in isolated fetal type II cells, but exposure of fetal type II cells to medium from steroid-treated fetal lung fibroblasts results in full responsivity.[30, 137, 157] In response to glucocorticoid, the fetal lung fibroblast produces fibroblast-pneumonocyte factor (FPF). FPF is a heat-stable polypeptide with apparent molecular weight of 5 to 15 kDa. Its production of FPF is organ specific[156] but not species specific.[158] Induction of FPF is inhibited by cycloheximide and actinomycin D.[51] Floros et al.[51] isolated cellular mRNA from glucocorticoid-treated and control fetal lung fibroblasts followed by methylmercury gel separation. Each resulting fraction was translated and the products tested for FPF biologic activity with fetal type II cells. A band of approximately 400 bases yielded FPF bioactivity. This material, however, is not recognized by monoclonal antibodies against the native protein.[135] When the FPF mRNA is translated after microinjection into *Xenopus* oocytes, however, it has both biologic and immunologic activity.[50] FPF increases surfactant phospholipid production by the type II cell in vitro[134, 136, 137] and in vivo.[135, 157] It stimulates surfactant lipid synthesis in fetal type II cells,[156] with the peak response being seen at 20 days' gestation.[29] FPF activates phosphocholine cytidylyltransferase.[134, 197] The stimulation of enzyme activity is rapid. Zimmermann and Post[207] reported a shift of enzyme from cytosol to microsomes in type II cells during development, indicating that such a regulatory mechanism for phosphocholine cytidylyltransferase may exist in fetal type II cells. Batenburg et al.[16] reported that fibroblast-conditioned cortisol-containing medium that probably contains FPF increases fatty acid synthesis in fetal type II cells. Morphologic studies are in keeping with these observations.

As noted earlier, fibroblasts adjacent to type II cells have increased GR.[18] Caniggia et al.[29] report that the fibroblasts close to the epithelium produce more FPF activity than distal fibroblasts. The physiologic role of FPF is suggested by the observation that in utero injection of partially purified FPF increases the synthesis of surfactant phosphatidylcholine in fetal rat lung[157] and that in ovo injection of monoclonal antibodies against FPF decreases the synthesis of phosphatidylcholine in the chick lung.[135] FPF bioactivity can be detected in human amniotic fluid near term.[153] FPF has also been isolated from a wide variety of species.[158] Torday and Kourembanas[184] report that in an earlier developmental time fetal lung fibroblasts produce an inhibitor of type II cell maturation whose programmed loss as lung development proceeds may allow FPF to start the maturational program.

Glucocorticoids have also been shown to affect lung surfactant protein (SP-A, SP-B, SP-C) synthesis. Glucocorticoid response elements are found in the 5' flanking region of the human SP-B[81] and human and rabbit SP-A[22, 23, 203] genes. In keeping with these observations, exposure of organ cultures from fetal rabbit[100] and rat[114] lung to glucocorticoids increases the amount of SP-A protein and of the corresponding mRNA. In human lung, a biphasic dose response to glucocorticoids has been observed with respect to SP-A protein and mRNA levels.[94, 121] In contrast, rats do not show this biphasic response.[114] Liley et al.[94] reported a biphasic time response to glucocorticoids with early stimulation and later loss of stimulation. Glucocorticoids have been shown to increase human SP-A gene transcription at low concentrations but to decrease mRNA stability at high concentrations.[23] Glucocorticoids also increase pulmonary SP-A mRNA and protein in fetal[126, 150] and adult rats[48, 126] in vivo. Human fetal lung explants have elevated mRNA and SP-B and SP-C protein when exposed to glucocorticoids.[95, 204] Fisher et al.[48] reported that steroid treatment enhances SP-B and SP-C mRNA in the adult rat.

THYROID HORMONES

Wu et al.[206] first observed that administration of thyroxine (T_4) to the fetal rabbit accelerates lung maturation. Hitchcock[72] presented morphologic evidence of accelerated lung maturation in fetal rats treated with T_4 or triiodothyronine (T_3). A challenge in studying thyroid hormones is the relative impermeability of the mammalian placenta to them. For this reason, Rooney et al.[145] administered thyrotropin-releasing hormone (TRH), which crosses the placenta, to pregnant rabbit does and observed enhanced lung maturation. TRH administration does not increase substrate incorporation into phosphatidylcholine[145] but does enhance morphologic indices of lung maturation.[43] In the lamb, TRH alone increases alveolar phosphatidylcholine but does not increase lung compliance, whereas in combination with glucocorticoids it markedly increases lung distensibility.[93] Ballard et al.[10] administered 3,5-dimethyl-3'-isopropylthyronine, a thyroid hormone analog that crosses the placenta in sufficient concentration to saturate receptors,[96] to pregnant rabbits and observed increased phosphatidylcholine synthesis and content in the fetal lungs. In fetal rabbits, T_3 and T_4 treatment accelerates thinning of the alveolar wall and alveolar stability.[33]

In mixed monolayer cultures of fetal rabbit lung, T_4 enhances the synthesis of phosphatidylcholine.[163] In organ cultures of fetal mouse lung, T_4 exposure results in morphologic evidence of enhanced maturation.[4] In a serum-free organ culture system with fetal rat lung, Gross and Wilson[66] observed only minor stimulation of phosphatidylcholine synthesis in the presence of T_3 alone, but supra-additive effects with other hormones. Similarly, Smith and Sabry[161] have shown that under serum-free conditions T_3 alone has little effect on phospholipid synthesis by dispersed fetal rat lung cells, but the thyroid hormone potentiates the glucocorticoid effect. Other studies with organ cultures of rabbit,[13] rat,[64] and human[60] fetal lung confirm relatively minor effects with thyroid hormones as compared with glucocorticoids. In fetal organ cultures, thyroid hormones do not appear to stimulate SP-A[12, 115,] SP-B,[95, 204] or SP-C[204] production. Indeed, T_3 reduces SP-A[114] and SP-B[113] mRNA levels in the rat fetal lung.

Thyroid hormone effects in vitro under serum-free (i.e., hormone-free) conditions are difficult to demonstrate, suggesting that in vivo they may be linked with the effects of other hormones. Gross and Wilson[66] reported that T_3 has a small effect on phospholipid synthesis alone, but that its effect is additive with dexamethasone in fetal rat lung organ cultures. Similar supra-additive effects of cortisol and T_3 have been reported for fetal rabbit and human lung.[13, 60] Synergistic interactions are seen in vivo in fetal rat[64] and lamb.[93, 149] Ballard et al.[13] reported that dexamethasone exposure of fetal rabbit lung explants enhances the T_3 effect but that T_3 pretreatment does not increase the response to dexamethasone. The hormones do not interact by effects on thyroid hormone receptors.[64] The dose response curve for T_3 in rabbit lung is similar in the presence or absence of dexamethasone.[13] Morishige[104] reported that thyroid hormones regulate the concentration of glucocorticoid receptors in rat newborn lung. Thyroid hormones increase the fetal type II cell response to FPF.[161] Similarly, addition of T_3 to fibroblast-conditioned medium causes increased stimulation of phosphocholine cytidylyltransferase activity in fetal type II cells.[197] T_3-treated cells contain more 3′, 5′–cyclic adenosine monophosphate (cAMP) after exposure to FPF.[161] Gross and Wilson[66] reported that T_3 enhances the response to theophylline. In contrast to synergistic effects of

these hormones on phospholipid synthesis, thyroid hormones do not potentiate glucocorticoid effects on the surfactant protein SP-A.[12] In the fetal rat, T_3 antagonizes the glucocorticoid effect on SP-A[114] and SP-B[113] gene expression. Thyroid hormones also oppose glucocorticoid effects on fatty acid synthesis in fetal rat lung.[141]

Circulating thyroid hormone levels are lower in infants with respiratory distress syndrome.[1, 36, 83] Hitchcock et al.[73] have shown that the perinatal rat lung accumulates T_3. Term newborn lambs made hypothyroid or athyroid during fetal life die of lung immaturity.[37, 45, 179] In neonatal rats, hypothyroidism induced by propylthiouracil is associated with reduced pulmonary surfactant.[147] Human fetal lungs are relatively enriched in T_3 receptors compared with other organs.[19] Gonzales and Ballard[59] found that nuclear T_3 receptors in rabbit lung rise during fetal life and peak on day 28. Maximal binding occurs more rapidly in fetal than adult lung cell nuclei.[59] Nuclear T_3 receptors have been demonstrated in adult type II cells[167]; clonally derived type II cells from adult rat[96]; and cell line A549, a type II cell–like line derived from a lung carcinoma.[96] Fetal rat type II cells convert T_4 to T_3.[151]

SEX DIFFERENCES IN LUNG MATURATION: ESTROGENS AND ANDROGENS

Premature male infants are at higher risk of respiratory distress syndrome than are female infants.[103] Lung maturation is delayed in male fetal rats.[5, 6] Male rabbit fetuses reach lung maturity later than females.[118] Human amniotic fluid indices of lung maturation are delayed in male fetuses.[186] In avian species, the female embryonic lung shows relatively delayed lung maturation.[119] This is only an apparent paradox because in avia the female is heterogametic and the male is homogametic, the reverse of mammals. Male rabbit fetuses respond less to glucocorticoids.[88] The largest study of glucocorticoid prevention of respiratory distress syndrome showed a better response in the female fetus.[34] Female fetuses with adjacent male littermates have less mature lungs than female fetuses bordered only by female littermates, implying that the difference is a hormonal one.[120]

Surfactant phospholipids in rabbit[79] and rat[180] fetal lung are increased after administration of estradiol. This is associated with increased synthesis of phosphatidylcholine[78] and morphologic precocity.[80] Possmayer et al.[131] reported positive effects of estrogen on phosphocholine cytidylyltransferase activity. Treatment of fetal rat[67, 99] and rabbit[77] lung organ cultures with estrogen enhances surfactant phospholipid synthesis. The estrogen effect is gestation dependent[98] and is accompanied by an increase in the number of cell-cell contacts between type II cells and fibroblasts.[3] Indeed, estradiol binding is localized in the fibroblast,[3] and estradiol does not directly affect surfactant lipid synthesis in fetal type II cells.[3] Estrogen binding activity is described in fetal rabbit,[77] rat,[99, 105] guinea pig,[123] and human lung.[102]

As already noted, in the fetal rabbit, the presence of male littermates slows lung maturation in adjacent female fetuses.[185] Administration of dihydrotestosterone to rabbit does delays lung maturation in female fetuses to the level seen in their male littermates.[120] Administration of an antiandrogen, flutamide, led to enhanced maturation in male fetal lungs to the level seen in female littermates.[120] Rat fetal lung contains receptors for androgen,[105] and their role in lung maturation has been shown in mice with testicular feminization syndrome, in which the surge of phosphatidylcholine in amniotic fluid of the male fetus is not delayed by androgens, as it is in the normal female littermates.[115] Androgens reduce phosphatidylcholine synthesis in rat female lung organ cultures to male levels.[98] Adamson and King[5] reported that the frequency of foot processes and basement membrane discontinuities is decreased in the male fetus, suggesting that the male delay is associated with reduced cell-cell communication. Androgen pretreatment of organotypic cultures followed by exposure to glucocorticoid reduces phosphatidylcholine synthesis, whereas androgens alone have no effect.[117] Fibroblasts of female fetal rats produce more FPF than their male counterparts, whereas there is no difference in phosphatidylcholine synthesis in response to FPF in type II cells from either sex.[182] Torday and others[49, 181]

also demonstrated that androgens inhibit the production of FPF by fetal lung fibroblasts and that this effect is pretranslational.

INSULIN AND MATERNAL DIABETES

The infant born to the mother with insulin-dependent diabetes is at significantly elevated risk for the occurrence of respiratory distress syndrome.[140] These infants are exposed to high glucose loads from the maternal compartment and resulting high insulin levels from the fetal pancreas.[125] A variety of animal models of maternal diabetes have been established. Rhoades et al.[138] induced maternal diabetes in rats on day 10 of gestation with streptozotocin. Fetal pulmonary total phospholipid synthesis was increased, but the production of surfactant phosphatidylcholine was decreased. In a similar animal model, differing in that the diabetic state was induced with streptozotocin before the onset of pregnancy, fetal pulmonary phosphatidylcholine synthesis was lowered.[193] In this model, Tsai et al.[191] observed no change in surfactant phosphatidylcholine synthesis, but the diabetic fetuses do not respond positively to dexamethasone as do those from control mothers. Lung slices from fetuses of rabbits made diabetic with alloxan 24 hours after mating failed to show differences from control animals with respect to surfactant synthesis,[41] but the lungs have less stability[172] and delayed morphologic maturation.[170] The changes are reversible with cortisol administration.[171] Others have shown biochemical changes with this model.[24]

Bourbon et al.[25] induced graded degrees of diabetes in rats with varying doses of streptozotocin. They observed that mild diabetes with fetal hyperinsulinemia delays surfactant lipid synthesis by impairing glycogen utilization, whereas severe diabetes without hyperinsulinemia decreases surfactant phosphatidylcholine formation owing to excessive glucose.[25] Continuous infusion of insulin in the fetal lamb delays the developmental appearance of surfactant.[200] Infusion of glucose in doses that make the sheep fetus hyperinsulinemic also decreases surfactant and reduces the response to cortisol.[199, 201] In the rat fetus, hyperinsulinemia and hyperglycemia impair surfactant lipid synthesis.[127] Patel and Rhodes[124] observed that hyperinsulinemia increases surfactant phosphatidylcholine synthesis in fetal rabbits. Exposure of fetal rat lung organ cultures[65] and organotypic cultures[44] to insulin decreases the synthesis of surfactant phosphatidylcholine. No inhibitory effects of insulin on surfactant synthesis were demonstrated in mixed monolayer cell cultures of fetal rabbit[160] and rat[30] lung. Exposure of mixed fetal rabbit lung cell cultures to insulin causes only a small increase in surfactant phosphatidylcholine synthesis, but insulin blocks the ability of the cells to respond to cortisol.[160] In fetal rat lung organ cultures, insulin reduces the response to dexamethasone.[65, 146] Insulin blocks the glucocorticoid-induced production of FPF by fetal lung fibroblasts.[30] In organ cultures, insulin inhibits SP-A accumulation.[169] SP-A levels are lower in the amniotic fluid of pregnant diabetic mothers.[168]

OTHER HORMONES

Lower cord blood levels of prolactin in infants with respiratory distress syndrome led to the hypothesis that prolactin may stimulate lung maturation.[71, 74] Conflicting reports on prolactin effects on lung maturation in fetal rabbits exist.[11, 35, 70] Prolactin, however, stimulates phospholipid synthesis in fetal rat lung explants[108] and in alveolar carcinoma A549 cells.[129] Inhibition of prolactin synthesis in the fetal rabbit with bromocriptine decreases phospholipids.[58] Combinations of prolactin and glucocorticoids stimulate phosphatidylcholine synthesis in human fetal lung,[101] which binds prolactin.[76]

Administration of epidermal growth factor (EGF) to the fetal rabbit[32] and lamb[174] accelerates lung maturation. EGF stimulates surfactant phospholipid and SP-A synthesis in organ explants of fetal human[205] and rat[63] lung. An additive interaction is seen between EGF and thyroid hormones[62] and retinoic acid[91] but not glucocorticoids.[63] EGF does not directly affect surfactant lipid synthesis by fetal type II cells[152] but appears to stimulate fetal lung fibroblasts

to produce FPF.[116, 152] EGF receptors are reported in the fetal rabbit[42] and human[111] lung.

CONCLUSIONS

The large amount of information that has accrued with respect to hormonal regulation of fetal lung maturation has, as with most medical research, given a dual benefit: Not only have new means to improve patient care (i.e., to prevent respiratory distress syndrome) resulted, but also new knowledge has accrued with respect to basic developmental processes.

REFERENCES

1. Abassi V, Merchant K, Abramson D. Postnatal triiodothyronine concentrations in healthy preterm infants and in infants with respiratory distress syndrome. Pediatr Res 1977;11:802.
2. Abramovitz M, Branchaud CL, Murphy BEP. Cortisol-cortisone conversion in human fetal lung: contrasting results using explant and monolayer cultures. Clin Invest Med 1981;4:18.
3. Adamson IYR, Bakowska J, McMillan EM, King GM. Accelerated fetal lung maturation by estrogen is associated with an epithelial-fibroblast interaction. In Vitro Cell Develop Biol 1990;26:784.
4. Adamson IYR, Bowden DH. Reaction of cultured adult and fetal lung to prednisolone and thyroxine. Arch Pathol 1975;99:80.
5. Adamson IYR, King GM. Sex differences in development of fetal rat lung. I. Autoradiographic and biochemical studies. Lab Invest 1984;50:456.
6. Adamson IYR, King GM. Sex-related differences in cellular composition and surfactant synthesis of developing fetal rat lungs. Am Rev Resp Dis 1984;129:130.
7. Aronson JF, McClaskey JW. Cortisone reductase activity levels in human lung and skin fibroblasts. In Vitro 1980;16:253.
8. Ballard PL, Ballard RA. Cytoplasmic receptor for glucocorticoids in lung of the human fetus and neonate. J Clin Invest 1974;53:477.
9. Ballard PL, Ballard RA, Gonzales LK, et al. Corticosteroid binding by fetal rat and rabbit lung in organ culture. J Steroid Biochem 1984;21:117.
10. Ballard PL, Benson BJ, Brehier A, et al. Transplacental stimulation of lung development in the fetal rabbit by 3,5-dimethyl-3′isopropyl-l-thyronine. J Clin Invest 1980;65:1407.
11. Ballard PL, Gluckman PDB, Brehier A, et al. Failure to detect an effect of prolactin on pulmonary surfactant and adrenal steroids in fetal sheep and rabbits. J Clin Invest 1978;62:879.
12. Ballard PL, Hawgood S, Liley H, et al. Regulation of pulmonary surfactant apoprotein SP 28-36 gene in fetal human lung. Proc Natl Acad Sci USA 1986;83:9527.
13. Ballard PL, Hovey ML, Gonzales LK. Thyroid hor-

mone stimulation of phosphatidylcholine synthesis in cultured fetal rabbit lung. J Clin Invest 1984;74:898.

14. Ballard PL, Mason RJ, Douglas WHJ. Glucocorticoid binding by isolated lung cells. Endocrinology 1978;102:1570.

15. Barrett CT, Sevanian A, Phelps DL. Effects of cortisol and aminophylline upon survival, pulmonary mechanics and secreted phosphatidylcholine of prematurely delivered rabbits. Pediatr Res 1978;12:38.

16. Batenburg JJ, Den Breejen JN, Geelen MJH, et al. Phosphatidylcholine synthesis in type II cells and regulation of the fatty acid supply. Prog Resp Dis 1990;25:96.

17. Bauer CR, Stern L, Colle E. Prolonged rupture of the membranes associated with decreased incidence of respiratory distress syndrome. Pediatrics 1974;53:7.

18. Beer DG, Butley MS, Cunha GR, Malkinson AM. Autoradiographic localization of specific (3H) dexamethasone binding in fetal lung. Develop Biol 1984;105:351.

19. Bernal J, Pekonen F. Ontogenesis of the nuclear 3,5,3′-triiodothyronine receptor in the human fetal brain. Endocrinology 1984;127:278.

20. Blackburn WR, Kelly JS, Dickman PS, et al. The role of the pituitary-adrenal thyroid axes in lung differentiation. II. Biochemical studies of developing lung in anencephalic rats. Lab Invest 1973;28:352.

21. Blackburn WR, Travers H, Potter M. The role of the pituitary-adrenal-thyroid axes in lung differentiation. I. Studies of the cytology and physical properties of anencephalic fetal rat lung. Lab Invest 1972;26:306.

22. Boggaram V, King K, Mendelson CR. The major apoprotein of rabbit pulmonary surfactant. Elucidation of primary sequence and cyclic AMP and developmental regulation. J Biol Chem 1988;263:2939.

23. Boggaram V, Smith ME, Mendelson CR. Regulation of expression of the gene encoding the major surfactant protein (SP-A) in human fetal lung in vitro. J Biol Chem 1989;264:11421.

24. Bose CL, Manne DN, D'Ercole AJ, Lawson EE. Delayed fetal pulmonary maturation in a rabbit model of the diabetic pregnancy. J Clin Invest 1980;66:220.

25. Bourbon JR, Pignol B, Marin L, et al. Maturation of fetal rat lung in diabetic pregnancies of graduated severity. Diabetes 1985;34:734.

26. Brehier A, Benson BJ, Williams MC, et al. Corticosteroid induction of phosphatidic acid phosphatase in fetal rabbit lung. Biochem Biophys Res Commun 1977;77:883.

27. Brehier A, Rooney SA. Phosphatidylcholine synthesis and glycogen depletion in fetal mouse lung. Developmental changes and the effects of dexamethasone. Exp Lung Res 1981;2:273.

28. Bronnegard M, Okret S. Characterization of the glucocorticoid receptor in fetal rat lung during development: influence of proteolytic activity. J Steroid Biochem 1988;31:809.

29. Caniggia I, Tseu I, Han R, et al. Spatial and temporal differences in fibroblast behaviour in fetal rat lung. Am J Physiol Lung Cell Mol Physiol 1991;5:L424.

30. Carlson KS, Smith BT, Post M. Insulin acts on the fibroblast to inhibit glucocorticoid stimulation of lung maturation. J Appl Physiol 1984;57:1577.

31. Carson S, Taeusch HW, Avery ME. The effects of cortisol injection on lung growth in fetal rabbits. J Appl Physiol 1973;34:660.

32. Catterton WZ, Escobedo MB, Sexson WR, et al. Ef-

33. Church J, Khafayan E, Chelani V, et al. Transplacental stimulation of fetal lung maturation: effect of tri-iodothyronine in the female and male rabbit fetus. Biol Neonate 1987;52:157.

34. Collaborative Group on Antenatal Steroid Therapy. Effect of antenatal dexamethasone administration on the prevention of respiratory distress syndrome. Am J Obstet Gynecol 1981;141:276.

35. Cox M, Torday JS. Pituitary oligopeptide regulation of phosphatidylcholine synthesis by fetal rabbit lung cells: lack of effect with prolactin. Am Rev Resp Dis 1981;123:181.

36. Cuestas RA, Lindall A, Engel RR. Low thyroid hormones and respiratory-distress syndrome of the newborn. N Engl J Med 1976;295:297.

37. Cunningham MD, Hollingsworth DR, Belin RP. Impaired surfactant production in cretin lambs. Obstet Gynecol 1980;55:439.

38. DeLemos RA, Diserens W, Halki J. Lung development after hypophysectomy in the goat fetus. Combined Abstracts of American Pediatrics Society and Society for Pediatric Research, 1971;272.

39. DeLemos RA, McLaughlin GW. Induction of the pulmonary surfactant in the fetal primate by the intrauterine administration of corticosteroids. Pediatr Res 1973;7:425.

40. DeLemos RA, Shermeta D, Knelson J, et al. Acceleration of appearance of pulmonary surfactant in the fetal lamb by administration of corticosteroids. Am Rev Resp Dis 1970;102:459.

41. Demottaz V, Epstein MF, Frantz ID. Phospholipid synthesis in lung slices from fetuses of alloxan diabetic rabbits. Pediatr Res 1980;14:47.

42. Devaskar UP. Epidermal growth factor receptors in fetal and maternal rabbit lung. Biochem Biophys Res Comm 1982;107:714.

43. Devaskar U, Nita K, Szewczyk K, et al. Transplacental stimulation of functional and morphologic fetal rabbit lung maturation: effect of thyrotropin-releasing hormone. Am J Obstet Gynecol 1987;157:460.

44. Engle M, Langan SM, Sanders RL. The effects of insulin and hyperglycemia on surfactant phospholipid synthesis in organotypic culture of type II pneumonocytes. Biochim Biophys Acta 1983;753:6.

45. Erenberg A, Rhodes ML, Weinstein MM, Kennedy RL. The effect of fetal thyroidectomy on ovine fetal lung maturation. Pediatr Res 1979;13:230.

46. Farrell PM, Zachman RD. Induction of choline phosphotransferase and lecithin synthesis in the fetal lung by corticosteroids. Science 1973;179:297.

47. Fencl M, Tulchinsky D. Total cortisol in amniotic fluid and fetal lung maturation. N Engl J Med 1975;292:133.

48. Fisher JH, McCormack F, Park SS, et al. In vivo regulation of surfactant proteins by glucocorticoids. Am J Resp Cell Mol Biol 1991;5:63.

49. Floros J, Nielsen HC, Torday JS. Dihydrotestosterone blocks fibroblast-pneumonocyte factor at a pretranslational level. J Biol Chem 1987;262:13592.

50. Floros J, Post M, Kay RM, Smith BT. Molecular basis for a pulmonary mesenchymal-epithelial interaction. In: Progress in developmental biology, Part B. New York: Alan R. Liss, 1986:333.

51. Floros J, Post M, Smith BT. Glucocorticoids affect the synthesis of pulmonary fibroblast-pneumonocyte

factor at a pretranslational level. J Biol Chem 1985;260:2265.

52. Gewolb IH, Hobbins JC, Tan Y. Amniotic fluid cortisol as an index of fetal lung maturity. Obstet Gynecol 1977;49:462.
53. Giannopoulos G. Glucocorticoid receptors in lung. I. Specific binding of glucocorticoids by cytoplasmic components of rabbit fetal lung. J Biol Chem 1973;248:3876.
54. Giannopoulos G. Variations in the levels of cytoplasmic glucocorticoid receptors in lungs of various species at different developmental stages. Endocrinology 1974;94:450.
55. Giannopoulos G, Mulay S, Solomon S. Cortisol receptors in rabbit fetal lung. Biochem Biophys Res Commun 1972;47:411.
56. Giannopoulos G, Mulay S, Solomon S. Glucocorticoid receptors in lung. II. Specific binding of glucocorticoids to nuclear components of rabbit fetal lung. J Biol Chem 1973;248:5016.
57. Gilden C, Sevanian A, Tierney DF, et al. Regulation of fetal lung phosphatidylcholine synthesis by cortisol: role of glycogen and glucose. Pediatr Res 1977;11:845.
58. Giussi GA, Ballejo G, Bustos R, Caldeyro-Barcia R. Effects of bromocriptine administration to pregnant rabbits upon fetal lung maturation. Pediatr Res 1981;15:850.
59. Gonzales L, Ballard PL. Nuclear 3,5,3'-triiodothyronine receptors in rabbit lung: characterization and developmental changes. Endocrinology 1982;111:542.
60. Gonzales LW, Ballard PL, Ertsey R, Williams MC. Glucocorticosteroids and thyroid hormones stimulate biochemical and morphological differentiation of fetal human lung in organ culture. J Clin Endocrinol Metab 1986;62:678.
61. Gross I, Ballard PL, Ballard RA, et al. Corticosteroid stimulation of phosphatidylcholine synthesis in cultured fetal rabbit lung. Evidence for de novo protein synthesis mediated by glucocorticoid receptors. Endocrinology 1983;12:829.
62. Gross I, Dynia DW. Do EGF and glucocorticoids act at the same metabolic sites in fetal rat lung? Pediatr Res 1984;18:392A.
63. Gross I, Dynia DW, Rooney SA, et al. Influence of epidermal growth factor on fetal rat lung development in vitro. Pediatr Res 1986;20:473.
64. Gross I, Dynia DW, Wilson CM, et al. Glucocorticoid-thyroid hormone interactions in fetal rat lung. Pediatr Res 1984;18:191.
65. Gross I, Walker Smith GJ, Wilson CM, et al. The influence of hormones on the biochemical development of fetal rat lung in organ culture. II. Insulin. Pediatr Res 1980;14:834.
66. Gross I, Wilson CM. Fetal lung in organ culture. IV. Supra-additive hormone interactions. J Appl Physiol 1982;52:1420.
67. Gross I, Wilson CM, Ingleson LD, et al. The influence of hormones on the biochemical development of fetal rat lung in organ culture. I. Estrogen. Biochim Biophys Acta 1979;575:375.
68. Guettari M, Dufour ME, Marin L. Effects of the antiglucocorticoid RU486 on the initiation of ultrastructural type II cell differentiation in fetal rat lung. Biol Neonate 1990;58:173.
69. Guettari M, Marin L, Bourbon J, et al. Effects of the antiglucocorticoid RU486 on the maturation of fetal rat lung surfactant. Exp Lung Res 1989;15:151.
70. Hamosh M, Hamosh P. The effect of prolactin on the lecithin content of fetal rabbit lung. J Clin Invest 1977;59:1002.
71. Hauth JC, Parker CR, MacDonald PC, et al. Role of fetal prolactin in lung maturation. Obstet Gynecol 1978;51:81.
72. Hitchcock KR. Hormones and the lung. I. Thyroid hormones and glucocorticoids in lung development. Anat Record 1979;194:15.
73. Hitchcock KR, Harney J, Reichlin S. Hormones and the lung. III. Thyroid hormone uptake kinetics of perinatal rat lung. Endocrinology 1980;107:294.
74. Ho Yuen BH, Phillips WD, Cannon W, et al. Prolactin, estradiol and thyroid hormones in umbilical cord blood of neonates with and without hyaline membrane disease: a study of 405 neonates from midpregnancy to term. Am J Obstet Gynecol 1982;142:698.
75. Honig LS, Smith BT, Slavkin HC, Donahue HG. Influence of the major histocompatibility complex (H-2) on glucocorticoid-stimulated pulmonary surfactant synthesis in two congenic mouse strains. Proc Soc Exp Biol Med 1984;176:419.
76. Josimovich JB, Merisko K, Boccella L, Tobon H. Binding of prolactin by fetal rhesus cell membrane fractions. Endocrinology 1977;100:557.
77. Khosla SS, Brehier A, Eisenfeld AJ, et al. Influence of sex hormones on lung maturation in the fetal rabbit. Biochim Biophys Acta 1981;750:112.
78. Khosla SS, Gobran LI, Rooney SA. Stimulation of phosphatidylcholine synthesis by 17beta-estradiol in fetal rabbit lung. Biochim Biophys Acta 1980;617:282.
79. Khosla SS, Rooney SA. Stimulation of fetal lung surfactant production by administration of 17beta-estradiol to the maternal rabbit. Am J Obstet Gynecol 1979;133:213.
80. Khosla SS, Walker Smith GJ, et al. Effects of estrogen on fetal rabbit lung maturation: morphological and biochemical studies. Pediatr Res 1981;15:1274.
81. Kister SE, Pilot-Matias TJ, Janis RS, et al. Characterization of the gene encoding the hydrophobic surfactant protein SPL(Phe). Pediatr Res 1988;23:512A.
82. Kitterman JA, Liggins GC, Campos GA, et al. Preparum maturation of the lung in fetal sheep: relation to cortisol. J Appl Physiol 1981;51:384.
83. Klein AH, Stinson D, Foley B, et al. Thyroid function studies in preterm infants recovering from the respiratory distress syndrome. J Pediatr 1977;91:261.
84. Klein GP, Baden M, Giroud CJP. Quantitative measurement and significance of five plasma corticosteroids during the perinatal period. J Clin Endocrinol Metab 1973;36:944.
85. Kling OR, Kotas RV. Endocrine influences on pulmonary maturation and the L/S ratio in the fetal baboon. Am J Obstet Gynecol 1975;121:664.
86. Kotas RV. Accelerated pulmonary surfactant after intrauterine infection in the fetal rabbit. Pediatrics 1973;51:655.
87. Kotas RV, Avery ME. Accelerated appearance of the pulmonary surfactant in the fetal rabbit. J Appl Physiol 1971;30:358.
88. Kotas RV, Avery ME. The influence of sex on fetal rabbit lung maturation and the response to glucocorticoid. Am Rev Resp Dis 1980;121:377.
89. Kotas RV, Kling OR, Block MF, et al. Response of immature baboon fetal lung to intra-amniotic betamethasone. Am J Obstet Gynec 1978;130:712.
90. Kotas RV, Mims L, Hart L. Reversible inhibition of lung cell number after glucocorticoid injection. Pediatrics 1974;53:358.

91. Leheup BP, Gray ME, Stahlman MT, LeQuire VS. Synergistic effect of epidermal growth factor and retinoic acid on lung phospholipid synthesis. Pediatr Res 1983;17:381A.

92. Liggins GC. Premature delivery of foetal lambs infused with glucocorticoids. J Endocrinol 1969;45:515.

93. Liggins GC, Schellenberg J, Manzai M, et al. Synergism of cortisol and thyrotropin-releasing hormone on lung maturation in fetal sheep. J Appl Physiol 1988;65:1880.

94. Liley HG, White R, Benson B, Ballard PL. Glucocorticoids both stimulate and inhibit production of pulmonary surfactant protein A in fetal human lung. Proc Natl Acad Sci USA 1988;85:9090.

95. Liley HG, White RT, Warr RG, et al. Regulation of messenger RNAs for the hydrophobic surfactant proteins in human lung. J Clin Invest 1989;83:1191.

96. Lindenberg JA, Brehier A, Ballard PL. Triiodothyronine nuclear binding in fetal and adult rabbit lung and cultured lung cells. Endocrinology 1978;103:1725.

97. Maniscalco WM, Finkelstein JN, Parkhurst AR. Dexamethasone increases de novo fatty acid synthesis in fetal rabbit lung explants. Pediatr Res 1985;19:1272.

98. McMillan EM, King GM, Adamson IYR. Sex hormones influence growth and surfactant production in fetal lung research. Exp Lung Res 1989;15:167.

99. Mendelson CR, Brown PK, MacDonald PC, Johnston JM. Characterization of a cytosolic estrogen-binding protein in lung tissue of fetal rats. Endocrinology 1981;109:210.

100. Mendelson CR, Chen C, Boggaram V, et al. Regulation of the synthesis of the major surfactant apoprotein in fetal rabbit lung tissue. J Biol Chem 1986;261:9938.

101. Mendelson CR, Johnston JM, McDonald P, Snyder JM. Multihormonal regulation of surfactant synthesis by human fetal lung in vitro. J Clin Endocrinol Metab 1981;53:307.

102. Mendelson CR, MacDonald PC, Johnston JM. Estrogen binding in human fetal lung tissue cytosol. Endocrinology 1980;106:368.

103. Miller HC, Futrakul P. Birth weight, gestational age, and sex as determining factors in the incidence of respiratory distress syndrome of premature infants. J Pediatr 1968;72:628.

104. Morishige WK. Thyroid hormone influence on glucocorticoid receptor levels in the neonatal rat lung. Endocrinology 1982;111:1017.

105. Morishige WK, Uetake CA. Receptors for androgens and estrogens in the rat lung. Endocrinology 1978;102:1827.

106. Motoyama E, Orzalesi M, Kikkawa Y, et al. Effect of cortisol on the maturation of fetal rabbit lungs. Pediatrics 1971;148:547.

107. Mulay S, Giannopoulos G, Solomon S. Corticosteroid levels in the mother and fetus of the rabbit during gestation. Endocrinology 1973;93:1342.

108. Mullon DK, Smith YF, Richardson LL, et al. Effect of prolactin on phospholipid synthesis in organ cultures of fetal rat lung. Biochim Biophys Acta 1983;751:166.

109. Murphy BEP. Cortisol and cortisone levels in the cord blood at delivery of infants with and without the respiratory distress syndrome. Am J Obstet Gynecol 1974;119:1112.

110. Naeye RL, Harcke HT, Blanc WA. Adrenal gland structure and the development of hyaline membrane disease. Pediatrics 1971;47:650.

111. Nexo E, Kryger-Baggesen M. The receptor for epidermal growth factor is present in human fetal kidney, liver and lung. Regulatory Peptides 1989;26:1.

112. Nicholas TE, Johnson RG, Lugg MA, Kim PA. Pulmonary phospholipid biosynthesis and the ability of the fetal rabbit lung to reduce cortisone to cortisol during the final ten days of gestation. Life Sci 1978;22:1517.

113. Nichols KV, Dynia DW, Floros J, et al. Hormonal regulation of fetal rat surfactant proteins A and B mRNA. A comparison. Pediatr Res 1989;25:57A.

114. Nichols KV, Floros J, Dynia DW, et al. Regulation of surfactant protein A mRNA by hormones and butyrate in cultured fetal lung. Am J Physiol Lung Cell Mol Physiol 1990;259:L488.

115. Nielsen HC. Androgen receptors influence the production of pulmonary surfactant in the testicular feminization mouse fetus. J Clin Invest 1985;76:177.

116. Nielsen HC. Epidermal growth factor influences the developmental clock regulating maturation of the fetal lung fibroblasts. Biochim Biophys Acta 1989;1012:201.

117. Nielsen HC, O'Kirk W, Sweezey N, Torday JS. Coordination of growth and differentiation in the fetal lung. Exp Cell Res 1990;188:89.

118. Nielsen HC, Torday JS. Sex differences in fetal rabbit pulmonary surfactant production. Pediatr Res 1981;15:1245.

119. Nielsen HC, Torday JS. Sex differences in avian embryo pulmonary surfactant production: evidence for sex chromosome involvement. Endocrinology 1985;117:31.

120. Nielsen HC, Zinman HM, Torday JS. Dihydrotestosterone inhibits fetal rabbit pulmonary surfactant production. J Clin Invest 1982;69:611.

121. Odom MJ, Snyder JM, Boggaram V, Mendelson CR. Glucocorticoid regulation of the major surfactant associated protein (SP-A) and its messenger ribonucleic acid and of morphological development of human lung in vitro. Endocrinology 1988;123:1712.

122. Oldenborg V, Van Golde LMG. The enzymes of phosphatidylcholine biosynthesis in the fetal mouse lung. Effects of dexamethasone. Biochim Biophys Acta 1977;489:454.

123. Pasqualini JR, Sumida C, Kelly C, Nguyen BL. Specific (3H) estradiol binding in the fetal uterus and testis of the guinea pig. Quantitative evolution of (3H) estradiol receptors in the different fetal tissues (kidney, lung, uterus and testis) during fetal development. J Steroid Biochem 1976;7:1031.

124. Patel DM, Rhodes PG. Effects of insulin and hydrocortisone on lung tissue phosphatidylcholine and disaturated phosphatidylcholine in fetal rabbits in vivo. Diabetologia 1984;27:478.

125. Pedersen J, Bojsen-Moller B, Poulsen H. Blood sugar in newborn infants of diabetic mothers. Acta Endocrinol 1954;15:33.

126. Phelps DS, Church S, Kourembanas S, et al. Increases in the 35 kDa surfactant-associated protein and its mRNA following in vivo dexamethasone treatment of fetal and neonatal rats. Electrophoresis 1987;8:235.

127. Pignol B, Bourbon J, Ktorza A, et al. Lung maturation in the hyperinsulinemic rat fetus. Pediatr Res 1987;21:436.

128. Pope TS, Rooney SA. Effect of glucocorticoid and thyroid hormones on regulatory enzymes of fatty acid synthesis and glycogen metabolism in developing fetal rat lung. Biochim Biophys Acta 1987;918:141.

129. Porreco RP, Merritt TA, Gluck L. Effect of prolactin on phospholipid synthesis by alveolar cell carcinoma (A549) in monolayer tissue culture. Am J Obstet Gynecol 1980;136:1071.

130. Possmayer F, Casola PG, Chan F. Glucocorticoid induction of pulmonary maturation in the rabbit fetus. The effect of maternal injection of betamethasone on the activity of enzymes in fetal lung. Biochim Biophys Acta 1979;574:197.

131. Possmayer F, Casola PG, Chan F, et al. Hormonal induction of pulmonary maturation in the rabbit fetus. Effects of maternal treatment with estradiol on the endogenous levels of cholinephosphate, CDP-choline, and phosphatidylcholine. Biochim Biophys Acta 1981;664:10.

132. Possmayer F, Duwe G, Metcalfe R. Cortisol induction of pulmonary maturation in the rabbit fetus. Its effects on enzymes related to phospholipid biosynthesis and on marker enzymes for subcellular organelles. Biochem J 1977;66:484.

133. Post M. Maternal administration of dexamethasone stimulates cholinephosphate cytidylyltransferase in fetal type II cells. Biochem J 1987;241:291.

134. Post M, Barsoumian A, Smith BT. The cellular mechanism of glucocorticoid acceleration of fetal lung maturation: fibroblast-pneumonocyte factor stimulates cholinephosphate cytidylyltransferase activity. J Biol Chem 1986;261:2179.

135. Post M, Floros J, Smith BT. Inhibition of lung maturation by monoclonal antibodies against fibroblast-pneumonocyte factor. Nature 1984;308:284.

136. Post M, Smith BT. Effect of fibroblast-pneumonocyte factor on the synthesis of surfactant phospholipids in type II cells from fetal rat lung. Biochim Biophys Acta 1984;793:297.

137. Post M, Torday JS, Smith BT. Alveolar type II cells isolated from fetal rat lung organotypic cultures synthesize and secrete surfactant-associated phospholipids and respond to fibroblast-pneumonocyte factor. Exp Lung Res 1984;7:53.

138. Rhoades RA, Filler DA, Vannata B. Influence of maternal diabetes on lipid metabolism in neonatal rat lung. Biochim Biophys Acta 1979;572:132.

139. Robert MF, Bator AT, Taeusch HW. Pulmonary pressure-volume relationships after corticotrophin (ACTH) and saline injections in fetal rabbits. Pediatr Res 1975;9:760.

140. Robert MF, Neff RK, Hubbell JP, et al. Association between maternal diabetes and the respiratory-distress syndrome in the newborn. N Engl J Med 1976;294:357.

141. Rooney SA, Gobran LI, Chu AJ. Thyroid hormones oppose some glucocorticoid effects on glycogen content and lipid synthesis in developing fetal rat lung. Pediatr Res 1986;20:545.

142. Rooney SA, Gobran L, Gross I, et al. Studies on pulmonary surfactant. Effects of cortisol administration to fetal rabbits on lung phospholipid content, composition and biosynthesis. Biochim Biophys Acta 1976;450:121.

143. Rooney SA, Gobran LI, Marino PA, et al. Effects of betamethasone on phospholipid content, composition and biosynthesis in the fetal rabbit lung. Biochim Biophys Acta 1979;572:64.

144. Rooney SA, Gross I, Gassenheimer LN, Motoyama EK. Stimulation of glycerophosphate phosphatidyltransferase activity in fetal rabbit lung by cortisol administration. Biochim Biophys Acta 1975;398:433.

145. Rooney SA, Gross I, Warshaw JB. Thyrotropin releasing hormone stimulates surfactant secretion in the fetal rabbit. Am Rev Resp Dis 1978;117:386.

146. Rooney SA, Ingelson LD, Wilson CM, Gross I. Insulin antagonism of dexamethasone-induced stimulation of cholinephosphate cytidylyltransferase in fetal rat lung in organ culture. Lung 1980;158:151.

147. Ruel J, Coulombe P, Dussault JH. Thyroid hormones, malnutrition and biochemical composition of developing rat lung. Am J Physiol Endocrinol 1982;242:E378.

148. Russel BJ, Nugent L, Chernick V. Effects of steroids on the enzymatic pathways of lecithin production in fetal rabbits. Biol Neonate 1974;24:306.

149. Schellenberg J, Liggins GC, Manzai M, et al. Synergistic hormonal effects on lung maturation in fetal sheep. J Appl Physiol 1988;65:94.

150. Schellhase DE, Shannon JM. Effects of maternal dexamethasone on expression of SP-A, SP-B and SP-C in the fetal rat lung. Am J Resp Cell Mol Biol 1991;4:304.

151. Segall-Blank M, Douglas W, Sanders R, Hitchcock K. Thyroxine metabolism in cultured cells from fetal rat lung. Pediatr Res 1983;17:596.

152. Sen N, Cake MH. Enhancement of disaturated phosphatidylcholine synthesis by epidermal growth factor in cultured fetal lung cells involves a fibroblast-epithelial cell interaction. Am J Resp Cell Mol Biol 1991;5:337.

153. Seybold W, Smith BT. Human amniotic fluid contains fibroblast pneumonocyte factor. Early Human Devel 1980;4:337.

154. Sharp-CaGeorge SM, Blicher BM, Gordon ER, Murphy BEP. Amniotic fluid cortisol and human fetal lung maturation. N Engl J Med 1977;296:89.

155. Smith BT. The role of pulmonary corticosteroid 11-reductase activity in lung maturation. Pediatr Res 1978;12:12.

156. Smith BT. Fibroblast-pneumonocyte factor: intercellular mediator of glucocorticoid effect on fetal lung. In: Stern L, Oh W, Friis-Hansen B, eds. Neonatal intensive care, vol. II. New York: Masson, 1978:25.

157. Smith BT. Lung maturation in the fetal rat: acceleration by the injection of fibroblast-pneumonocyte factor. Science 1979;20:1094.

158. Smith BT. Lack of species specificity in production of fibroblast-pneumonocyte factor by perinatal lung fibroblasts. In: Monset-Couchard M, Minkowski A, eds. Physiological and biochemical basis for perinatal medicine. New York: Karger, 1981:54.

159. Smith BT, Giroud CJP. Effects of cortisol on serially propagated fibroblast cell cultures derived from the rabbit fetal lung and skin. Can J Physiol Pharm 1975;53:1037.

160. Smith BT, Giroud CJP, Robert M, Avery ME. Insulin antagonism of cortisol action on lecithin synthesis by cultured fetal lung cells. J Pediatr 1975;87:953.

161. Smith BT, Sabry K. Glucocorticoid-thyroid synergism in lung maturation: a mechanism involving epithelial-mesenchymal interaction. Proc Natl Acad Sci USA 1983;80:1951.

162. Smith BT, Tanswell AK, Worthington D, Piercey WN. Local control of glucocorticoid levels by individual tissues in the fetus: commonality among foregut derivatives. In: Stern L, ed. Neonatal intensive care, vol III. New York: Masson, 1981:45.

163. Smith BT, Torday JS. Factors affecting lecithin syn-

thesis by fetal lung cells in culture. Pediatr Res 1974;8:848.

164. Smith BT, Torday JS, Giroud CJP. The growth promoting effect of cortisol on human fetal lung cells. Steroids 1974;22:515.

165. Smith BT, Worthington D, Maloney AHA. Fetal lung maturation. III. The amniotic fluid cortisol/cortisone ratio in preterm human delivery and the risk of respiratory distress syndrome. Obstet Gynecol 1977;49:527.

166. Smith BT, Worthington D, Piercey WN. The relationship of cortisol and cortisone to saturated lecithin concentration in ovine amniotic fluid and fetal lung liquid. Endocrinology 1977;101:104.

167. Smith DM, Hitchcock KR. Thyroid hormone binding to adult rat alveolar type II cells: an autoradiographic study. Exp Lung Res 1983;5:141.

168. Snyder JM, Kwun JE, O'Brien JA, et al. The concentration of the 35-KDa surfactant apoprotein in amniotic fluid from normal and diabetic pregnancies. Pediatr Res 1988;24:728.

169. Snyder JM, Mendelson CR. Insulin inhibits the accumulation of the major lung surfactant apoprotein in human fetal lung explants maintained in vitro. Endocrinology 1987;120:1250.

170. Sosenko IRS, Frantz ID, Roberts RJ, Meyrick B. Morphologic disturbance of lung maturation in fetuses of alloxan diabetic rabbits. Am Rev Resp Dis 1980;122:687.

171. Sosenko IRS, Hartig-Beecken I, Frantz ID. Cortisol reversal of functional delay of lung maturation in fetuses of diabetic rabbits. J Appl Physiol 1980;49:971.

172. Sosenko IRS, Lawson EE, Demottaz V, Frantz ID. Functional delay in lung maturation in fetuses of diabetic rabbits. J Appl Physiol 1980;48:643.

173. Sosenko IRS, Lewis PL, Frank L. Metyrapone delays surfactant and antioxidant enzyme maturation in developing rat lung. Pediatr Res 1986;20:672.

174. Sundell HW, Gray ME, Serenius FS, et al. Effects of epidermal growth factor on lung maturation in fetal lambs. Am J Pathol 1980;100:707.

175. Sweezey NB, Buch SJ, Li S, Post M. Feed-forward regulation of lung maturation: glucocorticoid receptor is stimulated by its ligand in maturing fetal rat lung. Pediatr Res 1990;27:306A.

176. Sweezey NB, Buch SJ, Rae S, et al. Glucocorticoid receptor and surfactant protein expression in maturing rat lung. Pediatr Res 1989;25:61A.

177. Taeusch HW, Brown E, Torday JS, Nielsen HC. Magnitude and duration of lung response to dexamethasone in fetal sheep. Am J Obstet Gynecol 1981;140:452.

178. Taeusch HW, Heitner M, Avery ME. Accelerated lung maturation and increased survival in premature rabbits treated with hydrocortisone. Am Rev Resp Dis 1972;105:971.

179. Thorburn GD. The role of the thyroid gland and kidneys in fetal growth. Ciba Foundation Symposia 1974;27:185.

180. Thuresson-Klein A, Moawad AH, Heldqvist P. Estrogen stimulates formation of lamellar bodies and release of surfactant in the fetal rat lung. Am J Obstet Gynecol 1985;151:506.

181. Torday JS. Dihydrotestosterone inhibits fibroblast-pneumonocyte factor mediated synthesis of saturated phosphatidylcholine by fetal rat lung cells. Biochim Biophys Acta 1985;835:23.

182. Torday JS. The sex difference in type II cell surfactant synthesis originates in the fibroblast. Exp Lung Res 1985;7:187.

183. Torday JS. Formal demonstration of glucocorticoid dependent fetal lung SPC synthesis. Pediatr Res 1985;19:164A.

184. Torday JS, Kourembanas S. Fetal rat lung fibroblasts produce a TGF beta homolog that blocks alveolar type II cell maturation. Develop Biol 1990;139:35.

185. Torday JS, Nielsen HC. The sex difference in fetal lung surfactant production. Exp Lung Res 1987;12:1.

186. Torday JS, Nielsen HC, Fencl M, Avery ME. Sex differences in fetal lung maturation. Am Rev Resp Dis 1981;123:205.

187. Torday JS, Olson EB, First NL. Production of cortisol from cortisone by the isolated, perfused fetal rabbit lung. Steroids 1976;27:869.

188. Torday JS, Post M, Smith BT. Compartmentalization of 11-oxidoreductase within the fetal lung alveolus. Am J Physiol Cell Physiol 1985;249:C173.

189. Torday JS, Smith BT, Giroud CJP. The rabbit fetal lung as a glucocorticoid target tissue. Endocrinology 1975;96:1462.

190. Torday JS, Zinman HM, Nielsen HC. Glucocorticoid regulation of DNA, protein and surfactant phospholipid in developing lung. Dev Pharmacol Ther 1986;9:124.

191. Tsai MY, Josephson MW, Brown DM. Fetal rat lung phosphatidylcholine synthesis in diabetic and normal pregnancies: a comparison of prenatal dexamethasone treatments. Biochim Biophys Acta 1981;664:174.

192. Tsao FHC, Gutcher GR, Zachman RD. Effect of hydrocortisone on the metabolism of phosphatidylcholine in maternal and fetal rabbit lungs and livers. Pediatr Res 1979;13:997.

193. Tyden O, Berne C, Eriksson U. Lung maturation in fetuses of diabetic rats. Pediatr Res 1980;14:1192.

194. Vidyasagar D, Chernick V. Effect of metopirone on the synthesis of lung surfactant in does and fetal rabbits. Biol Neonate 1975;27:1.

195. Vilos GA, Challis JRG, Lye SJ, et al. Accelerated prepartum maturation of the fetal sheep lung with physiological doses of adreno-corticotrophin. J Dev Physiol 1983;5:341.

196. Vilos GA, Challis JRG, Lye SJ, et al. Discordant accelerated pulmonary maturation after adrenocorticotrophic hormone-induced labor in twin sheep fetuses. Am J Obstet Gynecol 1988;159:1321.

197. Viscardi RM, Weinhold PA, Beals TM, Simons RH. Cholinephosphate cytidylyltransferase in fetal rat lung cells: activity and subcellular distribution in response to dexamethasone, triiodothyronine, and fibroblast-conditioned medium. Exp Lung Res 1989;15:223.

198. Wang NS, Kotas RV, Avery ME, Thurlbeck WM. Accelerated appearance of osmiophilic bodies in fetal lungs following steroid injection. J Appl Physiol 1971;30:362.

199. Warburton D. Chronic hyperglycemia with secondary hyperinsulinemia inhibits the maturational response of fetal lamb lungs to cortisol. J Clin Invest 1983;72:433.

200. Warburton D, Lew CD, Platzker ACG. Primary hyperinsulinemia reduces surface active material flux in tracheal fluid of fetal lambs. Pediatr Res 1981;15:1422.

201. Warburton D, Parton L, Buckley S, et al. Effects of glucose infusion on surfactant and glycogen regulation in fetal lamb lung. J Appl Physiol 1987;63:1750.

202. Weiss RR, Macri JN, Tejani N, et al. Antenatal diag-

nosis and lung maturation in anencephaly. Obstet Gynecol 1974;44:368.

203. White RT, Damm D, Miller J. Isolation and characterization of the human pulmonary surfactant apoprotein gene. Nature 1985;317:361.

204. Whitsett JA, Weaver TE, Clark JC, et al. Glucocorticoid enhances proteolipid Phe and pVal synthesis and mRNA in fetal lung. J Biol Chem 1987;262:15618.

205. Whitsett JA, Weaver TE, Lieberman MA, et al. Differ-ential effects of epidermal growth factor and transforming growth factor-beta on synthesis of $MR = 35,000$ surfactant-associated protein in fetal lung. J Biol Chem 1987;262:7908.

206. Wu B, Kikkawa Y, Orzalesi MM, et al. The effect of thyroxine on the maturation of fetal rabbit lungs. Biol Neonate 1973;22:161.

207. Zimmermann L, Post M. Regulation of phosphatidyl-choline synthesis in rat type II pneumocytes during development. Pediatr Res 1991;29:336A.

Carbohydrate Metabolism: Insulin and Glucagon

Mark A. Sperling

The fetus receives its glucose supply from the mother via placental transfer involving a noninsulin-responsive glucose transporter.[56, 78] Fetal glucose concentration is proportional to maternal glucose concentration, and fetal glucose production or gluconeogenesis is minimal as shown by isotope dilution experiments as well as by direct measurements of glucose and gluconeogenesis across the hepatic bed, mostly in the fetal sheep model.[15, 67, 159] Thus maternal hypoglycemia is associated with fetal hypoglycemia and hypoinsulinemia, with little evidence of compensatory glucose production.[3] Hypoxia, or the direct infusion of catecholamines, raises fetal glucose, reflecting the existence of appropriate catecholamine receptors that are coupled to their effector systems.[103] The dose-response effect of glucagon infusion on glucose levels is blunted in the fetus relative to the adult, suggesting a deficiency of glucagon receptors coupled to their respective effector systems.[34, 123] Maternal hyperglycemia is associated with fetal hyperglycemia and hyperinsulinemia. Glycogen deposits, reflecting glycogen synthesis, increase asymptomatically in the third trimester and fetal gluconeogenesis is evident close to term and is inducible by cortisol.[159] At birth, with the abrupt curtailment of nutrient supply on placental separation, a series of integrated signals involving hormones and their receptors mobilizes endogenous glucose via glycogenolysis and gluconeogenesis.[103] Insulin, glucagon, catecholamines, and their receptors are pivotal in these adaptations.[103, 146, 151] These normal adaptive events permit a rational framework for understanding the relatively frequent disturbances of glucose homeostasis in the newborn. Before discussing their roles in the fetus and neonate, a brief overview of insulin and glucagon secretion and action is provided. The critical role of these hormones in normal metabolism and in important disease states, such as hypoglycemia and diabetes, has made them the subject of in-depth reviews.[26, 42, 83, 86, 88, 145, 154, 160, 161]

SYNOPSIS OF INSULIN AND GLUCAGON: SECRETION AND ACTION

Insulin

Insulin is synthesized in the endoplasmic reticulum of β cells as proinsulin, a single-chain polypeptide in which the carboxy terminus of the B chain is linked to the amino end of the A chain by a connecting peptide, C-peptide. The C-peptide is split off in the Golgi apparatus, where insulin granules are packaged in membranes and align themselves along the microtubular, microfilamentous system of the cell.[86, 154, 155] This cell web provides a means of transporting the insulin granules from their site of manufacture toward the surface, where secretion occurs by emiocytosis, a process in which the membranes of insulin granules fuse with the cell membrane.[48, 86, 115, 154]

Stimuli to insulin secretion include carbohydrates, principally glucose, and amino acids and fatty acids. A specific glucose receptor exists on the cell surface of the β cell; evidence for this concept derives in part from the differential effects of anomeric forms of D-glucose (the α anomer being more potent in inducing insulin secretion than the β anomer) as well as the stimulating effects of nonmetabolizable sugars such as galactose.[64, 97] It has been proposed that subsequent intracellular glycolytic metabolism of glucose provides the energy source for further insulin synthesis. Thus insulin secretion in response to a glucose infusion is biphasic, as reflected in in vitro or in in vivo studies; the initial phase possibly represents preformed insulin already aligned on the cell web, whereas the second phase represents newly synthesized insulin. Translocation of ions, primarily affecting the transfer of calcium into the cell cytoplasm from extracellular and intracellular stores, is involved in the process of insulin secretion[93]; potassium ions as well as magnesium and phosphate ions also play a role.[46]

Insulin secretion is modulated by the autonomic nervous system; activation of α-adrenergic impulses inhibits, whereas activation of β-adrenergic stimuli promotes, insulin secretion via receptors of the β_2 type.[169] The insulin secretory system is linked to cyclic adenosine monophosphate (cAMP), so that theophylline or other phosphodiesterase inhibitors promote insulin secretion, as do substances such as glucagon that activate cAMP. The parasympathetic system, via the vagus, also stimulates insulin secretion.[12] Certain gastrointestinal hormones directly enhance insulin secretion, and, of these, glucose-potentiating, insulin-stimulating polypeptide (GIP) is likely to be of greatest physiologic importance.[36] Certain hormones, such as growth hormone, glucocorticoids, and sex steroids, enhance insulin secretion either directly or indirectly through antagonizing the metabolic effects of insulin.[145] Insulin action is initiated by specific binding to target cell receptors in tissues such as liver and fat cells and the subsequent translation into enzyme action, leading to glycogen and fat synthesis from glucose and protein synthesis from amino acids.[79, 132] The gene for insulin secretion has been mapped to chromosome 11 in humans.[122]

Glucagon

Glucagon, too, is synthesized in a larger prohormone form, and the mechanisms of synthesis and release are similar to those described for insulin.[36, 88] Glucagon secretion is stimulated by amino acids and hypoglycemia; hyperglycemia suppresses glucagon secretion.[54, 88] The autonomic nervous system also participates in glucagon release via the sympathetic and parasympathetic nervous systems.[49, 169] There is some controversy regarding the type of adrenergic receptor that modulates glucagon release, with evidence most likely favoring the β-adrenergic receptor.[169]

Proglucagon can be subject to different posttranslational cleavage products. The peptides emanating from the L cells of the gut increase after glucose (gut-glucagon, glicentin, glucagon-like peptides 1 and 2), whereas pancreatic glucagon is suppressed by glucose.[36]

Although the kidneys participate substantially in glucagon clearance,[74] glucagon action is primarily on the liver and is initiated by binding to receptors on cell membranes with stimulation of cAMP.[9, 160] In the liver, the stimulation of cAMP is responsible for glycogenol-

ysis. The effects of glucagon on increasing hepatic glucose output are transitory,[42, 160] although the liver appears to become dependent on a critical glucagon level to sustain hepatic glucose output.[26] Despite the downregulation of the effects of glucagon on hepatic glucose output, the contribution of gluconeogenesis steadily increases.[26] Thus the major function of glucagon appears to be prevention of hypoglycemia through activation of hepatic glucose output. The gene for glucagon has been cloned and mapped to chromosome 2, and its pancreatic expression has been reviewed.[122]

Somatostatin

This tetradecapeptide hormone, initially isolated from the hypothalamus by its action in inhibiting the release of growth hormone, also inhibits the release of a number of hormones, including insulin and glucagon.[42, 128, 161] Thus, with sustained somatostatin infusion, both insulin and glucagon concentrations in plasma fall markedly. Initially there is a fall in glucose, implying a predominant role for glucagon in maintaining glucose output. The possibility exists, however, that the fall in glucose represents a decrease in splanchnic blood flow together with impaired glucose absorption induced by somatostatin.[42] Later during somatostatin infusion, glucose production and its plasma levels rise, reflecting the prolonged absence of insulin.[42]

Somatostatin has also been localized to the D cells of the islets of Langerhans[127] in addition to the hypothalamus. Several secretogogues that promote the release of insulin and glucagon appear to promote the secretion of somatostatin from the pancreas,[160] and the authenticity of this material in plasma is now established.[30] The functional significance of pancreatic somatostatin may be to subserve local paracrine control of insulin and glucagon secretion.[122, 160]

EMBRYOLOGY AND ORGANIZATION OF THE ENDOCRINE PANCREAS

The pancreas appears approximately between the 20th and 25th somite in most species, including the human, in which this stage occurs during the fourth week following conception. Development of the pancreatic islets occurs in two phases. The first or primary transition involves the formation of the pancreatic diverticulum. Although cytodifferentiation of exocrine or endocrine β cells cannot be recognized, their specific secretory products—certain hydrolytic enzymes and insulin—can be recognized. In contrast, well-differentiated α cells containing glucagon granules in abundance are already present and account for approximately 5% of all cells. The D cells containing somatostatin also appear very early.[100] At this stage, mesenchymal cells accumulate around the primitive gut in proximity to the pancreatic diverticulum. Further epithelial development of the pancreas depends on this mesenchymal tissue or a factor extracted from it. This factor is not tissue or species specific because it can be extracted from chick embryos and used for rat pancreas, where it acts to stimulate DNA synthesis[89] via cAMP.[125] In addition, the mesenchymal factor influences differentiation because in its absence α cells predominate at the expense of acinar tissue; insulin and β cells remain constant. Thus the origin of α cells and acinar cells must be from a common stem cell, the differentiation of which can be shifted in one or another direction by this mesenchymal factor. The origin of the endocrine β cells is predominantly endodermal; although a neural crest origin for some of the islet endocrine cells has been suggested,[120] it does not appear to be valid for insulin or somatostatin, which are produced by fetal pancreas in culture in the absence of any innervation.[100, 126]

The second phase, or secondary transition, is characterized by an increase in the exocrine and endocrine β cells, which have morphologic and functional features similar to those of the mature cell. Thus α cells predominate early in gestation, whereas β cells and insulin synthesis occur later, from which it is inferred that insulin has no major role in early fetal development.[7, 70, 124] In neonates, the ratio of α cells to β cells is approximately 1:1, whereas in adults, the ratio is between 1:3 and 1:9.[105, 107] Because glucagon is so predominant in fetal life, in which along with somatostatin it appears before any other hormone and before specific target cells in liver and fat can re-

spond, a role in regulating early differentiation of the embryo via cAMP was proposed for it.[129]

The organization as well as the relative numbers of α and β cells also changes during gestation. Initially, α and β cells exist in adjacent clusters. Later the β cells become enveloped by α cells, which have a close relationship to the D cells,[160] and after 30 weeks, both cell types are mingled as they are in the adult. The possibility that the endocrine stem cells are pluripotent, permitting interconversion of α and β cells, has been suggested,[124] but apart from the mesenchymal factor, little is known of the regulation of these processes. The development of D cells containing somatostatin is in general closer to that of the β than the α cells in the rat pancreas.[100] The pancreatic content of somatostatin increases postnatally.[100]

In addition to the insulin-secreting β cells, glucagon-secreting α cells, and somatostatin-secreting D cells, another cell type has been characterized. This cell type contains pancreatic polypeptide.[71, 72] Gap junctions between adjoining cell membranes, identified by electron microscopy, provide a potential means of intercellular communication.[116, 117] The molecular size of these "pores" permits transfer of molecules, such as ions, but excludes substances with a molecular weight greater than 1900 daltons, thus effectively excluding direct transfer of the hormones themselves, which are of a larger molecular weight. Nevertheless, this organization of the islet allows for paracrine regulation in that somatostatin can inhibit the secretion of insulin, glucagon, and pancreatic polypeptide, whereas insulin inhibits glucagon secretion and possibly that of somatostatin also. Glucagon stimulates both insulin and somatostatin secretion.[122, 160] Failure of the appropriate organization and interrelationships between these cells may be a factor in the persistence of the budding-off process of islet cells from the ductule epithelium in neonatal life. This condition, termed *nesidioblastosis*, is an example of islet cell disorganization characterized by hyperinsulinemia as well as hypoglycemia.[71, 72]

FETAL INSULIN CONTENT AND SECRETION

The relative human pancreatic insulin content is higher in the fetus than in the adult, being

6.3 ± 1.1 U/g between 20 and 32 weeks and 12.7 ± 3.2 U/g between 34 and 40 weeks; adult values are 2.1 ± 0.3 U/g. This pattern of high insulin content that increases steadily with gestation has been confirmed in independent studies[8, 134] (Table 20–1).

In contrast to this high insulin content, fetal insulin secretion is obtunded, so release mechanisms rather than synthetic processes are responsible for low circulating levels. Glucose is a weak stimulus to acute insulin secretion in the fetus. Pancreatic islets isolated from human fetuses of 12 to 16 weeks' gestation fail to respond with a significant increase in insulin secretion during incubation with a high glucose medium[38]; modest increases were reported with pancreas slices of fetuses of 7 to 20 weeks' gestation.[134] Some maturation of this process exists, however, because there is a significant correlation between insulin response to glucose stimulation and gestational age or fetal body weight in the period of 15 to 24 weeks' gestation.[6, 123] The amino acids arginine and leucine are effective stimuli for fetal insulin secretion in vitro, as are glucagon, the phosphodiesterase inhibitor theophylline, and dibutyryl cAMP; the latter three compounds all raise cAMP levels and are effective even in the presence of low or no glucose in the incubating medium.[38, 93, 105] Tolbutamide is without effect, but certain ions, such as potassium and barium as well as ouabain, are effective.[105] Thus in vitro studies indicate that the β cell is functional from 14 to 24 weeks, responding to amino acids, ions, and factors that raise intracellular cAMP but not to glucose.

The in vivo situation is more difficult to define in humans because of the potential errors introduced by the stresses of experimental manipulation. In studies preceding hysterotomy, however, it was shown that glucose and arginine are without effect in promoting insulin secretion in the human fetus at midterm.[82] Similarly, by the use of the technique of fetal blood sampling via scalp capillaries, it was shown that before the onset of labor, the normal human fetus is relatively unresponsive to high glucose concentrations.[112] Neither glucose nor arginine were effective stimuli for insulin, but as in the in vitro studies, glucagon administration caused prompt insulin release. In this model, the administration of glucose and theophylline together into the monkey fetus in vivo resulted in a rise in fetal plasma insulin; glucose or theophylline alone was incapable of elevating insulin.[28]

These studies are compatible with the concept that the lack of insulin secretion in the intact fetus in vivo following glucose administration is related to a deficiency in the ability to generate cAMP or to its rapid destruction via phosphodiesterase. The phosphodiesterase that inactivates cAMP was reported to be very active,[131] and a twofold to threefold increase in islet cAMP occurs in newborn rat pups over the initial 72 hours of life.[63, 108] Thus transition from fetal to adult patterns of responsiveness may in part be due to maturation of cAMP systems and may account for the persistence of poor insulin secretion following glucose in the immediate newborn period in humans. As could be predicted, theophylline or glucagon in pharmacologic doses increases insulin secretion in newborn infants.[60] Note that insulin measured in the plasma of the fetus is of fetal origin because there is no transfer of insulin across the placenta in either the maternal to fetal or fetal to maternal directions[105] except

TABLE 20–1. Total Glucagon and Insulin in Human Fetal Pancreas

Gestational Age (Weeks)	Glucagon Concentration (ng/mg Tissue)*		Insulin (μU/mg Tissue)*
7–10.0	1.28 (n = 1)†	4.0 ± 1.2 (n = 7)‡	333 ± 64 (n = 7)‡
10.5–15.5	1.98 ± 0.5 (n = 2)†	9.7 ± 2.2 (n = 6)‡	1189 ± 359 (n = 6)‡
16–25	5.57 ± 01.86 (n = 4)†	66.0 ± 15.6 (n = 5)‡	4172 ± 1159 (n = 5)‡

*Mean ± SEM.

†Data adapted from Assan R., Boillot J. Pancreatic glucagon and glucagon-like material in tissues and plasmas from human fetuses 6–26 weeks old. In: Jonxis JH, Visser HK, Troelstra JA, et al, eds. Metabolic processes in the fetus and newborn infant. Nutricia Symposium. Baltimore: Williams & Wilkins, 1971:210.

‡Data adapted from Schaeffer LD, Wilder ML, Williams RH. Secretion and content of insulin and glucagon in human fetal pancreas slices in vitro. Proc Soc Exp Biol Med 1973;143:314.

when foreign insulin injected to the mother elicits an antibody response. Antibody-bound insulin can be transferred across the human placenta from mother to fetus and may be linked to fetal macrosomia, suggesting that the transferred insulin exerts biologic effects.[102]

Although the fetal insulin response to an acute glucose challenge is impaired, this is not true for islets chronically exposed to hyperglycemia. Thus hypertrophy and hyperplasia of fetal islets as well as an increased insulin content occur in infants of diabetic mothers exposed to the chronic hyperglycemia of maternal diabetes.[24] Such infants respond to glucose in utero with an adult type of biphasic insulin secretory response[112]; a similar hypersecretion of insulin relative to normal infants is seen in the immediate newborn period. The insulin responses of infants of gestationally diabetic mothers who do not require insulin therapy and therefore have less hyperglycemia are modestly elevated at delivery and following glucose administration or other stimuli.[163] These results suggest that chronic in utero hyperglycemia as well as other metabolic alterations consequent on inadequate insulin action in the mother may modify the developmental process of insulin secretion by accelerating the maturation of the secretory mechanisms.[45] Similar results have been reported in fetal and newborn rats, which serve as a convenient model, although extrapolation to the human must be made with caution.[53]

It is important to note that secretion, and not biosynthesis, is accelerated by chronic in utero hyperglycemia because even in normal pregnancy fetal insulin synthesis is comparable in rate to that of the neonatal period and can be stimulated by glucose. The level of glucose alone, however, cannot totally explain the maturation process because this seems to be independent of glucose after birth[51] and cannot be easily reproduced by prolonged culture of rat islets in a high-glucose medium.[7, 98] As previously pointed out, amino acids are potent stimuli in vitro but poor stimuli for insulin secretion in the fetus in vivo.[107, 134] In contrast, neonatal insulin responsiveness to amino acids is often striking, particularly when a mixture of amino acids is used.[59, 61, 130] These stimulatory effects are additive when glucose infusion is combined with amino acids.[59] Because the

infants studied were premature, it is inferred from the studies that insulin responsiveness to amino acids precedes that of glucose; as subsequently outlined, enhanced glucagon secretion to amino acids also occurs in the newborn period. The role of fatty acids in insulin secretion in the fetus and newborn is undefined.

The hormonal milieu may also affect the development of insulin secretion. Late in gestation, epinephrine inhibits insulin release, an effect mediated via stimulation of the α-adrenergic receptor because propranolol, a β-adrenergic blocker, mimics these effects, whereas phentolamine, an α-adrenergic blocker, results in enhanced insulin secretion (Fig. 20–1).[147] In anencephalic infants, the endocrine pancreas develops normally if the mother has unimpaired carbohydrate metabolism. If the mother's glucose tolerance is abnormal, however, hypertrophy and hyperplasia of fetal pancreatic β cells are found only if the fetal hypothalamic-pituitary system is functional.[162] Similar results have been reported in decapitated fetal rabbits, and growth hormone's role in this has been implicated.[73, 107] Although there is evidence that glucocorticoids may inhibit the proliferation of rat islets maintained in tissue culture, no effect of cortisol or growth hormone on β-cell replication in rat pancreas monolayer culture was reported in another study.[29] Because cortisol and growth hormone stimulate insulin secretion in vivo, any observed effects may be mediated by indirect rather than direct effects on pancreatic islets.

Two other clinical circumstances are known to be associated with hyperplasia and hypertrophy of pancreatic islets. Profoundly elevated plasma insulin concentrations have been reported in infants born to gestationally diabetic mothers treated with sulfonylureas.[107] These newborn infants show marked hypersecretion of insulin in response to oral glucose, and they may suffer severe and prolonged hypoglycemia. Infants with erythroblastosis fetalis may have islet cell hyperplasia, a high pancreatic insulin content, and hyperinsulinemia at birth that may be associated with severe hypoglycemia, particularly if the infant is premature.[107] The mechanism(s) responsible for this islet cell hyperplasia in erythroblastosis is not entirely clear. It has been suggested that the enlarged hyperplastic placenta in these infants

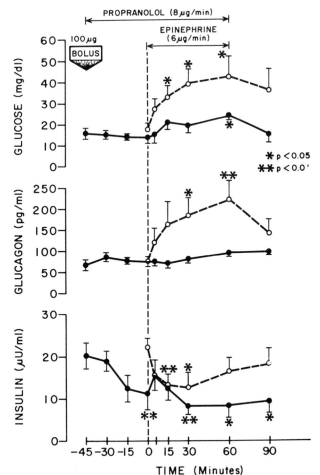

FIGURE 20–1. Effect of epinephrine infusion on plasma glucose, glucagon, and insulin concentration in fetal sheep late in gestation. Epinephrine alone stimulates glucose and glucagon but suppresses insulin. Propranolol alone has no effect on basal glucose and glucagon but suppresses basal insulin. In addition, propranolol blunts the stimulatory effects of epinephrine on glucose and glucagon and exaggerates the fall in insulin.
    ○——○ = Epinephrine alone; ●——● = propranolol ± epinephrine. (From Sperling MA, Christensen RA, Ganguli S, et al. Adrenergic modulation of pancreatic hormone secretion in utero: Studies in fetal sheep. Pediatr Res 1980;14:203. With permission.)

degrades insulin more actively than the normal placenta. Thus increased destruction would require compensatory hypersecretion of insulin. An alternate hypothesis suggests that hemolysis provides increased amounts of glutathione, which splits the disulfide bonds of the two insulin chains and thereby promotes compensatory hypersecretion of insulin.[156]

GLUCAGON IN THE FETUS

Immunoreactive pancreatic glucagon is detectable at about the eighth week of gestation but not before the sixth week (see Table 20–1). Thereafter a logarithmic increase in glucagon content per unit weight occurs; i.e., the increased content is not due simply to growth of the pancreatic mass. The pancreatic glucagon content at midgestation is 5 to 7 ng/mg of pancreas tissue, compared with 1 to 3 ng/mg in adult pancreas extracted under similar

conditions.[8, 134] Gastric and enteric tissues from these fetuses also contain material or materials that cross react with glucagon antisera and are said to possess glucagon-like immunoreactivity (GLI). The precise nature and function of these substances in humans are not completely known, but one of the components represents true glucagon with its full range of biologic activity.[36] Glucagon can be measured in human fetal plasma from 15 weeks' gestation onward, but no detectable rise followed intraperitoneal administration of arginine.[8] This plasma glucagon must be of fetal origin because the placenta is impermeable to glucagon transfer in either direction in humans early and late in gestation or in other mammals.[2, 27, 76, 109, 150] Reflecting the increased pancreatic glucagon content, plasma as well as amniotic fluid concentrations of this hormone appear to increase with gestational age.[44, 146]

    Amino acids such as arginine or alanine

stimulate release of glucagon in human pancreas slices in vitro[134] and in the rat or monkey fetus in vivo.[27, 53] In humans at term, the infusion of alanine into the mother during labor caused a significant increase in neonatal umbilical cord plasma as well as maternal plasma glucagon concentrations.[168] Because glucagon does not cross the placenta, whereas amino acids do, the findings imply that at term, human fetal α cells can respond to amino acids. Acute hypoglycemia cannot, but more prolonged hypoglycemia may, stimulate glucagon secretion in the rat fetus.[53] Catecholamines, such as norepinephrine or epinephrine, also can stimulate glucagon release in utero (see Fig. 20–1). This glucagon release is clearly mediated by the β-adrenergic receptor because propranolol blocks the stimulating effect of epinephrine.[147] The parasympathetic nervous system via acetylcholine is also capable of stimulating glucagon secretion in utero.[53] Hyperglycemia, however, which commonly suppresses glucagon in the normal adult organism, does not suppress fetal glucagon secretion in rats,[53] monkeys,[27] or lambs.[44]

The human fetal pancreatic glucagon content increases progressively throughout gestation. Secretion is not affected by acute changes in glucose, the substrate that is a major control of glucagon secretion in the normal mature organism, in which the major function of glucagon is maintenance of glucose supply. Amino acids, acetylcholine, and catecholamines are capable of stimulating glucagon release in the fetus in utero.

CARBOHYDRATE METABOLISM IN UTERO

Glucose in the fetus is obtained primarily by placental transfer from the mother.[10, 15, 50] Although the net flux of glucose is from mother to fetus, studies in sheep demonstrate that substantial quantities of glucose are transferred back from the fetus to the mother against the concentration gradient and in direct proportion to fetal glucose concentration.[4] These studies as well as studies with glucose analogs suggest that glucose transfer across the placenta occurs via a stereospecific facilitated diffusion system mediated by a glucose transporter.[4, 25, 56, 78, 153] The kinetics of glucose transfer across the placenta have been defined in the sheep.[4] In all species examined, fetal glucose concentration is lower than maternal glucose concentration but closely related to maternal glucose levels.[4, 10, 25, 50] Glucose uptake by the fetus is related to the maternal glucose concentration as well as to the maternal-fetal arterial glucose concentration difference.[4, 10, 25, 50] Late in gestation, fetal glucose turnover in the sheep is of the order of 6 to 10 mg/kg per minute.[4, 15]

Although the situation in sheep may not be applicable to that in humans, the remarkable similarity of total glucose turnover in the fetal sheep[4] and newborn human[13, 80] as well as the newborn sheep[32] and rhesus monkey[141] suggests that despite the differences between species in the plasma profiles of substrate concentrations, the quantitative aspects of glucose transfer, and possibly its utilization, may be similar.

Because the respiratory quotient is close to 1 in the human fetus near term, it has been suggested that glucose is the primary energy source of the fetus.[10, 15, 67, 77] Glucose may not, however, be the sole source of energy because indirect assessment via measurements of the glucose to oxygen quotient across the umbilical circulation of sheep suggests that glucose may contribute only 50% to fetal respiration, with the remainder derived from amino acids and lactate.[10] During maternal starvation, fetal glucose concentration and uptake fall, and the contribution of glucose to fetal respiration also falls, whereas the contribution from amino acids and lactate increases. It has been suggested that under conditions of maternal starvation, amino acids may be used for gluconeogenesis in the fetus, but direct evidence for this is lacking.[52, 144] Maternal insulin-induced hypoglycemia of 2 hours' duration results in no initiation of glucose production by the fetus, which remains completely dependent on the mother for its glucose supply.[3]

The constant supply of glucose under normal circumstances precludes the "need" for endogenous glucose production. Accordingly gluconeogenic enzymes are present in very low activity in fetal liver but mature rapidly after delivery in several species, including the human.[62, 95] Some in vitro gluconeogenesis and gluconeogenic enzymes in liver have been demonstrated in the fetuses of sheep, monkey, and human as well as in other species.[50] Cultured explants of human fetal liver, however, incorporated alanine-U-^{14}C into glucose at a rate of approximately 0.04 mg/kg per minute, a rate insufficient to meet known glucose requirements in the fetus or newborn.[137] The sequence of postpartum maturation of key gluconeogenic enzymes in the liver appears to be similar in rats and humans.[62, 95] The sharp increase of these enzyme activities after delivery correlates with the onset of postnatal gluconeogenesis and may be inducible by hormones, such as cortisol and glucagon.[66, 69, 159] The activity of the rate-limiting enzyme p-enolpyruvate carboxykinase (PEPCK), which normally appears after birth, can be induced to appear in utero through hormones such as glucagon that activate cAMP; insulin blocks this effect.[62, 65] As is subsequently detailed, a sharp increase in circulating glucagon and epinephrine concentrations occurs at delivery, whereas insulin remains low. These hormonal changes may therefore underlie the initiation of gluconeogenesis after delivery in part through the induction of key gluconeogenic enzymes.

In contrast to gluconeogenesis, glycogen synthesis and breakdown proceed actively in utero, particularly during the third trimester.[15, 55, 67, 77] Glycogen synthetase activity can be demonstrated in developing human and rat liver, and the activity of this enzyme is induced by cortisol and activated by insulin.[35, 136] A striking

increase in fetal liver glycogen content occurs during the third trimester; a spontaneous increase in cortisol levels also occurs late in the gestation.[159] Moreover, liver glucogen content as well as total body weight correlates closely with insulin concentrations in umbilical cord blood. Epinephrine and, to a lesser extent, glucagon induce a prompt increase in fetal plasma glucose levels, implying the existence of appropriate glycogenolytic mechanisms in utero.[77, 147]

ONTOGENY OF INSULIN AND GLUCAGON RECEPTORS

The ontogeny of insulin and glucagon receptors has been extensively studied over the past decade.[103] Insulin receptors of several fetal tissues are increased in number and affinity when compared with their adult counterparts (Table 20–2). These fetal/neonatal receptors are similar to adult in their physical-chemical properties. Although fetal insulin receptors do not always display down-regulation, their β subunits are capable of normal tyrosine kinase activity to produce autophosphorylation and the phosphorylation of other intracellular substrates. There is no correlation between fetal glycogen synthesis and fetal insulin receptors, whereas this is readily apparent for adult insulin receptors.[142] Because tyrosine kinase activity has been associated with various growth factors, such as insulin-like growth factor-1 (IGF-1), platelet-derived growth factor (PDGF), and

TABLE 20–2. Hepatic Fetal Receptors Compared with Corresponding Adult Receptors

Insulin	Glucagon	Epinephrine
Increased number (Ro)	Decreased number (Ro)	High β receptor number (Ro)
Increased affinity (K)	Decreased or equal affinity (K)	Decreased α receptor number (Ro)
Down-regulation—absent	Down-regulation—low Ro prevents assessment	
Autophosphorylation and tyrosine kinase activity—normal	Incomplete functional linkage to adenylate cyclase	Glycogenolysis—β mediated
Partial functional dissociation from some biologic actions	Functional linkage begins in late gestation	
Postnatally:	Postnatally:	Postnatally:
Decrease in Ro and K	Increase in Ro and perhaps K	Hepatic β receptors decrease in Ro
Functional linkage completed	Functional linkage completed	Hepatic α receptors increase in Ro
		Glycogenolysis gradually becomes α mediated

Data from Menon RK, Sperling MA. Carbohydrate metabolism in neonatal adaptation: the transition to post-natal life. Perinatol 1988;12:157.

certain oncogenes, insulin and its receptor may be important for fetal growth.[149]

In contrast to insulin receptors, fetal glucagon receptors are less in number compared with their adult counterparts and are poorly linked to cAMP production. Glucagon receptor number and linkage to cAMP increase markedly and rapidly after birth, associated with a rise in postnatal glucagon secretion[103] (Table 20–3). These maturational aspects and their potential physiologic significance are summarized in Tables 20–2 and 20–3. The insulin receptor gene has been cloned and extensively studied,[79] and the glucagon receptor gene has been isolated.[74a]

EVIDENCE FOR METABOLIC EFFECTS OF INSULIN AND GLUCAGON IN UTERO

Early in gestation, the pancreatic insulin content is low and, in the rat at least, is sufficient to raise plasma concentrations to approximately 10^{-12} M, a level too low to exert significant metabolic effects.[124] Thus growth during this early stage of gestation must be independent of any anabolic effects of insulin. If glucose were important during early gestation, its utilization and disposal would therefore have to be via insulin-independent enzyme systems. The isolated perfused canine liver can in fact switch from net glucose output to net glucose uptake when the perfusing glucose concentration is above a certain concentration and in the absence of any significant change in the perfusing insulin concentration.[22] Thus this

hepatic process appears to be essentially independent of insulin and implies at least some capacity for autoregulation of glucose uptake and output by liver. Similar results have been reported in rats and in the human fetal liver.[1]

Later in gestation, insulin possibly assumes an important role in fetal metabolism. There is evidence that insulin promotes an increase in cell size by stimulating protein synthesis. An increase in cell size does indeed occur after the 30th week of gestation, when pancreatic insulin content would be adequate to exert an influence. In vitro experiments with rhesus monkey fetal muscle demonstrate that insulin can increase glucose uptake, glucose oxidation, and incorporation of glucose into glycogen as early as 85 days' gestation, corresponding approximately to midterm.[19] Insulin, however, fails to exert a significant effect on glycogen synthesis in the isolated near-term fetal monkey liver.[55] More recent experiments using the fetal sheep preparation clearly demonstrate that insulin increases glucose utilization.[15, 143] Indeed, insulin may be considered to be a major anabolic growth hormone of the fetus.

This concept is further supported by the finding that the marked increase in fetal growth during the third trimester is largely due to fat deposition, which is exaggerated in infants of diabetic mothers who are hyperinsulinemic.[40] There is also a positive correlation between birth weight and serum insulin levels in normal infants as well as in infants of gestational diabetic mothers. Because infants of diabetic mothers are hyperinsulinemic at birth and because the transfer of free fatty acids

TABLE 20–3. Hypothesis for the Physiologic Significance of Insulin, Glucagon, and Epinephrine Levels and Receptor Characteristics in the Fetus and Newborn

Fetus	Newborn
Higher insulin receptor number (Ro) and affinity (K) should facilitate anabolic processes in some tissues leading to deposition of glycogen, protein, and fat despite low insulin levels. Low Ro and K and incomplete functional linkage of glucagon receptors and low glucagon levels limit glycogenolysis Fetus is dependent on maternal glucose supply but in emergency (hypoxia) can initiate endogenous glucose production, via β-adrenergic–mediated glycogenolysis	Following interruption of maternal nutrient supply, mobilization of glucose and other fuel stores is brought about by increase in epinephrine levels with functionally linked β receptors and increases in Ro of glucagon receptors, which are functionally linked to cAMP together with a surge in glucagon levels Falling insulin levels and decreasing insulin receptor Ro and K facilitate glycogenolysis and gluconeogenesis

Data from Menon RK, Sperling MA: Carbohydrate metabolism in neonatal adaptation: the transition to post-natal life. Semin Perinatol 1988;12:157.

across the human placenta is inadequate for deposition of fat by the fetus in the last trimester,[33] the data are compatible with the concept that insulin promotes lipogenesis during the period of rapid accumulation of fat in the fetus. Chronic infusions of glucose within the physiologic range evoke appropriate insulin secretion, and glucose concentrations correlate closely with insulin levels in the normal fetus.[67]

The metabolic functions of endogenously secreted glucagon in utero are less apparent. The high pancreatic glucagon concentrations in early gestation have prompted the suggestion that they might somehow influence organogenesis via their potent effect on raising cAMP levels.[129] In late gestation, direct infusions of glucagon into the fetal monkey raise the plasma glucose concentration, with the implication that glucagon can affect glycogenolytic mechanisms by activating phosphorylase.[27] This effect, as expected, is mediated via cAMP, as demonstrated in explants of fetal rat liver.[140] It is emphasized that only modest increments in fetal plasma glucose concentrations result from physiologic doses of administered glucagon.[34] This may be due partly to a delay in the maturation of the hepatic receptors of glucagon, a situation in striking contrast to the increase in the number and affinity of receptors for insulin.[103] The difficulty in demonstrating an effect of glucagon in vivo may be partly because it stimulates insulin release, thereby offsetting its ability to raise glucose concentrations. Consequently, when insulin concentrations decrease while glucagon concentrations increase, as occurs during epinephrine infusion to the fetus, a clear rise in glucose concentrations occurs[147] (see Fig. 20–1). It is important to note here that hypoxia in the fetal sheep results in an endogenous catecholamine release that is associated with an increase in plasma glucose.[77]

In nonphysiologic doses, glucagon can increase gluconeogenesis from alanine[137] as well as the early appearance of enzymes involved in gluconeogenesis, including glucose-6-phosphatase, pyruvate carboxylase, PEPCK, and tyrosine amino transferase (TAT).[62, 65] Similar enhancement by glucagon of human fetal liver enzyme activity of PEPCK and TAT in 20-week-old fetuses has been reported.[84] Note that in a variety of mammals these enzymes are not induced until the time of delivery.[62] Finally, glucagon in pharmacologic doses can stimulate DNA synthesis in the liver and exocrine pancreas.[94, 170]

Placental transfer of glucose resulting in anabolism of various tissues, including synthesis of glycogen, dominates fetal metabolism in utero. Insulin facilitates glucose utilization but may have greater effects on protein anabolism and on growth. Cortisol and growth hormone, both of which antagonize insulin's effect on glucose metabolism, are high in fetal plasma close to term. In addition, spontaneous epinephrine secretion can occur in response to hypoxia, and glucagon is also present. Thus hormonal mechanisms for countering insulin's effects and releasing glucose are present near term.

INSULIN AND GLUCAGON IN THE IMMEDIATE NEWBORN PERIOD

At birth, a number of dramatic changes in hormones and substrates permit the mobilization of endogenous glucose to compensate for the sudden interruption of placental supply. Glucagon concentrations rise threefold to fivefold within minutes to hours of delivery, not only in humans (Fig. 20–2),[148] but also in sheep (Fig. 20–3)[57] and other mammalian species.[51] Simultaneously plasma epinephrine and norepinephrine increase markedly at birth,[87, 118] while insulin concentrations remain in the low basal range (10 μU/mL or less) for several days (see Fig. 20–2).[148] The stimulus to the surge in glucagon while insulin levels remain low appears to be the dramatic rise in catecholamines because the events at birth can be simulated by infusions of catecholamines in utero (see Fig. 20–1).[147] The infusion of the potent inhibitor of glucagon release, somatostatin, begun in utero and continued into the neonatal period, cannot prevent the abrupt rise of glucagon immediately after cord cutting.[152]

On the basis of their known metabolic effects, the high concentrations of epinephrine and glucagon in conjunction with low levels of insulin, acting in concert, would be expected

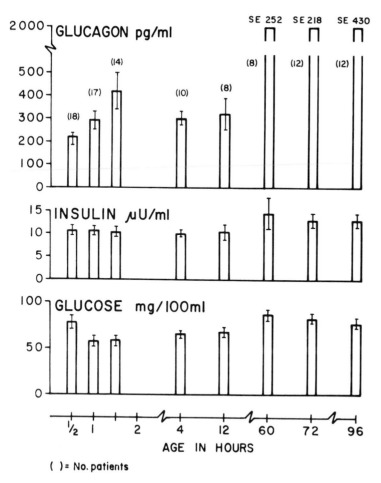

FIGURE 20–2. Plasma glucagon and insulin and glucose in normal human newborn infants. Note the brisk rise in glucagon, whereas insulin remains low, and the stabilization of glucose in the first 2 hours of life. The high glucagon concentrations from 60 hours onward reflect glucagon-like immunoreactivity rather than pancreatic glucagon. (From Sperling MA, DeLamater PV, Phelps D, et al. Spontaneous and amino acid stimulated glucagon secretion in the immediate postnatal period: Relation to glucose and insulin. J Clin Invest 1974; 53:1159. With permission.)

to mobilize glucose via glycogenolysis, to induce lipolysis, and to activate ketogenesis. Both the ratio and the absolute levels of glucagon and insulin are in the range shown to enhance markedly the ketogenic capacity of the liver in experimental animals.[99] Indeed, in normal human neonates, after a transitory fall, glucose concentrations stabilize at levels of 40 to 50 mg/dL within 3 to 4 hours after birth, whereas free fatty acid concentrations and also ketone bodies rise sharply in both plasma and urine. Thus, although glycogen reserves remain adequate in the first few hours of life, glucose could be provided for brain metabolism that does not depend on insulin, whereas fatty acids and ketones provide an alternate fuel source for muscles as well as other tissues.

Liver glycogen is rapidly depleted within several hours to approximately one-tenth of its original concentration in normal human newborns; in premature or dysmature infants, in whom liver glycogen stores are diminished, depletion occurs more rapidly.[139] A second rise in glucagon, while insulin remains low, occurs between the first and third days of life (Fig. 20–4).[148] This period corresponds to the time of rapid maturation of gluconeogenic enzymes as well as of the onset of gluconeogenesis.[95]

That the hormonal changes are critical for these adaptive events is amply demonstrated by experimental manipulations altering the hormonal concentrations. Thus infusion of somatostatin into neonatal lambs aged between

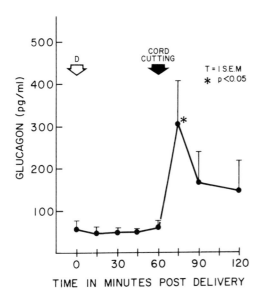

FIGURE 20–3. Glucagon concentrations in newborn sheep. Delivery alone while the cord remains intact (D ↓) has no effect, whereas cord cutting results in a prompt rise in glucagon. (From Grajwer LA, Sperling MA, Sack J, et al. Possible mechanisms and significance of the neonatal surge in glucagon secretion: Studies in newborn lambs. Pediatr Res 1977;11:833. With permission.)

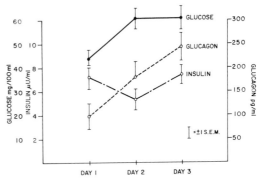

FIGURE 20–4. Sequential changes in glucose, glucagon, and insulin during the first 3 days of life in normal human newborns. Ten infants had fasting blood withdrawn serially. Note the rise in glucagon, which correlates to the rise in glucose, whereas insulin concentrations remain low and unchanged. (From Sperling MA, DeLamater PV, Phelps D, et al. Spontaneous and amino acid stimulated glucagon secretion in the immediate postnatal period: Relation to glucose and insulin. J Clin Invest 1974;53:1159. With permission.)

24 and 27 hours suppresses both insulin and glucagon concentrations and results in a fall in plasma glucose (Table 20–4).[152] Reinfusion of exogenous glucagon to simulate physiologic levels while maintaining low insulin concentrations through the infusion of somatostatin restores glucose concentrations to normal.[152] In contrast, reinfusion of insulin while maintaining low glucagon concentrations through the infusion of somatostatin results in profound hypoglycemia[152] (Fig. 20–5). Similar results are seen in human experiments of nature in which glucagon deficiency[164] or insulin excess is present.[165] Because it is possible to raise glucose concentrations by infusions of glucagon, even in the presence of high circulating insulin levels (Fig. 20–6), it appears that both the absolute concentrations and the ratios of these two hormones are important for neonatal glucose homeostasis. In addition, normal adaptive events clearly depend on the availability of adequate reserves of substrates: glycogen in liver, muscle as a source of amino acids for gluconeogenesis, and lipid stores for the release of fatty acids.

FACTORS AFFECTING INSULIN AND GLUCAGON SECRETION IN THE NEWBORN INFANT

Glucose

Glucose is a poor stimulus to insulin secretion in the newborn period. Because insulin secretion following a bolus of glucagon is normal, the poor insulin secretory response to glucose appears to reflect continuing immaturity of secretory mechanisms, related in part to imma-

TABLE 20–4. Changes During Somatostatin (SRIF) Infusion in Newborn Lambs*

	0–5 Minutes	0–60 Minutes
Δ Glucagon, pg/mL	−42.8	54.2
± SEM	10.5†	9.5†
Δ Insulin, μU/mL	− 7.2	− 9.0
± SEM	1.9‡	3.3‡
Δ Glucose, mg/dL	− 4.0	−11.5
± SEM	3.1	3.9‡

*The lambs were aged 1 to 3 days.
†P < 0.01 | compared to 0 time.
‡P < 0.05 | by paired t-test analysis for the change in each variable. (Data from Grajwer LA, Sperling MA, Sack J, et al. Possible mechanisms and significance of the neonatal surge in glucagon secretion: studies in newborn lambs. Pediatr Res 1977; 11:833.)

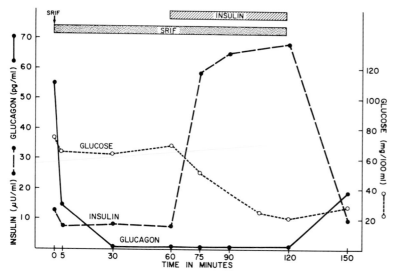

FIGURE 20–5. Effect of somatostatin (SRIF) infusion on glucose, insulin, and glucagon in newborn lambs. With SRIF alone, glucose, insulin, and glucagon all fall. Reinfusion of insulin results in profound hypoglycemia when glucagon is low. Cessation of infusion results in a return toward normal. (From Sperling MA, Grajwer L, Leake RD, et al. Effects of somatostatin (SRIF) infusion on glucose homeostasis in newborn lambs: Evidence for a significant role of glucagon. Pediatr Res 1977;11:962. With permission.)

turity of cAMP generation or its rapid destruction. A striking insulin secretory response can be achieved through a chronic glucose infusion of several hours' duration preceding a further bolus of glucose.[58] These findings clearly have implications for the interpretation of enhanced insulin secretion in infants born to diabetic mothers, in whom fetal β cells may have been "primed" by chronic hyperglycemia in utero. As for the fetus in utero, glucose does not inhibit glucagon secretion in the newborn period.[92] Simultaneous infusion of glucose with insulin, however, results in the suppression of glucagon release.[96] Thus it appears that insulin is required for the suppressive effects of glucose on glucagon secretion, possibly by facilitating the entry of glucose into the α cell. Again these findings have implications for glucagon secretion in infants born to

diabetic mothers, in whom prolonged hyperglycemia and hyperinsulinemia coexist in utero.

Amino Acids

Mixtures of amino acids can stimulate insulin release, particularly when combined with glucose as demonstrated in premature infants.[59, 130] In addition, amino acids, such as arginine or alanine, whether administered intravenously or orally, elicit prompt and significant glucagon secretion in the term fetus and in the initial hours of neonatal life (see Fig. 20–6).[148, 166] The glucagon secretory response to amino acids is obtunded when levels of glucose are elevated.[166] Similarly, the hyperglycemic effect of endogenous glucagon is also

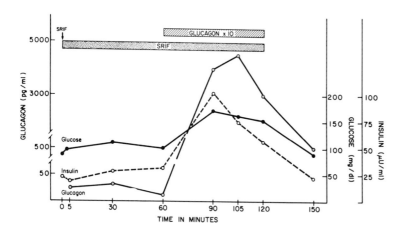

FIGURE 20–6. Effects of glucagon during somatostatin (SRIF) infusion in newborn lambs. Note that glucose rises despite insulin levels comparable to those in Figure 20–5 when glucagon levels are high. (From Sperling MA, Grajwer L, Leake RD, et al. Effects of somatostatin (SRIF) infusion on glucose homeostasis in newborn lambs: Evidence for a significant role of glucagon. Pediatr Res 1977;11:962. With permission.)

blunted when plasma glucose levels are >60 mg/dL, an effect that can also be demonstrated with exogenously administered glucagon.

Catecholamines

Infants with perinatal asphyxia demonstrate higher glucagon concentrations than do normal infants.[75] This is most likely due to enhanced catecholamine release because induction of experimental hypoxia in utero and in the newborn period can stimulate endogenous catecholamine release.[77, 118]

GLUCOSE HOMEOSTASIS IN THE NEWBORN PERIOD

In adults, it is well established that brain metabolism accounts for approximately 80% of the total daily glucose requirements.[41] Similar considerations apply to infants in whom the brain mass contributes a relatively greater proportion to total body mass.[13] Studies of cerebral metabolism in in vivo conditions indicate that the brain of infants can use glucose at a rate in excess of approximately 5 mg/100 g brain weight per minute.[121, 138] The brain of a full-term neonate, which is approximately 420 g in a 3.5-kg infant, would require glucose at a rate of 20 mg per minute or more, representing a glucose production of some 5 to 6 mg/kg per minute. Measurements of endogenous glucose production rates in infants, using stable isotopes, demonstrate values of 5 to 8 mg/kg per minute.[13, 81] Thus a large proportion of endogenous glucose production in infants can be accounted for by brain metabolism, and there is a remarkable correlation between glucose production and estimated brain weight at all ages.[13] In addition, the brain of infants and children, similar to that of adults, can adapt to use ketones as an alternate source of energy.[66, 121, 138]

Because brain growth is most rapid in the first year of life and because the larger proportion of glucose turnover is used for brain metabolism, the major impact of disturbances of energy homeostasis that fail to maintain glucose supply (hypoglycemia) or ketones in the newborn period is on brain development and function. These considerations underscore the importance of the hormonal patterns at birth, which permit a rational explanation of normal perinatal energy homeostasis in the context of catecholamine-glucagon-insulin-glucose interrelationships. The framework of these key adaptive processes is prepared in utero, where, in the last trimester, insulin facilitates deposition of glycogen and fat. In addition, disturbances in perinatal carbohydrate homeostasis can be explained more rationally, although not entirely, on the basis of these hormone substrate interrelationships.

CLINICAL CORRELATIONS
Premature and Small-for-Gestational-Age Infants

Infants who are small at birth because of prematurity or because of intrauterine growth retardation have an increased incidence of hypoglycemia.[31] Hormonal abnormalities are not responsible for this disturbance in energy balance because insulin and glucagon secretion both in the basal state and in response to stimuli such as amino acids is normal.[166] In addition, concentrations of cortisol and growth hormone also are normal.[166] Rather it appears that the substrate and enzymes for hepatic gluconeogenesis as well as the glycogen reserves are inadequate because plasma lactate and alanine levels are increased in small-for-gestational-age (SGA) infants in comparison with normal infants.[68, 104, 166] Moreover, the rise in glucagon induced by amino acids does not elicit a rise in glucose in SGA infants, although, with a similar stimulus, a rise in glucose is seen in premature and normal infants.[166] Observations made during experimental intrauterine growth retardation in the fetal and neonatal rat confirm the impaired gluconeogenesis and diminished glycogen reserves,[114] although some studies suggest that prolonged starvation in utero can accelerate the appearance of gluconeogenic mechanisms.[52, 113]

Infants of Diabetic Mothers

In contrast to the transient hypoglycemia of the SGA infant or the premature infant whose

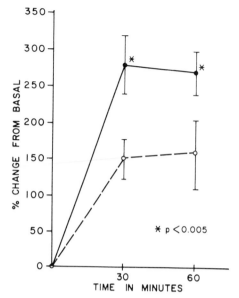

FIGURE 20–7. Effects of arginine infused via the umbilical vein in normal human newborns within the first 6 hours of life. Both glucagon and insulin secretion rise promptly although the glucagon response is greater. (From Sperling MA, DeLamater PV, Phelps D, et al. Spontaneous and amino acid stimulated glucagon secretion in the immediate postnatal period: Relation to glucose and insulin. J Clin Invest 1974;53:1159. With permission.)

body size and tissue nutrient content are diminished, infants of diabetic mothers are examples of nutrient surfeit; their body stores of glycogen, protein, and fat are replete.[40, 45] The hypoglycemia to which infants of diabetic mothers are prone, and which occurs in approximately 50% of infants born to insulin-dependent diabetic mothers, is clearly related to hyperinsulinemia. The pancreatic islets of these patients demonstrate hypertrophy and hyperplasia[24] as well as an increased insulin content. In addition, these infants in utero respond to glucose with an adult type of biphasic insulin secretory response.[21] The state of functional hyperinsulinism prevailing in utero results in metabolic effects, which are reflected in the increased fat, liver glycogen content, and total body size.[40] At delivery, the umbilical cord plasma insulin concentration is higher than in normal newborns and correlates with total body size.

Through the use of the C-peptide assay, it has been possible to confirm the basal hyperinsulinemia at birth as well as the excessive insulin secretory response following nutrient challenge after delivery. The state of func-

tional hyperinsulinemia in the newborn period is further supported by the findings of lower than normal plasma free fatty acid concentrations and an accelerated glucose disappearance rate following intravenous glucose challenge.[21]

Additional insights into understanding the disturbed carbohydrate metabolism of infants of diabetic mothers have been obtained from studies of spontaneous and amino acid–stimulated glucagon secretion in the immediate newborn period (Fig. 20–7). The spontaneous rise in plasma glucagon observed in normal infants in the first 2 hours of life is markedly impaired in infants of diabetic mothers.[16, 167] In addition, glucagon secretion in response to the intravenous administration of amino acid is also significantly inhibited in infants of diabetic mothers, and there is no rise in blood glucose such as occurs in normal infants following amino acid challenge[167] (Fig. 20–8).

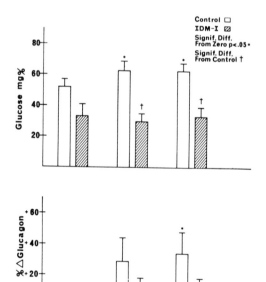

FIGURE 20–8. Glucose and glucagon following alanine infusion (1 mM/kg) at 1 hour of life in normal (control) infants and in infants born to insulin-dependent diabetic mothers (IDM-I). The infants born to diabetic mothers have an obtunded glucagon response, compared with the significant rise in controls. Similarly, IDM-I infants have no significant rise in glucose, which remains low, whereas in control infants, blood glucose rises significantly. (From Williams PR, Sperling MA, Racasa Z. Blunting of spontaneous and alanine-stimulated glucagon secretion in newborn infants of diabetic mothers. Am J Obstet Gynecol 1979;133:51. With permission.)

Thus the suppressed glucagon secretion may contribute significantly to the hypoglycemia in these infants. The mechanisms responsible for the hypoglucagonemia probably relate to the suppression of pancreatic α cell function by coexistent hyperglycemia and hyperinsulinemia in utero, although this could not be demonstrated in the fetal monkey.[37] Finally, these infants may have impaired or exhausted catecholamine secretion after birth, as reflected in a decrease of urinary excretion of epinephrine.[5, 90] Thus, despite the abundance in these infants of tissue stores of available substrate, the normal plasma hormonal patterns of low insulin, high glucagon, and high catecholamines are reversed, and their capacity for endogenous glucose production is significantly diminished when compared with normal infants.[80] In addition, the generation of ketone bodies is also inhibited so alternate fuel supplies cannot be mobilized for brain or muscle.

Nesidioblastosis and Islet Cell Hyperplasia

Similar to infants of diabetic mothers, these infants are large at birth, reflecting the anabolic effects of insulin in utero. Hypoglycemia, with insulin concentrations that are inappropriate (>10 μU/mL) for the level of glucose (≤40 mg/dL) may occur in the initial days of life.[71] This condition cannot be clinically distinguished from islet cell hyperplasia or adenoma; each is characterized by autonomous insulin secretion. Consequently, the term *islet cell dysmaturation syndrome* has been proposed to encompass this spectrum of islet cell abnormalities. The disorganization of the islet cell types and relationships has been demonstrated and accounts for their abnormal hormone secretion.[69]

Erythroblastosis Fetalis

These infants also have high pancreatic insulin contents, hyperinsulinemia at birth, neonatal hypoglycemia, and large body size similar to infants of diabetic mothers.[105] Plasma glucagon levels, however, have been found to be higher than normal before exchange transfusion.

During exchange transfusion, with blood preserved with acid citrate and glucose, plasma glucagon levels decline, and net glucagon balance is negative, while insulin secretion is prominent, and plasma insulin concentrations rise. Thus, with regard to both insulin and glucagon secretion, infants with erythroblastosis fetalis are similar to infants of diabetic mothers in having insulin stimulated and glucagon suppressed by glucose. They differ, however, in that spontaneous glucagon secretion appears to be high in erythroblastotic infants,[106] whereas it is low in infants of diabetic mothers.[16, 167] The addition of glucagon to the donor blood used for exchange transfusion may exert a protective effect on posttransfusion rebound hypoglycemia, despite the concurrent hyperinsulinemia.[106]

Transient Diabetes of the Newborn

A transient diabetic state with onset during the first week of life but with limited duration and spontaneous resolution after several weeks to months has been described by several groups.[43, 107, 119, 135] It occurs almost invariably in SGA infants. It is characterized by hyperglycemia and pronounced glycosuria, resulting in severe dehydration but with minimal or absent ketonemia or ketonuria. Although basal insulin concentrations are normal, the response to glucose or tolbutamide is low to absent. This syndrome, which may be familial, probably represents the extension of intrauterine and neonatal immaturity of insulin secretory mechanisms related to delayed maturation of the cAMP system.[119] It is not yet clear whether the underlying defect in humans is due to deficiency in the β cell adenyl cyclase, which generates cAMP, or to increased activity of the nucleotide phosphodiesterase, which destroys cAMP. Although insulin secretion in response to the stimulus of glucose or tolbutamide is absent, it can be augmented by theophylline, which inhibits phosphodiesterase.[119] The glucagon secretory profiles have not been determined in this condition.

This rare syndrome should be distinguished from the entity of transient hyperglycemia seen in association with electrolyte disturbance, acidosis, and abnormalities of the central nervous system.[20, 157] In the last-mentioned condition, euglycemia is rapidly restored by hydration and correction of acid-base balance. In transitory diabetes of the newborn, insulin treatment is required. Spontaneous recovery by several months of age is the rule, however, when insulin responses to a variety of stimuli can be demonstrated.[135]

CONCLUSIONS

This chapter has reviewed the normal development and secretory patterns of insulin and glucagon and the function of these hormones both in utero and in the immediate newborn period. The role of these hormones early in development is not defined nor is the developmental regulation of gene expression in the pancreas. It appears that carbohydrate metabolism during the first two trimesters is independent of insulin or glucagon action. In the third trimester, insulin assumes the dominant role in directing the disposition of nutrients, including glucose and amino acids, for anabolic storage in the form of glycogen, fat, and protein in anticipation of their utilization immediately after delivery. In contrast, glucagon appears to have little functional role with regard to controlling glucose production in utero, and the development of its receptors on target tissue is delayed when compared with the development of insulin receptors. At birth, there is a surge in glucagon, whereas insulin secretion remains obtunded. These events may be mediated via a surge in catecholamine secretion at birth, accompanied by rapid increase and coupling to the effector of glucagon receptors. Together these events appear to be important for the transition to extrauterine life, activating glycogenolysis, gluconeogenesis, and ketogenesis.

These considerations permit rational understanding of the adaptation in normal infants and provide a framework for understanding the departures from the norm in terms of insulin and glucagon secretion and action, as exemplified in infants of diabetic mothers or in infants with islet cell dysmaturation. The physiologic role of endogenously secreted somatostatin in these adaptive events is yet to be defined.

Further understanding of the secretion and action of these hormones is likely to emerge from the application of molecular biology to analyzing develomental and tissue-specific regulation of their genes, which should provide insight into the control of energy homeostasis in the perinatal period.

REFERENCES

1. Adam PAJ, Kekomaki M, Rahiala EL, et al. Autoregulation of glucose production by the isolated perfused human liver. Pediatr Res 1972;6:396.
2. Adam PAJ, King KC, Schwartz R, et al. Human placental barrier to ^{125}I-glucagon early in gestation. J Clin Endocrinol Metab 1972;34:772.
3. Anand RS, Ganguli S, Sperling MA. Effect of insulin-induced maternal hypoglycemia on fetal maternal glucose production, utilization and placental transfer in sheep. Am J Physiol 1980;238:E524.
4. Anand RS, Sperling MA, Ganguli S, et al. Bidirectional placental transfer of glucose and its turnover in fetal (and maternal) sheep. Pediatr Res 1979;13:783.
5. Artal R, Doug N, Wu P, Sperling MA. Circulating catecholamines and glucagon in infants of strictly controlled diabetic mothers. Biol Neonate 1988;53:121.
6. Ashworth MA, Leach FN, Milner RDG. Development of insulin secretion in the human fetus. Arch Dis Child 1973;48:151.
7. Asplund K, Andersson A, Jarrousse C, et al. Function of the fetal endocrine pancreas. Isr J Med Sci 1975;11:581.
8. Assan R, Boillot J. Pancreatic glucagon and glucagon-like material in tissues and plasmas from human fetuses 6–26 weeks old. In: Jonxis JH, Visser HK, Troelstra JA, et al, eds. Metabolic processes in the fetus and newborn infant. Nutricia Symposium. Baltimore: Williams & Wilkins, 1971:210.
9. Bataille D, Freychet P, Rosselin G. Interactions of glucagon, gut glucagon, vasoactive intestinal polypeptide and secretin with liver and fat cell plasma membranes: binding to specific sites and stimulation of adenylate cyclase. Endocrinology 1974;95:713.
10. Battaglia FC, Meschia G. Principal substrates of fetal metabolism. Physiol Rev 1978;58:499.
11. Berelowitz M, Kronheim S, Pimstone B, et al. Somatostatin-like immunoreactivity in rat blood. Characterization, regional differences and responses to oral and intravenous glucose. J Clin Invest 1978;61:1410.
12. Bergman RN, Miller RE. Direct enhancement of insulin secretion by vagal stimulation of the isolated pancreas. Am J Physiol 1973;225:481.
13. Bier DM, Leake RD, Haymond MW, et al. Measurement of "true" glucose production rates in infancy and childhood with 6,6-dideuteroglucose. Diabetes 1977;26:1016.
14. Blazquez E, Rubalcava B, Montesano R, et al. Development of insulin and glucagon binding and the adenylate cyclase response in liver membranes of the prenatal, postnatal and adult rat: evidence for glucagon "resistance." Endocrinology 1976;98:1014.
15. Bloch CA, Sperling MA. Sources and disposition of

fetal glucose: studies in the fetal lamb. Am J Perinatol 1988;5:344.

16. Bloom SR, Johnston DI. Failure of glucagon release in infants of diabetic mothers. BMJ 1972;4:453.

17. Bloom SR, Vaughan NJA, Russell RCG. Vagal control of glucagon release in man. Lancet 1974;2:546.

18. Bloomgarden ZT, Liljenquist JE, Cherrington AD, et al. Persistent stimulatory effect of glucagon on glucose production despite down regulation. J Clin Endocrinol Metab 1978;47:1152.

19. Bocek RM, Young MK, Beatty CH. Effect of insulin and epinephrine on the carbohydrate metabolism and adenylate cyclase activity of rhesus fetal muscle. Pediatr Res 1973;7:787.

20. Boulware SD, Tamborlane WV. Not all severe hyperglycemia is diabetes. Pediatrics 1992;89:330.

21. Brudenell M, Beard R. Diabetes in pregnancy. J Clin Endocrinol Metab 1972;1:673.

22. Bucolo RJ, Bergman RN, Marsh DJ, Yates FE. Dynamics of glucose autoregulation in the isolated, blood-perfused canine liver. Am J Physiol 1974;227:209.

23. Cahill GF Jr. Physiology of insulin in man. Diabetes 1971;20:785.

24. Cardell BS. Hypertrophy and hyperplasia in the pancreatic islets in newborn infants. J Pathol Bacteriol 1953;66:335.

25. Carstensen M, Leichweiss HP, Molsen G, et al. Evidence for a specific transport of d-hexoses across the human term placenta in vitro. Arch Gynaekol 1977;222:187.

26. Cherrington AD, Stevenson RW, Steiner KE, et al. Insulin, glucagon, and glucose as regulators of hepatic glucose uptake and production in vivo. Diab Metab Rev 1987;3:307.

27. Chez RA, Mintz DH, Epstein MF. Glucagon metabolism in nonhuman primate pregnancy. Am J Obstet Gynecol 1974;120:690.

28. Chez RA, Mintz DH, Hutchinson DL. Effect of theophylline on glucagon and glucose-mediated plasma insulin responses in subhuman primate fetus and neonate. Metabolism 1971;20:805.

29. Chick WL. Beta cell replication in rat pancreatic monolayer culture. Diabetes 1973;22:687.

30. Conlon JM, Strikant CB, Ipp E, et al. Properties of endogenous somatostatin-like immunoreactivity and synthetic somatostatin in dog plasma. J Clin Invest 1978;62:1187.

31. Cornblath M, Schwartz R. Disorders of carbohydrate metabolism in infancy, ed 2. Philadelphia: WB Saunders, 1976.

32. Cowett RM, Susa JB, Oh W, et al. Endogenous glucose production during constant glucose infusion in the newborn lamb. Pediatr Res 1978;12:853.

33. Dancis J, Jansen V, Kayden HJ, et al. Transfer across perfused human placenta. II. Free fatty acids. Pediatr Res 1973;7:192.

34. Devaskar SU, Ganguli S, Styer D, et al. Glucagon and glucose dynamics in sheep: evidence for glucagon resistance in the fetus. Am J Physiol 1984;246:E256.

35. Eisen HJ, Goldfine ID, Glinsman WH. Regulation of hepatic glycogen synthesis during fetal development: roles of hydrocortisone, insulin, and insulin receptors. Proc Natl Acad Sci USA 1973;70:3454.

36. Ensinck JW, D'Alessio DA. The entero-insular axis revisited. N Engl J Med 1992;326:1352.

37. Epstein M, Chez RA, Oakes GK, et al. Fetal pancreatic glucagon responses in glucose-intolerant nonhuman primate pregnancy. Am J Obstet Gynecol 1977;127:268.

38. Espinosa MMA, Driscoll SG, Steinke J. Insulin release from isolated human fetal pancreatic islets. Science 1970;168:1111.

39. Exton JH. Gluconeogenesis. Metabolism 1972;21:945.

40. Fee BA, Weil WB Jr. Body composition of infants of diabetic mothers by direct analysis. Ann NY Acad Sci 1963;110:869.

41. Felig P. The glucose-alanine cycle. Metabolism 1973;22:179.

42. Felig P, Wahren J, Sherwin R, et al. Insulin, glucagon, and somatostatin in normal physiology and diabetes mellitus. Diabetes 1976;25:1091.

43. Ferguson AW, Milner RDG. Transient neonatal diabetes mellitus in sibs. Arch Dis Child 1970;45:80.

44. Fiser RH Jr, Erenberg A, Sperling MA, et al. Insulin-glucagon substrate interrelations in the fetal sheep. Pediatr Res 1974;8:951.

45. Freinkel M. Of pregnancy and progeny. Diabetes 1980;29:1023.

46. Freinkel N, Younsi CE, Bonnar J, et al. Rapid transient efflux of phosphate ions from pancreatic islets as an early action of insulin secretagogues. J Clin Invest 1974;54:1179.

47. Gabbay KH, Gang DL. Hypoglycemia in a three month old girl. N Engl J Med 1978;299:241.

48. Gabbay KH, Korff J, Schneeberger EE. Vesicular binesis: glucose effect on insulin secretory vesicles. Science 1975;187:177.

49. Gerich JE, Langlois M, Noacco C, et al. Adrenergic modulation of pancreatic glucagon secretion in man. J Clin Invest 1974;53:1441.

50. Girard JR. Metabolic fuels of the fetus. Isr J Med Sci 1975;11:591.

51. Girard JR, Cuendet GS, Marliss EB, et al. Fuels, hormones, and liver metabolism at term and during the early postnatal period in the rat. J Clin Invest 1973;52:3190.

52. Girard JR, Guillet I, Marty J, Marliss EB. Plasma amino acid levels and development of hepatic gluconeogenesis in the newborn rat. Am J Physiol 1975;229:466.

53. Girard JR, Kervran A, Soufflet E, et al. Factors affecting the secretion of insulin and glucagon by the rat fetus. Diabetes 1974;23:310.

54. Girard J, Sperling MA. Glucagon in the fetus and newborn. In: Lefebvre PJ, ed. Handbook of experimental pharmacology, Vol 66/11. Heidelberg: Springer-Verlag, 1982:251.

55. Glinsman WH, Eisen HJ, Lynch A, et al. Glucose regulation by isolated near-term fetal monkey liver. Pediatr Res 1975;9:600.

56. Gould GW, Bell GI. Facilitative glucose transporters: an expanding family. Trends Biochem Sci 1990;15:18.

57. Grajwer LA, Sperling MA, Sack J, et al. Possible mechanisms and significance of the neonatal surge in glucagon secretion: studies in newborn lambs. Pediatr Res 1977;11:833.

58. Grasso S, Distefano G, Messina A, et al. Effect of glucose priming on insulin response in the premature infant. Diabetes 1975;24:291.

59. Grasso S, Messina A, Distefano G, et al. Insulin secretion in the premature infant. Response to glucose and amino acids. Diabetes 1973;22:349.

60. Grasso S, Messina A, Saporito N, et al. Effect of theophylline, glucagon and theophylline plus glucagon on insulin secretion in the premature infant. Diabetes 1970;19:837.

61. Grasso S, Palumbo G, Messina A, et al. Human mater-

nal and fetal serum insulin and growth hormone (HGH) response to glucose and leucine. Diabetes 1976;25:545.

62. Greengard O. Enzymic differentiation of human liver: comparison with the rat model. Pediatr Res 1977;11:669.

63. Grill V, Asplund K, Hellerstrom C, et al. Decreased cyclic AMP and insulin response to glucose in isolated islets of neonatal rats. Diabetes 1975;24:746.

64. Grodsky GM, Fanska R, West L, et al. Anomeric specificity of glucose-stimulated insulin release: evidence for a glucoreceptor? Science 1974;186:536.

65. Hanson RW, Reshef L, Ballard J. Hormonal regulation of hepatic P-enolpyruvate carboxykinase (GTP) during development. Fed Proc 1975;34:166.

66. Harding JE, Evans PC. β hydroxybutyrate is an alternative substrate for the fetal sheep brain. J Dev Physiol 1991;16:293.

67. Hay WW Jr. Fetal and neonatal glucose homeostasis and their relation to the small for gestational age infant. Semin Perinatol 1984;8:101.

68. Haymond MW, Karl IE, Pagliara AS. Increased gluconeogenic substrates in the small-for-gestational-age infant. N Engl J Med 1974;291:322.

69. Heitz PU, Kloppel G, Hacki WH, et al. Nesidioblastosis: the pathologic basis of persistent hyperinsulinemic hypoglycemia in infants. Diabetes 1977;26:632.

70. Hellman B. The development of the mammalian endocrine pancreas. Biol Neonate 1966;9:263.

71. Hirsch HJ, Loo S, Evans N, et al. Hypoglycemia of infancy and nesidioblastosis: studies with somatostatin. N Engl J Med 1977;296:1323.

72. Hirsch HJ, Loos SW, Gabbay KH. The development and regulation of the endocrine pancreas. J Pediatr 1977;91:518.

73. Jack PMB, Milner RDG. Effect of decapitation on the development of insulin secretion in the foetal rabbit. J Endocrinol 1973;57:23.

74. Jaspan JB, Rubenstein AH. Circulating glucagon. Plasma profiles and metabolism in health and disease. Diabetes 1977;26:887.

74a. Jelinek LJ, Lok S, Rosenberg GB. Expression cloning and signaling properties of the rat glucagon receptor. Science 1993;259:1614.

75. Johnston DI, Bloom SR. Plasma glucagon levels in the term human infant and effect of hypoxia. Arch Dis Child 1973;48:451.

76. Johnston DI, Bloom SR, Greene KR, et al. Failure of the human placenta to transfer pancreatic glucagon. Biol Neonate 1972;21:375.

77. Jones CT. Control of glucose metabolism in the perinatal period. J Dev Physiol 1991;15:81.

78. Kahn BB. Facilitative glucose transporters: regulatory mechanisms and dysregulation in diabetes. J Clin Invest 1992;89:1367.

79. Kahn CR, White MF. The insulin receptor and the molecular mechanism of insulin action. J Clin Invest 1988;82:1151.

80. Kalhan SC, Savin SM, Adam PAJ. Measurement of glucose turnover in the human newborn with glucose-I-^{13}C. J Clin Endocrinol Metab 1976;43:704.

81. Kalhan SC, Savin SM, Adam PAJ. Attenuated glucose production rate in newborn infants of insulin-dependent diabetic mothers. N Engl J Med 1977;296:375.

82. King KC, Butt J, Raivio K, et al. Human maternal and fetal insulin response to arginine. N Engl J Med 1971;285:607.

83. Kipnis DM. Nutrient regulation of insulin secretion in human subjects. Diabetes 1972;21:606.

84. Kirby L, Hahn P. Enzyme responses to prednisolone and dibutyryl adenosine 3'5'-monophosphate in human fetal liver. Pediatr Res 1974;8:37.

85. Kitabchi AE. Proinsulin and C-peptide: a review. Metabolism 1977;28:547.

86. Lacy PE. Beta cell secretion—from the standpoint of a pathologist. Diabetes 1970;19:895.

87. Lagercrantz H, Bistoletti P. Catecholamine release in the newborn infant at birth. Pediatr Res 1977;11:889.

88. Lefebvre PJ, Unger RH. Glucagon: molecular physiology, clinical and therapeutic implications. Oxford: Pergamon Press, 1972.

89. Levine S, Pictet R, Rutter WJ. Control of cell proliferation and cytodifferentiation by a factor reacting with the cell surface. Nature (Lond) New Biol 1973;246:49.

90. Light IH, Sutherland JM, Loggie JM, et al. Impaired epinephrine release in hypoglycemic infants of diabetic mothers. N Engl J Med 1967;277:394.

91. Loubatieres A, Marianna MM, Sorel G, et al. The action of β-adrenergic blocking and stimulating agents on insulin secretion characteristic of the type of B receptor. Diabetologia 1971;7:127.

92. Luyckx AS, Massi-Benedetti F, Falorni A, et al. Presence of pancreatic glucagon in the portal plasma of human neonates. Differences in the insulin and glucagon responses to glucose between normal infants and infants from diabetic mothers. Diabetologia 1972;8:296.

93. Malaisse WJ. Insulin secretion: multifactorial regulation for a single process of release. Diabetologia 1973;9:167.

94. Malamud D, Perrin L. Stimulation of DNA synthesis in mouse pancreas by triiodothyronine and glucagon. Endocrinology 1974;94:1157.

95. Marsac C, Saudubray JM, Moncion A, et al. Development of gluconeogenic enzymes in the liver of human newborns. Biol Neonate 1976;28:317.

96. Massi-Benedetti F, Falorni A, Luyckx A, et al. Inhibition of glucagon secretion in the human newborn by simultaneous administration of glucose and insulin. Horm Metab Res 1974;6:392.

97. Matschinsky FM, Pagliara AS, Hover BA, et al. Differential effects of α- and β-D-glucose on insulin and glucagon secretion from the isolated perfused rat pancreas. Diabetes 1975;24:369.

98. McEvoy RC, Hegre OD. Foetal rat pancreas in organ culture. Effects of media supplementation with various steroid hormones on the acinar and islet components. Differentiation 1976;6:105.

99. McGarry JD, Wright PH, Foster DW. Hormonal control of ketogenesis. J Clin Invest 1975;55:1202.

100. McIntosh N, Pictet RL, Kaplan SL, et al. The developmental pattern of somatostatin in the embryonic and fetal rat pancreas. Endocrinology 1977;101:825.

101. Menon RK, Chernausek SD, Sperling MA. Ontogeny of insulin-like growth factor I and insulin receptor kinase activity in rat liver. J Dev Physiol 1991;16:87.

102. Menon RK, Cohen RM, Sperling MA, et al. Transplacental passage of insulin in pregnant women with insulin-dependent diabetes mellitus. N Engl J Med 1990;323:309.

103. Menon RK, Sperling MA. Carbohydrate metabolism in neonatal adaptation: the transition to post-natal life. Sem Perinatol 1988;12:157.

104. Mestyan J, Soltesz G, Schultz K, et al. Hyperaminoacidemia due to the accumulation of gluconeogenic amino acid precursors in hypoglycemic small-for-gestational-age infants. J Pediatr 1975;87:409.

105. Milner RDG. The development of insulin secretion in man. In: Jonxis JH, Visser HK, Troelstra JA, et al, eds. Metabolic processes in the foetus and newborn infant. Nutricia Symposium. Baltimore: Williams & Wilkins, 1971:193.

106. Milner RDG, Chouksey SK, Assan R. Metabolic and hormonal effects of glucagon infusion in erythroblastotic infants. Arch Dis Child 1973;48:885.

107. Milner RDG, Ferguson AW, Naidu SH. Aetiology of transient neonatal diabetes. Arch Dis Child 1971;46:724.

108. Mintz DH, Levey GS, Schenk A. Adenosine 3',5'-cyclic monophosphate and phosphodiesterase activities in isolated fetal and neonatal rat pancreatic islets. Endocrinology 1973;92:614.

109. Moore WMO, Ward BS, Gordon C. Human placental transfer of glucagon. Clin Sci Mol Med 1974;46:125.

110. Neufeld ND, Kaplan SA, Lippe BM. Insulin binding studies in normal infants (NI) and infants of diabetic mothers (IDM). Pediatr Res 1978;12:397.

111. Noe BD, Bauer GE. Evidence for sequential metabolic cleavage of proglucagon to glucagon in glucagon biosynthesis. Endocrinology 1975;97:868.

112. Oakley NW, Beard RW, Turner RC. Effect of sustained maternal hyperglycemia on the fetus in normal and diabetic pregnancies. BMJ 1972;1:466.

113. Ogata ES. Carbohydrate metabolism in the fetus and neonate and altered neonatal glucoregulation. Pediatr Clin North Am 1986;33:25.

114. Oh W, D'Amodio MD, Yap LL, et al. Carbohydrate metabolism in experimental intrauterine growth retardation in rats. Am J Obstet Gynecol 1970;108:415.

115. Orci L, Gabbay KH, Malaisse WJ. Pancreatic beta-cell web: its possible role in insulin secretion. Science 1972;175:1128.

116. Orci L, Malaisse-Lagae F, Amberdt M, et al. Cell contacts in human islets of Langerhans. J Clin Endocrinol Metab 1975;41:841.

117. Orci L, Unger RH, Renold AE. Structural coupling between pancreatic islet cells. Experientia (Basel) 1973;29:1015.

118. Padbury JF, Martinez AM. Sympathoadrenal system activity at birth: integration of postnatal adaptation. Sem Perinatol 1988;12:163.

119. Pagliara AS, Karl IE, Kipnis DB. Transient neonatal diabetes: delayed maturation of the pancreatic beta cell. J Pediatr 1973;82:97.

120. Pearse AG, Polak JM, Heath CM. Development, differentiation and derivation of the endocrine polypeptide cells of the mouse pancreas. Diabetologia 1973;9:120.

121. Persson B, Settergren G, Dahlquist G. Cerebral arterio-venous difference of acetoacetate and D-B hydroxybutyrate in children. Acta Paediatr Scand 1972;61:273.

122. Philippe J. Structure and pancreatic expression of the insulin and glucagon genes. Endo Rev 1991;12:252.

123. Philipps AF, Rosenkrantz RS, et al. Effects of fetal insulin deficiency on growth in fetal lambs. Diabetes 1991;40:20.

124. Pictet P, Rutter WJ. Development of the embryonic endocrine pancreas. In: Steiner D, Freinkel N, eds. Handbook of physiology. Sec 7: Endocrinology. Vol 1. The endocrine pancreas. American Physiological Society. Baltimore: Williams & Wilkins, 1972:25.

125. Pictet RL, Filosa S, Phelps P, et al. Control of DNA synthesis in the embryonic pancreas: interaction of the mesenchymal factor and cyclic AMP. In: Slavkin HC, Greulich RC, eds. Extracellular matrix. New York: Academic Press, 1975:531.

126. Pictet RL, Rall LB, Phelps P, et al. The neural crest and the origin of the insulin-producing and other gastrointestinal hormone-producing cells. Science 1976;191:191.

127. Polak JM, Pearse AGE, Grimelius L, et al. Growth-hormone release-inhibiting hormone in gestational and pancreatic D-cells. Lancet 1975;1:1220.

128. Pozo Del E, Gomez-Pan A. Somatostatin: recent advances in basic research and clinical applications. Horm Res 1988;29:50.

129. Rall LB, Pictet RL, Williams RH, et al. Early differentiation of glucagon-producing cells in embryonic pancreas: a possible developmental role of glucagon. Proc Natl Acad Sci USA 1973;70:3478.

130. Reitano G, Distefano G, Vigo R, et al. Effect of priming of amino acids on insulin and growth hormone response in the premature infant. Diabetes 1978;27:334.

131. Renold AE. Insulin biosynthesis and secretion: a still unsettled topic. N Engl J Med 1970;282:173.

132. Roth J, Kahn CR, Lesniak MA, et al. Receptors for insulin, NSILA-s, and growth hormone: application to disease states in man. Rec Prog Horm Res 1975;31:95.

133. Sasaki H, Rubalcava B, Baetens D, et al. Identification of glucagon in the gastrointestinal tract. J Clin Invest 1975;56:135.

134. Schaeffer LD, Wilder ML, Williams RH. Secretion and content of insulin and glucagon in human fetal pancreas slices in vitro. Proc Soc Exp Biol Med 1973;143:314.

135. Schiff D, Colle E, Stern L. Metabolic and growth patterns in transient neonatal diabetes. N Engl J Med 1972;287:119.

136. Schwartz AL, Rall TW. Hormonal regulation of glycogen metabolism in human fetal liver. II. Regulation of glycogen synthase activity. Diabetes 1975;24:1113.

137. Schwartz AL, Rall TW. Hormonal regulation of incorporation of alanine-U-14C into glucose in human fetal liver explants. Diabetes 1975;24:650.

138. Settergren G, Lindblad BS, Persson B. Cerebral blood flow and exchange of oxygen, glucose, ketone bodies, lactate, pyruvate and amino acids in infants. Acta Paediatr Scand 1976;65:343.

139. Shelley HJ. Glycogen reserves and their changes at birth and in anoxia. Br Med Bull 1961;17:137.

140. Sherline P, Eisen H, Glinsman W. Acute hormonal regulation of cyclic AMP content and glycogen phosphorylase activity in fetal liver in organ culture. Endocrinology 1974;94:935.

141. Sherwood WG, Hill DE, Chance GW. Glucose homeostasis in preterm rhesus monkey neonates. Pediatr Res 1977;11:874.

142. Sinha M, Miller JD, Sperling MA, et al. Possible dissociation between insulin binding and insulin action in isolated fetal rat hepatocytes. Diabetes 1984;33:864.

143. Simmons MA, Jones MD, Battaglia FC, et al. Insulin effect on fetal glucose utilization. Pediatr Res 1978;12:90.

144. Simmons MA, Meschia G, Makowski EL, et al. Fetal metabolic response to maternal starvation. Pediatr Res 1974;8:830.

145. Sperling MA. Control of insulin secretion. Calif Med 1973;119:17.

146. Sperling MA. Integration of fuel homeostasis by insulin and glucagon in the newborn. In: Zoppi G, ed.

Monographs in pediatrics. Vol 16: Metabolic-endocrine responses to food intake in infancy. Basal: S Karger, 1982:39.

147. Sperling MA, Christensen RA, Ganguli S, et al. Adrenergic modulation of pancreatic hormone secretion in utero: studies in fetal sheep. Pediatr Res 1980;14:203.

148. Sperling MA, DeLamater PV, Phelps D, et al. Spontaneous and amino acid stimulated glucagon secretion in the immediate postnatal period: relation to glucose and insulin. J Clin Invest 1974;53:1159.

149. Sperling MA, Devaskar S. Insulin action in the fetal-placental unit. Insulin Action 1989;18:203.

150. Sperling MA, Erenberg A, Fisher RH, et al. Placental transfer of glucagon in sheep. Endocrinology 1973;93:1435.

151. Sperling MA, Ganguli S. Pre- and post-natal development of insulin and glucagon receptors: potential role in energy storage and utilization. In: Symposium on infant nutrition and the development of the gastrointestinal tract. J Pediatr Gastroentrol Nutr 1983; 2(suppl 1):S51.

152. Sperling MA, Grajwer L, Leake RD, et al. Effects of somatostatin (SRIF) infusion on glucose homeostasis in newborn lambs: evidence for a significant role of glucagon. Pediatr Res 1977;11:962.

153. Stacey TE, Weedon AP, Haworth C, et al. Fetomaternal transfer of glucose analogues by sheep placenta. Am J Physiol 1978;234:E32.

154. Steiner DF. Insulin today. Diabetes 1977;26:322.

155. Steiner DF, Chan SJ. An overview of insulin evolution. Horm Metab Res 1988;20:443.

156. Steinke J, Gries FA, Driscoll SG. In vitro studies of insulin inactivation in infants with reference to erythroblastosis fetalis. Blood 1967;30:359.

157. Stevenson RE, Bowyer FP. Hyperglycemia with hyperosmolar dehydration in nondiabetic infants. J Pediatr 1970;77:818.

158. Thorsson AV, Hintz RL. Insulin receptors in the newborn: increase in receptor affinity and number. N Engl J Med 1977;297:908.

159. Townsend SF, Rudolph D, Rudolph A. Cortisol induces perinatal hepatic gluconeogenesis in the lamb. J Dev Physiol 1991;16:71.

160. Unger RH, Orci L, Lelio MD. Glucagon and the A cell. N Engl J Med 1981;304:1518.

161. Vale W, Brazeau P, Rivier C, et al. Somatostatin. Rec Prog Horm Res 1975;31:365.

162. Van Assche FA, Gepts W, DeGasparo M. The endocrine pancreas in anencephalics: a histological, histochemical and biological study. Biol Neonate 1970;14:374.

163. Velasco MS, Paulsen EP. The response of infants of diabetic women to tolbutamide and leucine at birth and to glucose and tolbutamide at 2 years of age. Pediatrics 1969;43:546.

164. Vidnes J, Oyasaeter S. Glucagon deficiency causing severe neonatal hypoglycemia in a patient with normal insulin secretion. Pediatr Res 1977;11:943.

165. Vidnes J, Oyasaeter S. Reduced gluconeogenesis due to hyperinsulinism. Hormonal and metabolic studies in an infant with hypoglycemia. Pediatr Res 1978;12:619.

166. Williams PR, Fiser RH, Sperling MA, et al. Effects of oral alanine feeding on glucose, plasma glucagon and insulin concentrations in small-for-gestational-age infants. N Engl J Med 1975;292:612.

167. Williams PR, Sperling MA, Racasa Z. Blunting of spontaneous and alanine-stimulated glucagon secretion in newborn infants of diabetic mothers. Am J Obstet Gynecol 1979;133:51.

168. Wise JK, Lyall SS, Hendler R. Evidence of stimulation of glucagon secretion by alanine in the human fetus at term. J Clin Endocrinol Metab 1973;37:345.

169. Woods SC, Porte D Jr. Neural control of the endocrine pancreas. Physiol Rev 1974;54:596.

170. Yeoh GC, Oliver IT. Glucagon stimulation of DNA synthesis in neonatal rat liver. Eur J Biochem 1973;34:474.

Perinatal Mineral Metabolism

Francis Mimouni

Reginald C. Tsang

Mineral metabolism in fetal and neonatal life is tightly connected to maternal mineral metabolism, and a complex system regulates this interaction. This chapter addresses the homeostasis of perinatal mineral metabolism as well as the pathophysiology of its major disorders.

MINERAL HOMEOSTASIS

Mineral Homeostasis in Nonpregnant Adults

A description of mineral homeostasis in nonpregnant adults is required to understand the unique changes specific to the perinatal period. We first describe the regulation of calcium (Ca) and phosphorus (P), then that of magnesium (Mg) metabolism.

Regulation of Calcium and Phosphorus Metabolism

BODY CALCIUM AND PHOSPHORUS DISTRIBUTION

Ninety-nine per cent of the body's Ca and 85% of the body's P are contained in *bone*.[51] A small percentage, mostly present in the well-vascularized trabecular bone, is rapidly mobilizable and crucial in the regulation of blood Ca concentration.[51] By contrast, cortical bone mostly plays the role of supporting body weight and has little action in the regulation of calcemia.[51] In normal circumstances in adults, there are equal rates of bone formation and bone resorption (*coupling*), and bone remodeling is a continuous event.[13] Only 1% of total body Ca is found in blood, extracellular fluid, and various soft tissue.[51] In blood, Ca exists in three forms: (1) protein-bound Ca (40 to 45%); (2) complexed Ca (5 to 10%), bound to major anions, such as lactate, citrate, sulfate, bicarbonate, and phosphate; and (3) ionized Ca (iCa) (45 to 50%).[99] The last form is considered to be the active biologic form, which is involved in feedback regulation. For clinical purposes, most laboratories can measure routinely total Ca concentration, using colorimetric or atomic absorption spectrophotometric methods.[160] The latter method is highly specific and sensitive but does not give a direct

estimate of the active, ionized fraction. Measurements of the ultrafilterable fraction (including complexed Ca and iCa) are relatively cumbersome and also do not measure directly iCa.[97] Technology for direct measurement of iCa using ion-specific electrodes has become simple to use and is very accurate.[19] We believe that in the next decade direct measurement of iCa should largely replace that of total Ca.

Phosphorus also exists in blood in three forms: (1) protein bound (10%); (2) complexed, in the form of Ca, Mg, and sodium (Na) salts (approximately 40%); and (3) ionized (approximately 50%).[51] Only total inorganic P, however, can routinely be measured in body fluids.

CALCIUM AND PHOSPHORUS INTESTINAL ABSORPTION

The main sources of Ca in the Western diet are milk and its products. Ca is absorbed throughout the small intestine but mostly in its proximal part (duodenum and proximal jejunum), where pH is lowest.[143] Importantly, digestive juices contain significant amounts of Ca, which are only in part reabsorbed. Therefore fecal Ca losses comprise exogenous (dietary) and endogenously secreted fractions.[79] Traditional balance studies do not allow for this differentiation, in contrast to stable (nonradioactive) isotope methods, which involve two different Ca isotopes, one given orally and one given intravenously.[79] It is likely that only Ca in solution and probably only ionized Ca can be absorbed.[143] Thus the bioavailability of Ca varies among salts and depends on the interaction with dietary constituents. As an example, excess dietary phosphate inhibits Ca absorption and may induce hypocalcemia.[155] Dietary protein, lactose, and other carbohydrates appear to facilitate Ca absorption through the formation of soluble complexes,[181, 187] although this is not accepted by all.[152]

Both facilitated diffusion and vitamin D–dependent active transport play a role in intestinal Ca absorption. The vitamin D–dependent mechanism appears to be saturated or near saturated by low-Ca meals.[151] All increments in Ca absorption that occur when low or normal Ca meals are supplemented with extra Ca appear to be mediated by the vitamin D–independent mechanism.[151] Intestinal P absorption also occurs in the small intestine, preferentially in the jejunum.[30] It requires an active transport system under vitamin D control.[30]

ROLE OF THE KIDNEY

Although fecal Ca varies widely as a function of Ca intake, urinary Ca is influenced by diet in a more modest fashion.[94] This has led to the opinion that renal regulation of calcemia is of relatively low impact when compared with intestinal regulation.[94] With this in mind, it has been demonstrated that urinary Ca rises when Ca intake increases.[94] Both parathyroid hormone (PTH) and 1,25-dihydroxyvitamin D (1,25-[OH]$_2$ D) may play a role in the regulation of urinary Ca, as their production increases when dietary Ca is low, and they both stimulate reabsorption of Ca in the renal tubule.[136, 153] Dietary Na plays an important role because urinary Ca increases about 0.6 mmol/100 mEq increment in urinary Na, apparently owing to depression of both proximal and distal tubular reabsorption of Ca.[94] Urinary Ca also increases when fixed acid production increases or when dietary phosphate falls to very low levels.[94]

By contrast to Ca, P homeostasis is primarily controlled by the kidney.[61] P is filtered at the glomerulus, and up to 95 to 97% of it is reabsorbed in both the proximal and the distal tubule.[61] PTH has a major inhibitory role of P reabsorption because it causes urinary phosphate losses even in the face of total body P depletion.[61] Growth hormone, 1,25-dihydroxycholecalciferol, and insulin increase tubular phosphate reabsorption, but their exact role is unknown.[61]

ROLE OF THE BONE

As previously stated, trabecular bone represents a large reservoir of rapidly mobilizable Ca. During acute hypocalcemia (or hypercalcemia), acute release (or deposition) of Ca into (or from) bone plays a major role in the correction of blood Ca.[51] Major hormones releasing Ca from bone are PTH[42] and 1,25-(OH)$_2$ D,[22] and calcitonin (CT) has a major

hypocalcemic effect through inhibiting Ca release and favoring Ca entry into bone.[28, 47, 85, 108] Hyperphosphatemia has a potent hypocalcemic effect through precipitation of Ca salts into bone,[74, 157] induction of relative PTH resistance at the bone,[74, 157] and inhibition of 1,25-(OH)$_2$ D production from 25-hydroxycholecalciferol (25[OH]D) in the kidney.[68] Mg and hydrogen ion (H$^+$) compete with bone Ca, and both hypermagnesemia[103] and acidosis[40] lead to Ca release from bone.

ROLE OF PARATHYROID HORMONE

PTH is a polypeptide hormone of 84 amino acids and a molecular weight of 9500 daltons synthesized in the parathyroid glands located in the neck. The amino terminal sequence 1–34 contains the full biologic activity of the hormone.[120] Its half-life is short in the circulation, in the order of 20 minutes or less, with appearance of multiple PTH fragments.[120] A Mg-dependent adenylate cyclase is involved in both the secretion and the action of PTH[95]; thus Mg deficiency has the potential for inducing both a reduced secretion of PTH and PTH resistance.[95] PTH action on bone is to mobilize Ca and P by stimulating osteoclastic bone resorption.[42] At the kidney, PTH stimulates distal tubular reabsorption of filtered Ca.[153] A potent phosphaturic effect of PTH is achieved by inhibition of proximal P reabsorption.[61] PTH is not known to act directly on intestinal Ca or P absorption, but it indirectly increases their absorption by stimulating renal 1 hydroxylase[153] and enhancing the production of 1,25-(OH)$_2$ D at the kidney.[153] The combined effects of PTH are hypercalcemic.[153] PTH production and secretion are triggered predominantly by a decrease in serum iCa concentration.[95] Other factors are known to influence PTH secretion, but their exact physiologic role is unknown. These factors include serum Mg, β-adrenergic stimulation, cortisol, 1,25-(OH)$_2$ D, and CT.[95]

PTH is routinely measured by radioimmunoassay. Assays specific for the whole molecule are often preferred to assays specific for the midmolecule and even more to assays specific to the C- or the N-terminal fragment.[120] An assay involving a two-site immunoradiome-

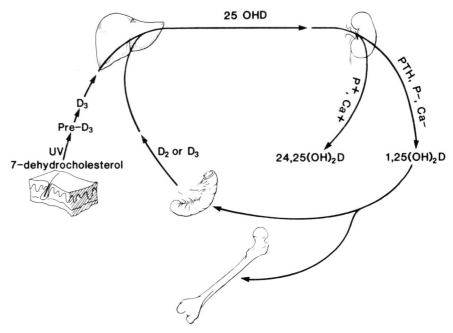

FIGURE 21–1. Pathway of vitamin D metabolism. Vitamin D is produced in the skin or absorbed from the intestine. Vitamin D is metabolized in the liver to 25 OHD. Under the regulation of PTH, and low P and Ca, 1,25(OH)₂ D is produced in the kidney. 1,25(OH)₂ D targets to the intestine, bone, and kidney to raise serum calcium and phosphate concentrations. (From Tsang RC, Noguchi A, Steichen JJ. Pediatric parathyroid disorders. Pediatr Clin North Am 1979;26:223. With permission.)

tric method measuring the whole molecule has been developed[120]; this assay appears to be highly accurate and specific, allowing clear segregation of normal subjects from patients with parathyroid disorders.[17, 120]

A PTH-related peptide (PTHrP) has been identified.[1, 17, 42, 90] This molecule, released from certain solid tumors, is believed to play a major role in hypercalcemia of malignancy, by increasing bone resorption and tubular reabsorption of Ca.[1, 17, 42, 90] It is related to PTH, as 8 of the first 13 amino acids are identical. PTHrP does not, however, cross react with PTH in radioimmunoassay, although it does in various bioassay systems. A possible physiologic role of PTHrP has been suggested because it is synthesized by normal keratinocytes, lactating breast tissue, and placenta.[42]

ROLE OF CALCITONIN

CT is secreted by the C cells of the thyroid gland. It is a 32 amino acid polypeptide and has a molecular weight of 3200 daltons. CT secretion is primarily stimulated by hypercal-

cemia, although β-adrenergic stimuli, Mg, gastrin, and glucagon are also known secretagogues.[109] CT has a potent hypocalcemic effect mediated by an inhibitory effect on bone resorption.[47] In addition, CT enhances urinary Ca excretion.[132] Despite abundant research, the exact physiologic role of CT in blood Ca regulation is still unclear. Indeed, patients with medullary carcinoma of the thyroid may have considerable elevations of serum CT concentrations without detectable hypocalcemia.[32] Further, patients with thyroid dysgenesis have abnormal calcemic curves when submitted to a calcium load but do not have significant baseline elevation of serum Ca.[25] There is no disease state caused by isolated CT deficiency, although it has been suggested that such deficiency might lead to hypercalcemia in Williams' syndrome.[37]

VITAMIN D ENDOCRINE SYSTEM

The pathway of vitamin D metabolism is illustrated in Figure 21–1. Vitamin D is derived from cholesterol in skin.[80, 81] Under the influence of ultraviolet B (UVB) irradiation, 7-dehydrocholesterol is converted into cholecalciferol, or vitamin D_3.[80, 81] Vitamin D may also originate from dietary sources under the form of D_3 (from animal origin) or D_2 (ergocalciferol, from plant origin).[80, 81] Vitamin D is liposoluble and requires intact bile salt secretion for micelle formation and absorption with fats.[118] Vitamin D_2 and D_3 undergo similar metabolic changes, after transport to the liver and the kidney by the vitamin D–binding protein.[34] For maximum potency, vitamin D must be hydroxylated in the liver at carbon 25 and in the kidney at carbon 1, to form $1,25\text{-}(OH)_2$ D.[21] Control of $1,25\text{-}(OH)_2$ D production takes place essentially at the level of the renal 1α-hydroxylation.[139] Low serum Ca and P concentrations stimulate directly 1α-hydroxylase activity.[83, 139] PTH, and possibly growth hormone insulin, estrogens, and prolactin also enhance $1,25\text{-}(OH)_2$ D formation at this level.[52, 76, 77, 135]

The catabolism of vitamin D occurs mostly in the liver and involves the p450 cytochrome system.[66] Therefore vitamin D catabolism and elimination may be enhanced by various substances stimulating this system, such as some anticonvulsants.[66] As shown with other steroid hormones, $1,25\text{-}(OH)_2$ D binds to an intracellular receptor protein, which involves the translocation of $1,25\text{-}(OH)_2$ D to the target cell nucleus.[56] This leads to mRNA induction, with subsequent synthesis of specific proteins, such as the calcium-binding protein.[119] Owing to its combined effect on stimulating intestinal calcium absorption[119] and bone resorption,[21, 22] $1,25\text{-}(OH)_2$ D has a potent hypercalcemic effect. It also enhances intestinal absorption of P.[89]

Vitamin D stores are best assessed by measurement of 25-(OH)D, the major circulating form of vitamin D.[54] Measurements of $1,25\text{-}(OH)_2$ D do not reflect reliably vitamin D status because serum $1,25\text{-}(OH)_2$ D concentrations may be elevated, normal, or low in vitamin D–deficiency rickets, depending on the degree and the duration of deficiency.[54, 139, 176] Measurements of vitamin D itself are also not useful to determine vitamin D stores because serum concentrations of vitamin D are acutely influenced by *recent* exposure to UVB.[81]

Regulation of Magnesium Homeostasis

Mg is distributed in the mineral phase of the skeleton (65%), in intracellular space (34%), and in extracellular fluid (1%).[3] Mg is therefore primarily an intracellular cation. Mg is an activator of multiple enzymatic systems, in particular, those connected with energy production and cell membrane function.[95] It also plays a role in regulation of mitochondrial function and in protein and DNA synthesis.[95] In plasma, Mg is present in three forms: (1) protein bound (25 to 30%); (2) ionized (55 to 60%); and (3) complexed as salts. There is no routinely available ion-selective electrode directly measuring the active, ionized fraction; one must rely for clinical purposes on the measurement of total Mg by colorimetry or, preferably, by atomic absorption spectrophotometry.[160] Measurements of serum Mg, however, may not accurately reflect intracellular Mg stores because a wide range of serum Mg concentration overlap exists between Mg deficiency and Mg sufficiency.[148] Measurements of intraerythrocyte or intraleukocyte Mg have not proved to be superior to serum Mg measurements and remain a research tool.[44, 141]

Mg is actively absorbed in the intestine[3] and actively reabsorbed (after glomerular filtration) in the renal tubule.[3, 95] Contrary to that of Ca, however, regulation of serum Mg concentration occurs mainly in the kidney.[95] A tight relationship exists between dietary Mg intake and urinary Mg.[95] Normally 95 to 97% of filtered Mg is reabsorbed.[95] An increase in serum Mg concentration leads to decreased renal reabsorption, whereas when Mg is deficient in the body or when diet is low in Mg, urinary excretion nearly disappears.[95] The hormonal regulation of serum Mg is difficult to study owing to complex relationships with serum Ca. PTH increases serum Mg concentration by increasing Mg mobilization from bone, decreasing renal Mg excretion, and increasing intestinal Mg absorption.[86, 102] Acute hypomagnesemia inhibits PTH secretion[148]; however, as stated previously, in chronic Mg deficiency, PTH secretion is impaired,[95, 148] presumably owing to decreased parathyroid gland Mg-dependent adenylcyclase activity,[95] and Mg replenishment leads to a paradoxic PTH release.[148]

MINERAL HOMEOSTASIS IN PREGNANCY

Mineral Homeostasis in the Mother

The human fetus accretes approximately 25 g of elemental Ca during pregnancy[59]; most of this accretion occurs in the last trimester.[59] Understandably significant changes in mineral metabolism occur during pregnancy and are likely aimed at meeting the increasing mineral needs of the fetus as well as in preparation for lactation.

During pregnancy, total Ca concentrations in maternal serum decrease, but there are few or no changes in serum iCa concentrations.[57, 115, 130] In fact, the decrease in total Ca is probably explained exclusively by the decrease in serum albumin, which occurs as a result of hemodilution of pregnancy.[130] Regardless of the mammalian species studied, the intestinal absorption of Ca was found to increase significantly during pregnancy.[55] This increase is not completely understood in that it seems to precede a rise in serum $1,25\text{-}(OH)_2$ D concentration, observed mainly in the last trimester of pregnancy.[38, 55, 73, 115] Stable Ca isotope studies in pregnancy show an increase in bone accretion and in bone resorption.[73] Bone accretion rate, however, seems to predominate.[73] Understanding these changes in bone accretion and bone resorption is not easy because changes in calciotropic hormone concentration do not correlate temporally well with changes in bone metabolism.[115] It is therefore possible that other factors, such as placental hormones, may have a direct effect on these changes. Studies of serum $1,25\text{-}(OH)_2$ D, PTH, or CT concentration during pregnancy are inconsistent. Most studies demonstrate an increase in serum $1,25\text{-}(OH)_2$ D during pregnancy.[115] Serum PTH, measured using C- or N-terminal fragments, was reported to increase during pregnancy.[18, 38, 131] In contrast, studies of bioactive PTH or of whole molecule immunoradioactive concentration show little or no change in pregnancy.[39, 115] Similarly, serum concentrations of CT are reported to be elevated in pregnancy[131] or unchanged.[88] In addition to technical differences in assays, studies may have differed by dietary Ca, which is known to influence serum concentrations of PTH, CT, or $1,25\text{-}(OH)_2$ D.

Placenta

PTH and CT do not appear to cross the placenta in either direction.[87, 88] Vitamin D metabolites (except vitamin D itself), however, appear to do so, and there is usually a good correlation between maternal and fetal values of 25-hydroxy D, and 1,25-dihydroxyvitamin D, especially when sensitive and accurate assays are employed.[82] Vitamin D status of the fetus appears to be largely determined by maternal vitamin D status through transfer of 25-(OH)D.[82]

The presence of an active transport mechanism of Ca from the mother to the fetus was suggested many years ago by the fact that from midpregnancy fetal serum Ca concentrations are consistently higher than those of the mother.[144] In support of this theory are several studies of placental Ca transport in the in situ perfused rat placenta, which show that maternal fetal Ca transport is greater than that of molecules that cross the placenta by simple diffusion.[159] Also, metabolic poisons, such as dinitrophenol or cyanide, inhibit Ca transport.[159] Bidirectional fluxes (mother to fetus and fetus to mother), however, have been demonstrated and vary considerably in magnitude in different species.[134, 159] From studies in the rhesus monkey, in which more than 80% of the calcium transferred from the mother returns from the fetus, it has been inferred that bidirectional fluxes of this extent also exist in the human.[134]

The exact mechanism of placental Ca transport and its regulation are the subject of intense research. From studies supporting the role of the Ca-binding protein, it has been suggested that vitamin D may be involved.[174, 180] Also, the placenta is the only organ other than the kidney to have 1-hydroxylase activity.[162] Various adenosine triphosphatases have been isolated from the placenta.[184] Their function and regulation, however, are still unclear.

Infants of chronically hypocalcemic mothers are at risk for developing hyperparathyroidism,[101] which may indicate that they were hypocalcemic in utero as well (presumably fetal hypocalcemia stimulates fetal parathyroid gland).[154] Infants of hypercalcemic mothers may develop neonatal hypoparathyroidism, which may indicate that they were hypercalcemic in utero.[16, 24, 46, 69] Thus the human fetus appears to be unprotected against chronic maternal hypercalcemia or hypocalcemia. In various animal models, however, acute maternal hypocalcemia or hypercalcemia did not have major effects on placental Ca transport.[8, 12, 27]

Within the duration of a term pregnancy, the human fetus accretes approximately 1 g of elemental Mg.[59] Most of it is transferred toward the end of pregnancy, when a daily amount of 4.5 to 6.0 mg per day is transferred.[59] As for Ca, fetal serum Mg concentration (assessed from cord blood values) is greater than maternal concentration at delivery.[65, 127] This is usually interpreted as in support of an active transport mechanism. Shaw et al.[149] using an in situ perfused rat placenta model, showed that the unidirectional maternal-fetal clearance of Mg was (1) higher than that of a diffusional marker of similar diffusion coefficient and (2) significantly lowered by cyanide, an inhibitor of energy-dependent mechanisms of transport. This study further supported the theory of an active transport mechanism of Mg across the placenta. This transport system is probably independent from that of Ca, as we showed that neither maternal acute hypermagnesemia nor chronic maternal Mg deficiency in the rat influenced the placental clearance of Ca.[36, 110] As it is suspected for Ca, both hypomagnesemia and hypermagnesemia on the maternal side lead to fetal hypomagnesemia and hypermagnesemia.[31, 35, 36, 43, 45, 107, 110, 149]

The Fetus

When the fetal and maternal calciotropic hormone concentrations are compared, fetal PTH and $1,25\text{-}(OH)_2$ D concentrations are lower and $24,25\text{-}(OH)_2$ D is higher.[82, 58, 167] This is interpreted as being secondary to the relative hypercalcemia observed during fetal life. This situation, combining a relative decrease of the bone resorptive hormones, PTH and $1,25\text{-}OH_2$ D, and a relative increase of the bone forming protective hormones, CT[15, 49, 78] and possibly $24,25\text{-}(OH)_2$ D,[125] appears to be aimed at maintaining a high bone formation rate, consistent with the high growth rate of the fetus. Reports using cytochemical bioassay measurements of PTH in maternal and cord blood, however, indicate that the bioactivity of PTH was extremely high in the fetus.[2] These studies are highly discordant with those using PTH values obtained by radioimmunoassay; the discordance might be due to a high PTHrP concentration during fetal life, as PTHrP can be produced by the placenta.[137]

NEONATAL MINERAL HOMEOSTASIS

Considerable changes in mineral metabolism occur after birth. Subsequent to cord clamping, placental transfer of mineral immediately ceases. It is gradually replaced by dietary sources. There is limited milk production during the first few days of lactation, however, and thus there is relatively limited milk intake in the first few days of life.[26] Within a few hours after birth, the infant's serum Ca concentration drops abruptly to reach a nadir at about 24 hours of age.[99] Thereafter serum Ca concentration remains stable above 8 mg/dL in the term healthy infant; it slowly rises by 1 week of age as the enteral mineral supply increases to reach early childhood values.[29, 156] At the same time, within hours after birth, both serum PTH and $1,25\text{-}(OH)_2$ D concentration dramatically increase,[98, 158] presumably in an attempt to maintain extracellular calcium homeostasis through Ca mobilization from bone and, possibly, through reduction of bone formation.[98] Serum osteocalcin concentration, a known index of bone formation,[72] undergoes an abrupt drop within the first 24 hours of life.[98] Two facts remain relatively poorly understood: (1) Despite the decreasing serum Ca concentration that follows cord clamping, a surge in serum CT concentration occurs at birth.[78] The serum CT values reached with the surge are higher than at any other period in life.[78] The significance and potential physiology of this apparently paradoxic CT surge are unknown. (2) Despite cessation of placental transport of Mg after birth and despite limited Mg supply through diet, serum Mg concentrations are known to rise slowly over the first few days of life.[148, 166] This phenomenon is also not understood.

DISORDERS OF MINERAL HOMEOSTASIS IN THE PERINATAL PERIOD

Neonatal Hypocalcemia

Decreased (or Absent) Parathyroid Hormone Secretion or Action

HYPOCALCEMIA OF PREMATURITY

The PTH response to decreasing serum Ca concentration at birth is a function of both gestational age and postnatal age, as demonstrated by (1) studies of serum PTH concentrations after birth and (2) studies of serum PTH concentrations following the decrease of serum iCa concentrations generated by exchange transfusions using citrate-treated blood.[41] The lower the gestational age and the lower the postnatal age, the lower will be the PTH response to hypocalcemia.[41, 167] PTH administration to preterm infants, however, leads to a calcemic response similar to that observed in full-term infants, which indicates that preterm infants have a normal bone sensitivity to PTH.[170]

MAGNESIUM DEFICIENCY

Neonatal Mg deficiency may impair both PTH secretion[95, 100, 148] and action.[103] This is discussed in more detail later in this chapter.

CONGENITAL HYPOPARATHYROIDISM

Congenital hypoparathyroidism may be primary or secondary. When it is primary, it may be inherited according to an X-linked mode[129] or an autosomal dominant mode[10]; it may also occur in association with a chromosome 16 or 18 ring[171] or as one of the components of the DiGeorge sequence.[71, 171] When complete, the sequence involves congenital thymic aplasia or hypoplasia (with various degrees of cellular immune deficiency) and cardiovascular malformations (mostly left-sided heart disease).[71, 171] The DiGeorge sequence is due to abnormal

development of pharyngeal pouches III and IV[71]; when pouch II is also involved, facial anomalies may coexist.[71] Much emphasis has been placed on partial DiGeorge sequences, in which one or two elements of the triad were found in different patients or within the same family.[11] It is therefore advisable to investigate carefully immune function and cardiac anatomy of all infants born with primary congenital hypoparathyroidism.

In transient congenital hypoparathyroidism, neonatal hypocalcemia (NHC) associated with very low or undetectable PTH concentrations is of transient duration (several weeks to months).[5] Such patients have an improvement in PTH function; this improvement may not be complete with time, even in the face of normocalcemia, as an infant with such a disease was reported at 2 years of age to have an abnormal PTH response to ethylenediamine-tetra-acetic acid (EDTA)–induced hypocalcemia.[5]

Congenital hypoparathyroidism may also develop secondary to maternal hypercalcemia[92]; in such cases, the mother is most often affected by primary hyperparathyroidism,[92] but any other cause of maternal hypercalcemia, such as benign, familial hypocalciuric hypercalcemia, may have the same consequences.[127] Presumably chronic exposure to maternal hypercalcemia leads to fetal hypercalcemia and secondary hypoparathyroidism. Two points are important: (1) In such cases, the prognosis is good because neonatal parathyroid gland function will resume in a few days to a few weeks and will attain normalcy[92]; (2) the mother may be totally asymptomatic, and the presence of neonatal hypocalcemia is the reason for discovery of her disease.[92] It is therefore important to obtain maternal serum Ca measurements in all infants with congenital hypoparathyroidism.

END-ORGAN RESISTANCE TO PARATHYROID HORMONE

Hereditary end-organ resistance to PTH (pseudohypoparathyroidism) may lead to hypocalcemia but usually not in the perinatal period because the disease appears to develop within the first 2 to 3 years of life.[173] Functional end-organ resistance to PTH, however, has been described in both Mg deficiency[103] and P intoxication[133] in neonates and may have played a role in their hypocalcemia.

Increased Calcitonin Production

Increased CT concentrations have been reported in asphyxiated infants, and their serum CT correlated inversely with the 1-minute and 5-minute Apgar scores.[179] Moreover, their serum Ca at 24 hours of age correlated inversely with their serum CT.[179] This relationship supports the theory of a role of CT in NHC but does not prove a causal relationship. As described previously, CT rises after birth in normal newborns.[78] CT secretion, however, might be "loosely" regulated at that time because a similar increase is observed in preterm infants and in infants[78] of diabetic mothers[112] despite frankly decreased serum Ca concentrations.

Vitamin D Disorders

It has been suggested that disorders of vitamin D metabolism may play a causative role in NHC in the following circumstances.

MATERNAL VITAMIN D DEFICIENCY

Infants born to Indian subcontinent immigrants to the United Kingdom have been shown to have a high rate of NHC as well as secondary hyperparathyroidism.[75, 123, 124, 128, 182] These infants and their mothers have very low serum 25(OH)D concentrations at the time of birth.[128] A similar observation was made of Bedouin infants in Saudi Arabia.[161]

ANTICONVULSANTS IN PREGNANCY

Epileptic patients treated with phenobarbital or phenytoin are at risk for vitamin D deficiency and osteomalacia[66]; the cause of vitamin D deficiency relates to increased vitamin D catabolism in the liver, as described previously.[66] Hypocalcemia has been reported in neonates born to epileptic mothers taking these drugs in pregnancy[50] and is prevented by maternal vitamin D supplementation.[104]

RESISTANCE TO 1,25-DIHYDROXYVITAMIN D

Resistance to $1,25-(OH)_2 D$ does not appear to be a major cause of NHC.[6, 23] Small preterm infants, who are at high risk for NHC, however, have been shown to be relatively resistant to exogenous $1,25-(OH)_2 D$.[91, 178] The role of this relative resistance in the genesis of NHC is unknown.

Decreased Mineral Intake or Absorption

In sick neonates (e.g., preterm, asphyxiated), the delay in initiating enteral feeds further limits their exogenous Ca supply.[150] In addition, Ca absorption appears to mature with postnatal age,[58, 122, 150, 163] being mostly intake dependent; this Ca absorption is consistent with passive diffusion early after birth[9, 58, 79] and acquires active transport characteristics later on.[9, 58, 121, 122, 145, 150, 163]

Hyperphosphatemia

Hyperphosphatemia may occur as a consequence of immature kidney function,[33] increased cell breakdown due to hypoxic-ischemic injury,[33, 179] or intake of high P content formula (which produces "late" hypocalcemic tetany occurring at the end of the first week of age).[177] In such cases, hypocalcemia may develop as a consequence of deposition of Ca in bone and soft tissue,[9] PTH resistance and augmentation of CT action at the bone,[96] and inhibition of $1,25-(OH)_2 D$ formation in the kidney.[83]

Ionized Calcium Chelation

A decrease in iCa (but not in total Ca) has been described when iCa is chelated by citrate (present in blood products),[41] bicarbonate[84, 168] (given to correct acidosis), and free fatty acids[183] (which may be elevated in lipid-intolerant infants receiving intravenous lipids). Alkalosis of any kind may also increase Ca binding to protein[84] and decreases Ca flux from bone.[70] Also, phosphate salts may bind directly to iCa.[93]

Phototherapy

The mechanism by which phototherapy used to treat neonatal hyperbilirubinemia could lead to NHC is complex.[138] Phototherapy decreases melatonin secretion[138]; in rats, melatonin inhibits bone Ca uptake by a permissive action on glucocorticoids.[67] Thus, phototherapy would indirectly depress Ca release from bone.[67]

Neonatal Hypercalcemia

Primary Hyperparathyroidism

Congenital primary hyperparathyroidism is a rare disorder.[62] Most often, the hyperparathyroidism is due to parathyroid hyperplasia rather than to adenomas.[62] Most cases are sporadic, although familial cases compatible with autosomal recessive inheritance have been described.[62] A high incidence of congenital primary hyperparathyroidism has been described in families affected by the so-called benign hypocalciuric hypercalcemia and may represent a homozygous form of the disease.[105] In such infants, hypercalcemia may be strikingly high with severe hypophosphatemia, hypercalciuria, and hyperphosphaturia.[62, 105] Massive bone resorption, evidenced by osteopenia and spontaneous fractures, may be seen on skeletal x-ray films.[62, 105] Renal ultrasonography often reveals nephrocalcinosis. Treatment is usually surgical and consists of subtotal parathyroidectomy.[62, 105]

Congenital Secondary Hyperparathyroidism

This condition is usually caused by chronic maternal hypocalcemia[101]; in most cases, the mother is hypocalcemic because of hypoparathyroidism, which may be idiopathic or secondary to surgical removal of the parathyroid glands.[101] Rarely the mother is hypocalcemic because of another condition, such as pseudohypoparathyroidism.[60] Neonatal hyperparathyroidism secondary to maternal hypocalcemia has a highly variable presentation.[101] At one end of the spectrum, severe bone disease similar to that observed in primary hyperparathyroidism is found.[101] At the other end of the spectrum, hyperparathyroidism may be asymptomatic clinically and even radiologically, and bone demineralization assessed by photon absorptiometry together with elevated serum PTH concentrations makes the diagnosis.[101] It is likely that the severity of maternal hypocalcemia determines the severity of the neonatal clinical signs.[101]

Idiopathic Infantile Hypercalcemia

Idiopathic infantile hypercalcemia is a disorder of mineral metabolism with large overlap with the so-called Williams' syndrome.[117] In this syndrome, elfin facies, mental retardation, and supravalvular aortic stenosis are the major features.[117] Some patients with Williams' syndrome do not appear to be hypercalcemic, whereas some patients with idiopathic infantile hypercalcemia have none of the morphologic features of Williams' syndrome. The cause of this syndrome is unknown, and multiple theories have been developed in the past 20 years. Increased sensitivity to vitamin D[14] or increased production of $1,25\text{-}(OH)_2 D$[53] both have been suggested. Culler et al.[37] have proposed that calcitonin deficiency is at the origin of this condition.

Subcutaneous Fat Necrosis

Subcutaneous fat necrosis may develop after birth, in particular when there is combination of trauma (areas of pressure) and hypoxic ischemic injury or cold stress.[113, 147, 165, 175] These areas tend to calcify. Some patients with extensive subcutaneous fat necrosis in the following weeks develop sometimes severe hypercalcemia of unknown cause.[147, 165, 175] Several mechanisms have been suggested, which include sudden release of a large amount of Ca from the subcutaneous fat, abnormal sensitivity to $1,25\text{-}(OH)_2 D$, or increased $1,25\text{-}(OH)_2 D$ production.[48, 113, 147, 165, 175]

Bartter's Syndrome

This renal tubular disorder leading to electrolyte and water wastage may be complicated by hypercalcemia and hypercalciuria.[146] Metabolic alkalosis usually is present, mostly owing to potassium wastage.[146] These patients often are born prematurely with a history of polyhydramnios (owing to intrauterine polyuria), failure to thrive, and episodes of fever, vomiting, and diarrhea.[146] Osteopenia with nephrocalcinosis may complicate the syndrome.[146]

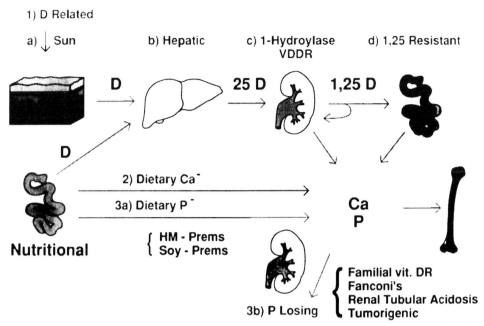

FIGURE 21–2. Rickets can result from (1) (a) low sunshine exposure and poor production of vitamin D and low intake of vitamin D, (b) hepatic hydroxylation defect, (c) 1-hydroxylase deficiency in the kidney, (d) 1,25-dihydroxyvitamin D resistance; (2) nutritional calcium deficiency; (3) (a) nutritional phosphate deficiency, (b) phosphate losing syndromes.

The pathophysiology of this form of Bartter's syndrome is not well understood but may involve prostaglandin metabolism.[146] Indeed, hyperprostaglandinuria E_2 has been documented, and indomethacin suppression has led to significant improvement in both the clinical and the biochemical features of this syndrome.[146]

Severe Hypophosphatasia

This rare inherited disorder is caused by deficient alkaline phosphatase activity in bone, liver, and intestine.[164] The inheritance is autosomal recessive.[164, 185] Patients have a combination of severe rickets at birth and hypercalcemia with hypercalciuria.[164, 185] Supranormal blood and urine concentrations of phosphoethanolamine and inorganic pyrophosphate indicate that these compounds are natural substrates for tissue-nonspecific alkaline phosphatase.[183] It has been suggested that the biochemical features of the syndrome result from the failure of Ca to deposit in bone.[164, 185]

Hypercalcemic, Hypophosphatemic Rickets of Prematurity

This condition is almost exclusive to preterm infants of very low birth weight who are breast-fed with non–mineral-fortified breast milk (Fig. 21–2).[63, 64, 140, 142] These patients are deficient in P, which leads to rickets and elevated $1,25\text{-}(OH)_2$ D production with subsequent increased bone resorption, hypercalcemia, and hypercalciuria. This condition is rarer since the introduction of high P–content breast milk fortifiers for premature infants.[63]

Familial Hypocalciuric Hypercalcemia

This disease, also called *benign familial hypocalcemia,* is transmitted in an autosomal dominant manner.[105] Its benign denomination is justified by the usual lack of complications.[105] The pathogenesis is unknown, and it is generally considered that this is a benign form of hyperparathyroidism.[105] Some offspring of those families, however, develop severe neonatal hyperparathyroidism (see section on congenital secondary hyperparathyroidism) and it has been suggested that these patients represent a homozygous form of the disease.[105]

Neonatal Hypomagnesemia

In normal healthy infants, the PTH response to the physiologic drop of serum Ca correlates with Mg status at birth.[100] Mg deficiency may have an impact on neonatal metabolism, as evidenced in infants of diabetic mothers.[111, 114, 116, 169, 172] In diabetes, glucosuria leads to urinary Mg wastage and subsequent Mg deficiency. When a pregnant diabetic women is Mg deficient, her fetus will also be Mg deficient, as demonstrated by decreased amniotic fluid Mg concentration[114] or decreased cord blood or neonatal serum Mg concentration.[111, 114, 116, 169, 172] Infants of diabetic mothers have decreased PTH response to decreasing serum Ca after birth,[169, 172] and their PTH response to hypocalcemia correlates with their serum Mg concentration.[169, 172] In these patients, serum Mg and Ca are tightly correlated.[116]

Other situations than maternal diabetes have been described to be associated with Mg deficiency–induced NHC. They include (1) infants with primary, lifelong congenital renal Mg wastage[7, 186] or Mg malabsorption,[166] (2) infants with short-gut due to surgical resection,[166] and (3) infants with acute tubular necrosis at the polyuric stage or infants who have received nephrotoxic agents such as gentamicin.[106]

Neonatal Hypermagnesemia

Neonatal hypermagnesemia is mostly iatrogenic and is due to maternal treatment with Mg sulfate salts given for either prevention of prematurity as a tocolytic agent[45] or for prevention of seizures in preeclampsia.[35, 107] In these infants, hypermagnesemia suppresses neonatal parathyroid function[43]; however, serum Ca concentration appears to be normal or even increased compared with control infants[43]; this is possibly related to direct effects of Mg, which facilitates the release of Ca from bone.[103] Also, displacement of Ca from blood protein or salts may increase serum iCa concentrations.[97]

Acknowledgments

Supported in part by NIH HD 18505, NIH HD 11, NIH P5 OHD20748, Bristol-Myers Laboratories, the Gerber Product Company, the Twenty-Five Club of Magee–Women's Hospital, and the Magee–Women's Hospital Research Fund.

We wish to thank Maureen Davis and Diane Frazier for help in the typing and preparation of this manuscript.

REFERENCES

1. Akatsu T, Takahashi N, Udagawa N, et al. Parathyroid hormone (PTH)-related protein is a potent stimulator of osteoclast-like multinucleated cell formation to the same extent as PTH in mouse marrow cultures. Endocrinology 1989;125:20.
2. Allgrove J, Adami S, Manning RM, O'Riordan JLH. Cytochemical bioassay of parathyroid hormone in maternal and cord blood. Arch Dis Child 1985;60:110.
3. Anast CS, Gardner DW. Magnesium metabolism. In: Bronner F, Coburn JW, eds. Disorders of mineral metabolism: pathophysiology of calcium, phosphorus, and magnesium. New York: Academic Press, 1981:423.
4. Atchley DW. On diabetic acidosis: detailed study of electrolyte balance following withdrawal and re-establishment of insulin therapy. J Clin Invest 1933;12:297.
5. Bainbridge R, Mughal Z, Mimouni F, Tsang RC. Transient congenital hypoparathyroidism: how transient is it? J Pediatr 1987;3:866.
6. Balsan S, Garabedian M, Courtecuisse V, et al. Long-term therapy with 1 alpha hydroxyvitamin D_3 in children with pseudodeficiency rickets. Clin Endocrinol 1977;7:2255.
7. Bar RS, Wilson HE, Mazza Ferri EL. Hypomagnesemia-hypocalcemia secondary to renal magnesium wasting. Ann Intern Med 1975;82:646.
8. Barlet JP, Davicco MJ, LeFaivre J, et al. Fetal blood calcium induced in the cow by calcium infusion or by solanium glaucophyllum ingestion. Horm Metab Res 1979;11:57.
9. Barltrop D, Mole RH, Sutton A. Absorption and endogenous faecal excretion of calcium by low birth-weight infants on feeds with varying contents of calcium and phosphate. Arch Dis Child 1977;52:41.
10. Barr DGD, Prader A, Esper U, et al. Chronic hypoparathyroidism in two generations. Helv Paediatr Acta 1971;26:507.
11. Barrett DJ, Ammann AJ, Cowan MJ, et al. Clinical and immunologic spectrum of the DiGeorge syndrome. J Clin Lab Immunol 1981;6:1.
12. Bawden JW, Wolkoff AS. Fetal blood calcium responses to maternal calcium infusion in sheep. Am J Obstet Gynecol 1967;99:55.
13. Baylink DJ, Lin CC. The regulation of endosteal bone volume. J Periodontol 1979;50:43.
14. Becroft DMO, Chambers D. Supravascular aortic stenosis—infantile hypercalcemia syndrome: in vitro hypersensitivity to vitamin D_2 and calcium. J Med Genet 1976;13:223.
15. Bergman L. Studies on early neonatal hypocalcemia. Acta Paediatr Scand 1974;248(suppl):1.
16. Better OS, Levi J, Grief E, et al. Prolonged neonatal parathyroid suppression: a sequel to asymptomatic maternal hyperparathyroidism. Arch Surg 1973;106:722.
17. Blind E, Schmidt-Gayk H, Scharla S, et al. Two-site assay of intact parathyroid hormone in the investigation of primary hyperparathyroidism and other disorders of calcium metabolism compared with a midregion assay. J Clin Endocrinol Metab 1988;67:353.

18. Bouillon R, DeMoor P. Pathophysiological data obtained with a radioimmunoassay for human parathyroid hormone. Ann Endocrinol 1973;34:657.

19. Bowers GN, Brassard C, Sena SF. Measurement of ionized calcium in serum with ion-selective electrodes: a mature technology that can meet the daily service needs. Clin Chem 1986;32:1437.

20. Boyle IT, Gray RW, DeLuca HF. Regulation by calcium of in vivo synthesis of 1,25-dihydroxycholecalciferol and 21,25-dihydroxycholecalciferol. Proc Natl Acad Sci USA 1971;68:2131.

21. Brommage R, DeLuca HF. Evidence that 1,25-dihydroxyvitamin D_3 is the physiologically active metabolite of vitamin D_3. Endocr Rev 1985;6:491.

22. Brommage R, Neuman WF. Mechanism of mobilization of bone mineral by 1,25-dihydroxyvitamin D_3. Am J Physiol 1979;237:E113.

23. Brooks MH, Bell NH, Love L, et al. Vitamin D dependent rickets type II: resistance of target organs to 1,25-dihydroxyvitamin D. N Engl J Med 1978;298:996.

24. Bruce J, Strong JA. Maternal hyperparathyroidism and parathyroid deficiency in the child with an account of the effect of parathyroidectomy on renal function, and of an attempt to transplant part of the tumor. Q J Med 1955;24:307.

25. Carey DE, Jones KL, Parthemore JG, Deftos LJ. Calcitonin secretion in congenital nongoitrous cretinism. J Clin Invest 1980;65:892.

26. Casey CE, Neifert MR, Seacat JM, Neville MC. Nutrient intake by breast-fed infants during the first five days after birth. Am J Dis Child 1986;140:933.

27. Chalon S, Garel JM. Plasma calcium control in the rat fetus. III. Influence of alterations in maternal plasma calcium on fetal plasma calcium levels. Biol Neonate 1985;48:329.

28. Chambers TJ, McSheehy PM, Thomson BM, Fuller K. The effect of calcium-regulating hormones and prostaglandins on bone resorption by osteoclasts disaggregated from neonatal rabbit bones. Endocrinology 1985;60:234.

29. Chan GM, Nordmeyer FR, Richter BE, et al. Comparison of serum total calcium, dialyzable calcium, and dialyzable magnesium in well and sick neonates. Clin Physiol Biochem 1984;2:154.

30. Chen TC, Castillo L, Korychadahl M, DeLuca HF. Role of vitamin D metabolism in phosphate transport of rat intestine. J Nutr 1974;104:1056.

31. Cholst IN, Steinberg SF, Tropper PJ, et al. The influence of hypermagnesemia on serum calcium and parathyroid hormone levels in human subjects. N Engl J Med 1984;310:1221.

32. Clemens TL, Holick MF. Recent advances in the hormonal regulation of calcium and phosphorus in adult animals and humans. In: Holick MF, Gray TK, Anast CS, eds. Perinatal calcium and phosphorus metabolism. Amsterdam: Elsevier, 1983:1.

33. Connelly JP, Crawford JD, Watson J. Studies of neonatal hyperphosphatemia. Pediatrics 1962;43:425.

34. Cooke NE, Haddad JG. Vitamin D binding protein (Gc-Globulin). Endocr Rev 1989;10:294.

35. Cruikshank DP, Pitkin RM, Reynolds WA, et al. Effects of magnesium sulfate treatment on perinatal calcium metabolism. I. Maternal and fetal responses. Am J Obstet Gynecol 1979;134:243.

36. Cruz M, Mimouni F, Tsang RC, Hammond G. Is calcium (Ca) transported independently of magnesium (Mg) across in-situ perfused rat placenta? Pediatr Res 1990;27:281A.

37. Culler FL, Jones KL, Deftos LJ. Impaired calcitonin secretion in patients with Williams syndrome. J Pediatr 1985;107:720.

38. Cushard WG, Creditor MA, Canterbury JM, et al. Physiologic hyperparathyroidism in pregnancy. J Clin Endocrinol Metab 1972;34:767.

39. Davis OK, Hawkins DS, Rubin LP, et al. Serum parathyroid hormone (PTH) in pregnant women determined by an immunoradiometric assay for intact PTH. J Clin Endocrinol Metab 1988;67:850.

40. Delling G, Donath K. Morphometrische, electronenmikroskopische und physikalisch-chemische Untersuchungen über die experimentelle Osteoporose bei chronischer Acidose. Virchows Arch (Pathol Anat) 1973;358:321.

41. Dincsoy MY, Tsang RC, Laskarzewski P, et al. The role of postnatal age and magnesium on parathyroid hormone responses during "exchange" blood transfusion in the newborn period. J Pediatr 1982;100:277.

42. Donahue HJ, Fryer MJ, Heath H III. Structure-function relationships for full-length recombinant parathyroid hormone-related peptide and its amino-terminal fragments: effects of cytosolic calcium ion mobilization and adenylate cyclase activation in rat osteoblast-like cells. Endocrinology 1990;126:1471.

43. Donovan EF, Tsang RC, Steichen JJ, et al. Neonatal hypermagnesemia: effect on parathyroid hormone and calcium homeostasis. J Pediatr 1980;96:305.

44. Elin RJ, Hosseini JM. Magnesium content of mononuclear blood cells. Clin Chem 1985;31:377.

45. Elliot JP. Magnesium sulfate as a tocolytic agent. Am J Obstet Gynecol 1983;147:277.

46. Ertel NH, Reiss JS, Spergel G. Hypomagnesemia in neonatal tetany associated with maternal hyperparathyroidism. N Engl J Med 1969;280:260.

47. Feldman RS, Krieger NS, Tashjian AH. Effects of parathyroid hormone and calcitonin on osteoclast formation in vitro. Endocrinology 1980;107:1137.

48. Finne PH, Sanderrud J, Aksnes L, et al. Hypercalcemia with increased and unregulated 1,25-dihydroxyvitamin D production in a neonate with subcutaneous fat necrosis. J Pediatr 1988;112:792.

49. Friedman J, Raisy LG. Thyrocalcitonin: inhibitor of bone resorption in tissue culture. Science 1965;150:1465.

50. Friis B, Sardeman H. Neonatal hypocalcemia after intrauterine exposure to anticonvulsant drugs. Arch Dis Child 1977;52:239.

51. Fourman P. Calcium metabolism and the bone. Oxford: Blackwell, 1960:27.

52. Garabedian M, Holick MF, DeLuca HF, Boyle IT. Control of 25-hydroxycholecalciferol metabolism by parathyroid glands. Proc Natl Acad Sci USA 1972;69:1673.

53. Garabedian M, Jocoz E, Guillozo H, et al. Elevated plasma 1,25-dihydroxyvitamin D concentrations in infants with hypercalcemia and an elfin facies. N Engl J Med 1985;213:948.

54. Garabedian M, Vainsel M, Mallet E, et al. Circulating vitamin D metabolite concentrations in children with nutritional rickets. J Pediatr 1983;103:381.

55. Garel JM. Hormonal control of calcium metabolism during the reproductive cycle in mammals. Physiol Rev 1987;67:1.

56. Gerstenfeld LC, Kelly CM, VonDeck M, Lian JB. Effects of 1,25-dihydroxyvitamin D_3 on induction of chondrocyte maturation in culture: extracellular matrix gene expression and morphology. Endocrinology 1990;126:1599.

57. Gertner JM, Coustan DR, Kliger AS. Pregnancy state

of physiologic absorptive hypercalciuria. Am J Med 1986;81:451.

58. Giles MM, Fenton MH, Shaw B, et al. Sequential calcium and phosphorus balance studies in preterm infants. J Pediatr 1987;110:591.

59. Givens MH, Machy IG. The chemical composition of the human fetus. J Biol Chem 1933;102:7.

60. Glass EJ, Barr DGD. Transient neonatal hyperparathyroidism secondary to maternal pseudohypoparathyroidism. Arch Dis Child 1981;56:565.

61. Gmaj P, Murer H. Cellular mechanisms of inorganic phosphate transport in kidney. Physiol Rev 1986;66:36.

62. Goldbloom RB, Gillies DA, Prasad M. Hereditary parathyroid hyperplasia: a surgical emergency. Pediatrics 1972;49:514.

63. Greer FR, McCormick A. Improved bone mineralization and growth in premature infants fed fortified own mother's milk. J Pediatr 1988;112:961.

64. Greer FR, Steichen JJ, Tsang RC. Calcium and phosphate supplements in breast milk-related rickets. Am J Dis Child 1982;136:581.

65. Gupta MM, Kuppuswamy G, Subramanian AR. Transplacental transfer of 25-hydroxycholecalciferol. Postgrad Med 1982;58:408.

66. Hahn TJ, Birge SJ, Scharp CR, Avioli LV. Phenobarbital-induced alterations in vitamin D metabolism. J Clin Invest 1972;51:741.

67. Hakanson DO, Bergstrom WH. Prevention of light-induced hypocalcemia by melatonin. In: Norman AW, ed. Vitamin D, chemical, biochemical and clinical endocrinology of calcium metabolism. Berlin: Walter deGruyter, 1982:1163.

68. Halloran BP, Spencer EM. Dietary phosphorus and 1,25-dihydroxyvitamin D metabolism: influence of insulin-like growth factor I. Endocrinology 1988;123:1225.

69. Hanukoglu A, Chalew S, Kowarski AA. Late onset hypocalcemia, rickets and hypoparathyroidism in an infant of a mother with hyperparathyroidism. J Pediatr 1988;112:751.

70. Harrison HE. Tetany. In: Behrman R, Vaughn VC III, eds. Nelson textbook of pediatrics, ed 12. Philadelphia: WB Saunders, 1983:249.

71. Harvey JC, Dungan WT, Elders MJ, Hughes ER. Third and fourth pharyngeal pouch syndrome, associated with vascular anomalies and hypocalcemic seizure. Clin Pediatr 1970;9:496.

72. Hauscka PV. Osteocalcin. The vitamin K–dependent Ca^{2+}-binding protein of bone matrix. Hemostasis 1986;16:258.

73. Heaney RP, Skillman TG. Calcium metabolism in normal human pregnancy. J Clin Endocrinol Metab 1971;33:66.

74. Hebert LA, Lemann J Jr, Petersen JR, Lennon EJ. Studies of the mechanism by which phosphate infusion lowers serum calcium concentration. J Clin Invest 1966;45:1886.

75. Heckmatt JZ, Peacock M, Davies AE, et al. Plasma 25-hydroxyvitamin D in pregnant Asian women and their babies. Lancet 1979;2:546.

76. Henry HL. Regulation of the hydroxylation of 25-hydroxyvitamin D_3 in vivo and in primary cultures of chick kidney cells. J Biol Chem 1979;254:2722.

77. Henry HL. Insulin permits parathyroid hormone stimulation of 1,25-dehydroxyvitamin D_3 production in cultured kidney cells. Endocrinology 1981;108:733.

78. Hillman LS, Rojanasathit S, Slatopolsky E, Haddad JG. Serial measurements of serum calcium, magnesium, parathyroid hormone, calcitonin and 25-hydroxyvitamin D in premature and term infants during the first week of life. Pediatr Res 1977;11:739.

79. Hillman LS, Tack E, Covell DG, et al. Measurement of true calcium absorption in premature infants using intravenous ^{46}Ca and oral ^{46}Ca. Pediatr Res 1988;23:589.

80. Holick MF. The cutaneous photosynthesis of previtamin D_3: a unique photoendocrine system. J Invest Dermatol 1981;76:51.

81. Holick MF, Uskovic M, Henley JW, et al. The photoproduction of 1α,25-dihydroxyvitamin D_3 in skin. An approach to the therapy of vitamin D-resistant syndromes. N Engl J Med 1980;303:349.

82. Hollis BW, Pittard WB. Evaluation of the total feto-maternal vitamin D relationships at term. Evidence for racial differences. J Clin Endocrinol Metab 1986;59:652.

83. Hughes MR, Brumbaugh PF, Haussler MR, et al. Regulation of serum 1α 25-dihydroxyvitamin D_3 by calcium and phosphate in the rat. Science 1975;190:578.

84. Hughes WS, Aurbach GD, Sharp ME, Marx SJ. The effect of the bicarbonate anion on serum ionized calcium concentration in vitro. J Lab Clin Med 1984;103:93.

85. Jaros GG, Belonje PC, van Hoorn-Hickman R, Newman E. Transient response of the calcium homeostatic system: effect of calcitonin. Am J Physiol 1984;246:R693.

86. Jones KH, Fourman P. Effects of infusions of magnesium and calcium in parathyroid insufficiency. Clin Sci 1966;30:139.

87. Kaplan EL, Burrington JD, Klementschitsch P, et al. Primary hyperparathyroidism, pregnancy and neonatal hypocalcemia. Surgery 1984;96:717.

88. Kichura TS, Horst RL, Beitz DC, et al. Relationship between prepartal dietary calcium and phosphorus, vitamin D metabolism and parturient paresis in dairy cows. J Nutr 1982;112:480.

89. Kikuchi T, Arab NL, Kikuchi K, Ghishan FK. Intestinal maturation: characterization of mitochondrial phosphate transport in the rat and its regulation by 1,25-$(OH)_2$ vitamin D_3. Pediatr Res 1989;25:605.

90. Klein-Nulend J, Fall PM, Raisz LG. Comparison of the effects of synthetic human parathyroid hormone (PTH)-(1-34)-related peptide of malignancy and bovine PTH-(1-34) on bone formation and resorption in organ culture. Endocrinology 1990;126:223.

91. Koo WWK, Tsang RC, Poser JW, et al. Elevated serum calcium and osteocalcin levels from calcitriol in preterm infants: A prospective randomized study. Am J Dis Child 1986;140:1152.

92. Kristoffersson A, Dahlgren S, Lithner F, Jarhult J. Primary hyperparathyroidism in pregnancy. Surgery 1985;97:326.

93. Lehmmann M, Mimouni F, Tsang RC. Effect of phosphate concentration on ionized calcium concentration in vitro. Am J Dis Child 1989;143:1340.

94. Lemon J Jr, Adams ND, Gray RW. Urinary calcium excretion in human beings. N Engl J Med 1979;301:535.

95. Levine BS, Coburn JW. Magnesium, the mimic/antagonist of calcium. N Engl J Med 1984;310:1253.

96. Lineralli LG. Newborn urinary cAMP and developmental renal responsiveness to parathyroid hormone. Pediatrics 1972;50:14.

97. Liu CL, Mimouni F, Ho M, Tsang RC. In vitro effects of magnesium on ionized calcium concentration in serum. Am J Dis Child 1988;142:837.

98. Loughead JL, Mimouni F, Ross R, Tsang RC. Postnatal changes in serum osteocalcin and parathyroid hormone concentrations. J Am Coll Nutr 1990;9:358.

99. Loughead JL, Mimouni F, Tsang RC. Serum ionized calcium concentration in the neonate. Am J Dis Child 1988;142:516.

100. Loughead JL, Mimouni F, Tsang RC, Khoury JC. A role for magnesium in neonatal parathyroid gland function? J Am Coll Nutr 1991;10:123.

101. Loughead JL, Mughal Z, Mimouni F, et al. The spectrum and natural history of congenital hyperparathyroidism secondary to maternal hypocalcemia. Am J Perinatol 1990;74:350.

102. MacIntyre I, Boss S, Troughton VA. Parathyroid hormone and magnesium homeostasis. Nature 1963;198:1058.

103. MacManus J, Heaton FW. The influence of magnesium on calcium release from bone in vitro. Biochim Biophys Acta 1970;215:360.

104. Markestad T, Ulstein M, Strandjord RE, et al. Anticonvulsant drug therapy in human pregnancy. Effects on serum concentration of vitamin D metabolites in maternal and cord blood. Am J Obstet Gynecol 1984;150:254.

105. Marx SJ, Fraser D, Rapoport A. Familial hypocalciuric hypercalcemia: mild expression of the gene in heterozygotes and severe expression in homozygotes. Am J Med 1985;78:15.

106. Massry SG, Seelig MC. Hypomagnesemia and hypermagnesemia. Clin Nephrol 1977;7:147.

107. McGuinness GA, Weinstein MM, Cruikshank DP, Pitkin RM. Effects of magnesium sulfate treatment on perinatal calcium metabolism. II. Neonatal responses. Obstet Gynecol 1980;56:595.

108. Messer HH, Armstrong WD, Singer L. Characteristics of calcium uptake by calcitonin-treated mouse calvaria in vitro. Calc Tiss Res 1974;15:85.

109. Metz SA, Deftos LJ, Baylink D, Robertson RP. Neuroendocrine modulation of calcitonin and parathormone secretion in normal man. J Clin Endocrinol Metab 1978;47:159.

110. Mimouni F, Hammond G, Mughal Z, et al. Independent transport mechanisms for calcium (Ca) and magnesium (Mg) across in situ perfused placentas of rat fetuses? Pediatr Res 1998;23:248A.

111. Mimouni F, Loughead J, Miodovnik M, et al. Early neonatal predictors of neonatal hypocalcemia in infants of diabetic mothers: an epidemiologic study. Am J Perinatol 1990;7:203.

112. Mimouni F, Loughead JL, Tsang RC, Khoury J. Postnatal surge in serum calcitonin concentrations: no contribution to neonatal hypocalcemia in infants of diabetic mothers. Pediatr Res 1990;28:493.

113. Mimouni F, Merlob P, Metzker A, Reisner SH. Supraventricular tachycardia: the icebag technique may be harmful in newborn infants. J Pediatr 1983;103:337.

114. Mimouni F, Miodovnik M, Tsang RC, et al. Decreased amniotic fluid magnesium concentration in diabetic pregnancy. Obstet Gynecol 1987;69:12.

115. Mimouni F, Tsang RC, Hertzberg VS, et al. Parathyroid hormone and calcitriol changes in normal and insulin-dependent diabetic pregnancies. Obstet Gynecol 1989;74:47.

116. Mimouni F, Tsang RC, Hertzberg V, Miodovnik M. Polycythemia, hypomagnesemia, and hypocalcemia in infants of diabetic mothers. Am J Dis Child 1986;140:798.

117. Morris CA, Demsey SA, Leonard CO, et al. Natural history of Williams syndrome: physical characteristics. J Pediatr 1988;113:318.

118. Nechama H, Holf D, Harell A. The intestinal absorption of vitamin D and its metabolites. J Mol Med 1977;2:413.

119. Nemere I, Norman AW. 1,25-dihydroxyvitamin D_3–mediated vesicular transport of calcium in intestine: time course studies. Endocrinology 1988;122:2962.

120. Nussbaum SR, Zahradnik RJ, Lavigne JR, et al. Highly sensitive two-site immunoradiometric assay of parathyrin, and its clinical utility in evaluating patients with hypercalcemia. Clin Chem 1987;33:1364.

121. Oh W. Renal function and clinical disorders in the neonate. Clin Perinatol 1981;8:215.

122. Okamoto E, Muttart C, Zucker C, Heird W. Use of medium chain triglycerides in feeding the low-birth-weight infant. Am J Dis Child 1982;136:428.

123. Okonojua F, Menon RK, Houlder S, et al. Parathyroid hormone and neonatal calcium homeostasis: evidence for secondary hyperparathyroidism in the Asian neonate. Metabolism 1986;35:803.

124. Okonojua F, Menon RK, Houlder S, et al. Calcium, vitamin D and parathyroid hormone relationships in pregnant Caucasian and Asian women and their neonates. Ann Clin Biochem 1987;24:22.

125. Ornoy A, Goodwin D, Noff D, et al. 24,25 dihydroxyvitamin D is a metabolite of vitamin D essential for bone formation. Nature 1978;276:517.

126. Page LA, Haddow JE. Self-limited neonatal hypoparathyroidism in familial hypocalciuric hypercalcemia. J Pediatr 1987;111:261.

127. Paunier L, Girardin NE, Brioschi PA, Beguin F. Maternal-fetal relationship of extra and intracellular magnesium and potassium concentration. In: Altura BM, Durlach J, Seelig MS, eds. Magnesium in cellular processes and medicine. Basel: Karger, 1987:151.

128. Paunier L, LaCourt G, Pilloud P, et al. 25-hydroxyvitamin D and calcium levels in maternal, cord and infant serum in relation to maternal vitamin D intake. Helv Pediatr Acta 1978;33:95.

129. Peden VH. True idiopathic hypoparathyroidism as a sex linked recessive trait. Am J Hum Genet 1960;12:323.

130. Pitkin RM. Calcium metabolism in pregnancy: a review. Am J Obstet Gynecol 1975;121:724.

131. Pitkin PM. Calcium metabolism in pregnancy and the perinatal period: a review. Am J Obstet Gynecol 1985;151:99.

132. Potts JT Jr, Deftos LJ. Parathyroid hormone, calcitonin, vitamin D, bone, and bone mineral metabolism. In: Bondy PK, Rosenberg LE, eds. Duncan's diseases of metabolism, ed 7. Philadelphia: WB Saunders, 1988:1225.

133. Raisz LG, Niemann I. Effect of phosphate, calcium and magnesium on bone resorption and hormonal responses in tissue culture. Endocrinology 1969;85:446.

134. Ramberg CF, Delivoria-Papadopoulos M, Crandall ED, et al. Kinetic analysis of calcium transport across the placenta. J Appl Physiol 1973;35:662.

135. Rasmussen H, Wong M, Bikle D, Goodman DBP. Hormonal control of the renal conversion of 25-hydroxycholecalciferol to 1,25-dihydroxycholecalciferol. J Clin Invest 1972;51:2502.

136. Reichel H, Koeffler HP, Norman AW. The role of the vitamin D endocrine system in health and disease. N Engl J Med 1989;320:980.

137. Rodda CP, Kubota M, Heath JA, et al. Evidence for a novel parathyroid hormone-related protein in fetal

lamb parathyroid glands and sheep placenta: comparisons with a similar protein implicated in humoral hypercalcemia of malignancy. J Endocrinol 1988;117:261.

138. Romagnoli C, Polidori G, Cataloli L, et al. Phototherapy induced hypocalcemia. J Pediatr 1979;94:815.

139. Rosen JF, Chesney RW. Circulating calcitriol concentrations in health and disease. J Pediatr 1983;103:1.

140. Rowe J, Rowe D, Spackman T, et al. Hypophosphatemia and hypercalciuria in small premature infants fed human milk: evidence for inadequate dietary phosphorus. J Pediatr 1984;104:112.

141. Ryzen E, Servis KL, Rude RK. Effect of intravenous epinephrine on serum magnesium and free intracellular red blood cell magnesium concentrations measured by nuclear magnetic resonance. J Am Coll Nutr 1990;9:114.

142. Sann L, David L, Loras B, et al. Neonatal hypercalcemia in preterm infants fed with human milk. Helv Paediatr Acta 1985;40:117.

143. Schachter D, Dowdle EB, Schenker H. Active transportation of calcium by the small intestine of the rat. Am J Physiol 1960;198:263.

144. Schauberger CW, Pitkin RM. Maternal-perinatal calcium relationships. Obstet Gynecol 1979;53:74.

145. Senterre J, Salle B. Calcium and phosphorus economy of the preterm infants and its interaction with vitamin D and its metabolites. Acta Paediatr Scand 1982;296(suppl):85.

146. Seyberth HW, Rascher W, Schweer H, et al. Congenital hypokalemia with hypercalciuria in preterm infants: a hyperprostaglandinuric tubular syndrome different from Bartter syndrome. J Pediatr 1985;107:694.

147. Sharlin DN, Koblenzer P. Necrosis of subcutaneous fat with hypercalcemia. Clin Pediatr 1970;9:290.

148. Shaul PW, Mimouni F, Tsang RC, Specker BL. Role of magnesium in neonatal calcium homeostasis: effects of magnesium infusion on calciotropic hormones and calcium. Pediatr Res 1987;22:319.

149. Shaw AJ, Mughal MZ, Mohammed T, et al. Evidence for active maternofetal transfer of magnesium across the in situ perfused rat placenta. Pediatr Res 1990;27:622.

150. Shaw JCL. Evidence for defective skeletal mineralization in low birthweight infants: the absorption of calcium and fat. Pediatrics 1976;57:16.

151. Sheikh MS, Ramirez A, Emmett M, et al. Role of vitamin D–dependent and vitamin D–independent mechanisms in absorption of food calcium. J Clin Invest 1988;81:126.

152. Sheikh MS, Santa Ana CA, Nicar MJ, et al. Calcium absorption: effect of meal and glucose polymer. Am J Clin Nutr 1988;48:312.

153. Slovik DM, Daly MA, Potts JT Jr, Neer RM. Renal 1,25-dihydroxyvitamin D, phosphaturic, and cyclic-amp responses to intravenous synthetic human parathyroid hormone-(1-34) administration in normal subjects. Clin Endocrinol 1984;20:369.

154. Smith FG, Alexander DP, Buckle RM, et al. Parathyroid hormone in fetal and adult sheep: the effect of hypocalcemia. J Endocrinol 1972;53:339.

155. Smith RH, McAllan AB. Binding of magnesium and calcium in the contents of the small intestine of the calf. Br J Nutr 1966;20:703.

156. Specker BL, Lichtenstein P, Mimouni F, et al. Calcium-regulating hormones and minerals from birth to 18 months of age: a cross-sectional study. II. Effects of sex, race, age, season and diet on serum minerals, parathyroid hormone, and calcitonin. Pediatrics 1986;77:591.

157. Stamp TCB. The hypocalcaemic effect of intravenous phosphate administration. Clin Sci 1971;40:55.

158. Steichen JJ, Tsang RC, Gratton TL, et al. Vitamin D homeostasis in the perinatal period. 1,25 dihydroxyvitamin D in maternal, cord, and neonatal blood. N Engl J Med 1980;302:315.

159. Stulc J, Stulcova B. Transport of calcium by the placenta of the rat. J Physiol 1986;371:1.

160. Sunderman TW, Carrol JE. Measurements of serum calcium and magnesium by atomic absorption spectrometry. Am J Clin Pathol 1965;43:302.

161. Taha SA, Dost SM, Sedrani SH. 25-hydroxyvitamin D and total calcium: extraordinarily low plasma concentrations in Saudi mothers and their neonates. Pediatr Res 1984;18:739.

162. Tanaka Y, Halloran B, Schnoes HK. In vitro production of 1,25-dihydroxyvitamin D_3 by rat placental tissue. Proc Natl Acad Sci USA 1979;76:5033.

163. Tantibhedhyangkul P. Hashim S. Medium chain triglycerides feeding in premature infants: effects on calcium and magnesium absorption. Pediatrics 1978;61:537.

164. Teree TM, Klein LR. Hypophosphatasia: clinical and metabolic studies. J Pediatr 1968;72:41.

165. Thomsen RJ. Subcutaneous fat necrosis of the newborn and idiopathic hypercalcemia. Arch Dermatol 1980;116:1155.

166. Tsang RC. Neonatal magnesium disturbances. Am J Dis Child 1972;124:282.

167. Tsang RC, Chen IW, Friedman MA, Chen I. Neonatal parathyroid function: role of gestational age and postnatal age. J Pediatr 1973;83:728.

168. Tsang RC, Chen I, Hayes W, et al. Neonatal hypocalcemia in infants with birth asphyxia. J Pediatr 1974;84:428.

169. Tsang RC, Kleinman L, Sutherland JM, Light IJ. Hypocalcemia in infants of diabetic mothers: studies in Ca, P, and Mg metabolism and in parahormone responsiveness. J Pediatr 1972;80:384.

170. Tsang RC, Light IJ, Sutherland JM, Kleinman LI. Possible pathogenetic factors in neonatal hypocalcemia of prematurity. The role of gestation, hyperphosphatemia, hypomagnesemia, urinary calcium loss, and parathyroid responsiveness. J Pediatr 1973;82:423.

171. Tsang RC, Noguchi A, Steichen JJ. Pediatric parathyroid disorders. Pediatr Clin North Am 1979;26:223.

172. Tsang RC, Strub R, Brown DR, et al. Hypomagnesemia in infants of diabetic mothers: perinatal studies. J Pediatr 1976;89:115.

173. Tsang RC, Venkataraman P, Ho M, et al. The development of pseudohypoparathyroidism. Involvement of progressively increasing serum parathyroid hormone concentrations, increased 1,25-dihydroxyvitamin D concentrations, and ''migratory'' subcutaneous calcifications. Am J Dis Child 1984;138:654.

174. Tuan RS. Calcium-binding protein of the human placenta: characterization, immunohistochemical localization and functional involvement in Ca^{2+} transport. Biochem J 1985;227:317.

175. Veldhuis JD, Kulin HE, Demers IM, Lambert PW. Infantile hypercalcemia with subcutaneous fat necrosis: endocrine studies. J Pediatr 1979;95:460.

176. Venkataraman PS, Tsang RC, Buckley DD, et al. Elevation of serum 1,25-dihydroxyvitamin D response to physiologic doses of vitamin D in vitamin-D deficient infants. J Pediatr 1983;103:416.

177. Venkataraman PS, Tsang RC, Greer FR, et al. Late

infantile tetany and secondary hyperparathyroidism in infants fed humanized cow milk formula: longitudinal follow-up. Am J Dis Child 1985;139:664.

178. Venkataraman PS, Tsang RC, Steichen JJ, et al. Early neonatal hypocalcemia in extremely preterm infants. High incidence, early onset, and refractoriness to supraphysiologic doses of calcitriol. Am J Dis Child 1986;140:1004.

179. Venkataraman PS, Tsang RC, Wen Chen I, Sperling MA. Pathogenesis of early neonatal hypocalcemia: studies of serum calcitonin, gastrin, and plasma glucagon. J Pediatr 1987;110:599.

180. Warembourg M, Pernet C, Thomasset M. Distribution of vitamin D–dependent calcium-binding protein messenger ribonucleic acid in rat placenta and duodenum. Endocrinology 1986;119:176.

181. Wasserman RH, Lengemann FW. Further observation on lactose stimulation of the gastrointestinal absorption of calcium and strontium in the rat. J Nutr 1960;70:377.

182. Watney PJM, Chance GW, Scott P, Thompson JM. Maternal factors in neonatal hypocalcemia: a study in 3 ethnic groups. BMJ 1971;2:432.

183. Whitsett J, Tsang RC. In vitro effects of fatty acids on serum ionized calcium. J Pediatr 1977;91:233.

184. Whitsett JA, Tsang RC. Calcium uptake and binding by membrane fractions of the human placenta. Pediatr Res 1980;14:769.

185. Whyte MP, Magill HL, Fallon MD, Herrod HG. Infantile hypophosphatasia: normalization of circulating bone alkaline phosphatase activity followed by skeletal remineralization. J Pediatr 1986;108:82.

186. Zelikovic I, Dabbagh S, Friedman AL, et al. Severe renal osteodystrophy without elevated serum immunoreactive parathyroid hormone concentrations in hypomagnesemia due to renal magnesium wasting. Pediatrics 1987;79:403.

187. Zheng JJ, Wood RJ, Rosenberg IH. Enhancement of calcium absorption in rats by coadministration of glucose polymer. Am J Clin Nutr 1985;41:243.

Newborn Adaptation: Adrenocortical Hormones and Adrenocorticotropic Hormone

Mark A. Sperling

The structure, biosynthetic pathways, and function of the fetal adrenal and its relation to the maternal adrenal as well as placental function have been previously reviewed (see Chapter 14). Following birth, the function of the fetal adrenal changes dramatically from that of providing dehydroepiandrosterone sulfate (DHEAS) as a precursor for placental estrogen synthesis to a major role in subserving fluid and electrolyte balance. A role for a fetal adrenal surge in cortisol secretion as a signal for parturition and as a factor inducing lung maturation is also gaining recognition. Major advances have occurred in the past decade in understanding the molecular basis of these effects as well as the molecular genetic basis for abnormalities in hormone synthesis and action. One practical benefit of these fundamental discoveries is the ability to diagnose suspected disease in utero precisely and initiate available remedial treatment in utero or immediately at birth. Clinically disorders of adrenal function in the newborn period produce abnormalities of fluid and electrolyte balance, vomiting, hypoglycemia, vasomotor collapse, or ambiguous genitalia representing inborn defects of steroidogenesis that may affect the gonad as well as the adrenal.

POSTNATAL CHANGES IN ADRENAL

At birth, the mean weight of both adrenals is approximately 6.5 g, a mass that is 10 to 20 times larger than the adult gland relative to body size.[114] About 70 to 85% of the adrenal is occupied by the fetal zone, which involutes rapidly so 50% of the total weight of the gland is lost within 3 weeks. By 3 months, the mean weight of the adrenal is less than 3.5 g, and thereafter there is a gradual increase to a value of 5.2 g at 2 years. The involution of the fetal zone parallels the initial fall in total weight, and the fetal zone composes less than 10% of the gland after 4 to 5 months. Patterns of involution are similar in full-term and premature infants.[62] The fetal zone is markedly reduced or absent in anencephalic infants, in whom cord blood 17-ketosteroid (DHEAS) levels are also markedly diminished, further documenting the now-established role of the fetal adrenal zone as a source of DHEAS.[9, 102] Residual, although diminished, capacity of the adrenals of anencephalics to secrete steroids may reflect in part the effects of human chorionic gonadotropin (hCG) as a factor regulating the fetal zone of the fetal adrenal (see also Chapter 14). A detailed review of the regulation of the primate fetal adrenal cortex and its physiologic significance can be found in the work of Ducsay et al.[21] and Pepe and Albrecht.[88]

PLASMA ADRENOCORTICOTROPIC HORMONE AT BIRTH

Corticotropin-releasing factor (CRF), initially isolated in 1981,[119] can stimulate the release of adrenocorticotropic hormone (ACTH) by human fetal pituitary tissue as early as 14 weeks' gestation, suggesting that regulation of the CRF-ACTH axis is well established at the time of birth.[12] Similarly, CRF can stimulate the release of other products of proopiomelanocortin, the prototype precursor molecule that gives rise to multiple different peptides via alternative processing pathways in pituitary tissues[49] by midgestation.[37, 40] Studies using precise radioimmunoassay (RIA)[15, 105, 127] or the redox bioassay[46] clearly demonstrate ACTH in fetal and neonatal plasma. The levels in full-term infants at birth tend to be lower than concentrations in cord blood before 34 weeks' gestation and maternal levels during labor[127] but higher than the afternoon levels of normal adults. There were no reported differences in cord ACTH levels between term infants born vaginally after spontaneous labor, by cesarean section after or before spontaneous labor, or vaginally after oxytocin-induced labor. These results suggest that fetal ACTH does not rise with spontaneous labor, implying that an increased ACTH concentration in fetal plasma is not essential for initiation of labor in the human.

Qualitatively similar but quantitatively disparate results have been reported from Finland.[105] In these studies, maternal and umbilical cord levels of ACTH were similar; ACTH fell by 30 to 50% within an hour of birth and remained stable over the ensuing 24 hours in the newborn. Both maternal and fetal-newborn levels were higher than those of nonpregnant women. No effect of gestational age, duration of labor, duration of ruptured membranes, birth weight, or Apgar score on cord blood ACTH was noted.

The fall in newborn ACTH values during the initial hours of life has been confirmed.[15] Although values remain higher than those of prepubertal children throughout the first 3 to 5 days of life, ACTH values are equivalent to those of older children by 1 week of life. ACTH values of infants born to diabetic mothers are indistinguishable from those of normal infants during the first week of life despite the hypoglycemia of the former.[15]

The ultrasensitive redox bioassay confirms the higher ACTH levels of normal neonates compared with adult levels.[46] In view of controversy regarding the nature of circulating ACTH as measured by RIA and its relation to β-lipotropin,[69] the redox bioassay or a radioreceptor assay[128] probably reflects authentic ACTH activity. The latter, however, has not been applied to the newborn period. Because ACTH does not cross the placenta, measurement of this hormone in fetal and neonatal plasma reflects the secretion of this hormone by the fetal pituitary.[75]

The time at which the now well-established circadian periodicity of ACTH secretion and its relation to the sleep-wake cycle[60] become established in the newborn is now known.[94, 121] A change in plasma 17-hydroxycorticosteroids (17-OHCS) between 8:00 AM and 8:00 PM, similar to the adult pattern of high morning and low nocturnal levels, appears to be established by 3 months of life,[121] although previously it could not be shown to exist before 1 to 3 years of age.[30] Studies indicate that in 1-year-old infants, cortisol secretion, as reflected in urinary free cortisol excretion, decreases during episodes of daytime sleep and increases before and after the period of sleep.[115] The significance of decreased cortisol secretion with daytime sleep in infants remains unknown; a role for rapid eye movement (REM) sleep or sleep-related hormone levels in stimulating brain growth remains conjectural.[115] Thus the establishment of the ACTH-cortisol diurnal rhythm after birth appears by 3 months of life.[121] Postnatal development of this rhythm may reflect postnatal maturation of the central nervous system. The mechanism of action of ACTH with regard to stimulating steroidogenesis has been extensively reviewed.[32, 39]

CORTICOSTEROID-BINDING GLOBULIN

Cortisol circulates in plasma bound to a high-affinity, specific binding protein, corticosteroid-binding globulin (CBG-transcortin), which is in equilibrium with the free, biologically active fraction. In addition, some cortisol is bound with a lower affinity to serum albumin. Although albumin is present in similar concentrations in maternal and fetal plasma, CBG concentrations in maternal plasma (1.2×10^{-6} M) are approximately fivefold higher than fetal CBG levels (0.25×10^{-6} M).[16, 44] Thus transcortin is not transferred across the placenta, resulting in a large concentration gradient between maternal and fetal transcortin levels. Because studies show that the affinity constants (Ka) of fetal and maternal transcortin are similar, as is its behavior on polyacrylamide gel electrophoresis, physicochemical differences do not explain the different binding capabilities in the maternal versus fetal plasma. It is possible that there is differential expression during growth and development of the genes coding for CBG and that subtle differences, such as point mutations, may alter function without affecting physicochemical properties. New insights have been obtained from studies of the molecular properties and novel functions of CBG and related binding proteins.[45, 99]

The differences in transcortin explain in part the concentration gradient of total plasma cortisol between mother and fetus.[44] About 80% of maternal cortisol is converted to cortisone by the placenta, indicating that the free cortisol, or diffusible fraction, may be higher in the fetus than could be accounted for by the transfer of free cortisol from the mother[16] (see later; see also Chaper 14). Transcortin has also been found in amniotic fluid.[16]

Transcortin-binding capacity remains low during the first month of life and then increases at a variable rate so transcortin levels after 1 year of life are in the adult range of the order of 0.5×10^{-6} M. This adult binding capacity is less (50%) than that of pregnancy because estrogens stimulate the formation of various protein-binding globulins, such as CBG-transcortin or thyroxine-binding globulin (TBG).[45, 99]

Adult transcortin concentrations are quite constant throughout the day, vary little from day to day, and are unaffected by the levels of cortisol. When transcortin levels are increased by estrogens, which are then withdrawn, transcortin levels fall, with a half-life of 4 to 5 days. Progesterone, deoxycorticosterone (DOC) corticosterone, and certain synthetic corticosteroid analogs have high affinity for transcortin, but their secretion rates are low in comparison to cortisol; aldosterone and androgenic steroids have little affinity for transcortin. A genetically determined absence or increase of transcortin resulting in extremely low or high levels of plasma cortisol has been described.[67, 68] Apart from its recognition and avoidance of excessive investigation for adrenal insufficiency, these entities have no functional significance because free, biologically active cortisol levels remain normal. CBG-transcortin has also been identified in human milk, which suggests a potential means of supplying the infant with CBG after delivery.[100]

PLASMA CORTISOL IN NEONATES

The placental transfer of glucocorticoids has been reviewed in Chapter 14. Studies by Migeon et al.[71] as well as others had suggested that cortisol was transferred across the placenta from mother to fetus. These conclusions were based in part on the following observations:

1. Maternal cortisol levels were always higher than those of the infant at birth.
2. The ratio of maternal to newborn cord levels of cortisol always remained within a narrow range. Thus infants born vaginally to mothers after labor had higher cortisol levels at birth than infants born by elective cesarean section; mothers of the former had higher plasma cortisol levels than the latter.
3. Increased cortisol levels induced by the administration of ACTH or cortisol to mothers undergoing cesarean section resulted in higher cortisol levels in their infants at birth.

4. Labeled cortisol administered to mothers during labor could be identified in newborn plasma.

In the light of the observations of Murphy and others[16, 77, 79] demonstrating that 80% of maternal cortisol reaching the placenta is converted to cortisone and that previously determined cord cortisol levels overestimated the actual values because of interference in the assays by the high levels of cortisone and progesterone, earlier conclusions regarding the degree of placental transfer of cortisol require modification. When allowance is made for the placental conversion of cortisol to cortisone, for the greater transcortin concentrations in maternal plasma, and for the use of specific assays for cortisol, it appears that the concentration of free unbound cortisol (diffusible cortisol) in fetal cord plasma is considerable.[16, 88] Cord arterial levels are higher than cord venous levels, indicating that the bulk of circulating cord cortisol is of fetal origin. A resistance to the placental diffusion of cortisol therefore seems to exist[6, 8] (Table 22–1). The earlier cited studies concerning ACTH levels in the mother, fetus, and newborn do not reflect this fetal cortisol surge, perhaps owing to methodologic difficulties with ACTH assay.[26]

Thus, under normal physiologic conditions, the fetal adrenal may be relatively autonomous and suppression of the fetal pituitary-adrenal axis prevented by the mechanisms limiting transfer of maternal cortisol, as described earlier. This does not preclude, however, the pla-

TABLE 22–1. Serum Cortisol Levels in Mother and Fetus (μg/dL)

	Mother (Spontaneous Labor)	Cord Arterial	Cord Venous
Total mean ±SEM	41.1	7.4	5.1
	3.3	0.6	0.4
% Free* ±SEM	26.2	75.3	71.1
	1.7	2.8	2.6
Diffusible (Free)†	10.7	5.6	3.6
±SEM	1.1	0.6	0.6

*Transcortin levels are fivefold higher in mother than fetus; fetal levels are approximately half of adult nonpregnant levels.

†Only 20% of this diffusible cortisol crosses the placenta as such because 80% is converted to cortisone by the placenta.

Adapted from Campbell AL, Murphy BEP. The maternal-fetal cortisol gradient during pregnancy and delivery. J Clin Endocrinol Metab 1977; 45:435.

cental transfer of substantial quantities of glucocorticoids and suppression of the fetal pituitary-adrenal axis through the administration of pharmacologic doses to the mother or when the mother has Cushing's syndrome. Some transient suppression of fetal adrenal cortisol secretion may occur following the use of synthetic glucocorticoids to induce fetal lung maturation.[3] No long-term sequelae in terms of growth, size at 1 year of age, rate of infection, or immune competence have been noted with the use of cortisol injected on day 1 of life.[27] The typical circadian rhythm of cortisol appears to be established by 3 months of life.[121] Adrenal insufficiency, presenting with vascular collapse, hyponatremia, and hyperkalemia in the immediate newborn period with spontaneous resolution by age 7 weeks, has been reported in an infant born to a mother with Cushing's syndrome due to an adrenocortical adenoma.[59]

Plasma concentrations of cortisol fall in the first few hours of life, reaching a nadir by 24 to 36 hours.[118, 125] Plasma concentrations of free cortisol also fall transiently after birth and are higher in premature compared with full-term infants at 3 to 5 days of life.[94, 125] The response to exogenous ACTH is normal immediately after birth, but there is a smaller response in the initial days of life corresponding to the period of low plasma cortisol levels.[10] Beyond 5 days of life, administration of synthetic ACTH to infants results in a pronounced increase of serum cortisol as well as certain androgens, such as androstenedione. It is surprising that testosterone levels fall in newborn males after administration of ACTH, whereas they rise in females, which suggests that high cortisol levels suppress testicular secretion of testosterone.[28] There is some evidence that the half-life of cortisol may be prolonged in the immediate newborn period, but this has not been consistently observed.[10] Because of immaturity in glucuronyl-transferase activity, plasma levels of conjugated 17-OHCS are low in the first 5 days of life, after which they appear to rise to the normal values observed in later childhood.

Cortisol secretion rates estimated by the single isotope dilution technique and determination of the specific activity of two metabolites of cortisol (tetrahydrocortisone and tetrahydrocortisol) collected in a 48-hour sample of urine were higher in the first 5 days of life than in older infants, children, and adults when corrected for surface area.[53] Urinary excretion of 17-OHCS when corrected for surface area is lower in the first 5 days of life than subsequently, suggesting a difference in the metabolic fate of cortisol in the initial days of life and a possible mechanism for the apparent high secretion rates during this period. From age 5 days, cortisol secretion per square meter of surface area is similar in infants, children, and adults.[53] Cortisol production in the first 5 days of life is similar in infants born vaginally, those delivered by cesarean section, and those born to diabetic mothers.[54] Average values of cortisol production in the first 5 days of life have been estimated as 18 ± 4 mg/M^2 per 24 hours; beyond 5 days of life, values are 14 ± 3 mg/M^2 per 24 hours.

OTHER GLUCOCORTICOIDS IN THE IMMEDIATE NEWBORN PERIOD

The plasma concentrations of several steroids at birth and in the initial hours and days of life are summarized in Table 22–2. These data are based on a longitudinal study involving sequential sampling of 12 newborn infants.[20, 106, 107] There appears to be a significant maternal-umbilical gradient for each of the reported steroids. Those steroids originating predominantly from the fetoplacental unit, such as DOC, progesterone, and 17-hydroxyprogesterone (17-OHP), disappear rapidly from newborn plasma. Cortisol and corticosterone levels display a transient dip between 2 and 12 hours of life but rapidly return to levels that are higher than later in infancy. These values provide reference standards with which to assess adrenal function in the newborn period.[20, 106, 107, 125] Although traditionally considered a predominantly adrenal steroid in infancy, 17-OHP levels in male infants at 1 to 2 months of age and in female infants at 6 to 9 months of age may respectively reflect testicular and ovarian activity during these periods of infancy.[29, 108]

PLASMA 17-KETOSTEROIDS IN NEONATES

Total plasma 17-ketosteroids are higher in umbilical cord plasma than in simultaneously ob-

TABLE 22–2. Plasma Corticosteroids in Normal Newborn Infants

Source/Time	Corticosterone (μg/dL)	Deoxy-corticosterone (μg/dL)	Proges-terone (μg/dL)	Hydroxy-progesterone (μg/dL)	Cortisol (μg/dL)	Cortisone (μg/dL)	11 Desoxy-cortisone Compound-S (ng/dL)	Aldosterone (ng/dL)
MV	3.6	0.29	12.0	1.1	54.8	6.1	6.20	0.40
UV	1.1	0.63	27.1	3.3	7.0	13.8	5.41	0.37
2 hours	0.9	0.55	5.7	0.89	10.4	8.3	8.12	0.17
4 hours	0.3	0.45	6.8	0.60	4.9	8.7	—	—
6 hours	0.28	0.30	4.6	0.40	2.8	7.5	4.20	0.19
12 hours	0.52	0.12	2.4	0.20	7.6	5.7	3.88	0.20
24 hours	0.08	0.12	1.25	0.09	2.7	4.1	3.33	0.17
4 days	0.19	0.01	0.09	0.08	5.7	2.3	2.94	0.16
7 days	0.25	0.01	0.05	0.12	3.5	2.2	1.83	0.06

MV = Maternal vein; UV = umbilical vein. All other samples from peripheral blood.

Data adapted from Sippell WG, Becker H, Versmold HT, et al. Longitudinal studies of plasma aldosterone, corticosterone, deoxycorticosterone, progesterone, 17-hydroxyprogesterone, cortisol and cortisone determined simultaneously in mother and child at birth and during the early neonatal period. I. Spontaneous delivery. J Clin Endocrinol Metab 1978;46:971; Dorr HG, Sippell WG, Versmold HT, et al. Plasma aldosterone and 11-deoxycortisol in term neonates: a reevaluation. J Clin Endocrinol Metab 1987;65:208.

tained maternal samples. Concentrations fall precipitously in the first 5 days.[34] Compared with those in normal adults, plasma concentrations of 17-ketosteroids are twofold to threefold elevated in normal full-term neonates, sixfold to eightfold higher in neonates with congenital adrenal hyperplasia, and 10-fold higher in premature infants in whom they persist at higher levels for longer than in full-term infants. The predominant ketosteroids are dehydroepiandrosterone (DHEA) and its sulfate (DHEAS).[34]

Application of precise RIAs confirms that DHEAS is the predominant 17-ketosteroid in newborn plasma, is higher in the serum of prematures, and decreases over the first 3 weeks of life to levels that remain higher than those of prepubertal children.[57] In full-term infants at a mean age of 7 days, concentrations were approximately 100 μg/dL (range 23 to 296 μg/dL); in premature infants at a mean age of 12 days, concentrations were 272 μg/dL (range 26 to 967 μg/dL).[57]

The predominance of DHEA and DHEAS in neonatal life and its longer persistence in premature infants reflect the persistence of underactivity of the enzyme Δ^5-3β-ol-dehydrogenase (3β-01) in the immediate newborn period, which may last for up to a month.[34] The predominance and persistence of other Δ^5-3β-ol-hydroxysterols and sterols in the immediate newborn period, their decline in parallel to the decline in 17-ketosteroids (DHEA and DHEAS), and the high urinary excretion of 16α-hydroxysteroids for up to a month in pre-

mature infants are all in accord with the concept that these steroids are derived from the fetal adrenal cortex deficient in 3β-ol enzyme activity.[34] Further, deficiency of this enzyme system has been demonstrated directly by in vitro incubation of fetal zone adrenal tissue[17] and indirectly through histochemical distribution of enzyme activity throughout gestation.[42] Finally, the high urinary excretion of 17-ketosteroids in the early newborn period is positively correlated to the plasma levels of DHEAS. Excretion of 5 to 10 mg of 17-ketosteroids per day corresponds to plasma levels of 100 to 300 μg/dL in childhood.[57] In the first 2 weeks of life, urinary 17-ketosteroid excretion is up to 2 mg per 24 hours. From 1 month to 5 years of age, the excretion is less than 2 mg per 24 hours.

MINERALOCORTICOIDS IN THE NEWBORN PERIOD

Human fetal adrenals can synthesize aldosterone from progesterone in vitro[22] or following perfusion of the fetus at midterm with corticosterone.[87] In addition to fetal synthesis, small amounts of aldosterone cross the placenta from mother to fetus.[5] Plasma concentrations in the first 3 days of life remain high, with a mean of 25.9 ± 3.5 ng/dL.[7]

The appropriate responsiveness of aldosterone secretion by the fetus and neonate to changes in maternal sodium intake or maternal use of diuretics has been demonstrated.[7]

Thus, with low sodium intake or use of diuretics by the mother, umbilical cord levels of aldosterone are 75 ± 13.3 ng/dL, and levels remain high (80 ± 15 ng/dL) for the initial 3 days of life. These levels must be compared with normal adult supine levels of approximately 5 and 20 ng/dL, respectively, on a normal and low sodium intake.

Infants born after normal labor have higher aldosterone levels than those born after elective cesarean section. Similar high cord aldosterone values with progressive decline over the initial days of life have been reported by others.[58, 92] In these studies, a highly significant negative correlation was found between the day of sampling and the aldosterone level and between the aldosterone level and the sodium:potassium ratio in urine. These and other studies,[104] however, suggest a relative insensitivity of the newborn renal tubule to the sodium-conserving effects of aldosterone or antagonism to its effects by atrial natriuretic hormone, progesterone, and 17-OH-progesterone, the levels of which decline after the first 3 days of life. Although a relationship between sodium intake, urinary excretion, and plasma aldosterone levels appears to exist in the newborn period, it was demonstrable only at high sodium intake; over the range of normal sodium intake, these relationships were not apparent. Plasma aldosterone levels in full-term, premature, or small-for-gestational age infants are equally high and not related to gestational age.[104]

Urinary aldosterone excretion is relatively low in the newborn period. Thus, when related to surface area, urinary excretion of metabolites of aldosterone by newborns is threefold that of control adults, although plasma concentrations may be up to eightfold those of adults. These data suggest that the metabolic clearance of aldosterone is lower in the newborn period.[92]

In view of the close relation of aldosterone secretion to the renin-angiotensin system of humans,[47, 83] it is not surprising that plasma renin activity, measured by RIA of the amount of angiotensin generated per unit of time, is highest in the newborn period (approximately 450 μg/L per minute) and falls rapidly and progressively with increasing age, reaching the adult range (approximately 25 μg/L per min-

ute) after 1 year of life. Thus the entire renin-angiotensin-aldosterone system is hyperactive in the immediate newborn period and is associated with renal sodium retention and an increase in exchangeable sodium. It has been proposed that the overactivity of this system in the newborn period subserves volume expansion and maintenance of blood pressure to compensate for relative immaturity of the autonomic nervous system.[101] The levels of renin-angiotensin in newborn cord-plasma cannot entirely explain the high aldosterone levels because maternal activity and renin substrate always exceed paired cord values whereas, as noted, cord aldosterone levels tend to exceed paired maternal values. This relative dissociation between newborn levels of aldosterone and its stimulating hormone renin suggests that fetal aldosterone secretion is more sensitive to renin-produced angiotensin, may be under the control of different stimuli such as ACTH, or reflects altered fetal metabolism of renin.[50]

DISORDERS OF THE ADRENAL IN THE NEWBORN PERIOD

The clinical manifestations of disordered adrenal function in the immediate newborn period result predominantly from inadequate secretion or action of glucocorticoids, mineralocorticoids, or both (Table 22–3). In addition, as a consequence of enzyme defects of steroidogenesis that affect the gonad as well as the adrenal, overproduction or underproduction of potent androgens can occur, depending on the site of blockade (Figs. 22–1 and 22–2). Thus there may be progressive virilization of the external genitalia in females and males or undervirilization in males. Ambiguity of the external genitalia is therefore a common manifestation of disordered adrenal function. Despite clinical manifestations that are highly similar, precise diagnosis is essential for appropriate therapy, long-term outlook, and genetic counseling. Excessive formation of glucocorticoids or mineralocorticoids is extremely rare in infancy. The mechanism(s) of action of glucocorticoids[116] and aldosterone[47] has been ex-

TABLE 22–3. Clinical Manifestations of Adrenal Insufficiency in Infancy

Cortisol Deficiency
Hypoglycemia
Inability to withstand stress
Vasomotor collapse
Hyperpigmentation (ACTH excess)
Apneic spells
Seizure

Adolesterone Deficiency
Vomiting
Hyponatremia
Urinary salt wasting
Hyperkalemia
Failure to thrive
Volume depletion
Hypotension
Dehydration
Cyanosis
Shock

Androgen Excess or Deficiency
Ambiguous genitalia

tensively reviewed. Table 22–4 presents a classification of adrenal insufficiency in infancy.

Congenital Adrenal Hypoplasia

Anencephaly, or congenital hypoplasia of the pituitary gland, is regularly associated with adrenal hypoplasia[93] (see also Chapter 12). This affects primarily the fetal adrenal zone with a well-differentiated but small permanent cortex. Congenital adrenal hypoplasia may also occur as an isolated defect with or without a familial tendency. In the familial forms, autosomal recessive as well as X-linked forms have been described.[84, 111] The histology of the adrenal gland in the autosomal recessive form resembles that seen with pituitary hypoplasia. In the X-linked form, the adrenal cortex is disorganized and composed of large cells resembling the cells of the fetal cortex. Occasionally adrenal tissue has been identified in conjunction with ovary or testis or diffusely scattered throughout the retroperitoneum; rarely no adrenal is found.[111] External genitalia are normal in both males and females because the defect is restricted to the absence of an adrenal.[84, 111] Clinical features of adrenal insufficiency are severe (see Table 22–2) and may result in death within 72 hours of life if unrecognized and untreated. Some affected individ-

uals, however, may be seen later in infancy with feeding difficulties, vomiting, hypoglycemia, and hyperpigmentation of skin and buccal mucosa.

A clue to the antenatal existence of this condition may be extremely low maternal serum levels and excretion of estrogens, particularly estriol, reflecting lack of fetal provision of DHEAS as precursor substrate.[84] This clue is particularly useful in mothers with a history of sudden unexplained death of a newborn. In anticipation of delivery of an affected infant, prompt replacement of glucocorticoid and mineralocorticoid at birth can be lifesaving. Parenthetically many of the infants have been born after spontaneous labor at term, thereby by implication denying the importance of a fetal cortisol surge for the onset of labor.

Laboratory findings reveal low or undetectable plasma levels or urinary excretion of cortisol, aldosterone, total 17-OHCS, and 17-ketosteroids. In those without pituitary hypoplasia, endogenous ACTH levels are elevated, and there is no response to exogenous ACTH, restriction in sodium, and change in posture.[111] Pituitary secretion of other hormones, including growth hormone, follicle-stimulating hormone (FSH), and luteinizing hormone (LH), is normal. Differential diagnosis includes adrenal hemorrhage, calcification, or cysts, which may be excluded by radiologic techniques. With one exception, none of the defects in steroidogenesis will have such low plasma levels or urinary excretion of all adrenal steroids. The exception is the earliest step in steroid biosynthesis—20,22-desmolase deficiency—which may mimic all the biochemical features (see Figs. 22–1 and 22–2 and further details later). In this latter circumstance, however, the adrenals are large and lipid laden, and the defect also involves the gonads, causing ambiguity of external genitalia in males.

The locus for congenital adrenal hypoplasia of the X-linked type has been mapped to a microdeletion on the short arm of the X chromosome in the Xp-21 region. Deletions of contiguous loci in this region are also associated with Duchenne's muscular dystrophy and glycerol kinase deficiency, which may occur together with congenital adrenal hypoplasia as a symptom complex. Such patients may have milder muscular dystrophy, which may not be

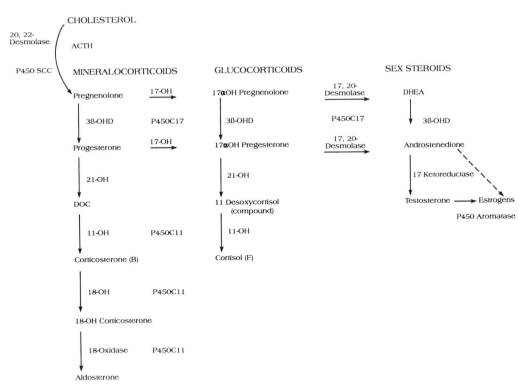

FIGURE 22–1. Simplified scheme of steroidogenesis in the adrenal gland. The broken arrow to estrogens indicates that estrogen formation occurs in the periphery rather than by direct secretion from the adrenal. 17-OH = 17α-hydroxylase; 3β-OHD = 3β-hydroxysteroid dehydrogenase, Δ⁵ to Δ⁴ isomerase; 21-OH = 21-hydroxylase; 11-OH = 11-hydroxylase; 18-OH = 18-hydroxylase; DOC = deoxycorticosterone. Note P450C17 catalyzes both. 17-hydroxylase. and 17,20-desmolase (lyase) activity; P450C11 catalyzes 11-hydroxylase, 18-hydroxylase, and 18-oxidase.

detectable in the newborn period. Glycerol kinase deficiency is detectable by spurious elevation of triglyceride levels, the measurement of which is based on liberated glycerol.[70] The availability of DNA probes enable antenatal diagnosis in suspected cases.

Adrenal Hemorrhage

The cause of this condition is unknown, but birth trauma to the large and rapidly involuting newborn adrenal is the widely accepted theory. The onset is usually between the second and seventh day of life,[11] and the clinical findings may be severe, as outlined in Table 22–2. Unexplained jaundice and a palpable abdominal mass that requires differentiation from neuroblastoma may provide diagnostic clues.[61, 95, 112] Calcification of the adrenal gland may become radiologically evident within a month and usually persists for life.[61] Treatment is with replacement of glucocorticoids

and mineralocorticoids and is commonly lifelong, although resolution and spontaneous recovery may occur.

Congenital Adrenal Hyperplasia

The syndromes of congenital adrenal hyperplasia result from a defect in one of the enzymatic steps of adrenal steroidogenesis as outlined in Figs. 22–1 and 22–2. As a consequence of the enzyme block and depending on the severity of enzyme deficiency, there is diminished or less efficient production of the end products, cortisol or aldosterone (or both), and accumulation of the products immediately proximal to the blocked step. Commencing in utero and persisting into postnatal life, lack of cortisol stimulates pituitary secretion of ACTH (melanocyte-stimulating hormone [MSH]), adrenal hyperplasia, and overproduction of steroids proximal to the blocked step.

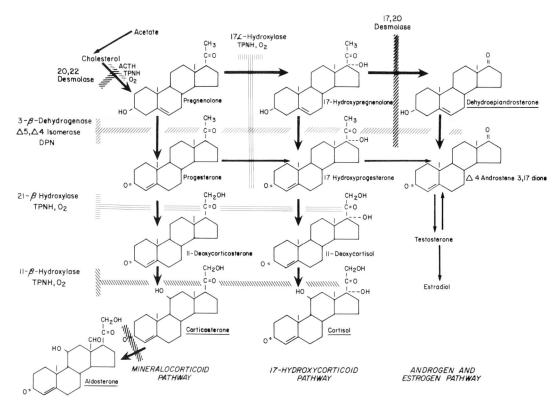

FIGURE 22–2. Biosynthetic pathways in the adrenal gland showing the structure of the major steroids. The shaded lines indicate the potential site of a block in the appropriate enzymatic step. See text for details.

Overproduction or underproduction of potent androgens can also occur, depending on the site of blockade in steroidogenesis (see Figs. 22–1 and 22–2). Similar steps govern gonadal steroidogenesis. Because masculinization of the external genitalia is controlled by circulating androgens regardless of chromosomal or gonadal sex, progressive virilization of the external genitalia in males and females or undervirilization in males may result. Ambiguity of the external genitalia may ensue: thus the term *adrenogenital syndrome*.

The pathophysiology of all of these enzyme deficiencies and their diagnosis can be understood in the context of:

1. Site and severity of the enzyme defect.
2. Overproduction of precursors.
3. Impact of androgens on virilization, differentiation of external genitalia, and somatic growth.
4. Impact of impaired glucocorticoid synthesis on glucose homeostasis and the ability to withstand stress.
5. Impact of mineralocorticoid deficiency on fluid and electrolyte homeostasis.

Only brief descriptions of the defects are provided here, with emphasis on their presen-

TABLE 22–4. Causes of Adrenal Insufficiency in the Neonatal Period

Congenital adrenal hypoplasia
 Secondary to ACTH deficiency
 Autosomal recessive
 X-linked
Adrenal hemorrhage
Congenital adrenal hyperplasia
 Deficiency of enzymes before pregnenolone—P450scc
 3β-hydroxysteroid dehydrogenase deficiency
 21-hydroxylase deficiency—P450c21
 11β-hydroxylase deficiency—P450c11
 17-hydroxylase deficiency—P450c17
Isolated deficiency of aldosterone synthesis
 18-hydroxylase deficiency—P450c11
 18-hydroxysteroid dehydrogenase deficiency—P450c11
Pseudohypoaldosteronism—end organ
 unresponsiveness to aldosterone
Congenital adrenal unresponsiveness to ACTH

Note: P450c11 catalyzes 11-hydroxylase as well as 18-hydroxylase and 18-oxidase activity. P450c17 catalyzes both 17-hydroxylase and 17-20 desmolase (lyase) activity.

tation in the newborn period. In-depth reviews of the biochemistry and pathophysiology of congenital adrenal hyperplasia may be found in standard texts[81] and in reviews.[73, 74, 124] Inheritance of all of these enzyme defects is compatible with an autosomal recessive model; the genes regulating each involved enzyme have been cloned and mapped to the chromosomal location as summarized in Table 22–5.

Deficiency of Enzymes Proximal to Pregnenolone

This rare defect was initially considered to involve the cleavage of the cholesterol side chain between carbons 20 and 22, which is the initial reaction in the conversion of cholesterol to pregnenolone[65, 73, 74, 81, 124] (see Figs. 22–1 and 22–2). The entire cleavage process, although termed a *desmolase,* may represent a series of enzyme reactions shared by the adrenal and gonad.[56, 65] Because of the early site in the assembly of all steroids, features of glucocorticoid and mineralocorticoid deficiency are severe (see Table 22–2), and genetic males have ambiguous genitalia or may be phenotypically female. The syndrome was considered to be incompatible with life because most patients have died shortly after birth. Several long-term survivors, however, have now been reported.[56, 65]

Laboratory investigation reveals virtual absence of all plasma or urinary steroids, including pregnenolone, although urinary cholesterol excretion may be increased.[56, 65] Early recognition and appropriate replacement with

adequate mineralocorticoid and glucocorticoid is essential for survival. In those who die, a presumptive diagnosis can be made if the adrenals are markedly enlarged and the cells typically distended with cholesterol, from which the synonym *congenital adrenal lipoid hyperplasia* is derived. Without demonstrating enlarged adrenals by radiographic or radioisotopic techniques, it may be impossible to distinguish this entity from congenital aplasia or hypoplasia of the adrenals. After an index case has been identified, antenatal diagnosis of future pregnancies may be possible through monitoring of maternal estriol levels or excretion, as in the case of congenital adrenal hypoplasia. Plastic reconstruction of external genitalia in line with those of a female may be necessary for survivors who are genetic males.

Aminoglutethimide, a toxic drug used rarely to inhibit steroidogenesis in adrenal carcinoma, acts by inhibiting the desmolase system and can experimentally simulate lipoid adrenal hyperplasia.

3β-Hydroxysteroid Dehydrogenase Deficiency

In this rare form of congenital adrenal hyperplasia, the enzyme defect occurs early in adrenal (and gonadal) steroidogenesis and affects the mineralocorticoid, glucocorticoid, and sex steroid pathways (see Fig. 22–1; Fig. 22–3).[73, 74, 81, 124] Thus, in severe enzyme deficiency, salt loss, hyponatremia, hyperkalemia, vomiting, and shock are characteristic, and six of the seven originally reported patients died despite adequate glucocorticoid and salt replacement. In those cases, the adrenals were hypertrophied and histologically were laden with lipid. In patients with partial enzyme defects, mineralocorticoid deficiency may not become apparent without stress; hyponatremia and hyperkalemia may become manifest during salt deprivation, particularly during withdrawal of supplemental glucocorticoid.[13, 55, 130] There may be gradation in the severity of salt loss even in affected siblings, emphasizing the clinical heterogeneity in this syndrome, which may not be apparent in infant females.[13, 55, 130] As a result of this enzyme deficiency, there is excessive accumulation of DHEA, a weak androgen, and defective conversion to the more potent

TABLE 22–5. Congenital Adrenal Hyperplasia Enzyme and Gene Location

Enzyme	Location	Chromosome
P450scc (20–22 desmolase)	Mitochondria	15
3β-HSD	Endoplasmic reticulum	1
P450c17 (17-hydroxylase) (17-20 desmolase)	Endoplasmic reticulum	10
P450c21	Endoplasmic reticulum	6
P450c11 (11-hydroxylase) (18-hydroxylase) (18-oxidase)	Mitochondria	8

P450scc: Side-chain cleavage.
3β-HSD: Hydroxysteroid dehydrogenase $\Delta^5 \rightarrow \Delta^4$ isomerase.
P450c17: Catalyzes both 17-hydroxylase and 17-20 desmolase (lyase) activity.
P450c21: 21-Hydroxylase.
P450c11: Catalyzes 11-hydroxylase as well as 18-hydroxylase–18-oxidase.

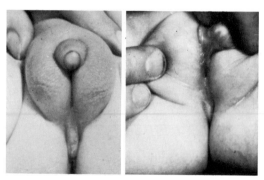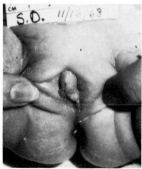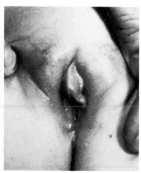

FIGURE 22–3. 3β-Hydroxysteroid dehydrogenase deficiency in a male (left panel) and a female (right panel). Note the bifid scrotum and third degree hypospadias in the male and the clitoral hypertrophy with pubic hair development in the female. See text for details.

adrogens androstenedione and testosterone (see Figs. 22–1 and 22–2). Consequently, the external genitalia show variable degrees of abnormality in both males and females. Males have hypospadias, often perineal or second-degree in type, and bifid scrotum with or without cryptorchidism; females have labial fusion, clitoral hypertrophy, which may be mild but progressive, and mild but progressive hirsutism (see Fig. 22–3). Thus both males and females have "partial" virilization.

Laboratory tests reveal high plasma levels and urinary excretion of 17-ketosteroids in which DHEA or its metabolites predominate. 17-OHCS and aldosterone levels and urinary excretion are typically low but may be normal in those with partial defects in whom plasma cortisol and cortisol production rates have been shown to be within the normal range.[55] Pregnenolone and its derivatives (Δ⁵-pregnanetriol, 17α-OH pregnenolone) rather than progesterone derivatives (pregnanetriol) predominate in urine, reflecting the lack of enzyme isomerase activity required to shift the double bond from the C5-C6 position in the B-ring to the C4-C5 position of the A-ring in the steroid nucleus.[13, 55, 130] Because the enzyme defects also occur in the gonad, the response to exogenous and presumably endogenous gonadotropin is subnormal. In individuals with partial defects, there is evidence for increasing 3β-ol activity with age, the enzyme activity being extra-adrenal, and probably hepatic in origin.[13, 55] Consequently, with increasing age, a large amount of pregnanetriol may appear in urine, but this does not represent the coex-

istence of a double enzyme defect in 3β-ol and 21-hydroxylase deficiency.

In addition to replacement with glucocorticoid and mineralocorticoids, surgical correction of hypospadias or clitoromegaly may be required.

21-Hydroxylase Deficiency

This is the most common variant of congenital adrenal hyperplasia, resulting from a defect in the enzyme catalyzing the conversion of progesterone and 17-OHP to DOC and 11-deoxycortisol, a step requiring hydroxylation of the carbon at the 21 position of the steroid nucleus (see Figs. 22–1 and 22–2). Because the androgenic pathway is unaffected, the fetus is exposed to excessive androgens from about the third month of intrauterine life. Consequently, newborn females show variable degrees of masculinization of the external genitalia, ranging from mild clitoral hypertrophy to complete labioscrotal fusion simulating a scrotum, a male phallus with a urethral opening at its tip, and no palpable gonads within the scrotal sac (Figs. 22–4 and 22–5). Excessive pigmentation may be present around the genitalia or nipples, reflecting increased ACTH with its inherent MSH activity. In newborn males, no genital abnormality is present. In both sexes, however, progressive virilization results in rapid initial growth, accelerated bone age development with premature fusion of epiphyses, progressive clitoral or penile enlargement, premature appearance of pubic and axillary hair, acne, hirsutism, deepening of the voice, and male gender identification.

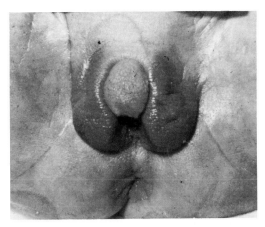

FIGURE 22–4. Moderately severe virilization in a genetic female infant with 21-hydroxylase deficiency. Clitoral hypertrophy is prominent, with some fusion of the labioscrotal folds. Note the hyperpigmentation of the labia, indicating excessive ACTH with its inherent MSH-like activity.

Severe 21-hydroxylase deficiency manifests within days to weeks of life with the classic features of adrenal insufficiency (see Table 22–2). Plasma and urinary cortisol and aldosterone as well as their metabolites are decreased; salt restriction is poorly tolerated and does not result in increased aldosterone secretion. Females with ambiguous external genitalia are readily diagnosed. In females with complete virilization of the external genitalia and in genetic males, the diagnosis may be missed. Bilateral undescended and impalpable testes and a small scrotum should be viewed with a high index of suspicion for the possibility of 21-hydroxylase defect. The death of an older sibling in infancy, particularly during stress, is often recorded. Vomiting is often attributed to pyloric stenosis, although the serum electrolyte profiles are quite distinct (see later).

In patients with milder defects, serum electrolytes are normal; cortisol and aldosterone levels and production may be normal, increasing appropriately during salt restriction. The response to exogenous ACTH may be subnormal, indicating existing maximal stimulation by endogenous ACTH. Many of these patients develop the classic features of hyponatremia, hyperkalemia, salt loss, dehydration, and vascular collapse during stress or during diagnostic sodium restriction. There is no direct correlation between the degree of virilization of the external genitalia and the severity of enzyme deficiency. Evidence demonstrating a close genetic linkage between histocompatibility leukocyte antigen (HLA) and both severe and mild forms of 21-hydroxylase deficiency[23, 63] led to the recognition that the responsible genes were located on chromosome 6. The cloning of these genes and detailed studies of the relation between genotypic and phenotypic abnormalities have markedly enhanced understanding of this group of disorders and provided precision in establishing antenatal diagnosis.[18, 24, 76, 80, 86] Molecular analysis of DNA from chorionic villi can establish the diagnosis as well as the sex of the fetus, thereby enabling attempts at prevention of masculinization of external genitalia in a female by provision of dexamethasone to mothers in the first trimester, in anticipation that this potent steroid, after crossing the placenta, would suppress fetal ACTH over secretion.[24, 86] This approach requires that treatment of a pregnancy at risk (by virtue of known previous outcome in the birth of an affected child) begin as early as 5 weeks' gestation, followed by chorionic villous sampling to establish the diagnosis. If the female fetus is not affected or if the fetus is male, treatment can be discontinued, whereas a fe-

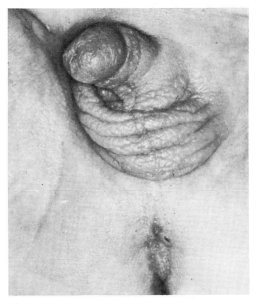

FIGURE 22–5. Complete virilization in a genetic female infant with 21-hydroxylase deficiency. The labia have completely fused to simulate a scrotum in which no gonads were palpable. The clitoris is enlarged to simulate a small phallus that has undergone circumcision. The infant had vascular collapse, hyponatremia, and hyperkalemia.

male infant would have had the benefit of therapy during the critical period of maturation of the fetal pituitary-adrenal axis and the differentiation of the external genitalia, generally completed by the 12th to 14th week of gestation.

Whether or not patients manifest salt loss and other features of adrenal insufficiency after birth, clinically affected patients have elevated plasma levels of 17-OHP[18, 48, 66, 81] as well as various androgens, including testosterone, derived from peripheral conversion of androgenic precursors.[48, 81, 85] Markedly elevated levels of 17-OHP are the sine qua non of this condition. Although plasma levels normally are high in umbilical cord blood, they fall rapidly during the first day of life (see Table 22–4), so values above 2 ng/mL after the first day of life are virtually diagnostic; values as high as 395 ng/mL have been obtained in affected neonates within the first week of life.[85] A micro method using eluates of filter paper impregnated with blood permits easy mailing of test samples to laboratories performing the assay, if required.[18, 81, 85]

The excretory product of 17-OHP in urine is pregnanetriol, and its urinary excretion in those affected with 21-hydroxylase deficiency exceeds the normal value of less than 1 to 2 mg per 24 hours in the newborn period. Although equally valid, this determination is more time-consuming and more difficult because of ensuring adequate collection of a 24-hour urine specimen in an infant. Urinary 17-ketosteroid excretion is also increased above the upper limit of approximately 2 mg per 24 hours. Characteristically urinary excretion of 17-OHCS, as measured by the Glenn-Nelson procedure using the Porter-Silber reaction that measures only those compounds with a hydroxyl (OH) group at carbons 17 and 21 and a ketone group (C = O) at carbon 20 (cortisol, cortisone, and 11-deoxycortisol and their tetrahydroderivatives), is low in 21-hydroxylase deficiency as well as all enzyme defects above this level (see Fig. 22–1).

Several points are worthy of mention. First, determination of urinary 17-OHCS by this method underestimates cortisol secretion in the newborn period. This is because the method measures glucuronides of the tetrahydroderivatives of cortisol and cortisone, but

glucuronyl transferase activity is deficient in the initial days of life. Normal urinary excretion of 17-OHCS is approximately 1.0 mg/M² per 24 hours the first 5 days of life; when corrected per gram of urinary creatinine per 24 hours, 17-OHCS excretion is 2 to 6 mg per 24 hours.[113] Second, in the incomplete forms of 21-hydroxylase deficiency, plasma levels as well as urinary excretion of cortisol may be normal despite increased plasma levels and urinary excretion of precursors above the block. Third, determination of 17-OHCS as 17-ketogenic steroids markedly overestimates the actual contribution of cortisol because 17-OHP is oxidized to a 17-ketosteroid, indicating no deficiency or excess of cortisol, when in actuality there is deficiency. To circumvent some of these problems, it has been suggested that urinary free cortisol excretion be used as an index of plasma cortisol and its secretion rate. Normal values of urinary free cortisol are 75 ± 18 μg/g creatinine per 24 hours.[31]

The recognition of this condition is essential not only for the lifesaving replacement of glucocorticoids and mineralocorticoids as well as supplementation of dietary sodium chloride in the newborn period, but also for appropriate sex assignment to permit appropriate sex rearing and gender identification. These and other considerations relating to management beyond the newborn period are discussed in detail elsewhere.[18, 73, 74, 124] The incidence of this enzyme defect has been estimated to be 1 in 12,000 live births in whites and 1 in 500 live births in certain Eskimos.

11-Hydroxylase Deficiency

A defect of this enzymatic step blocks the conversion of 11-deoxycortisol (compound-S) to cortisol (compound-F) in the glucocorticoid pathway and the conversion of 11-DOC to corticosterone (compound-B) in the mineralocorticoid pathway (see Figs. 22–1 and 22–2). Consequently, the plasma concentrations of compound-S and DOC are elevated, as are their respective urinary excretion products, whereas plasma and urinary cortisol and aldosterone are diminished. Appropriate caution is required in interpreting the results of urinary 17-OHCS excretion, which is markedly elevated because compound-S and its urinary metabolite tetrahydro-S both contain the 17, 21-dihydroxy, 20-keto grouping reacting in standard 17-OHCS assay.

Plasma androgens and urinary 17-ketosteroid excretion are both elevated, reflecting excessive adrenal androgen production, which is unaffected by the enzyme block and stimulated by excessive ACTH as a result of inadequate cortisol secretion (see Figs. 22–1 and 22–2). Consequently, this condition is characterized by all the sequelae of excessive androgen formation, including ambiguity of the external genitalia in genetic and gonadal females, and by progressive postnatal virilization in both sexes as described for 21-hydroxylase deficiency. Salt loss, hyponatremia, and hyperkalemia, however, do not occur because DOC is a potent mineralocorticoid, so the dramatic sequelae of adrenal insufficiency do not occur. Indeed, hypertension may appear later in childhood as a result of excessive DOC, with salt and volume expansion. Reflecting this expanded extracellular volume, plasma renin levels are low. Replacement with glucocorticoids suppresses ACTH and its effects on excessive androgen and DOC formation; mineralocorticoid replacement also may be necessary after the production of excess DOC is curtailed because aldosterone cannot be adequately produced.[81] Specific diagnosis of this entity requires precise assays for compound-S; 17-OHP cross reacts with many of the antisera used in the standard plasma RIA for compound-S. Normal compound-S values in plasma are <1 $\mu g/dL$; levels with 11-hydroxylase deficiency are commonly >5 $\mu g/dL$.

The gene for 11-hydroxylase is located on chromosome 8 (see Table 22–5). Based on studies of animal adrenal glands, it had been suggested that the last three steps in aldosterone biosynthesis (11-hydroxylation, 18-hydroxylation, and 18-oxidation) are mediated by the same cytochrome P-450 enzyme, termed *P450c11* and formerly considered to mediate only 11-hydroxylation. It has now been confirmed in humans that the enzyme catalyzes all three oxidation-reduction steps in aldosterone biosynthesis and that the distinct clinical symptom entities of 11-hydroxylase deficiency and isolated aldosterone deficiency due to 18-hydroxylation (corticosterone methyl oxidase type I) or 18-oxidation (corticosterone methyl

oxidase Type II) may be caused by different mutations in the single gene for this multifunctional enzyme.[41, 120] Accordingly it is appropriate to consider isolated deficiency of aldosterone caused by 18-hydroxylase or 18-oxidase deficiency in the context of abnormalities of the 11-hydroxylase gene complex.

Isolated Deficiency of Aldosterone

The penultimate and ultimate steps in the formation of aldosterone appear to consist of a hydroxylation of corticosterone at carbon 18 to 18-hydroxycorticosterone and its subsequent dehydrogenation (oxidation) to aldosterone. Because both steps are beyond the formation of cortisol (see Fig. 22–1), there is no adrenal hyperplasia owing to ACTH excess and no disturbance in sex steroid synthesis. Accordingly there is no ambiguity of external genitalia. The defective steps are beyond the formation of potent mineralocorticoids, such as DOC. Therefore in the immediate newborn period, affected patients have features of mineralocorticoid deficiency (see Table 22–2): vomiting, dehydration, hyponatremia, hyperkalemia, metabolic acidosis, and failure to thrive.

More recently, the traditional concepts concerning the final two steps of aldosterone biosynthesis from corticosterone have been challenged. Although a two-step mixed oxidation-reduction reaction is likely, the actual intermediate may not be 18-hydroxycorticosterone itself.[117] Thus the suggested terminology for the defects in the two final biosynthetic steps for aldosterone are corticosterone methyloxidase defects types 1 and 2. When corticosterone only is elevated (and not suppressible by exogenous glucocorticoid to distinguish it from the elevation of this steroid found in 17-hydroxylase deficiency) the defect is type 1.[123] When the defect is characterized by overproduction of both corticosterone and 18-hydroxycorticosterone, the defect is type 2.[117]

The original report on 18-hydroxylase deficiency was of three cousins from an inbred family. Urinary excretion of 17-OHCS and of 17-ketosteroids was normal and increased appropriately following administration of ACTH. Aldosterone excretion was undetectable, with no rise following ACTH or salt restriction. The urinary excretion of corticosterone and its metabolites was markedly increased, whereas 18-hydroxycorticosterone and its metabolites were absent, thus pinpointing the defective locus.

Salt restriction is poorly tolerated, but marginal sodium balance can be maintained on a normal sodium intake, and the clinical response to administered salt and a mineralocorticoid is excellent. Milder forms of this entity exist because biochemical features of this defect have been reported in young adults.[41, 96, 97, 123]

The clinical pattern in those affected by a defect in the final step of aldosterone biosynthesis is identical to that already described. Biochemically the defect involves the final dehydrogenation (oxidation) of 18-hydroxycorticosterone to aldosterone. Thus the steroid patterns differ only in that 18-hydroxycorticosterone and its metabolites are increased, whereas aldosterone remains low. The inheritance of both defects is compatible with an autosomal recessive pattern.[41, 96, 97, 120]

A transient form of isolated hypoaldosteronism in infancy has been described, and it has been suggested that affected infants have a maturational defect in one or both of the final steps of aldosterone biosynthesis. Definitive steroid studies have not been performed, so an enzyme block in aldosterone biosynthesis has not been excluded. In all forms of congenital aldosterone deficiency, the clinical severity of symptoms and urinary salt wasting tends to improve with increasing age. Thus the apparent transient nature of hypoaldosteronism in infancy may represent the amelioration of an inadequately documented enzyme deficiency.[81]

Pseudohypoaldosteronism (End-Organ Unresponsiveness to Aldosterone)

Pseudohypoaldosteronism is the name given to the salt-wasting syndrome of infancy and early childhood characterized by renal tubular unresponsiveness to the metabolic effects of aldosterone. Severe hyponatremia, hyperkalemia, urinary sodium wasting, vomiting, and circulatory collapse are universal findings in early infancy. Renal function and adrenal function are otherwise normal, as determined by cortisol levels, which are normal or high and which respond appropriately to ACTH. Plasma androgens and 17-ketosteroid excretion are also normal. Plasma aldosterone levels and secretion rate are markedly elevated, to 10-fold normal; plasma renin concentrations are also extraordinarily high. Mineralocorticoid therapy does not correct urinary salt loss.

The syndrome is explicable on the basis of renal tubular unresponsiveness to the action of aldosterone, with secondary stimulation of the renin-angiotensin-aldosterone system owing to salt loss, dehydration, and volume depletion.[91] As such, this syndrome represents a further example of end-organ unresponsiveness to a hormone owing to a complete or partial defect in the type I, mineralocorticoid-like receptor.[2, 25, 82] Complete unresponsiveness is not always present because in some cases spironolactone, an aldosterone inhibitor, aggravated salt loss, and a partial response to high doses of mineralocorticoids has been observed. These cases appear to be sporadic, although affected first cousins have been reported, suggesting autosomal recessive transmission.[2]

A variant of this syndrome had been proposed in which plasma aldosterone levels were normal or only modestly elevated and in which there was good clinical response to mineralocorticoids.[96–98] In this form, consanguinity had been a prominent feature in the families of affected individuals, suggesting an autosomal recessive pattern of inheritance. Reinvestigation of these patients demonstrated that their defect actually was in the ultimate step of aldosterone biosynthesis (type II corticosterone methyloxidase defect with elevated 18-hydroxycorticosterone relative to aldosterone)[117] rather than a defect in end-organ responsiveness.[96] Pseudohypoaldosteronism is a distinct entity in which mineralocorticoid therapy is ineffective or only partially effective. Supplemental salt replacement of up to 5 g per day is compatible with survival, correction of serum electrolyte patterns, and normal growth. Although clinically the defect ameliorates with increasing age, the defective response to aldosterone persists.[2, 90]

17α-Hydroxylase Deficiency, 17,20-Desmolase Deficiency: P450c17

A defect in this enzyme complex prevents the formation of cortisol or any of its 17-hydroxylated precursors as well as the formation of all sex steroids; the enzyme defect is also shared by the gonad. Mineralocorticoid formation is not affected (see Figs. 22–1 and 22–2). Only recently has it become apparent that 17α-hydroxylase and 17, 20-desmolase activity represents the spectrum of the same enzyme (P450c17) encoded by a single gene located on chromosome 10.[89, 129] Yanase et al.[129] have extensively reviewed the molecular basis of the various clinical manifestations and biochemical abnormalities noted in this syndrome.

As could be predicted from a defect interfering with adrenal and testicular androgen formation and thereby male sexual differentiation, genotypic males appear as complete phenotypic females or have ambiguous genitalia at birth. The penis is small or rudimentary; hypospadias may be present; labioscrotal folds fail to fuse, creating a shallow vagina; and cryptorchidism may be present. Genetic females show no ambiguity of external genitalia at birth, but secondary sexual characteristics, including menarche, fail to appear.

Because cortisol synthesis is impaired, ACTH levels are elevated, and adrenal hyperplasia results. Administration of exogenous ACTH causes no rise or a subnormal response in existing low levels and excretion of cortisol, 17-OHCS, or 17-ketosteroids. Because mineralocorticoid formation is not affected, however, features of adrenal insufficiency do not occur. Indeed, corticosterone and DOC concentrations usually are elevated, whereas plasma renin and aldosterone levels are subnormal, suggesting salt and water retention and volume expansion by DOC with suppression of the renin-angiotensin-aldosterone system. Hypokalemic alkalosis and hypertension characteristically occur later in childhood. Genetic females or males with complete, pheno-

typically female, external genitalia are usually not diagnosed until failure of pubertal development, unless hypertension and hypokalemia are recognized earlier. Males with the partial defect are recognized earlier by virtue of ambiguous external genitalia. Therapy with glucocorticoids corrects the hypertension and hypokalemic alkalosis by suppressing ACTH and its effects on DOC synthesis. Sex steroid therapy is required in older patients to achieve the appropriate secondary sexual characteristics.[19, 51, 89, 129]

Hereditary Adrenocortical Unresponsiveness to Adrenocorticotropic Hormone

Individuals affected by this entity are seen in later infancy or early childhood with recurrent episodes of hypoglycemia, often manifesting as seizures, and hyperpigmentation of the skin and buccal mucosa. Serum electrolytes are normal, and there are no other manifestations of mineralocorticoid deficiency.[35, 72] Sudden death can occur during episodes of stress, such as infection or surgery in untreated patients; a history of sudden death in one or more siblings frequently has been recorded.[52, 72]

The hyperpigmentation in association with hypoglycemia and in the absence of electrolyte disturbance suggests glucocorticoid deficiency and overproduction of ACTH, with its inherent MSH activity, but sparing of mineralocorticoid production. Indeed, plasma concentration and production rate of cortisol are low or undetectable, whereas aldosterone and corticosterone levels or production rates are normal or elevated, suggesting a selective defect in ACTH responsiveness. Similarly, urinary excretion of 17-OHCS or 17-ketosteroids is low or undetectable, whereas aldosterone excretion is high.[52, 72] Endogenous plasma ACTH concentration is strikingly elevated, and there is no response in plasma or urinary cortisol, 17-OHCS, 17-ketosteroids, and aldosterone to acute or prolonged administration of ACTH in pharmacologic doses.[110] In contrast, following the institution of salt restriction, aldosterone level and excretion increase promptly, accompanied by renal conservation of sodium.[52, 72, 110] Antibodies to adrenal tissue are not present in affected patients.[72]

The adrenal glands in affected patients are usually small and histologically demonstrate atrophy of the adrenal cortex with relative sparing of zona glomerulosa responsible for mineralocorticoid production. Genetic analysis of affected pedigrees suggests that inheritance of this disorder may be either autosomal recessive or X-linked recessive.[52, 72]

The high endogenous concentration of ACTH and lack of response in any adrenal steroid to administered ACTH, but with normal mineralocorticoid production to salt restriction, implicate end-organ unresponsiveness to ACTH and retention of normal mineralocorticoid responsiveness to the stimulus of angiotensin II.[110] The mechanism of action of ACTH involves binding to a specific cell membrane receptor, activation of cyclic 3′, 5′-adenosine monophosphate (cAMP), and initiation of a subsequent series of intracellular events culminating in steroidogenesis.[39] Theoretically a defect in any of these sites is possible. In vitro incubation of adrenal slices from an affected individual in the presence of added cAMP resulted in no changes of cortisol production, implying that in this patient, at least, the defect resided in steps beyond the membrane activation of cAMP.[52] In contrast, cortisol production increased after intravenous administration of theophylline in a patient with the syndrome variant associated with achalasia and alacrima.[35] Plasma cortisol increments following ACTH have been reported to be subnormal in the parents and some siblings of affected individuals, thereby providing a potential means for identifying the heterozygote state.[52, 72] A point mutation in the adrenocorticotropin receptor has been described in patients with the familial[16a] glucocorticoid deficiency.

Treatment consists of appropriate replacement with glucocorticoids; supplemental salt with or without mineralocorticoid administration is not necessary.

A variant of this syndrome, associated with achalasia of the cardia and disturbed autonomic function, including deficient lacrimation, has been described. Seizures occurred in childhood, with no recognizable anomalies in the immediate newborn period.[1, 35]

SYNDROMES THAT MIMIC ADRENAL INSUFFICIENCY
Bartter's Syndrome

This syndrome commonly occurs in late infancy or early childhood and is characterized by hypokalemia, hypochloremia, alkalosis, normal blood pressure, hyperaldosteronism, and hyperplasia of the juxtaglomerular apparatus. Other features include growth retardation, muscle weakness, mental retardation, polyuria, and inability to concentrate urine. Plasma renin and angiotensin levels are elevated, but the pressor and aldosterone response to infused angiotensin is diminished.[4]

Chronic abuse of diuretics, laxatives, or any cause of sodium depletion may simulate the features by stimulating the renin-angiotensin-aldosterone system. Consequently, the term *Bartter's syndrome* should be restricted to those patients with hypokalemic alkalosis, normotension, hyperaldosteronism, and juxtaglomerular hyperplasia without a primary renal, gastrointestinal, or drug-induced cause. The precise pathogenesis of Bartter's syndrome is unknown, but impaired reabsorption of sodium in the ascending limb of Henle's loop is a possibility.[33] A role for prostaglandins in the genesis of this syndrome is supported by the substantial correction of electrolyte disturbances with the use of prostaglandin synthetase inhibitors, such as indomethacin.[122] This treatment is not always efficacious, and prostaglandin synthetase inhibitors do not completely normalize serum potassium concentrations, so potassium supplements may be required.[14] Expansion of plasma volume by sodium loading does not lower aldosterone levels in Bartter's syndrome, although they are lowered by this maneuver when the syndrome is simulated by renal, gastrointestinal, or drug-induced causes. A variant of Bartter's syndrome with hypercalcinuria and nephrocalcinosis has been described.[103]

ADRENAL INSUFFICIENCY IN NEWBORN INFANTS: DIAGNOSTIC AND THERAPEUTIC CONSIDERATIONS

In the newborn period, the features that suggest adrenal insufficiency are predominantly

TABLE 22–6. Clinical and Biochemical Features in Newborn Adrenal Insufficiency

	Electrolyte Disturbance	Ambiguous Genitalia		Serum					Urine	
		Virilized Female	Incomplete Male	Cortisol	Aldosterone	17-Hydroxy-progesterone	Dehydroepi-androsterone	17-Hydroxy-corticosteroids	17-Ketosteroids	Pregnanetriol
Hypoplasia	Severe	No	No	Decrease	Decrease	Decrease	Decrease	Decrease	Decrease	Decrease
Hemorrhage	Moderate-Severe	No	No	Decrease	Decrease	Decrease	Decrease	Decrease	Decrease	Decrease
Desmolase (20, 22)	Severe	No	Yes	Decrease	Decrease	Decrease	Decrease	Decrease	Decrease	Decrease
3β-HSD	Severe	Yes	Yes	Decrease	Decrease	Decrease	Increase	Decrease	Increase	Decrease
21-Hydroxylase	Moderate-Severe	Yes	No	Decrease	Decrease	Increase	Increase	Decrease	Increase	Increase
Aldosterone synthesis block*	Severe	No	No	Normal	Decrease	Normal	Normal	Normal	Normal	Normal
Pseudohypoaldosteronism	Severe	No	No	Normal	Increase	Normal	Normal	Normal	Normal	Normal
11-Hydroxylase	None	Yes	No	Decrease	Decrease	Normal-Sl. Increase	Normal	Increase	Increase	Normal-Sl. Increase
17-Hydroxylase	None	No	Yes	Decrease	Normal-Decrease	Decrease	Decrease	Decrease	Decrease	Decrease
Unresponsiveness to ACTH	None	No	No	Decrease	Normal-Low	Normal	Normal	Decrease	Decrease	Decrease

*Aldosterone synthesis block is mediated by P450c11, which catalyzes 18-hydroxylase and 18-oxidase activity as well as 11-hydroxylase activity. 17-hydroxylase (P450c17) also catalyzes 17-20 desmolase (lyase) activity.

437

those of mineralocorticoid deficiency (Table 22–6), with or without ambiguous external genitalia. The vomiting, combined with electrolyte disturbances of adrenal insufficiency, is often confused with pyloric stenosis, although the electrolyte patterns in serum and urine are quite distinct. Thus, in pyloric stenosis, there is hypochloremic alkalosis as a result of the loss of gastric juice containing hydrochloric acid; serum potassium is normal to low, and serum sodium is usually normal. By contrast, in mineralocorticoid insufficiency, serum concentration of sodium is low, that of potassium is elevated, and that of chloride is normal; there may be metabolic acidosis, and urinary sodium loss is prominent. Ambiguous genitalia provide a major clue, and the determination of genetic sex via karyotyping or the more rapid determination of nuclear chromatin should precede sex assignment despite parental or other pressure for a rapid decision. Intravenous infusion of normal saline can be begun while the diagnostic plan is being formulated; in severe cases, mineralocorticoids should not be withheld before establishing the diagnosis. Usually the diagnosis can be established by the disturbances in serum or urinary steroids as outlined in Table 22–6.

Because of the concern regarding the absorption of orally administered steroids, therapy in the newborn period must be given parenterally. Glucocorticoids may be given as hydrocortisone, 25 mg/M² per 24 hours intravenously during the acute phase; cortisone acetate may be given intramuscularly every third day at 3 times the daily dose. Mineralocorticoid therapy is given as DOC acetate (DOCA), 1 to 2 mg intramuscularly daily. In an acutely ill infant with clinical features of adrenal insufficiency, DOCA should be given along with normal saline infusion even before the diagnosis is established. Depending on the severity of the condition, oral therapy with cortisone acetate as glucocorticoid (20 to 25 mg/M² per 24 hours) and 9α-fluorocortisol (Florinef), a synthetic mineralocorticoid, at a dose of 0.05 to 0.1 mg per 24 hours along with additional salt, 10 to 20 mEq per 24 hours, can be given as early as 1 month of age. Details of therapy beyond the immediate newborn period can be found elsewhere.[81]

CUSHING'S SYNDROME IN INFANCY

The endogenous secretion of excessive glucocorticoids owing to any adrenal cause is rare in the first year of life and virtually never occurs in the immediate newborn period.[38] One patient diagnosed at 1 month of age had bilateral hyperplasia of the adrenal glands; most affected patients in the first year have adenoma, carcinoma, or occasionally nodular hyperplasia or multiple adenoma.[38] Classic cushingoid features or obesity with failure of longitudinal growth is seen; short stature or failure to grow may be the major clinical manifestation.[109] Elevated glucocorticoids and sex steroids in plasma and urine, nonsuppressible by standard doses of exogenous glucocorticoid (dexamethasone), establish the diagnosis; precise localization by radiologic or catheterization techniques may be required before surgery.[38, 109, 126] Parenteral glucocorticoids are necessary both before and immediately after surgery to avoid a crisis of adrenal insufficiency. Subsequent replacement therapy may be lifelong.

REFERENCES

1. Allgrove J, Clayden GS, Grant DB, Macaulay JC. Familial glucocorticoid deficiency and achalasia of the cardia and deficient tear production. Lancet 1978;1:1284.
2. Armanini D, Kuhnle U, Strasser T, et al. Aldosterone-receptor deficiency in pseudohypoaldosteronism. N Engl J Med. 1985; 313:1178.
3. Ballard PL, Granberg P, Ballard RA. Glucocorticoid levels in maternal and cord serum after prenatal betamethasone therapy to prevent respiratory distress syndrome. J Clin Invest 1975;56:1548.
4. Bartter FC, Pronove P, Gill JR, MacCardle RD. Hyperplasia of the juxtaglomerular complex with hyperaldosteronism and hypokalemic alkalosis: a new syndrome. Am J Med 1962;33:811.
5. Bayard F, Ances IG, Tapper AJ, et al. Transplacental passage and fetal secretion of aldosterone. J Clin Invest 1970;49:1389.
6. Beitins IZ, Bayard F, Ances IG, et al. The metabolic clearance rate, blood production, interconversion and transplacental passage of cortisol and cortisone in pregnancy near term. Pediatr Res 1973;7:509.
7. Beitins IZ, Bayard F, Levitsky L, et al. Plasma aldosterone concentration at delivery and during the newborn period. J Clin Invest 1972;51:386.
8. Beitins IZ, Kowarske A, Shermeta DW, et al. Fetal maternal secretion rate of cortisol in sheep: diffusion resistance of the placenta. Pediatr Res 1970;4:129.

9. Benirschke K. Adrenals in anencephaly and hydrocephaly. Obstet Gynecol 1956;8:412.

10. Bertrand J, Gilly R, and Loras B. Neonatal adrenal function: free and conjugated plasma 17-hydroxycorticosteroids in the newborn during the first 5 days of life. Effect of hydrocortisone and ACTH administration. In: Currie AR, Symington T, Grant JK, eds. The human adrenal cortex. Baltimore: Williams & Wilkins, 1962:608.

11. Black J, Williams DI. Natural history of adrenal hemorrhage in the newborn. Arch Dis Child 1973;48:173.

12. Blumenfeld Z, Jaffe RB. Hypophysiotropic and neuromodulatory regulation of adrenocorticotropin in the human fetal pituitary gland. J Clin Invest 1986;78:288.

13. Bongiovanni AM, Eberlein WR, Moshang T Jr. Urinary excretion of pregnanetriol and Δ5 pregnanetriol in two forms of congenital adrenal hyperplasia. J Clin Invest 1971;50:2751.

14. Brouhard BH. Prostaglandins and hypokalemia. J Pediatr 1985;107:738.

15. Cacciari E, Cicognani A, Pirazzoli P, et al. Plasma ACTH values during the first seven days of life in infants of diabetic mothers. J Pediatr 1975;87:943.

16. Campbell AL, Murphy BEP. The maternal-fetal cortisol gradient during pregnancy and delivery. J Clin Endocrinol Metab 1977;45:435.

16a. Clark AJL, McLoughlin L, Grossman A. Familial glucocorticoid deficiency with point mutation in the adrenocorticotropin receptor. Lancet 1993;341:461.

17. Cooke BA, Taylor PD. Site of dehydroepiandrosterone sulphate biosynthesis in the adrenal gland of the previable fetus. J Endocrinol 1971;51:547.

18. Cutler GB Jr, Laue L. Congenital adrenal hyperplasia due to 21-hydroxylase deficiency. N Engl J Med 1990;323:1806.

19. Dean HJ, Shackleton CHL, Winter JSD. Diagnosis and natural history of 17-hydroxylase deficiency in a newborn male. J Clin Endocrinol Metab 1984;59:513.

20. Dorr HG, Sippell WG, Versmold HT, et al. Plasma aldosterone and 11-deoxycortisol in term neonates: a reevaluation. J Clin Endocrinol Metab 1987;65:208.

21. Ducsay CA, Hess DL, McLellan MC, et al. Endocrine and morphological maturation of the fetal and neonatal adrenal cortex in baboons. J Clin Endocrinol Metab 1991;73:385.

22. Dufau M, Villee DB. Aldosterone biosynthesis by human fetal adrenals in vitro. Biochim Biophys Acta 1969;176:637.

23. Dupont B, Oberfield SE, Smithwick EM, et al. Close genetic linkage between HLA and congenital adrenal hyperplasia (21-hydroxylase deficiency). Lancet 1977;2:1309.

24. Editorial. Prenatal treatment of congenital adrenal hyperplasia. Lancet 1990;335:510.

25. Evans RM. The steroid and thyroid hormone receptor superfamily. Science 1988;240:889.

26. Fehm HL, Voigt KH, Pfeiffer EF. Problems and artefacts in ACTH assay. Horm Metab Res 1972;4:477.

27. Fitzhardinge PM, Eisen A, Lejtenyi C, et al. Sequelae of early steroid administration to the newborn infant. Pediatrics 1974;53:877.

28. Forest MG. Age-related response of plasma testosterone, Δ₄-androstenedione and cortisol to adrenocorticotropin in infants, children and adults. J Clin Endocrinol Metab 1978;47:931.

29. Forest MG, Cathiard AM. Ontogenic study of plasma 17α-hydroxyprogesterone in the human. I. Postnatal study: evidence of a transient ovarian activity in infancy. Pediatr Res 1978;12:6.

30. Franks RC. Diurnal variation of plasma 17-hydroxycorticosteroids in children. J Clin Endocrinol Metab 1967;27:75.

31. Franks RC. Urinary 17-hydroxycorticoid and cortisol excretion in childhood. J Clin Endocrinol Metab 1973;36:702.

32. Ganong WF, Alpert LC, Lee TC. ACTH and the regulation of adrenocortical secretion. N Engl J Med 1974;290:1006.

33. Gardner JD, Simopoulos AP, Lapey A, Shibolet S. Altered membrane sodium transport in Bartter's syndrome. J Clin Invest 1972;51:1565.

34. Gardner LI. Development of the normal fetal and neonatal adrenal. In: Gardner LI, ed. Endocrine and genetic diseases of childhood and adolescence. Philadelphia: WB Saunders, 1975:460.

35. Geffner ME, Lippe BM, Kaplan SA, et al. Selective ACTH insensitivity, achalasia, and alacrima: a multisystem disorder presenting in childhood. Pediatr Res 1983;17:532.

36. Gemzell CA, Heijkenskjold F, Strom L. A method for demonstrating growth hormone activity in human plasma. J Clin Endocrinol Metab 1955;15:537.

37. Gibbs DM, Stewart RD, Liu JH, et al. Effects of synthetic corticotropin-releasing factor and dopamine on the release of immunoreactive β-endorphin/β-lipotropin and α-melanocyte-stimulating hormone from human fetal pituitaries in vitro. J Clin Endocrinol Metab 1982;55:1149.

38. Gilbert MG, Cleveland WW. Cushing's syndrome in infancy. Pediatrics 1970;46:217.

39. Gill GN. Mechanism of ACTH action. Metabolism 1972;21:571.

40. Gillies G, Grossman A. The CRFs and their control: chemistry, physiology and clinical implications. Clin Endocrinol Metab 1985;14:821.

41. Globerman H, Rosler A, Theodor R, et al. An inherited defect in aldosterone biosynthesis caused by a mutation in or near the gene for steroid 11-hydroxylase. N Engl J Med 1988;319:1193.

42. Goldman AS, Yakovac WC, Bongiovanni AM. Development of activity of 3β-hydroxysteroid dehydrogenase in human fetal tissues and in two anencephalic newborns. J Clin Endocrinol Metab 1966;26:14.

43. Gutai JP, Kowarski AA, Migeon CJ. The detection of the heterozygous carrier for congenital adrenal hyperplasia. J Pediatr 1977;90:924.

44. Hadjian AJ, Chedin M, Cochet C, Chambaz, EM. Cortisol binding to proteins in plasma in the human neonate and infant. Pediatr Res 1975;9:40.

45. Hammond GH. Molecular properties of corticosteroid binding globulin and the sex-steroid binding protein. Endocr Rev 1990;11:65.

46. Holdaway IM, Rees LH, Landon J. Circulating corticotropin levels in severe hypopituitarism and in the neonate. Lancet 1973;2:1170.

47. Horton R. Aldosterone: review of its physiology and diagnostic aspects of primary aldosteronism. Metabolism 1973;22:1525.

48. Hughes IA, Winter JSD. The relationship between serum concentrations of 17-OH-progesterone and other serum and urinary steroids in patients with congenital and adrenal hyperplasia. J Clin Endocrinol Metab 1978;46:98.

49. Imura H. ACTH and related peptides: molecular biology, biochemistry and regulation of secretion. Clin Endocrinol Metab 1985;14:845.

50. Katz FH, Beck P, Makowski EL. The renin-aldosterone system in mother and fetus at term. Am J Obstet Gynecol 1974;118:51.

51. Kaufman FR, Costin G, Goebelsmann U, et al. Male pseudohermaphroditism due to 17,20-desmolase deficiency. J Clin Endocrinol Metab 1983;57:32.

52. Kelch RP, Kaplan SL, Biglieri EG, et al. Hereditary adrenocortical unresponsiveness to adrenocorticotropic hormone. J Pediatr 1972;81:726.

53. Kenny FM, Preeyasombat C, Migeon CJ. Cortisol production rate. II. Normal infants, children and adults. Pediatrics 1966;37:34.

54. Kenny FM, Preeyasombat C, Spaulding JS, Migeon CJ. Cortisol production rate. IV. Infants born of steroid-treated mothers and of diabetic mothers. Infants with trisomy syndrome and with anencephaly. Pediatrics 1966;37:960.

55. Kenny FM, Reynolds JW, Green OC. Partial 3β-hydroxysteroid dehydrogenase (3β-HSD) deficiency in a family with congenital adrenal hyperplasia: evidence of increasing 3β-HSD activity with age. Pediatrics 1971;48:756.

56. Kirkland RT, Kirkland JL, Johnson CM, et al. Congenital lipoid adrenal hyperplasia in an eight-year-old phenotypic female. J Clin Endocrinol Metab 1973;36:488.

57. Korth-Schutz S, Levine LS, New MI. Dehydroepiandrosterone sulfate (DS) levels, a rapid test for abnormal adrenal androgen secretion. J Clin Endocrinol Metab 1976;42:1005.

58. Kowarski A, Katz H, Migeon CJ. Plasma aldosterone concentration in normal subjects from infancy to adulthood. J Clin Endocrinol Metab 1974;38:489.

59. Kreines K, DeVaux WD. Neonatal adrenal insufficiency associated with maternal Cushing's syndrome. Pediatrics 1971;47:516.

60. Krieger DT. Rhythms of ACTH and corticosteroid secretion in health and disease, and their experimental modification. J Steroid Biochem 1975;6:785.

61. Kuhn J, Jewett T, Munschauer R. The clinical and radiographic features of massive neonatal adrenal hemorrhage. Radiology 1971;99:647.

62. Lanman JT. The fetal zone of the adrenal gland. Its developmental course, comparative anatomy, and possible physiologic functions. Medicine 1953;32:389.

63. Levine LS, Zachmann M, New MI, et al. Genetic mapping of the 21-hydroxylase-deficiency gene within the HLA linkage group. N Engl J Med 1978;299:911.

64. Lieberman E, Rosler A, Cohen T, et al. Absence of linkage between C-11 OH-deficient congenital adrenal hyperplasia and HLA (abstr). Pediatr Res 1978;12:1088.

65. Lin D, Gitelman SE, Saenger P, Miller WL. Normal genes for the cholesterol side chain cleavage enzyme, P450scc, in congenital lipoid adrenal hyperplasia. J Clin Invest 1991;88:1955.

66. Lippe BM, LaFranchi SH, Lavin N, et al. Serum 17-alpha-hydroxyprogesterone, progesterone, estradiol and testosterone in the diagnosis and management of congenital adrenal hyperplasia. J Pediatr 1974; 85:782.

67. Lohrenz F, Doe RP, Seal US. Idiopathic or genetic elevation of corticosteroid binding globulin? J Clin Endocrinol Metab 1968;28:1073.

68. Lohrenz FN, Seal US, Doe RP. Adrenal function and serum protein concentrations in a kindred with decreased corticosteroid-binding globulin (CBG) concentration. J Clin Endocrinol Metab 1967;27:966.

69. Mains RE, Eipper BA, Ling N. Common precursor to corticotropins and endorphins. Proc Natl Acad Sci USA 1977;74:3014.

70. McCabe ERB, Towbin J, Chamberlain F, et al. Complementary DNA probes for the Duchenne muscular dystrophy locus demonstrate a previously undetectable deletion in a patient with dystrophic myopathy, glycerol kinase deficiency and congenital adrenal hypoplasia. J Clin Invest 1989;83:95.

71. Migeon CJ, Bertrand J, Gemzell CA. The transplacental passage of various steroid hormones in mid-pregnancy. Rec Prog Horm Res 1961;17:207.

72. Migeon CJ, Kenny FM, Kowarski A, et al. The syndrome of congenital adrenocortical unresponsiveness to ACTH: report of six cases. Pediatr Res 1968;2:501.

73. Miller WL. Molecular biology of steroid hormone synthesis. Endocr Rev 1988;9:295.

74. Miller WL, Levine LS. Molecular and clinical advances in congenital adrenal hyperplasia. J Pediatr 1987;111:1.

75. Miyakawa I, Ikeda I, Maeyama M. Transport of ACTH across human placenta. J Clin Endocrinol Metab 1974;39:440.

76. Morel Y, Andre J, Uring-Lambert B, et al. Rearrangements and point mutations of P450c21 genes are distinguished by five restriction endonuclease haplotypes identified by a new probing strategy in 57 families with congenital adrenal hyperplasia. J Clin Invest 1989;83:527.

77. Murphy BEP. Non-chromatographic radio transinassay for cortisol: application to human adult serum, umbilical cord serum and amniotic fluid. J Clin Endocrinol Metab 1975;41:1050.

78. Murphy BEP. Chorionic membrane as an extra-adrenal source of human fetal cortisol in human amniotic fluid. Nature 1977;266:179.

79. Murphy BEP, Clark SJ, Donald IR, et al. Conversion of maternal cortisol to cortisone during placental transfer to the fetus. Am J Obstet Gynecol 1974;118:538.

80. New MI, Speiser PW. Genetics of adrenal steroid 21-hydroxylase deficiency. Endocr Rev 1986;7:331.

81. New MI, White PC, Pang S, et al. The adrenal hyperplasias. In: Scriver CR, Beaudet AL, Sly WS, Valle D, eds. The metabolic basis of inherited disease, ed 6. New York: McGraw-Hill, 1989:1881.

82. Oberfield SE, Levine LS, Carey RM, et al. Pseudohypoaldosteronism: multiple target organ unresponsiveness to mineralocorticoid hormones. J Clin Endocrinol Metab 1979;48:228.

83. Oparil S, Haber E. The renin-angiotensin system. N Engl J Med 1974;291:389.

84. Pakravan P, Kenny FM, Depp R, Allen AC. Familial congenital absence of adrenal glands: evaluation of glucocorticoid, mineralocorticoid, and estrogen metabolism in the perinatal period. J Pediatr 1974;84:74.

85. Pang S, Hotchkiss J, Drash AL, et al. Microfilter paper method for 17α-hydroxprogesterone radioimmunoassay: its application for rapid screening for congenital adrenal hyperplasia. J Clin Endocrinol Metab 1977;45:1003.

86. Pang S, Pollack MS, Marshall RN, Immken L. Prenatal treatment of congenital adrenal hyperplasia due to 21-hydroxylase deficiency. N Engl J Med 1990;322:111.

87. Pasqualini JR, Wiqvist N, Diczfalusy E. Biosynthesis of aldosterone by human fetuses perfused with corticosterone at mid-term. Biochim Biophys Acta 1966;121:430.

88. Pepe GF, Albrecht ED. Regulation of the primate fetal adrenal cortex. Endocr Rev 1990;11:151.

89. Peterson RE, Imperato-McGinley J, Gautier T, Shackleton C. Male pseudohermaphroditism due to multiple defects in steroid-biosynthetic microsomal mixed-function oxidases: a new variant of congenital adrenal hyperplasia. N Engl J Med 1985;313:1182.

90. Postel-Vinay MC, Alberti GM, Ricour C, et al. Pseudohypoaldosteronism: persistence of hyperaldosteronism and evidence for renal tubular and intestinal responsiveness to endogenous aldosterone. J Clin Endocrinol Metab 1974;39:1038.

91. Proesmans W, Geussens H, Corbeel L, Eeckels R. Pseudohypoaldosteronism. Am J Dis Child 1973; 126:510.

92. Raux-Eurin MC, Pham-Huu-Trung MT, Marrec, D, Girard, F. Plasma aldosterone concentrations during the neonatal period. Pediatr Res 1977;11:182.

93. Reid JD. Congenital absence of the pituitary gland. J Pediatr 1960;56:658.

94. Rokicki W, Forest MG, Loras B, et al. Free cortisol of human plasma in the first three months of life. Biol Neonate 1990;57:21.

95. Rose J, Berdon, WE, Sullivan T, Baker DH. Prolonged jaundice as presenting sign of massive adrenal hemorrhage in the newborn. Radiology 1971;98:263.

96. Rosler A, Rabinowitz D, Theodor R, et al. The nature of the defect in a salt-wasting disorder in Jews in Iran. J. Clin Endocrinol Metab 1977;44:279.

97. Rosler A, Theodor R, Boichis H, et al. Metabolic response to the administration of angiotensin II, K and ACTH in two salt-wasting syndromes. J Clin Endocrinol Metab 1977;44:292.

98. Rosler A, Theodor R, Gazit E, et al. Salt wastage, raised plasma-renin activity, and normal or high plasma aldosterone: a form of pseudohypoaldosteronism. Lancet 1973;1:959.

99. Rosner W. The function of corticosteroid-binding globulin and sex-steroid binding globulin: recent advances. Endocr Rev 1990;11:80.

100. Rosner W, Beers PC, Awan T, Khan S. Identification of corticosteroid-binding globulin in human milk: measurement with a filter disk assay. J Clin Endocrinol Metab 1976;42:1064.

101. Sassard J, Sann L, Vincent M, et al. Plasma renin activity in normal subjects from infancy to puberty. J Clin Endocrinol Metab 1975;40:524.

102. Seron-Ferre M, Lawrence CC, Jaffe LB. Role of hCG in regulation of the fetal zone of the human fetal adrenal gland. J Clin Endocrinol Metab 1978;46:834.

103. Seyberth HW, Rascher W, Schweer H, et al. Congenital hypokalemia with hypercalciuria in preterm infants: a hyperprostaglandinuric syndrome different from Bartter syndrome. J Pediatr 1985;107:694.

104. Siegel SR, Fisher DA, Oh W. Serum aldosterone concentrations related to sodium balance in the newborn infant. Pediatrics 1974;53:410.

105. Simila S, Kauppila A, Ylikorkala O, et al. Adrenocorticotrophic hormone during the first day of life. Eur J Pediatr 1977;124:173.

106. Sippell WG, Becker H, Versmold HT, et al. Longitudinal studies of plasma aldosterone, corticosterone, deoxycorticosterone, progesterone, 17-hydroxyprogesterone, cortisol and cortisone determined simultaneously in mother and child at birth and during the early neonatal period. I. Spontaneous delivery. J Clin Endocrinol Metab 1978;46:971.

107. Sippell WG, Dorr HG, Becker H, et al. Simultaneous determination of seven unconjugated steroids in maternal venous and umbilical arterial and venous serum in elective and emergency cesarean section at term. Am J Obstet Gynecol 1979;135:530.

108. Sippell WG, Dorr HG, Bidlingmaier F, Knorr D. Plasma levels of aldosterone, corticosterone, 11-deoxycorticosterone, progesterone, 17-hydroxyprogesterone, cortisol and cortisone during infancy and childhood. Pediatr Res 1980;14:39.

109. Solomon IL, Schoen EJ. Juvenile Cushing's syndrome manifested primarily by growth failure. Am J Dis Child 1976;130:200.

110. Spark RF, Etzkorn JR. Absent aldosterone response to ACTH in familial glucocorticoid deficiency. N Engl J Med 1977;297:917.

111. Sperling MA, Wolfsen AR, Fisher DA. Congenital adrenal hypoplasia: an isolated defect of organogenesis. J Pediatr 1973;82:44.

112. Stevens RC, Tomsykoski AJ. Bilateral adrenal hemorrhage and calcification. Am J Dis Child 1954;87:475.

113. Streeten DHP, Faas FH, Elders MJ, et al. Hypercortisolism in childhood: shortcomings of conventional diagnostic criteria. Pediatrics 1975;56:797.

114. Tähkäh H. On the weight and structure of the adrenal glands and the factors affecting them in children of 0–2 years. Acta Paediatr 1951;40(suppl 81):1.

115. Tennes K, Vernadakis A. Cortisol excretion levels and daytime sleep in one-year-old infants. J Clin Endocrinol Metab 1977;44:175.

116. Thompson EB, Lippman ME. Mechanism of action of glucocorticoids. Metabolism 1974;23:159.

117. Ulick S. Diagnosis and nomenclature of the disorders of the terminal portion of the aldosterone biosynthetic pathway. J Clin Endocrinol Metab 1976;43:92.

118. Ulstrom RA, Colle E, Reynolds JW, Burley J. Adrenocortical steroid metabolism in newborn infants. IV. Plasma concentrations of cortisol in the early neonatal period. J Clin Endocrinol Metab 1961;21:414.

119. Vale W, Spiess J, Rivier C, Rivier J. Characterization of a 41-residue ovine hypothalamic peptide that stimulates secretion of corticotropin and β-endorphin (abstr). Science 1981;213:1394.

120. Veldhuis JD, Kulin HE, Santen RJ, et al. Inborn error in the terminal step of aldosterone biosynthesis: corticosterone methyl oxidase type II deficiency in a North Amercian pedigree. N Engl J Med 1980; 303:117.

121. Vermes I, Dohanics J, Toth G, Pongracz F. Maturation of the circadian rhythm of the adrenocortical functions in human neonates and infants. Horm Res 1980;12:237.

122. Vinci JM, Gill JR Jr, Bowden RE, et al. The kallikrein-kinin system in Bartter's syndrome and its response to prostaglandin synthetase inhibition. J Clin Invest 1978;61:1671.

123. Waldhausl W, Herkner K, Nowotny P, Bratusch-Marrain P. Combined 17α-and 18-hydroxylase deficiency associated with complete male pseudohermaphroditism and hypoaldosteronism. J Clin Endocrinal Metab 1978;46:236.

124. White PC, New MI, Dupont B. Congenital adrenal hyperplasia. N Engl J Med 1987;316:1519 (Part 1), 1580 (Part 2).

125. Wiener D, Smith J, Dahlem S, et al. Serum adrenal steroid levels in healthy full-term 3 day old infants. J Pediatr 1987;110:122.

126. Winter JSD. Cushing's syndrome in childhood. In: Gardner LI, ed. Endocrine and genetic diseases of childhood and adolescence. Philadelphia: WB Saunders, 1975:500.

127. Winters AJ, Oliver C, Colston C, et al. Plasma ACTH levels in the human fetus and neonate as related to age and parturition. J Clin Endocrinol Metab 1974;39:269.
128. Wolfsen AR, McIntyre HB, Odell WD. Adrenocorticotropin measurement by competitive binding receptor assay. J Clin Endocrinol Metab 1972;34:684.
129. Yanase T, Simpson ER, Waterman MR. 17 alpha-hydroxylase/17,20-lyase deficiency: from clinical investigation to molecular definition. Endocr Rev 1991;12:91.
130. Zachmann M, Vollmin JA, Murset G, et al. Unusual type of congenital adrenal hyperplasia probably due to deficiency of 3β-hydroxysteroid dehydrogenase: case report of a surviving girl with steroid studies. J Clin Endocrinol Metab 1970;30:719.

Index

———

Note: Page numbers in *italics* refer to illustrations; page numbers followed by (t) indicate tables.

A cells, 48, *49*, 49t
  glucagon synthesis and secretion by, 58–59
Abortion, lutectomy and, 5–6
ACE (angiotensin-converting enzyme), 100, 158
Acid-labile aldosterone, 159
Acromegaly, 127
ACTH. See *Adrenocorticotropic hormone (ACTH)*.
Actin, 358, *358*
Activin, autocrine/paracrine action of, on gonadal
    steroidogenesis, 225
Adenohypophysis. See also *Pituitary gland*.
  cells of, 120
  embryogenesis of, 198–203, *199–202*
  hormones of. See also specific hormone, e.g.,
    Growth hormone (GH).
    ontogeny of, 207–233
    maternal, 120–128
      function of, throughout pregnancy, 120–121
Adenosine triphosphate (ATP), in glucose
    metabolism, 51
ADH (antidiuretic hormone). See *Vasopressin*.
Adhesion, in blastocyst implantation, 343–344, *344*
Adipose tissue, brown, thermogenesis of, 328
    thyroid hormone effects on, 328–330, *329*
Adrenal gland, biosynthetic pathways in, 152, 276,
    428
  congenital hyperplasia of, 286–287, *288*, 289
    clinical manifestations of, 287, 427–434
    deficiency of enzymes proximal to pregneno-
      lone in, *427–428*, 429
    enzyme and gene location in, 429t
    11-hydroxylase deficiency in, 289, *427–428*,
      432–433
    21-hydroxylase deficiency in, 287, 430–432,
      431
    3β-hydroxysteroid dehydrogenase deficiency
      in, 287, *427*, 429–430, *430*

Adrenal gland *(Continued)*
    isolated aldosterone deficiency in, *427*, 433–
      434
    pathophysiology of, 428
  congenital hypoplasia of, 289
  clinical manifestations of, 426–427
  cortex of, 152–160
    aldosterone synthesis and secretion in, 106,
      157–158, *158*
      mechanism of action of, 106, 158–159
      metabolism of, 159
    glucocorticoid synthesis in, 152–153, *152–153*
      classification, control, and effects of, 152t
      diurnal rhythm of, 154
      feedback regulation of, 154
      mechanism of action of, 155
      metabolism of, 155–156, *156*
      plasma binding and, 154–155
      regulation of, 153–154
      stress and, 154, *154*
    morphology of, 152
    steroid biosynthesis in, 4, *5*
    zona fasciculata of, *152–153*, 152–156, 277
    zona glomerulosa of, 157–159, 277
    zona reticularis of, 159–160, 277–278
  DHA/DHS production by, 8
  fetal, 276–291
    DHA/DHS production by, 8–9
    embryology and development of, 276–277,
      276–277
    functions of, 278–282
    histology of, *176*, 277–278
    interaction of placenta with, 280
    pathology of, 286–290
    regulation of, 282–286
    steroidogenesis in, 278, *279*, 279t, 280, 284t,
      284–285
    vs. adult adrenal gland, 276, *276*

ISBN 0-7216-4232-2

90038